Cardiac Arrhythmias 1999 - Vol. 1

Springer-Verlag Italia Srl.

Cardiac Arrhythmias 1999
Vol. 1

Edited by
Antonio Raviele

Proceedings of the
6th International Workshop
on Cardiac Arrhythmias

(Venice, 5-8 October 1999)

Lectures and Structured Symposia

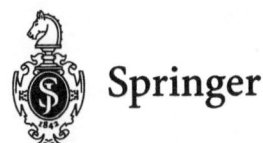 Springer

ANTONIO RAVIELE, MD
Divisione di Cardiologia
Ospedale Umberto I
Via Circonvallazione 50
I-30174 Venezia Mestre

© Springer-Verlag Italia 2000
Originally published by Springer-Verlag Italia, Milan in 2000
Softcover reprint of the hardcover 1st edition 2000
ISBN 978-88-470-2178-5   ISBN 978-88-470-2139-6 (eBook)
DOI 10.1007/978-88-470-2139-6
Library of Congress Cataloging-in-Publication Data: Applied for

Cover design: Simona Colombo, Milan
Typesetting: Graphostudio, Milan

SPIN: 10744185

Preface

This book, consisting of two volumes, contains the Proceedings of the 6th International Workshop on Cardiac Arrythmias held in Venice, Italy at the Fondazione Giorgio Cini, on 5-8 October 1999. Over the four days of the meeting, practically all aspects of heart rhythm disorders were addressed and discussed by internationally renowned experts and by the numerous participants coming from all around the world. Volume 1 – which will be distributed by the international book trade – comprises the contributions of the structured symposia, while Volume 2 contains those of the satellite symposia. This second volume will exclusively be available to the participants of the workshop. On the whole, I believe the book represents the state of our present knowledge about cardiac arrhythmias and antiarrhythmic therapy.

The main topics dealt with in the two volumes include: molecular pathology of cardiac arrhythmias; atrial fibrillation with its different pathophysiological, electrophysiological, clinical and therapeutic aspects; atrial flutter and other supraventricular tachyarrhythmias; ventricular arrhythmias, with particular focus on malignant, idiopathic and uncommon forms; non-antiarrhythmic and antiarrhythmic measures for prevention of sudden death; technological advances and clinical aspects of ICD therapy; modern evaluation of patients with syncope; and, finally, cardiac pacing with practical issues, controversial indications, usefulness of different pacing modes and sites of stimulation and, in particular, usefulness of left ventricular or biventricular pacing for treatment of heart failure.

Many individuals have contributed to the realization of this book. First of all, I am indebted to the numerous Authors who dedicated a significant part of their invaluable time in preparing excellent manuscripts. Without their enthusiasm and personal effort this book would not have been possible. Then, I am sincerely grateful to the Publisher, Springer-Verlag, who provided the means for early publication of the Proceedings, with a high quality of reproduction and clarity of content. Donatella Rizza, Executive Editor, worked with me diligently and tirelessly to collect and review the manuscripts. A special word of thanks goes to my teacher, Professor Eligio Piccolo, who transmitted to me a passion for the medical profession and for scientific research. I also wish to acknowledge the important contributions of my colleagues, Drs. De Piccoli, Di

Pede, Bonso, Rigo, Zuin, Gasparini, Giada and Themistoclakis. Rita Reggiani and Cristina Imola of Adria Congrex are thanked for preparing and realizing the workshops. Their support and encouragement were essential for me. Finally, my deepest gratitude goes to my family, Carmen, Francesca and Michele, for their patience, personal sacrifice and continuous help.

Antonio Raviele

Table of Contents

VENTRICULAR ARRHYTHMIAS

List of Contributors

ADAM M., 50
ADINOLFI E., 509, 530
AEBISCHER N., 514
ALBONI P., 419, 522
ALMENDRAL J., 202
ALONSO C., 569
ANDREWS M.L., 299
APOLLONI R., 50
ARENA G., 485
ARENAL A., 202
ASCHIERI D., 80
AVELLA A., 530
BAGLIANI G., 50
BALDI N., 198
BARTOLETTI A., 423
BARTOLI P., 449
BASSO C., 6, 262
BENDINI M.G., 50
BENDITT D.G., 463
BERTAGLIA E., 268
BETTIOL K., 419
BIANCHI S., 212
BLANC J.J., 565
BOCHIARDO M., 136
BONGIORNI M.G., 386, 485
BONSO A., 85, 120, 131, 176, 475
BOTTONI N., 423, 449
BRACCHETTI D., 70
BREITHARDT G., 285
BRIGNOLE M., 386, 423, 449
BRUGADA J., 44, 255
BRUGADA P., 255
BRUGADA R., 44, 255
BUJA G., 262

CALABRESE F., 6
CALÒ L., 136
CANNOM D.S., 319
CAPPATO R., 386
CAPRIOGLIO F., 99
CAPUCCI A., 80, 386
CARBUCICCHIO C., 149
CARRERAS G., 50
CATTAFI G., 169
CAZZIN R., 534
CHEN C.H., 70
CHEN S.-A., 167
CHIARIELLO M., 494
CLÉMENTY J., 545
CODA L., 136
COLELLA A., 551
CONNOLLY S., 403
CORO L., 176
CORRADO A., 85, 120, 475
CORRADO D., 262
COSTA S., 423, 449
COSTANZO A., 494
COSTOLI A., 551
CRESTA R., 494
CRIJNS H.J.G.M., 105
CROTTI L., 291
CUTAIA V., 99
D'AVILA A., 341
DAUBERT J.C., 569
DE CRISTOFARO M., 268
DE PICCOLI B., 91, 99
DE PONTI R., 185, 216
DEHARO J.C., 551
DEL ROSSO A., 423, 449

LECTURES

Sudden Ischemic Cardiac Death: The Clinical Approach

A. Maseri

Introduction

Sudden ischemic cardiac death (SICD) is a collective, descriptive term for unexpected, natural cardiac death occurring as a result of some of the consequences of either acute myocardial ischemia and necrosis or of post-infarction scarring, hypertrophy and cardiac failure. It is responsible for about 85% of sudden death cases in adults; about 50% of cases occur in individuals without known ischemic heart disease (IHD), and the other 50% occur in patients with known IHD [about 75% with history of myocardial infarction (MI) and about 50% with history of heart failure]. The incidence of SICD increases markedly in the successive classes of the New York Heart Association (NYHA) functional classification of symptoms, but the percentage of cardiac deaths represented by SICD is, on average, about 50% in each of the four classes.

Pathogenetic Mechanisms

In individuals without known IHD and in patients with known IHD the most common cause of SICD is cardiac arrest due to either ventricular tachycardia (VT) or ventricular fibrillation (VF) and, much more rarely, to severe brady-arrhythmias.

An acute ischemic origin is common because in cases of SICD examined at autopsy the prevalence of both fresh thrombi, suggestive of acute ischemia, or signs of recent necrosis is over 75%, a percentage comparable to the prevalence of acute MI or persistent ST-T wave changes suggestive of severe ischemia in survivors resuscitated out of hospital.

There is increasing evidence that the most common causes of SICD (i.e. VT and VF) result from a combination of either acute ischemia and necrosis or of chronic myocardial scar, which favor disorganization of the sequence of electrical

Istituto di Cardiologia, Università Cattolica del Sacro Cuore, Rome, Italy activation with multiple re-entrant circuits, or with premature ventricular impulses. Thus, frequent and complex premature ventricular contractions (PVCs) may be innocuous in the absence of myocardial vulnerability.

Warning Symptoms

The possible warning symptoms of SICD are vague. About 40% of patients dying suddenly out of hospital had consulted a doctor in the previous 4 weeks; in less than 25% of cases this was because of angina, the usual cause being fatigue. A similar finding was reported in patients who had been resuscitated from cardiac arrest.

Predictive Value of Tests

As indicated in the introduction, on average, the risk of SICD is about half that of total IHD mortality, as in each ischemic syndrome about 50% of deaths are sudden. However, it is difficult to identify the 50% of patients who are likely to die suddenly:

In high risk patients a high predictive value is provided by heart failure, reduced ejection fraction (EF), prolongation of the QT interval, frequent PVCs (more than 10 per hour), reduced heart rate variability and ventricular after-potentials, but most of these variables are interrelated and their interdependence and incremental predictive roles need to be more accurately established.

In low risk patients the predictive accuracy of tests is very low according to the Bayesian theory.

Preventive strategies vary according to the different risk groups.
1. Patients in whom prevention of sudden death is unlikely to substantially prolong life expectancy should be treated only with the aim of improving the quality of life.
2. High-risk patients in whom prevention of sudden death can substantially prolong life expectancy can be considered for implantation of defibrillators, pacemakers.

However, about 70% of SICD occur in low risk patients and in previously healthy individuals. In such low risk groups the preventive approach cannot be based on a "blanket" treatment applied indiscriminately. A rational, effective strategy should be based on knowledge of the specific predisposing and precipitating causes in each of the homogeneous groups of patients which is easily identifiable clinically.

A Rational Clinical Approach to SICD

The development of specific preventive strategies can only begin by gathering detailed knowledge of three fundamental aspects:

First, the distinction of SICD in terms of time from onset of symptoms (instantaneous or within 6 h) is useful to physicians because only noninstantaneous death can give patients some time to seek immediate medical assistance.

Second, the distinction of patients in whom fatal arrhythmias develop in the presence of chronic myocardial scar tissue, but in the absence of a new episode of ischemia (type 1), from those in whom fatal arrhythmias are triggered by either new episodes of ischemia, as in patients with variant angina (type 2A), or of acute infarction (type 2B).

Third, the frequency with which tachy- or bradyarrhythmias precipitate SICD (type 1 or type 2A or type 2B), the contributory role of neurohumoral and of other determinants of risk and the incremental predictive value of specific tests in each of the easily identifiable clinical subgroups described below.

Therefore a clinically useful registry for SICD should be organized to include:
1. The time of occurrence of SICD after the onset of symptoms:
   (a) Instantaneous
   (b) Delayed up to 1 or to 6 h
2. The specific trigger of SICD that must be prevented [coronary spasm (type 2A), acute infarction (type 2B) or primary tachy- or bradyarrhythmias occurring in the absence of ischemia (type 1)], the role and the predictive value of indices of neurohumoral imbalance and other markers of risk. Whether occurrence of SICD is caused by an acute ischemic episode or occurs in the absence of ischemia can be defined clinically by the occurrence of the following:
   (a) Anginal pain and its duration before cardiac arrest, indicative of acute ischemia or of acute MI
   (b) SICD death occurring in the absence of symptoms of acute ischemia or necrosis (this definition, however, also includes cases precipitated by myocardial ischemia or necrosis occurring without chest pain)
3. The clinical syndromes in which SICD develops, with severity indicated by Canadian or New York Heart Association class, easily recognizable by any practising physician:
   (a) No previously known IHD in individuals with high, intermediate or low levels of coronary risk factors
   (b) Chronic IHD, with or without cardiac failure (NYHA class)
      - Recent MI (< 6 months)
      - Recent unstable angina (< 6 months)
      - Old MI (> 6 months)
      - Resolved unstable angina (> 6 months)
      - Chronic stable angina (Canadian class)
      - Variant angina

In order to acquire this information, which is necessary for the development of specific, preventive strategies, the time has come to set up a systematic prospective, multicenter data collection in a common registry.

Suggested Reading

Maseri A (1995) Ischemic Heart Disease. Rational basis for clinical practice and clinical research. Churchill Livingstone, New York, pp 673-683

Molecular Pathology of Cardiac Diseases Liable to Cause Sudden Death

F. Calabrese, C. Basso, G. Thiene and M. Valente

A sudden death (SD) always has a tragic impact both on families and on the general community. Although cardiac diseases liable to result in SD are mostly well identified, the etiopathogenetic understanding of most of these disorders is poor. To improve presymptomatic diagnosis, prevention and treatment, we need to define these disorders at the molecular and cellular levels.

This chapter will address the general principles of molecular pathology in cardiovascular medicine. The most common pathological substrates of SD and the current knowledge of the molecular basis of cardiovascular diseases liable to result in cardiac arrest will be reviewed as well.

Molecular Biology in Cardiovascular Medicine

The field of molecular biology was considered to have started in the 1950s, with the discoveries of the structure of DNA, the structure and mechanism of tRNA and the breaking of the genetic code [1-3]. The field has now entered its golden era with the development of recombinant technologies which are now utilized in virtually every subspeciality of diagnostic medicine and pathology [4]. Wide application of these techniques results from their sensitivity, specificity, speed, and relatively inexpensive cost. Although the ethics and economics of some molecular tests will spark intensive discussion, recombinant DNA technologies are likely to play an ever-increasing role in disease diagnosis and pathogenesis.

Unfortunately these new technologies were not immediately adopted in the field of cardiovascular disease. The reasons for this reluctance were mainly due to some organic features of the heart: (1) adult myocytes are differentiated cells, no longer capable of proliferating and thus not of primary interest in molecular biology; (2) most genomic mutations associated with hereditary cardiopathy usually cause lethal diseases, giving little access for future molecular approaches; (3) tumors, which are uncontrolled forms of proliferation and quite useful for pro-

Istituto di Anatomia Patologica, Università di Padova, Padua, Italy

viding information regarding development, are very rare in the heart; (4) it has only recently become possible to obtain intact DNA and RNA using fresh cardiac tissue for in vivo studies through endomyocardial biopsy. Since the 1980s molecular biology techniques have been used more and more accurately, offering unprecedented opportunities for improved diagnosis, detection, prevention and treatment of various forms of cardiovascular disease [5].

The most important subfields in which these techniques are successfully used are summarized in Table 1.

Table 1. Recombinant DNA technologies: major applications in cardiovascular fields

In vivo morpho-functional analysis of protein

Production of proteins present in low quantity and generation of new specific drugs

Sensitive and specific detection of different pathological processes using molecular hybridization assays and new molecular techniques

Identification and isolation of disease-causing genes (molecular genetic)

Better understanding of molecular cardiac development

Structural-Functional Analysis of Protein and Generation of New Specific Drugs

Before the widespread use of recombinant DNA technologies the protein function was tested only in an indirect way: protein isolation from tissue, purification and in vitro evaluation of its biochemical kinetics (studying its affinity for the substrate and production of each new protein).

Up to today the function of a specific protein could not be tested precisely. Nowadays using recombinant DNA technologies (such as molecular cloning and gene sequencing) it is possible to modify the gene which codes the specific protein to produce a non-functioning protein or on the contrary, to induce greater expression using a promoter. Cultured cells have typically been used to study in vivo mutant forms of proteins. However, for some proteins, adequate cell culture expression systems do not exist, and their expression in transgenic animals has now become an attractive alternative.

Other studies, conducted to perform structural-functional analysis of proteins in vivo, addressed the ionic sodium, calcium and potassium channels. The specific mRNA for the proteins of a given ionic channel is isolated, cloned and injected in the oocyte and then the ionic flow monitored using the "path clumping" technique.

Recombinant DNA technologies can quickly develop specific drugs with minimal or no collateral effects by transforming and specifically defining the biological properties of a protein or part of one in vivo. Tissue plasminogen activator (t-PA), used for thrombolysis in myocardial infarction, represents just one of the most important and well-known examples. It is the result of the genetic fusion of three genes: one codes a portion of the antibody (Fab) against fibrin, a second codes the Fab of antibodies against the tissue type plasminogen inhibitor (t-PA), also known as PA1, and a third codes the catalytic unit of recombinant tissue type plasminogen activator (rt-PA) [6]. More than 40 different forms of t-PA have been produced in attempts to reduce its side effects and inprove its therapeutic efficiency.

Sensitive and Specific Detection of Different Pathological Processes Using New Molecular Assays

The principle of all molecular hybridization assays is the complementary base pairing between two nucleic acid strands. In situ hybridization (ISH) provides the direct detection of nucleic acid in cellular material in which simultaneous morphological analysis can be performed.

Since its introduction in 1985, the polymerase chain reaction (PCR) has led to a veritable revolution in molecular biology [7]. It has been referred to as the "molecular biologist's photocopying machine" as it allows millions of copies of any specific DNA sequence to be generated within a few hours. The reaction consists of an in vitro enzymatic amplification of a defined DNA sequence by repeated rounds of heat denaturation, primer annealing and DNA polymerase-mediated primer extension. The amplified DNA can then be seen as a distinct band after standard agarose gel electrophoresis, and the specificity of detection can be increased by subsequent hybridization or DNA sequencing. According to the nested PCR technique, a second pair of primers "internal" to the original primer pair is used in a subsequent series of amplification cycles. Using this strategy, the sensitivity is enhanced from 100 to 1000 times, to a such an extent that even a single copy target can be detected in a complex background of 300 000 cells or more. Recently a number of strategies have also been reported for carrying out nested PCR in a single tube [8, 9].

One of the most important and frequent applications of these novel techniques is for the identification of microbial pathogens. Given the extreme sensitivity of these techniques, particularly of PCR, a single copy of a gene can be readily detected from extremely small amounts of tissue, such as small fragments of endomyocardial biopsies. The significance of detection of viral genomes in heart tissue is reduced by latency, common to some viruses such as herpes viruses. Reverse transcriptase PCR of specific viral mRNA is usually performed to detect active viral replication, in other words the infective state of the virus. The decision to develop and apply PCR for routine diagnosis of myocarditis must be considered in relation to the low cost, speed, sensitivity and reliability of more conventional culture and/or serological methods [10]. PCR holds its greatest promise for extending diagnosis beyond simple infective agent detection. Important genetic characteristics such as virulence and responsiveness to chemotherapy are amenable to direct analysis by PCR. This area of endeavor is proceeding rapidly, and it is likely that many types of microrganisms will be categorized pathologically according to subtle genetic changes.

PCR may detect virtually all the common genetically inherited diseases in which the defective gene has been identified, such as Duchenne muscular dystrophy and hypertrophic cardiomyopathy [11, 12].

PCR can also trace the inheritance of diseases in which the defective locus has only been defined in terms of linkage to other cellular genes. Using PCR, allelic forms of many cellular genes can be identified by sizing selected introns between the coding exons [13]. This approach should provide much more detailed linkage studies than are presently possible using restriction fragment length polymorphism (RFLP) analysis.

Sequencing of PCR-amplified genes has led to the discovery of disease-associated single-nucleotide differences in the genes like those encoding histocompatibility antigens [14, 15] and various hormone and growth-factor receptor molecules. PCR-based analysis will undoubtedly lead to the identification of a vast array of genetically based diseases as well as provide insights into disease pathogenesis.

A variety of types of samples may be used in PCR. Extracted nucleic acid may be amplified with ease, even in a partially purified sample. Extracted DNA or RNA from formalin-fixed, paraffin-embedded samples obtained either at autopsy or at surgery are successfully used as templates for PCR. This could permit ever more frequent application, including in retrospective studies.

Apoptosis is a mechanism by which cells respond to damage by triggering a program of cell death [16-18]. Apoptosis has only recently been recognized as a component of many common cardiac pathologies such as chronic heart failure, viral myocarditis and ischemia [19-21]. Since apoptosis involves the fragmentation of chromatin, several researchers have used DNA polymerases or terminal transferases to end-label DNA strand breaks by the incorporation of biotinylated nucleotide in situ end labeling (ISEL) [22, 23]. Labeled nuclei are then identified by the addition of a streptavidin-peroxidase conjugate and an appropriate peroxidase substrate. These methods have several potential advantages: greater sensitivity (more nuclei are detected as being apoptotic), greater specificity (there is less equivocation since apoptotic nuclei are clearly marked); and easy quantitation (the labeled nuclei in tissue sections may be counted by automated image cytometry).

Identification and Isolation of Disease-Causing Genes

Through the application of recombinant DNA technology, the study of human genetic disorders has undergone a substantial surge in activity. Many cardiovascular diseases recognize genetic factors that can contribute to their pathogenesis. According to a survey of the human conditions caused largely by mutations in a single gene (currently more than 16,000 have been identified) [24], a large number (7-8%) affect the cardiovascular system. This suggests that potentially 5,000 or more genes are involved in the embryology, differentiation and maturation of cardiovascular structures and in all the processes that regulate cardiovascular function.

A genetic marker is a trait whose inheritance can be followed within a family. This trait becomes a marker for genes located within the neighboring chromosomal region. If an individual has inherited the marker from a given chromosomal region, by inference, the individual should have inherited all of the genes located within that chromosomal region.

DNA sequence variations between individuals are routinely ascertained using restriction enzymes. Each restriction enzyme recognizes and cleaves double-stranded DNA at a specific sequence of nucleotides. Variation in the presence of restriction enzyme sites results in the generation of different-size fragments of DNA (restriction fragment length polymorphism, RFLP). These fragments of DNA are detected by a procedure using gel electrophoresis, transfer of the separated DNA to a filter membrane, and hybridization to a radiolabeled probe (southern blotting) [25-27].

Genetic linkage may be defined as the nonrandom assortment of two DNA markers (defined as multiallelic polymorphic loci) within a family because of their physical proximity on the same chromosome. The closer two markers are within the same segment of chromosomal DNA, the less likely it is that a recombination event will occur between them and the more tightly linked they are. In any genetic linkage study, informative meioses are those that occur in an individual who is heterozygous at the marker loci. With their high level of polymorphism and their ability to detect both alleles in heterozygotes, RFLPs are particularly well suited for genetic studies. Linkage relationships (or the lack of them) are expressed mathematically as the logarithm of the odds (LOD score) in favor of linkage at given distance between the marker and the phenotype loci. LOD scores of 3.0 or greater are considered statistically significant, while LOD scores of ≤ 2.0 statistically exclude two markers as being linked. LOD scores between 2.0 and 3.0 are considered inconclusive. Several single-gene disorders have been linked to DNA markers over the last few years, such as those identified as causing dilated cardiomyopathy, arrhythmogenic right ventricular cardiomyopathy and long QT syndrome.

Better Understanding of Molecular Cardiac Development

Cardiogenesis is one of the most critical steps in embryonic development.

A large body of genetically based studies have elucidated the principles and pathways that guide cardiovascular development in both invertebrate and vertebrate species. Different transcriptional regulators (GATA factors, MEF-2 family, etc.) have been found in specific steps of cardiac morphogenesis [28, 29] from the establishment of left-right asymmetry in the primitive heart tube, looping morphogenesis, right and left ventricular chamber specification, trabeculation, outflow tract septation, conotruncal development, functional maturation of the ventricular chamber, expansion of the compact zone and endocardial cushion formation. In this regard, a variety of genetic systems, including fruit flies (Drosophila), zebrafish, frogs, chicks and mice are used to identify and better understand the complex stages of cardiovascular growth and development [30].

Molecular Basis of Cardiovascular Substrates at Risk of Sudden Death

Whereas SD in the adult is mostly due to atherosclerotic coronary artery disease often associated with previous myocardial infarction [31, 32], a large spectrum of cardiac substrates may underlie SD in the young [33-37]. We recently calculated an overall prevalence of SD of 0.8/100,000 per year in the young [38]. Based upon the Veneto region study project on juvenile SD, cardiovascular SD accounted for more than 80% of the collected cases, and about one third of SDs were due to a congenital heart defect present since birth [37]. As to the pathophysiologic mechanism, cardiac arrest may be mechanical or arrhythmic in nature. Table 2 reports the main causes of cardiovascular SD in our series of cases collected since 1979 [38].

Table 2. Causes of sudden death in people aged ≤ 35 years in the Veneto region of Italy, 1979 to 1996. (From [38], modified)

Cause	Total	
Arrhythmogenic right ventricular cardiomyopathy	29	(10.8%)
Atherosclerotic coronary artery disease	45	(16.7%)
Anomalous origin of coronary artery	7	(2.6%)
Disease of conduction system	24	(8.9%)
Mitral valve prolapse	26	(9.7%)
Hypertrophic cardiomyopathy	17	(6.3%)
Myocarditis	22	(8.2%)
Myocardial bridge	7	(2.6%)
Pulmonary thromboembolism	4	(1.5%)
Dissecting aortic aneurysm	12	(4.5%)
Dilated cardiomyopathy	10	(3.7%)
Other	66	(24.5%)
Total	269	

Arrhythmic Sudden Death with Structural Heart Disease

Heart Muscle Disease

Hypertrophic cardiomyopathy. The natural history of hypertrophic cardiomyopathy is often marked by SD [39, 40]. Heart dysfunction appears more in the form of electrical instability than of impaired contractility. The reported incidence of SD is 2-4% a year in adults and 4-6% a year in children and adolescents. Risk factors are considered to be young age, previous syncopal episodes, a malignant family history, myocardial ischemia, sustained ventricular tachycardia on electrophysiological test and ventricular tachycardia on Holter monitoring [39]. A complex interaction occurs between left ventricular hypertrophy, left ventricular outflow pressure gradient, diastolic dysfunction and myocardial ischemia, which accounts for the great variability of clinical findings. Myocardial disarray, with myocytes spatially arranged in a chaotic manner, and interstitial fibrosis, represent an ideal substrate of inhomogeneous intraventricular conduction with potential reentry phenomena [41]. Moreover, detailed pathologic studies on subjects dying suddenly demonstrated the superimposition of ischemic damage to the dysplastic myocardium, in the shape of myocyte necrosis and large fibrous scars mimicking healed infarction. The ischemic damage may occur in the absence of significant epicardial coronary artery disease, although small vessel disease as well as intramural course of the left anterior descending coronary artery have been noted [42]. The combination of myocardial disarray and replacement fibrosis has to be considered a highly malignant arrhythmogenic substrate in hypertrophic cardiomyopathy.

Recently, molecular genetic studies demonstrated that hypertrophic cardiomyopathy is a heterogeneous disease, with several missense mutations in genes encoding for proteins of the cardiac sarcomere [43]. Mutations in 7 sarcomeric protein genes have been identified in affected families (Table 3): β-myosin

Table 3. Genetic basis of cardiac diseases liable to cause sudden death

Disease	Locus	Gene	Reference
Hypertrophic cardiomyopathy	1q3	CTnT	Thierfelder et al. [48]
			Watkins et al. [55]
	3p	MELC	Poetter et al. [45]
	7q3*	?	MacRae et al. [50]
	11p11.2	MyPBC	Bonne et al. [53]
			Watkins et al. [54]
	12q23-q24.3	MRLC	Poetter et al. [45]
	14q11-q12	β-MHC	Jarcho et al. [44]
	15q2	α-TM	Thierfelder et al. [48]
			Watkins et al. [55]
	19p13.2-q13.2	CTn1	Kimura et al. [47]
Arrhythmogenic right ventricular cardiomyopathy	14q23-q24	?	Rampazzo et al. [64]
	1q42-q43	?	Rampazzo et al. [65]
	14q12-q22	?	Severini et al. [66]
	2q32.1-q32.2	?	Rampazzo et al. [67]
	3p23	?	Ahmad et al. [68]
Naxos disease	17q21	?	Coonar et al. [69]
Familial idiopathic VF	3p21-q23	SCN5A	Chen et al. [143]
X-linked dilated cardiomyopathy	Xp.21.2	Dystrophin	Muntoni et al. [81]
			Muntoni et al. [82]
			Milasin et al. [91]
			Ortiz Lopez et al. [92]
Barth syndrome	Xq28	G.4.5	Bione et al. [93]
Autosomal dominant dilated cardiomyopathy	1q32	?	Durand et al. [84]
	2p31	?	Siu [85]
	9q13-q21	?	Krajinovic et al. [86]
	10q21-q23	?	Bowles et al. [87]
	3p22-p25	?	Olson and Keating [89]
	15q14	Actin	Olson et al. [90]

Cont.

Cont. Table 3.

Disease	Locus	Gene	Reference
Conduction defect and dilated cardiomyopathy	1p1-1q1	?	Kass et al. [88]
LQTS (Romano Ward type)	3p21-p23	SCN5A	Wang et al. [131]
	4q25-q27	?	Schott et al. [135]
	7q35-q36	HERG	Curran et al. [132]
	11p15.5	KvLQT1	Wang et al. [133]
	21q22.1-q22	MinK	Splawski et al. [134]
LQTS (Jervell and Lange-Nielsen type)	11p15.5	KvLQT1	Neyroud et al. [136] Splawski et al. [137]
	21q22.1-q22	MinK	Schultze-Bahr et al. [138]
PFHB-I	19q13.2-q13.2	?	Brink et al. [97] De Meeus et al. [98]
Supravalvular aortic stenosis	7q11.23	Elastin	Ewart et al. [109] Curran et al. [110]
Marfan syndrome	15q15-q21.3	Fibrillin-1	Kainulainen et al. [145] Dietz et al. [146]

* associated with Wolff-Parkinson-White Syndrome

heavy chain on chromosome 14, cardiac essential myosin light chain on chromosome 3, cardiac regulatory myosin light chain on chromosome 12, cardiac troponin T on chromosome 1, cardiac troponin I on chromosome 19, α-tropomyosin on chromosome 15 and cardiac myosin-binding protein C on chromosome 11 [44-53]. Available data suggest that mutations in β-myosin heavy chain and myosin-binding protein C are more common than the others. Moreover, beside locus heterogeneity, there is marked allelic heterogeneity for all the identified genes and more than 80 different mutations have been reported, the majority being missense mutations. Mutations in different components of the sarcomere appear to produce the same phenotype expression. From the functional point of view, sarcomeric contractile performance becomes depressed, suggesting that myocyte hypertrophy could be a compensatory response. Some mutations have been reported to carry a benign significance, with a low risk for SD, whereas others are associated with a poor prognosis, thus explaining the existence of subgroups of families with a malignant history. Although data on genotype-phenotype correlations are still preliminary, it seems that the phenotype varies not only with the type of mutation but also within individuals carrying the same mutation. For instance, the arginine-to-glutamine mutation in 403 codon of β-myosin is associated with a poor prognosis, whereas the arginine-to-tryptophan mutation appears more benign [51, 52]. Moreover, the knowledge that myosin-binding protein C mutations appear to be associated with age-related penetrance in adulthood would have consequences for genetic counseling [53, 54]. As to the phenotype caused by troponin

T mutation, it appears to be associated with no or mild hypertrophy, up to 50% of nonpenetrance and a high risk of SD, even in the absence of severe left ventricular hypertrophy [55, 56].

Arrhythmogenic right ventricular cardiomyopathy. Also known as right ventricular dysplasia, this is one of the leading causes of SD in the young in our series [57-59]. Arrhythmogenic right ventricular cardiomyopathy may be a concealed abnormality in apparently healthy subjects. In terms of contractility, heart performance may be preserved since the left ventricle is usually spared. This explains why the disease is observed even in sports champions, manifesting only with minor symptoms like palpitations or lipothymia, and why the diagnosis is frequently missed in preparticipation screenings [38]. In these subjects the presence of ECG abnormalities, like an inverted T wave in the right precordial leads (V1-V3), increased QRS duration >110 ms, late potentials detected by high resolution electrocardiography and ventricular arrhythmias, even in the shape of single premature ventricular beats with left bundle branch block morphology, should raise suspicion of the disease and lead to further investigation. Imaging procedures, whether non-invasive or invasive, are useful in detecting structural and functional abnormalities of the right ventricle, such as bulging, wall motion abnormalities and dilatation [60]. Nuclear magnetic resonance, furthermore, is a very effective tool for tissue characterization and may help detect the fatty myocardial infiltration [60]. The disease is characterized pathologically by a peculiar myocardial atrophy with fibro-fatty substitution of the right ventricular free wall in an apparently normal heart. Histology reveals the disappearance (atrophy) of the right ventricular myocardium and the fibro-fatty or fatty replacement, with a wave-front extension from the epicardium towards the endocardium [59, 61]. The intraventricular conduction delay, resulting from the fibro-fatty replacement is a source of electrical instability, due to reentrant phenomena, in the shape of ventricular arrhythmias (premature ventricular beats, non-sustained or sustained ventricular tachycardia) with left bundle branch block morphology, indicating a right ventricular origin. Evidence of acquired, progressive cell death rules out a congenital heart disease. The disease is now listed among cardiomyopathies in the WHO revised classification [62].

A familial character has been demonstrated in nearly 50% of cases, with an autosomal dominant inheritance [63]. Even though a defective gene has not been identified so far, 5 different gene loci have been described, 2 of which are located in close proximity on chromosome 14 (14q23-q24 and 14q12-q22), a third locus located on chromosome 1 (1q42-q43), a fourth on chromosome 2 (2q32.1-q32.2) and the fifth on chromosome 3 (3p23) [64-68]. An autosomal recessive variant of arrhythmogenic right ventricular cardiomyopathy (ARVC) that is associated with woolly hair and palmoplantar keratoderma has been reported from the island of Naxos in Greece and linked to chromosome 17 (17q21), within the gene encoding a keratin, a reasonable candidate for this entity [69]. In the experience collected by Nava et al. in Padua, no linkage was found to the known chromosomal loci in 50% of families [70]. Thus, several genes seem to be involved, suggesting genetic heterogeneity. A genetically determined atrophy might explain this cardiomyopathy, which might then be considered a myocardial dystrophy. The histological similarities with some skeletal muscular dystrophies, like Duchenne and Becker, favor this hypothesis.

Recently, apoptosis (genetically determined cell death) has been postulated to account for cell death [71, 72]. Evidence supporting this view has been collected both at autopsy and from biopsy material (Fig. 1). Interestingly, the presence of

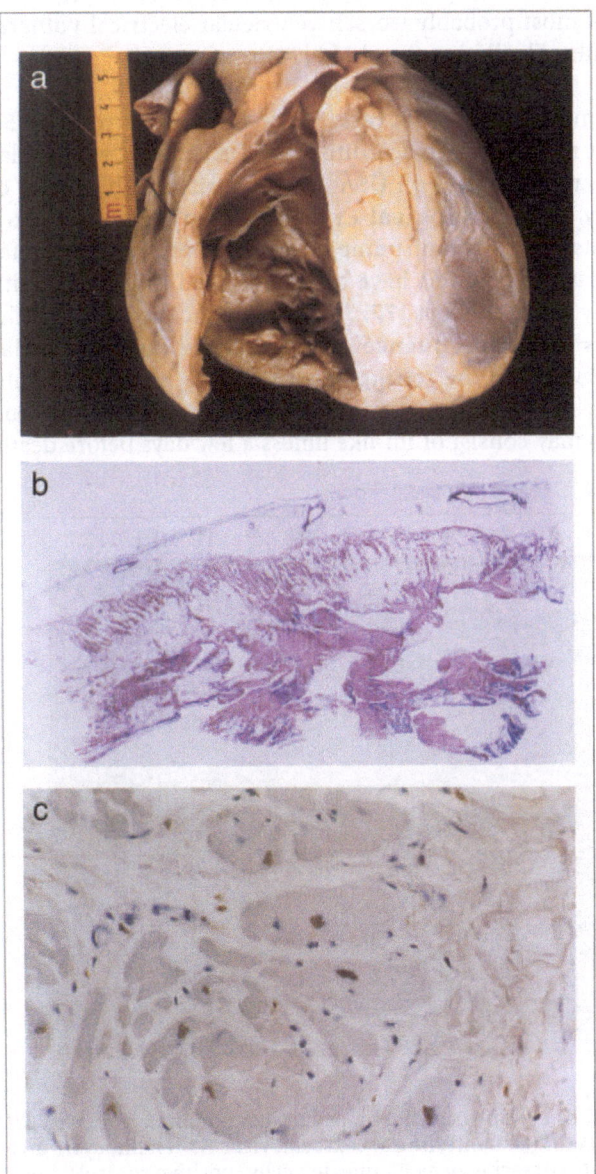

Fig. 1a-c. Sudden death due to arrhythmogenic right ventricular cardiomyopathy in a 28-year-old man with a previous history of syncopal episodes. a. Gross view: note the yellow appearance of the right ventricular free wall. b. Histology of the right ventricular freewall revealing massive fatty replacement. Azan Mallory, x 3. c. Photographs of TUNEL-stained myocardium: intensely dark stained nuclei of myocytes adjacent to adipose tissue. Original magnification x 300

apoptosis was found in the early and acute symptomatic phase of the disease [72].

Focal myocarditis with myocyte death was observed in all cases with fibro-fatty variant: whether inflammation is primary or secondary to cell death remains to be established [59, 73]. Recent analysis using nested PCR for enterovirus failed to detect any viral genome in biopsies of affected patients with both recent and chronic clinical onset of the disease (Fig. 2). Focal, progressive cell death may lead to either fibrous or fatty replacement, with adipocytes taking the place of dying myocytes. Focal myocarditis, bouts of apoptosis, right ventricular aneurysms and left ventricular involvement most probably worsen ventricular electrical vulnerability and lower the ventricular fibrillation threshold [74].

Myocarditis. SD caused by myocarditis is not rare, particularly in the young [75]. The strongest evidence that subclinical myocarditis can be a cause of ventricular fibrillation comes from an autopsy series on USA army recruits in which 40% of those who died suddenly had histological evidence of myocarditis [76]. Myocarditis usually presents with signs of pump failure and ventricular dilatation. Nonetheless, ventricular arrhythmias have been described in patients with myocarditis and apparently normal heart [77, 78]. SD may occur in either the active or the heale phases as a consequence of life-threatening ventricular arrhythmias that mostly develop in the setting of an unstable myocardial substrate, namely inflammatory infiltrate, interstitial edema, myocardial necrosis and fibrosis. Previous symptoms may consist of flu-like illness a few days before death,

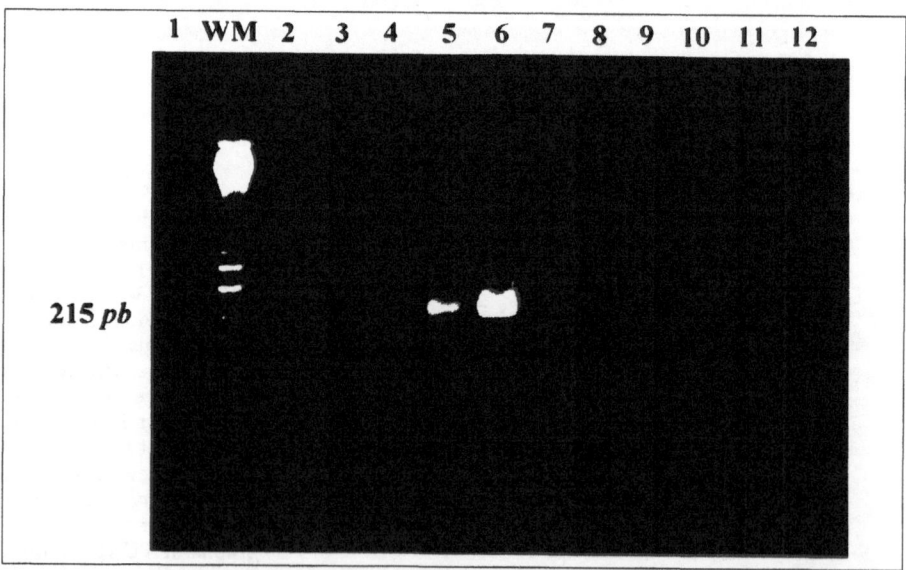

Fig. 2. Results of nested RT-PCR of endomyocardial biopsy tissues obtained from ARVC/D patients. Line 2,4,7-12: nine ARVC/D patients; line 5: coxsackievirus B3 lymphocytic myocarditis (positive control); line 6: coxsackievirus B3 infected cells (positive control); line 1: uninfected cells. (From [74] with permission)

syncopal episodes and premature ventricular beats. The gross appearance of the heart is not distinctive and its weight may be within normal values. Histology invariably discloses a patchy inflammatory infiltrate, sometimes no more than three foci at magnification x 6 and not necessarily associated with myocardial necrosis. The inflammatory infiltrate is usually polymorphous and less frequently purely lymphocytic. This subtle substrate, together with possible inflammatory involvement of the conduction system, is highly arrhythmogenic, accounting for unexpected arrhythmic cardiac arrest. Myocardial infection, whether bacterial or viral, has rarely been investigated. Noteworthy is the report of an increased sudden cardiac death rate among young Swedish elite orienteers with histopathological evidence of myocarditis and serologic demonstration of antibodies to *Chlamydia pneumoniae* [79].

Nonetheless, viral infections are the most plausible cause. Molecular biology techniques with PCR are now an essential tool and the gold standard for an etiological diagnosis. Application of gene amplification techniques is particularly useful in detecting viral nucleic acids in biopsies, especially when characteristic cytopathic changes cannot be observed on light microscopy, a rather frequent condition in acute fatal forms causing SD. Although enteroviruses are the most important causative agent in the pathogenesis of myocarditis, several studies have shown that various other viruses, such as adenovirus, herpesvirus (cytomegalovirus, herpes simplex virus, Epstein-Barr virus), parvovirus, influenza virus A and B, and hepatitis C virus can be involved in myocardial infective disease, particularly in the pediatric population (Fig. 3) [10, 80].

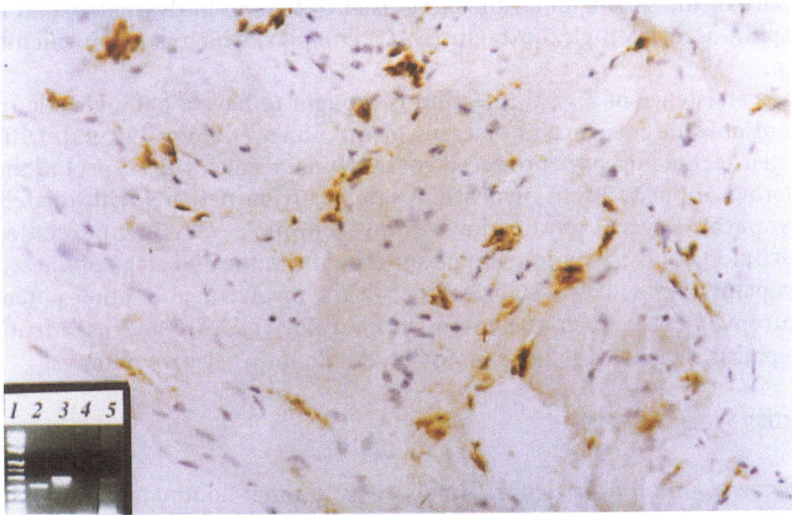

Fig. 3. Myocarditis in pediatric age. Numerous inflammatory cells stained strongly for UCHL-1 (CD45RO), demonstrating that the lymphocytes of the infiltrate are primarily T cells. *Insert:* PCR analysis for adenovirus: lane 1: molecular size marker, lane 2: β-globin amplimer ("housekeeping" gene), lane 3: adenovirus positive control, lane 4: negative control, lane 5: myocarditis

Dilated cardiomyopathy. Dilated cardiomyopathy is a genetically and clinically heterogeneous disease. The natural history demonstrates that death occurs not only due to progressive congestive heart failure or as a complication of thromboembolism, but also abruptly due to arrhythmic cardiac arrest. In these circumstances death is obviously expected and, according to definition, it should not be considered strictly as a true SD. However, in a few cases of dilated cardiomyopathy arrhythmic SD may be the first manifestation of the disease and the diagnosis achieved only at postmortem by observing a heavy heart with dilated ventricles and no inflammatory or coronary artery disease.

As to the molecular basis of dilated cardiomyopathy, at least 30% of cases are inherited, with a significant percentage of the remaining cases being acquired (i.e., myocarditis, autoimmune, etc.). Inherited forms may have autosomal dominant, autosomal recessive, X-linked, or mitochondrial transmission, with evident genetic heterogeneity [83].

Genes for the autosomal dominant form have been mapped to six different loci. Four of them are associated with "pure" dilated cardiomyopathy: 1q32, 2p31, 9q13, and 10q21-23 [84-87]; whereas the remaining two loci refer to dilated cardiomyopathy with conduction defects: 1p1-1q1 and 3p22-3p25 [88, 89]. Quite recently, cardiac actin gene mutation on chromosome 15q14 has been identified [90].

The genes for two X-linked cardiomyopathies have been identified and multiple mutations of both have been reported as well. They are the dystrophin gene (Xp.21.2), which is also responsible for Duchenne and Becker muscular dystrophy [91, 92], and the G 4.5 gene (Xq28) in the Barth syndrome [93]. Whereas the G 4.5 gene function is still unknown, dystrophin is a large cytoskeletal protein of the inner face of the sarcolemma, attaching itself to F-actin in the matrix and to the dystrophin-associated glycoprotein (DAG) complex, which is a transmembrane protein.

The persistence of a viral infection is thought to have a pathogenetic role in different chronic myocardial diseases of unknown etiology [94, 95]. Different molecular techniques have produced controversial results with respect to the rate of enteroviral positivity in myocardial samples from patients with dilated cardiomyopathy. Several studies have showed no or a very low percentage of enteroviral PCR positivity in patients suffering from the end stage of dilated cardiomyopathy (Fig. 4) [96]. Viral clearance or the involvement of other potentially cardiotropic viruses, such as human cytomegalovirus, coronavirus, adenovirus and hepatitis C virus, could explain the predominantly negative findings.

Conduction System Diseases

Progressive familial heart block. This is an autosomal dominant disease characterized by progression from a normal conduction pattern to bundle branch block and subsequently to complete heart block with wide QRS complexes [97]. Typical manifestations of the disease are syncope, SD and Morgagni-Stokes-Adams attacks. Treatment with pacemaker implantation is required. A study of 86 family members of three pedigrees, in which 34 members were affected, led to the

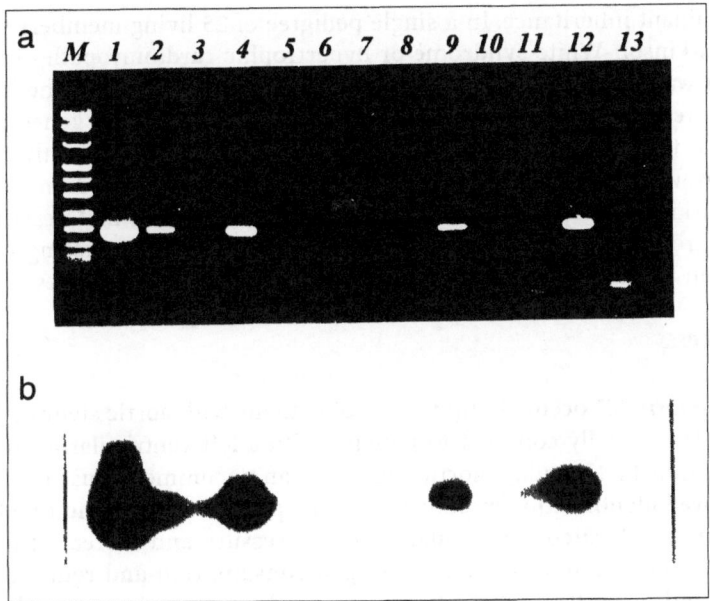

Fig. 4a,b. RT-PCR for enterovirus in native hearts of cardiac transplanted patients. Agarose gel electrophoresis (**a**) and its southern hybridization (**b**). M: molecular size marker Line 1: Coxsackievirus B3 infected cells (positive control), lane 2: case of DC (enterovirus +), lane 4: case of lymphocitic myocarditis (enterovirus +), lane 9 and 12: cases of lymphocitic myocarditis (coxsackievirus B3 + ,positive controls), lane3, 5-8 and 10,11 are cases of ischemic cardiopathy, dilated cardiomyopathy and valvular disease (enterovirus -), lane 13: uninfected cells (negative control). (From [96] with permission)

demonstration of genetic linkage to chromosome 19 (19q13.2-q13.3) and the gene was localized to within 10cM of the kallikrein locus [98].

Familial Wolff-Parkinson-White syndrome. Wolff-Parkinson-White syndrome is a disorder in which an aberrant myocardial fascicle joins the atria to the ventricles, beyond the specialized AV junction [99]. Known by the eponym of Kent's bundle, it consists of a 200- to 400-micron-thick structure, directly connecting the atrial with the ventricular musculature [100]. It is the smallest common congenital heart disease and affects 0.5-1‰ of live births [101]. Usually located in the lateral rings, especially the left AV one related to the attachment of the mural mitral leaflet, it consists of ordinary myocardium which does not possess decremental properties of specialized AV nodal conducting tissues. Due to the regular delay through the specialized AV junction tissue, the atrial impulse excites the ventricles earlier through the accessory pathway. The risk of SD in patients is low and mainly related to the occurrence of atrial fibrillation, which may convert into ventricular fibrillation due to the short refractoriness of the AV accessory pathway, which allows transmission of more than 300 impulses per minute to the ventricles [102]. In most of the cases, the disease is not hereditary, although some familial cases of Wolff-Parkinson-White have been reported, suggesting autosomal dominant inheritance. In a single pedigree of 25 living members with either Wolff-Parkinson-White syndrome or hypertrophic cardiomyopathy, or both, the disorder was linked to chromosome 7 (7q3) [50]. It is unknown whether a single defect is responsible for both clinical pictures or whether two genes are located very close to each other (contiguous gene syndrome), thus frequently cosegregating. However, other associations of familial hypertrophic cardiomyopathy and Wolff-Parkinson-White syndrome have been identified, like that described in the cardiac troponin I gene on chromosome 19 [47], thus suggesting that Wolff-Parkinson-White syndrome may have several different pathogeneses.

Valve Diseases

Aortic stenosis. SD occurs in up to 20% of patients with aortic stenosis [103]. The risk of SD is usually confined to patients with a left ventricular/aortic gradient above 50 mmHg. Nowadays aortic stenosis is an uncommon cause of SD, because of improved identification of patients at risk, sport restriction and timely surgical intervention. Elevated ventricular systolic pressure and increased myocardial mass may both account for raised oxygen consumption and reduced coronary reserve and provide a substrate for myocardial ischemia, particularly in the subendocardium, even in the absence of coronary artery disease. Pathologic study of these SD cases usually discloses subendocardial ischemia in terms of myocytolysis and scarring, both well-known arrhythmogenic substrates. Exercise increases oxygen demand and the blood perfusion discrepancy, with the onset of lethal ventricular tachyarrhythmias. Whereas in the elderly aortic stenosis is usually the result of senile dystrophic calcification of the aortic valve or of a calcified bicuspid valve [104, 105], in the young it is mostly related to congenital valve malformations, like unicuspid or bicuspid conditions with dysplastic cusp stiffness [106].

Bicuspid aortic valve occurs in about 1%-2% of the general population and can be a predisposing factor for SD not only due to the increased risk of aortic dissection (see below) but also the risk of development of aortic stenosis [107]. Familial cases with autosomal dominant inheritance have been reported [108].

Supravalvular aortic stenosis occurs with a frequency of 1/25,000. A familial pattern with autosomal dominant inheritance has been reported. The disease has been linked to chromosome 7 and results from a defect in the elastin gene which causes an hour-glass obstruction of the ascending aorta and left ventricular hypertrophy [109, 110]. The phenotype is thus linked to gross DNA rearrangements in elastin. It is marked by elastosis of the aortic tunica media, intimal thickening and dysplastic cusps [111, 112]. Isolation of the coronary ostia, because of fusion of semilunar cusps leaflets with the aortic wall, as well as a stenotic intra-arterial course of the coronary arteries further aggravate the coronary ischemia in these patients [113]. Williams syndrome is an autosomal dominant disorder that is characterized by supravalvular aortic stenosis, peripheral pulmonary stenosis, obstructive coronary lesions, abnormal facies and mental retardation. This syndrome was found to be associated with deletion of a region of chromosome 7 (7q11.23) that includes the elastin gene and is thought to be a contiguous gene disorder caused by the deletion of multiple adjacent genes.

Mitral valve prolapse. This has been reported to occur in 1% of the male and 6% of the female population. However, SD is rare, especially in people less than 20 years of age [114]. Unexpected death may rarely be a mechanical complication of valve function, with chordal rupture and pulmonary edema. More frequently it is a consequence of an abrupt electrical disorder in the form of ventricular tachycardia and fibrillation. It was postulated that elongated chordae or redundant valve leaflets, by rubbing against the ventricular endocardium, may elicit ventricular electrical instability and promote cardiac arrest. Hemodynamically significant mitral valve regurgitation, autonomic nervous system dysfunction, conduction system abnormalities as well as focal myocarditis have also been advanced as possible etiopathogenetic mechanisms [114]. Recently, histologic studies of the right ventricular myocardium disclosed significant fatty infiltration, especially at infundibular level, in a subset of patients dying suddenly [114, 115].

Familial mitral valve prolapse has been classified as an inherited connective tissue disorder and several studies suggest that the mode of inheritance is autosomal dominant. It may occur alone or in association with minor physical features such as pectus excavatum, straight back syndrome, long thin chest, long arms or joint hypermobility, but in the absence of other features of Marfan syndrome. Moreover, mitral valve prolapse is very frequent in patients affected by Marfan syndrome (see below), and it is also well recognized to occur in numerous other heritable disorders of connective tissue, such as Ehlers-Danlos syndrome, osteogenesis imperfecta and pseudoxanthoma elasticum [116, 117].

Coronary Artery Disease

The coronary artery pathology in SD adult victims consists of single, double or triple vessel atherosclerotic disease and usually includes a thrombotic occlusion of a coronary segment, which accounts for sharp interruption of the regional myocardial blood flow [31, 32]. By contrast, coronary SD in the young usually is due to a single subobstructive plaque, located at the first tract of the anterior descending coronary artery, mostly fibrocellular, devoid of atheroma, fissuring or thrombosis [36]. The preservation of the tunica media, the absence of thrombosis and the frequent occurrence of unexpected death at rest, following event of variant angina, are all features in keeping with a transient ischemic event, most probably ascribable to coronary vasospasm. In the setting of acute thrombosis, superficial erosion seems to be a peculiar mechanism precipitating plaque instability, unlike in the adult where it is mainly due to rupture of the thin fibrous cap [118]. Endothelial erosion may be the consequence of plaque inflammation and of intimal smooth muscle cell proliferation.

Several reports, using molecular hybridization assays, have shown a correlation between the incidence of atherosclerosis and the presence of infective microorganisms, like herpesviruses and *Chlamydia pneumoniae* [119-121]. Both organisms have been identified in atheromatous lesions in coronary arteries and in other organs obtained at autopsy. Increased titers of antibodies to these organisms have been used as a predictor of further adverse events in patients who have had a myocardial infection. Atherosclerotic lesions were not reproduced experimentally in animals by injection of these microorganisms, a fact that leaves their role questionable as etiologic agents, according to Koch postulates. However, the possibility that infection, combined with other factors, may be responsible for the genesis of atherosclerotic plaques in some patients cannot be ruled out.

Genetic studies have shown that different genes are expressed in the disease and this could be an interesting factor in deciphering the complex nature of atherogenesis [122]. Because atherosclerosis is a multigenic disease, understanding the patterns of gene expression may help to explain varying susceptibility to agents causing disease as well as response to therapy. Studies in transgenic mice have revealed that Lp(a) lipoprotein, cholesterol ester transfer protein, apolipoprotein A (the principal apoprotein of high density lipoprotein), and other molecules have little effect on atherogenesis, whereas macrophage colony- stimulating factor appears to be important in the regulation of the numbers of monocytes and macrophages and in lesion formation [123, 124].

Some authors, using ISEL or DNA gel electrophoresis, have shown that apoptosis may modulate the cellularity of lesions that produce human vascular obstruction, particularly those with evidence of more extensive proliferative activity [125].

Arrhythmic Sudden Death Without Structural Heart Disease ("Idiopathic" Arrhythmic Sudden Death)

There are patients who undergo a cardiac arrest due to ventricular fibrillation without clinical identification of even a subtle structural abnormality [126]. Overall, sudden cardiac death remains unexplained in 5%-10% of cases, even after a thorough macroscopic and microscopic examination, including the conduction system and cardiac innervation [127]. In other words, no apparent organic substrate is detected by traditional investigations ("mors sine materia") and death is ascribable merely to an abrupt, functional disorder. Whether these cases are truly idiopathic or unexplained because of a clinical inability to identify pathologic substrates, remains to be elucidated. It may be that the structural abnormality resides at a molecular level.

Long QT Syndrome

The long QT syndrome (LQTS) is the best known congenital cause of arrhythmic SD in the absence of gross structural cardiac pathology [128]. It is a familial disease with high cardiac electrical instability, presenting with syncope due to ventricular tachyarrhythmias or with cardiac arrest on exercise or emotional stress, often under the age of 15. The cause of death cannot be ascertained at necropsy unless there are prior ECG data.

Genetic analysis reveals multiple abnormalities in genes related both to potassium and sodium cardiac channels. Alterations of ion pumps and current account for the lengthened action potential and prolonged QT interval on ECG, and the propensity to ventricular fibrillation. The mortality in untreated symptomatic cases exceeds 60% within 15 years. Clearly ECG screening of surviving relatives is the only way to establish the diagnosis in asymptomatic carriers [128].

On the basis of pattern of transmission, two major clinical syndromes have been described: the more common autosomal dominant form with a pure cardiac phenotype (Romano-Ward) [129] and the rarer autosomal recessive form characterized by the association with congenital deafness (Jervell and Lang-Nielsen) [130].

Five loci have been associated with the Romano-Ward LQTS and they are located on chromosome 3 (3p21-p23), encoding for the cardiac sodium channel (SCN5A); chromosome 7 (7q35-q36), encoding for the Ikr potassium channel protein (HERG); chromosome 11 (11p15.5), encoding for the α-subunit of the Iks potassium channel protein (KvLQT1); chromosome 21 (21q22.1-q22), encoding an ancillary subunit for the Iks channel complex (MinK); and chromosome 4 (4q25-q27); but the defective protein is still unknown [131-135]. Moreover, families linked to none of these genes have been described, thus suggesting the existence of other disease genes. Apart from a few mutations which are "hotspots", most of the mutations identified are missense mutations which are not confined to a single location but are frequently found at various positions within each gene in different families. It seems that this remarkable genetic heterogeneity contributes to the high variability of the clinical picture. The autosomal recessive variant of LQTS (Jervell and Lange-Nielsen) arises in patients who inherit abnormal KvLQT1 or minK alleles from both parents and expresses itself with especially long QT intervals. The abnormal allele can be the same or different ("compound heterozygosity") [136-138]. As a consequence, parents of subjects with Jervell and Lange-Nielsen variant carry long QT syndrome mutations, although most are asymptomatic.

As to the functional consequences of LQTS mutations, if mutations in KvLQT1, KCNE1 or HERG are expressed alone or with wild-type alleles in oocytes or in other lines, they exhibit "loss of function", thus resulting in a reduction of the total current carried by the defective channel complexes. On the other hand, SCN5A channel mutations cause a "gain of function" with an increased sodium current. With respect to genotype-phenotype correlations, the different time and voltage dependence of the ionic currents may in some way explain the variable phenotype [139].

Brugada Syndrome

A clinical and ECG syndrome, characterized by right bundle branch block with right precordial ST segment elevation and an apparently normal heart, has been described in cases of SD by Brugada and Brugada, unfortunately without postmortem reports [140]. These ECG characteristics may depend on exaggerated transmural differences in action potential configuration, especially in the right ventricular outflow tract. Actually, Martini et al. [141] previously reported similar cases with apparent idiopathic ventricular fibrillation in which there was evidence of concealed right ventricular pathology. By studying a family with a case of SD, confirmation of an organic substrate was given recently by Corrado et al. [142], who reported not only fibro-fatty dystrophy in the right ventricular free wall but also involvement of the conduction system with sclerotic interruption of the right bundle branch. The coexistence of both "septal" and "parietal" right conduction defects might account for the ECG pattern of right bundle branch block and persistent ST segment elevation as well as ventricular electrical instability.

Conversely, in the absence of structural heart disease, the ECG abnormalities could arise from ion current dysfunction, such as I_{to}. L-type Ca^{2+} current [$I_{Ca(L)}$] and I_{Na}. Noteworthy is that at least one variant of the Brugada syndrome is caused by mutations in cardiac sodium channels gene SCN5A [143]. This is the same gene implicated in a form of long QT syndrome (LQT3), the mutation of which causes loss of function in the Brugada syndrome and gain of function in the LQT3. However, other families with Brugada syndrome have been tested showing no defects on the cardiac sodium channel, thus suggesting genetic heterogeneity analogous to that seen in other inherited heart diseases.

Mechanical Sudden Death: Aortic Rupture

This occurs as a consequence of spontaneous laceration of the ascending aorta with hemopericardium and cardiac tamponade. The basic defect consists of elastic disruption in the the tunica media and cystic medial necrosis leading to aortic wall fragility [144]. The disease is rarely isolated in the young, being usually associated with a genetic or congenital anomaly, like Marfan syndrome, isthmal coarctation or a bicuspid aortic valve [37].

Although many cases have an equal severity of tunica media degeneration, only in *Marfan syndrome* has a genetic defect been discovered, mapping to chromosome 15q15-q21.3 [145, 146]. The disease is familial in the majority of patients, whereas 30% are sporadic. The defective gene encodes fibrillin-1, which is the major constituent of microfibrils of the extracellular matrix. The heart in Marfan patients who die suddenly because of aortic dissection (usually type I-II with rupture within the pericardial cavity) exhibits typical cardiovascular features consisting of mitral valve prolapse, annulo-aortic ectasia, with or without fusiform aneurysm of the ascending aorta, and aortic incompetence. Nonetheless, aortic dissection in Marfan syndrome may also be observed without dilatation of the aorta, so that its occurrence may be unpredictable on clinical grounds.

Familial aortic dissection, in the absence of Marfan stigmata and hypertension, has been reported rarely and no defective gene has yet been identified [147].

The association between an isolated *bicuspid aortic valve* and dissection is not incidental. Indeed, the incidence of bicuspid aortic valve among those with aortic dissection is significantly higher than in the normal population (12% vs 1%) (148-150). The rupture involves a severely degenerated ascending aorta, with or without dilatation, in the setting of a normally pliable bileaflet valve [37]. Although dissections have been reported amongst the offspring of individuals with a bicuspid aortic valve, familial SD has not been proven. Considering the frequency of a bicuspid aortic valve amongst the general population, the risk of dissection is quite rare. Most probably, only in a subpopulation of patients with a bicuspid aortic valve is medial necrosis present. Echocardiographic monitoring of the aortic root in individuals with this anomaly may detect progressive aortic dilatation as a marker of underlying vessel wall degeneration and impending rupture, thus providing indirect evidence of aortic wall fragility [151, 152]. One may wonder whether a bicuspid aortic valve and medial necrosis are the phenotypic expressions of the same genetic disease or simply a congenital heart disease complex, in which the maldevelopment involves either the aortic valve or wall, which both derive from the neural crest [153, 154].

This seems to be the case in *isthmal coarctation* (so-called adult coarctation), which is also associated with a bicuspid aortic valve in 50% of cases and in which aortic dissection frequently occurs in the natural history. An equal severity of medial necrosis in spontaneous aortic rupture has been reported in Marfan syndrome, isolated bicuspid aortic valve or isthmal coarctation, with or without a bicuspid valve. A relationship between the development of the aortic arch and neural crest has been proven by experimental embryologists [154].

More recently, apoptosis has been demonstrated to play a role in the progressive loss of smooth muscle cells of the tunica media in patients with aortic dilatation and congenital aortic valve malformation (bicuspid aortic valve), thus suggesting that premature smooth muscle cell apoptosis in the medial layer could be a part of a genetic program underlying aortic disease in patients with aortic valve malformations [155].

Conclusions

In conclusion, the pathologist's role should not simply be to establish whether SD is due to natural or unnatural causes. A careful postmortem investigation can be the source of vital information for the community, relatives and future generations. An accurate diagnosis of the underlying morbid entity and ultimate cause of death is the prerequisite to establish whether the disease is hereditary, thus representing the starting point for a wide-ranging investigation of the family members, as well as to assess the possible role of acquired etiologic factors such as infectious agents.

Acknowledgements. Supported by Veneto Region, Venice, Italy

References

1. Watson JD, Crick FHC (1953) Molecular structure of nucleic acids: A structure for deoxyribose nucleic acid. Nature 171:737-738

2. Watson JD, Crick FHC (1953) Genetic implications of the structure of deoxyribonu- cleic acid. Nature 171:964-967
3. Wilkins MHF, Stokes AR, Wilson HR (1953) Molecular structure of structure of deoxypentose nucleic acids. Nature 171:748-750
4. Watson JD, Tooze J, Kurtz DT (1983) Recombinant DNA: a short course. Freeman, New York
5. Roberts R (l987) Integrated program for the training of cardiovascular fellows in molecular biology. In: Albertini A, Lenfant C, Paoletti R (eds) Biotechnology in clini- cal medicine. Raven Press, New York, pp 99-105
6. Haber E, Quertermous T, Matsueda GR et al (1989) Innovative approaches to plasmi- nogen activator therapy. Science 243:51-56
7. Saiki RK, Scharf S, Falona F et al (1985) Enzymatic amplification of β-globin genomic sequences and restriction site analysis for diagnosis of sickle cell anemia. Science 239:1350-1354
8. Erlich HA, Gelfand D, Sninsky JJ (1991) Recent advances in the polymerase chain reaction. Science 252:1643-1651
9. Yourno J (1992) A method for nested PCR with single closed reaction tubes. PCR Methods Appl 2:60-65
10. Martin AM, Webber S, Fricker J et al (1994) Acute myocarditis. Rapid diagnosis by PCR in children. Circulation 90:330-339
11. Chamberlain, JS, Gibbs RA, Ranier JE et al (1988) Deletion screening of the Duchenne muscular dystrophy locus via multiplex DNA amplification. Nucleic Acids Res 16:11141-11156
12. Tanigawa G, Jarcho JA, Kass A et al (1990) A molecular basis for familial hypertrophic cardiomyopathy: an α/β cardiac myosin heavy chain hybrid gene. Cell 62:991-998
13. Tautz D (1989) Hypervariability of simple sequences as a general source for poly- morphic DNA markers. Nucleic Acids Res 17:6463-6471
14. Kagnoff MF, Harwood JI, Bugawan TL et al (1989) Structural analysis of the HLA-DR, DQ and DP alleles on the celiac disease associated HLA-DR3 (DRw17) haplotype. Proc Natl Acad Sci USA 86:6274-6278
15. Scharf SJ, Friedmann A, Steinman L et al (1989) Specific HLA-DQB and HLA-DRB1 alleles confer sensitivity to pemphigus vulgaris. Proc Natl Acad Sci USA 86:6215- 6219
16. Steller H (1995) Mechanisms and genes of cellular suicide. Science 267:1445-1449
17. Tompson CB (1995) Apoptosis in the pathogenesis and treatment of disease. Science 267:1456-1462
18. Vaux DL, Strasser A (1996) The molecular biology of apoptosis. Proc Natl Acad Sci USA 93:2239-2244
19. Olivetti G, Abbi R, Quaini F et al (1997) Apoptosis in the failing human heart. N Engl J Med 336:1131-1141
20. Itoh G, Tamura J, Suzuki M et al (1995) DNA fragmentation of human infarcted myo- cardial cells demonstrated by the nick end labeling method and DNA agarose gel electrophoresis. Am J Pathol 146:1235-1331
21. Lane JR, Neuman DA, Lafond-Walker A et al (1993) Role of IL1 and tumor necrosis factor in coxsackie virus-induced autoimmune myocarditis. J Immunol 151:1682-1690
22. Gavrieli Y, Sherman Y, Ben-Sasson SA (1992) Identification of programmed cell death in situ via specific labeling of nuclear DNA fragmentation. J Cell Biol 119:493-501
23. Ansari B, Coates BD, Greenstein BD, Hall PA (1993) In situ end labeling detects DNA strand breaks in apoptosis and other physiological and pathological states. J Pathol 170:1-8

24. Schuler GD, Boguski MS, Stewart EA et al (1996) A gene map of the human genome. Science 274:540-546

25. Caskey CT (1987) Disease diagnosis by recombinant DNA methods. Science 236:1223-1228

26. Fenoglio-Preiser C, Willman CL (1987) Molecular biology and the pathologist. Arch Pathol Lab Med 111:601-619

27. Killen A, Orr HT (1990) Molecular basis of human genetic disease: clinical applications of genetic linkage analysis. In: Fenoglio-Preisier CM, Willman CL, Kaufman N (eds) Molecular diagnostics in pathology. Williams & Wilkins, Baltimore

28. Molkentin J, Firulli A, Black B et al (1996) MEF2B is a potent transactivator expressed in early myogenic lineages. Mol Cell Biol 16:3814-3824

29. Morrisey EE, Ip HS, Lu MM et al (1996) GATA 6: a zinc finger transcription factor that is expressed in multiple cell lineages derived from lateral mesoderm. Dev Biol 177:309-322

30. Fishman MC, Chien KR (1997) Fashioning the vertebrate heart: earliest embryonic decisions. Development 124:2099-3117

31. Baroldi G, Falzi G, Mariani F (1979) Sudden coronary death: a postmortem study in 208 selected cases compared to 97 "control" subjects. Am Heart J 98:20-31

32. Davies MJ, Thomas A (1984) Thrombosis and acute coronary artery lesions in sudden cardiac ischemic death. N Engl J Med 310:1137-1140

33. Lambert EC, Menon VA, Wagner HR et al (1974) Sudden unexpected death from cardiovascular disease in children. Am J Cardiol 34:89-96

34. Driscoll DJ, Edwards WD (1985) Sudden unexpected death in children and adolescents. J Am Coll Cardiol 5[Suppl B]:118B-121B

35. Topaz O, Edwards JE (1985) Pathologic features of sudden death in children, adolescents, and young adults. Chest 87:476-482

36. Corrado D, Basso C, Poletti A, Angelini A, Valente M, Thiene G (1994) Sudden death in the young. Is coronary thrombosis the major precipitating factor? Circulation 90:2315-2323

37. Basso C, Frescura C, Corrado D et al (1995) Congenital heart disease and sudden death in the young. Hum Pathol 26:1065-1072

38. Corrado D, Basso C, Schiavon M, Thiene G (1998) Screening for hypertrophic cardiomyopathy in young athletes. N Engl J Med 339:364-369

39. Spirito P, Seidman CE, McKenna WJ, Maron BJ (1997) The management of hypertrophic cardiomyopathy. N Engl J Med 336:775-785

40. Maron BJ, Roberts WC, McAllister HA, Rosing DR, Epstein SE (1980) Sudden death in young athletes. Circulation 62:218-229

41. Maron BJ, Roberts WC (1979) Quantitative analysis of cardiac muscle cell disorganization in the ventricular septum of patients with hypertrophic cardiomyopathy. Circulation 59:689-706

42. Maron BJ, Wolfson JK, Epstein SE, Roberts WC (1986) Intramural ("small vessel") coronary artery disease in hypertrophic cardiomyopathy. J Am Coll Cardiol 8:545-557

43. Bonne G, Carrier L, Richard P, Hainque B, Schwartz K (1998) Familial hypertrophic cardiomyopathy. From mutations to functional defects. Circulation Res 83:580-593

44. Jarcho JA, McKenna W, Pare JAP et al (1989) Mapping a gene for familial hypertrophic cardiomyopathy to chromosome 14q1. N Engl J Med 321:1372-1378

45. Poetter K, Jiang H, Hassanzadeh S et al (1996) Mutation in either the essential or regulatory light chains of myosin are associated with a rare myopathy in human heart and skeletal muscle. Nat Genet 13:63-69

46. Watkins H, MacRae C, Thierfelder L et al (1993) A disease locus for familial hypertrophic cardiomyopathy maps to chromosome 1q3. Nat Genet 3:333-337

47. Kimura A, Harada H, Park JE et al (1997) Mutations in the cardiac troponin I gene associated with hypertrophic cardiomyopathy. Nat Genet 16:379-382

48. Thierfelder L, Watkins H, MacRae C et al (1994) Alpha-tropomyosin and cardiac troponin T mutations cause familial hypertrophic cardiomyopathy: a disease of the sarcomere. Cell 77:701-712

49. Carrier L, Hengstenberg C, Beckmann JS et al (1993) Mapping of a novel gene for familial hypertrophic cardiomyopathy to chromosome 11. Nat Genet 4:311-313

50. MacRae CA, Ghaisas N, Kass S et al (1995) Familial hypertrophic cardiomyopathy with Wolff-Parkinson-White syndrome maps to a locus on chromosome 7q3. J Clin Invest 96:1216-1220

51. Watkins H, Rosenzweig A, Hwang DS et al (1992) Characteristics and prognostic implications of myosin missense mutations in familial hypertrophic cardiomyopathy. N Engl J Med 326:1108-1114

52. Epstein ND, Cohn GM, Cyran F, Fananapazir L (1992) Differences in clinical expression of hypertrophic cardiomyopathy associated with two distinct mutations in the beta-myosin heavy chain gene. A 908Leu-Val mutation and a 403Arg-Gln mutation. Circulation 86:345-352

53. Bonne G, Carrier L, Bercovici J et al (1995) Cardiac myosin binding protein-C gene splice acceptor site mutation is associated with familial hypertrophic cardiomyopathy. Nat Genet 11:438-440

54. Watkins H, Conner D, Thierfelder L et al (1995) Mutations in the cardiac myosin binding protein-C gene on chromosome 11 cause familial hypertrophic cardiomyopathy. Nat Genet 11:434-437

55. Watkins H, McKenna WJ, Thierfelder L et al (1995) Mutations in the genes for cardiac troponin T and tropomyosin in hypertrophic cardiomyopathy. N Engl J Med 332:1058-1064

56. Forissier JF, Carrier L, Farza H et al (1996) Codon 102 of the cardiac troponin T gene is a putative hot spot for mutations in familial hypertrophic cardiomyopathy. Circulation 94:3069-3073

57. Thiene G, Nava A, Corrado D, Rossi L, Pennelli N (1988) Right ventricular cardiomyopathy and sudden death in young people. N Engl J Med 318:129-133

58. Nava A, Rossi L, Thiene G (eds) (1997) Arrhythmogenic right ventricular cardiomyopathy/dysplasia. Elsevier, Amsterdam

59. Basso C, Thiene G, Corrado D, Angelini A, Nava A, Valente M (1996) Arrhythmogenic right ventricular cardiomyopathy: dysplasia, dystrophy, or myocarditis? Circulation 94:983-991

60. McKenna WJ, Thiene G, Nava A et al (1994) Diagnosis of arrhythmogenic right ventricular dysplasia/cardiomyopathy. Br Heart J 71:215-218

61. Angelini A, Basso C, Nava A, Thiene G (1996) Endomyocardial biopsy in arrhythmogenic right ventricular cardiomyopathy. Am Heart J 132:203-206

62. Richardson P, McKenna WJ, Bristow et al (1996) Report of the 1995 WHO/ISFC Task Force on the definition and classification of cardiomyopathies. Circulation 93:841-842

63. Nava A, Thiene G, Canciani B et al (1988) Familial occurrence of right ventricular dysplasia. A study involing nine families. J Am Coll Cardiol 12:1222-28

64. Rampazzo A, Nava A, Danieli GA et al (1994) The gene for arrhythmogenic right ventricular cardiomyopathy maps to chromosome 14q23-q24. Hum Molec Genet 3:959-62

65. Rampazzo A, Nava A, Erne P et al (1995) A new locus for arrhythmogenic right ventricular cardiomyopathy (ARVD2) maps to chromosome 1q42-q43. Hum Mol Genet 11:2151-2154

66. Severini GM, Krajinovic M, Pinamonti B et al (1996) A new locus for arrhythmogenic right ventricular dysplasia on the long arm of chromosome 14. Genomics 31:193-20
67. Rampazzo A, Nava A, Miorin M et al (1997) ARVD4, a new locus for arrhythmogenic right ventricular cardiomyopathy, maps to chromosome 2 long arm. Genomics 45:259-263
68. Ahmad F, Duanxiang Li, Karibe A et al (1998) Localization of a gene responsible for arrhythmogenic right ventricular dysplasia to chromosome 3p23. Circulation 98:2791-2795
69. Coonar AS, Protonotarios N, Tsatsopoulou A et al (1998) Gene for arrhythmogenic right ventricular cardiomyopathy with diffuse nonepidermolytic palmoplantar keratoderma and woolly hair (Naxos disease) maps to 17q21. Circulation 97:2049-2058
70. Nava A, Bauce B, Villanova C et al (1999) Arrhythmogenic right ventricular cardiomyopathy: long term follow-up of 37 families. J Am Coll Cardiol (Abst Suppl):497A
71. Mallat Z, Teddgui A, Fontaliran F, Frank R, Durigon M, Fontaine G (1996) Evidence of apoptosis in arrhythmogenic right ventricular dysplasia. N Engl J Med 335:1190-1196
72. Valente M, Calabrese F, Thiene G et al (1998) In vivo evidence of apoptosis in arrhythmogenic right ventricular cardiomyopathy. Am J Pathol 152:479-84
73. Thiene G, Corrado D, Nava A et al (1991) Right ventricular cardiomyopathy: is there evidence of an inflammatory aetiology? Eur Heart J 12 [suppl D]:22-25
74. Valente M, Calabrese F, Angelini A, Caforio ALP, Basso C, Thiene G (1997) Pathobiology. In: Nava A, Rossi L, Thiene G (eds) Arrhythmogenic right ventricular cardiomyopathy/dysplasia. Elsevier Science, Amsterdam
75. Neuspiel DR, Kuller LH (1985) Sudden and unexpected natural death in childhood and adolescence. JAMA 254:1321-1325
76. Phillips MP, Robinowtz M, Higgins JR et al (1986) Sudden cardiac death in Air Force recruits. JAMA 256:2696-2699
77. Frustaci A, Bellocci F, Olsen EGJ (1994) Results of biventricular endomyocardial biopsy in survivors of cardiac arrest with apparently normal hearts. Am J Cardiol 74:890
78. Basso C, Boffa G, Corrado D, Thiene G (1997) Myocarditis and sudden death in the young. Circulation 96:I-698
79. Wesslen L, Påhlson C, Lindquist O et al (1996) An increase in sudden unexpected cardiac deaths among young Swedish orienteers during 1979-1992. Eur Heart J 17:902-910
80. Akhtar N, Ni J, Stromberg D et al (1999) Tracheal aspirate as a substrate for polymerase chain reaction detection of viral genome in childhood pneumonia and myocarditis. Circulation 99:2011-2018
81. Muntoni F, Cau M, Fanau A, Congiu R et al (1993) Deletion of the dystrophin muscle-promoter region associated with X-linked dilated cardiomyopathy. N Engl J Med 329:921-925
82. Muntoni F, Wilson L, Marrosu G et al (1995) A mutation in the dystrophin gene selectively affecting dystrophin expression in the heart. J Clin Invest 96:693-699
83. Schultz KR, Garjarski RJ, Pignatelli R et al (1995) Genetic heterogeneity in familial dilated cardiomyopathy. Biochem Mol Med 56:87-93
84. Durand JB, Bachinski LL, Bieling LC et al (1995) Localization of a gene responsible for familial dilated cardiomyopathy to chromosome 1q32. Circulation 92:3387-3389
85. Siu BL (1997) A novel locus for familial dilated cardiomyopathy on chromosome 2p31. Proceedings of the second world congress of pediatric cardiology and cardiac surgery
86. Krajinovic M, Pinamonti B, Sinagra G et al (1995) Linkage of familial dilated cardiomyopathy to chromosome 9. Am J Hum Genet 57:846-52

87. Bowles KR, Gajarski R, Porter P et al (1996) Gene mapping of familial autosomal dominant dilated cardiomyopathy to chromosome 10q21-23. J Clin Invest 98:1355-60

88. Kass S, MacRae C, Graber HL et al (1994) A gene defect that causes conduction system disease and dilated cardiomyopathy maps to chromosome 1p1-1q1. Nat Genet 7:546-551

89. Olson TM, Keating MT (1996) Mapping a cardiomyopathy locus to chromosome 3p22-p25. J Clin Invest 97:528-532

90. Olson TM, Michels VV, Thibodeau SN, Tai YS, Keating MT (1998) Actin mutations in dilated cardiomyopathy: a heritable form of heart failure. Science 280:750-3

91. Milasin J, Muntoni F, Severini GM et al (1996) A point mutation in the 5' splice site of the dystrophin gene first intron responsible for X-linked cardiomyopathy. Hum Mol Genet 5:73-79

92. Ortiz Lopez R, Li H, Su J, Goytia V, Towbin JA (1997) Evidence for a dystrophin missense mutation as a cause of X-linked dilated cardiomyopathy. Circulation 95:2434-40

93. Bione S, D'Adamo P, Maestrini E, Gedeom AK, Bolhuis PA, Toniolo D (1996) A novel X-linked gene, G4.5, is responsible for Barth syndrome. Nat Genet 12:385-389

94. Giacca M, Severini GM, Mestroni L et al (1994) Low frequency of detection by nested polymerase chain reaction of Enterovirus ribonucleic acid in endomyocardial tissue of patients with idiopathic dilated cardiomyopathy. J Am Coll Cardiol 24:1033-1040

95. Andreoletti L, Hober D, Decoene C et al (1996) Detection of enteroviral RNA by polymerase chain reaction in endomyocardial tissue of patients with chronic cardiac diseases. J Med Virol 48:53-59

96. Calabrese F, Valente M, Thiene G et al (1999) Enteroviral genome in native hearts may influence outcome of patients who undergo cardiac transplantation. Diagn Mol Pathol (in press)

97. Brink PA, Ferreira A, Moolman JC, Weymar HW, van der Merve PL, Corfield VA (1995) Gene for progressive familial heart block type I maps to chromosome 19q13. Circulation 91:1633-40

98. De Meeus A, Stephan E, Debrus et al (1995) An isolated cardiac conduction disease maps to chromosome 19q. Circ Res 77:735-740

99. Wolff L, Parkinson J, White PD (1930) Bundle branch block with short PR interval in healthy young people prone to paroxysmal tachycardia. Am Heart J 5:685

100. Anderson RH, Becker AF, Brechenmacher C, Davies MJ, Rossi L (1975) Ventricular preexcitation. A proposed nomenclature for its substrates. Eur J Cardiol 3:27-36

101. Guize L, Soria R, Chaouat JC, Chretien JM, Houe D, le-Heuzey J (1985) Prevalence and course of Wolff-Parkinson-White syndrome in a population of 138,048 subjects. Ann Med Intern Paris 136:474-478

102. Wellens HJJ, Durrer D (1974) Wolff-Parkinson-White syndrome and atrial fibrillation. Am J Cardiol 34:777-782

103. Schwartz LS, Goldfischer J, Sprague GJ, Schartz SP (1969) Syncope and sudden death in aortic stenosis. Am J Cardiol 23:647-658

104. Turri M, Thiene G, Bortolotti U, Milano A, Mazzucco A, Gallucci V (1990) Surgical pathology of aortic valve disease. A study based on 602 specimens. Eur J Cardiothorac Surg 4:556-560

105. Angelini A, Basso C, Grassi G, Casarotto D, Thiene G (1994) Surgical pathology of valve disease in the elderly. Aging Clin Exp Res 6:225-237

106. Pomerance A (1972) Pathogenesis of aortic stenosis and its relation to age. Br Heart J 34:569-574

107. Giusti S, Cocco P, Thiene G (1991) Valvola aortica bicuspide: una cardiopatia congenita "minore" a rischio di catastrofiche complicanze. G Ital Cardiol 21:189-201

108. Gale AN, McKusick VA, Hutchins GM, Gott VL (1977) Familial congenital bicuspid aortic valve: secondary calcific aortic stenosis and aortic aneurysm. Chest 72:668-670

109. Ewart A, Morris C, Ensing G et al (1993) A human vascular disease, supravalvular aortic stenosis maps to chromosome 7. Proc Natl Acad Sci USA 90:3226-3230

110. Curran ME, Atkinson D, Ewart A, Morris C, Leppert M, Keating MT (1993) The elastin gene is disrupted by a translocation associated with supravalvular aortic stenosis. Cell 73:159-168

111. Williams JCP, Barratt Boyes BG, Lowe JB (1961) Supravalvular aortic stenosis. Circulation 24:1311-1318

112. Morrow AG, Waldhausen JA, Peters RL, Bloodwell RD, Braunwald E (1959) Supravalvular aortic stenosis. Clinical, hemodynamic and pathologic observations. Circulation 20:1003-1010

113. Thiene G, Ho SY (1986) Aortic root pathology and sudden death in youth: review of anatomical varieties. Appl Pathol 4:237-245

114. Corrado D, Basso C, Nava A, Rossi L, Thiene G (1997) Sudden death in young people with apparently isolated mitral valve prolapse. G Ital Cardiol 27:1097-1105

115. Martini B, Basso C, Thiene G (1995) Sudden death in mitral valve prolapse with Holter monitoring – documented ventricular fibrillation evidence of coexisting arrhythmogenic right ventricular cardiomyopathy. Int J Cardiol 49:274-278

116. Pyeritz RE, Wappel MA (1983) Mitral valve dysfunction in the Marfan syndrome. Am J Med 74:797-807

117. Jaffe AS, Geltman EM, Rodney GE, Uitto J (1981) Mitral valve prolapse. A consistent manifestation of type IV Ehlers-Danlos syndrome. The pathogenetic role of the abnormal production of type III collagen. Circulation 64:121-125

118. Davies MJ (1996) Stability and instability: two faces of coronary atherosclerosis. The Paul Dudley Withe Lecture 1995. Circulation 94:2013-2020

119. Libby P, Egan D, Skarlatos S (1997) Roles of infectious agents in atherosclerosis and restenosis: an assesment of evidence and need for future research. Circulation 96:4095-4103

120. Hendrix MG, Salimans MM, van Boven CP et al (1990) High prevalence of latently present cytomegalovirus in arterial walls of patients suffering from grade III atherosclerosis. Am J Pathol 136:23-28

121. Jackson LA, Campbell LA, Schmidt RA et al (1997) Specificity of detection of Chlamydia pneumoniae in cardiovascular atheroma: evaluation of the innocent bystander hypothesis. Am J Pathol 150:1785-90

122. Ramsay G (1998) DNA chips: state-of-the-art. Nat Biotechnol 16:40-44

123. Qiao J-H, Tripathi J, Mishra NK et al (1997) Role of macrophage colony-stimulating factor in atherosclerosis: studies of osteopetrotic mice. Am J Pathol 150:1687-99

124. de Villiers WJS, Smith JD, Miyata M et al (1998) Macrophage phenotype in mice deficient in both macrophage-colony-stimulating factor (op) and apolipoprotein E. Arterioscler Thromb Vasc Biol 18:631-640

125. Isner JM, Kearney M, Bortman S et al (1995) Apoptosis in human atherosclerosis and restenosis. Circulation 91:2703-2711

126. Consensus statement of the Joint Steering Committees of the UCARE and of the Idiopathic Ventricular Fibrillation Registry of the United States (1997) Survivors of out-of-hospital cardiac arrest with apparently normal heart. Need for definition and standardized clinical evaluation. Circulation 95:265-272

127. Corrado D, Basso C, Angelini A, Thiene G (1995) Sudden arrhythmic death in young people with apparently normal heart. J Am Coll Cardiol [Suppl]:188A (abstract)

128. Schwartz PJ, Locati EH, Napolitano C, Priori SG (1995) The long QT syndrome. In: Zipes DP, Jalife J (eds) Cardiac electrophysiology: from cell to bedside, 2nd ed. Saunders, Philadelphia

129. Romano C, Gemme G, Pongiglione R (1963) Aritmie cardiache rare dell'età pediatrica. Clin Pediatr 45:658-683

130. Jervell A, Lange-Nielsen F (1957) Congenital deaf-mutism, functional heart disease with prolongation of the QTc interval and sudden death. Am Heart J 54:59-68

131. Wang Q, Shen J, Splawski I et al (1995) SCN5A mutations associated with an inherited cardiac arrhythmia, long QT syndrome. Cell 80:805-11

132. Curran ME, Splawski I, Timothy KW, Vincent GM, Green ED, Keating MT (1995) A molecular basis for cardiac arrhythmia: HERG mutations cause long QT syndrome. Cell 80:795-803

133. Wang Q, Curran ME, Splawski I et al (1996) Positional cloning of a novel potassium channel gene: KVLQT1 mutations cause cardiac arrhythmias. Nat Genet 12:17-23

134. Splawski I, Tristani-Firouzi M, Lehmann MH, Sanguinetti MC, Keating MT (1997) Mutations in the hminK gene cause long QT syndrome and suppress Iks function. Nature Genet 17:338-340

135. Schott JJ, Peltier S, Foley P et al (1995) Mapping of a new gene for the LQT syndrome. Am J Hum Genet 57:1114-1122

136. Neyroud N, Tesson F, Denjoy I et al (1997) A novel mutation in the potassium channel gene KVLQT causes the Jervell and Lange-Nielsen cardioauditory syndrome. Nat Genet 15:186-189

137. Splawski I, Timothy KW, Vincent GM et al (1997) Molecular basis of the long QT syndrome associated with deafness. N Engl J Med 336:1562-1567

138. Schulze-Bahr E, Wang Q, Wedekind H, Haverkamp W, Chen Q, Sun Y (1997) KCNE1 mutations cause Jervell and Lange-Nielsen syndrome. Nature Genet 17:267-8

139. Priori S, Barhanin J, Hauer RNW et al (1999) Genetic and molecular basis of cardiac arrhythmias. Impact on clinical management. Eur Heart J 20:174-195

140. Brugada P, Brugada J (1992) Right bundle branch block, persistent ST segment elevation and sudden cardiac death: a distinct clinical and electrocardiographic syndrome. J Am Coll Cardiol 20:1391-1396

141. Martini B, Nava A, Thiene G et al (1989) Ventricular fibrillation without apparent heart disease: description of six cases. Am Heart J 118:1203-1209

142. Corrado D, Nava A, Buja G et al (1996) Familial cardiomyopathy underlies syndrome of right bundle branch block, ST segment elevation and sudden death. J Am Coll Cardiol 27:443-448

143. Chen Q, Kirsch GE, Zhang D et al (1998) Genetic basis and molecular mechanism for idiopathic ventricular fibrillation. Nature 392:293-296

144. Larson EW, Edwards WD (1984) Risk factors of aortic dissection: a necropsy study of 161 cases. Am J Cardiol 53:849-855

145. Kainulainen K, Pulkkinen K, Savolainen A et al (1990) Location on chromosome 15 of the gene defect causing Marfan syndrome. N Engl J Med 323:935-939

146. Dietz HC, Outting GR, Pyeritz RE et al (1991) Marfan syndrome caused by a recurrent de novo missense mutation in the fibrillin gene. Nature 352:337-339

147. Disertori M, Bertagnoli C, Thiene G et al (1992) Aneurisma dissecante dell'aorta a carattere familiare. G Ital Cardiol 21:849-853

148. Edwards WD, Leaf DS, Edwards JE (1978) Dissecting aortic aneurysm associated with congenital bicuspid aortic valve. Circulation 57:1022-1025

149. Roberts CS, Roberts WC (1991) Dissection of the aorta associated with congenital malformation of aortic valve. J Am Coll Cardiol 17:712-716

150. McKusick VA, Logue RB, Bahnson HT (1957) Association of aortic valvular disease and cystic medial necrosis of the ascending aorta. Report of four instances. Circulation 16:188-194

151. Pachulski RT, Weinberg AL, Chan KW (1991) Aortic aneurysm in patients with functionally normal or minimally stenotic bicuspid aortic valve. Am J Cardiol 67:781

152. Nistri S, Sorbo MD, Basso C, Scognamiglio R, Thiene G (1999) Aortic root size in patients with normally functioning bicuspid aortic valve. Proceedings of the World Symposium on Heart Valve Diseases, London UK

153. Lindsay J (1988) Coarctation of the aorta, bicuspid aortic valve and abnormal ascending aortic wall. Am J Cardiol 61:182-184

154. Kappetein AP, Gittenberger-de Groot AC, Zwinderman AH, Rohmer J, Poelmann RE, Huysmans HA (1991) The neural crest as a possible pathogenetic factor in coarctation of the aorta and bicuspid aortic valve. J Thorac Cardiovasc Surg 102:830-836

155. Bondermann D, Gharehbahi-Schnell E, Wollenek G, Maurer G, Baumgartner H, Lang IM (1999) Mechanisms underlying aortic dilatation in congenital aortic valve malformation. Circulation 99:2138-2143

ATRIAL FIBRILLATION

Are All Paroxysms of Atrial Fibrillation Focally Initiated?

D.C. Shah, M. Haïssaguerre and P. Jaïs

The most striking electrophysiologic characteristic of atrial fibrillation (AF) is the absence of discrete P waves along with irregular and asynchronous atrial activity [1]. It is perhaps therefore not surprising that the overwhelming majority of investigative efforts have been directed at analysing this characteristic of the arrhythmia and therefore involved the study of AF in the maintenance phase [2-6]. Additionally, there is no available model of spontaneous paroxysmal AF, and as a result the spontaneous debut of paroxysms of AF has not been analysed.

As emphasized above AF does not begin spontaneously in the commonly studied laboratory animals such as dog, pig, goat, sheep or rabbit. In man, until recently studies of spontaneous initiation have concentrated on relatively remote episodes of changes in heart rate or on the time course of recurrence of AF after DC cardioversion.

Two clinical groups lend themselves particularly to the study of spontaneous initiation-patients in whom paroxysms are both frequent and short lasting and those in whom paroxysms have been truncated by drugs/electrical cardioversion/surgical or catheter atriotomies. These groups are particularly suited to allow sequential mapping of events at initiation.

In our laboratory, we began by studying the initiation of AF in the selected situation of paroxysmal frequent and short lasting AF [7-9] and then confirmed these findings in a wider, unselected group of patients with paroxysmal AF. The results of mapping were verified by elimination of arrhythmias as a result of successful ablation. Since the results in these two groups are similar if not identical, they will be presented here together.

Patients and Methods

Patient Characteristics

The first 45 patients (group A) all had multidrug-resistant daily episodes of AF as well as more than 700 ectopic beats per 24 h (Holter recording). Their clinical details are summarized in Table 1.

Hôpital Cardiologique du Haut-Lévêque, Bordeaux-Pessac, France

Table 1. Patient characteristics: group A (45 patients)

Clinical characteristics	
Sex (M / F)	35 / 10
Age (years)	
Mean ± SD	54 ± 11
Range	18 – 78
Duration of AF (years)	6 ± 6
No. of unsuccessful drugs	5 ± 2
Structural heart disease (no. of patients)[a]	14
Previous embolic episode (no. of patients)	7
Pre-procedural duration of AF (min/24 h)[b]	
Mean ± SD	344 ± 326
Median	215
Range	15 – 1440
Echocardiographic parameters	
End-diastolic LV dimension (mm)	
Mean ± SD	51 ± 6
Median	51
Range	44 – 64
End-systolic LV dimension (mm)	
Mean ± SD	32 ± 5
Median	32
Range	24 – 45
Percentage of LV shortening	
Mean ± SD	36 ± 8
Median	35
Range	18 – 52
Anterior posterior LA dimension (mm)	
Mean ± SD	39 ± 7
Median	39
Range	28 – 50

AF, atrial fibrillation; LA, left atrium; LV, left ventricle
[a]Structural heart disease includes dilated or hypertrophic cardiomyopathy in five patients, myocardial infarction in four, mitral valve regurgitation in three, and atrial septal defect and cor pulmonale in one each
[b]All patients had > 700 ectopic beats/24 h

The next 65 patients (group B) also had resistant symptomatic paroxysmal AF but did not require any threshold ectopic frequency for inclusion. Their details are summarized in Table 2.

Table 2. Patient characteristics: group B (65 patients)

Clinical characteristics	
Sex (M/F)	53 / 12
Age (years)	51 ± 11
Duration of AF (years)	5 ± 5
Number of unsuccessful drugs	5 ± 2
Structural heart disease	16
Previous embolic episode	6
Hypertension	8
Diabetes	4
Pre-procedural duration of AF (min/24 h)	
Mean ± SD	460 ± 454
Median	300
Range	0 – 1440
Echocardiographic parameters	
End-diastolic LV diameter (mm)	
Mean ± SD	51 ± 5
Median	50
Range	42 – 64
End-systolic LV diameter (mm)	
Mean ± SD	32 ± 6
Median	32
Range	21 – 47
Percentage of LV shortening	
Mean ± SD	37 ± 8
Median	35
Range	22 – 57
Anterior-posterior LA dimension (mm)	
Mean ± SD	40 ± 7
Median	40
Range	25 – 55

Electrophysiologic Study

On admission, oral anticoagulants were replaced by heparin which was stopped 4-6 h before ablation, since trans-septal catheterization was required.

Three catheters were introduced percutaneously: two quadripolar roving ablation catheters with a thermocouple and a 4-mm tip into the left atrium; and one catheter in the right atrial appendage or coronary sinus to provide stable reference electrograms during mapping as well as for stimulation. Two roving catheters were used to map two pulmonary veins simultaneously. Surface ECG leads (I, II, III and V1) and bipolar intracardiac electrograms filtered at 30-500 Hz were recorded with a polygraph (model Midas, PPG).

If the arrhythmia did not spontaneously develop during electrophysiologic monitoring or was not sufficiently sustained, physiologic procedures (e.g., Valsalva's manoeuvre or carotid-sinus massage), atrial pacing, pharmacologic agents (e.g., isoproterenol, adenosine triphosphate, digoxin, propranolol, or verapamil), or all three methods were used.

Localization of Arrhythmogenic Triggers (Atrial Ectopic Beats)

The preliminary study involved intracardiac mapping of isolated ectopic beats. The ectopic focus was localized according to the earliest atrial activity relative to the reference electrogram or the onset of the ectopic P wave. Mechanically produced beats were prevented by avoiding catheter manipulation during the recordings, and such beats were excluded from analysis by comparing ECG pattern and intracardiac sequence with confirmed spontaneous ectopic beats. If no early sharp bipolar activity was recorded in the right atrium, the ectopic beats were considered to have originated in the left atrium. Direct mapping of the left atrium and pulmonary veins was performed by means of trans-septal catheterization. The role of ectopic beats in the initiation of AF was confirmed by on-site recording of a paroxysm of fibrillation.

Ablation Procedure

Angiography was performed before and after ablation. For ablation in the left atrium, an intravenous dose of 0.5 mg heparin per kilogram of body weight was administered during ablation, followed by an infusion to maintain a partial thromboplastin time of 60-90 s. Sedatives and nalbuphine were administered intravenously to control pain.

Ablation was performed at the site with the earliest recorded ectopic activity; if necessary within the pulmonary vein for the first group of 45, and at the pulmonary vein ostium instead in the next 65 patients. Temperature-controlled radiofrequency energy was delivered with a target temperature of 70 °C in the right atrium or 55-60 °C in the left atrium to minimize the risk of clot formation for 60-120s, except when there was a rise in impedance.

Subcutaneous heparin was administered after ablation to maintain the partial thromboplastin time. Successful ablation was defined as the elimination of atrial triggers during the 60 min after ablation and absence of the targeted ectopic beats during the subsequent 8 days (without antiarrhythmic drugs) as shown by telemetry and Holter monitoring.

The patients were discharged on a regime of oral anticoagulants for at least 3 months, but with no antiarrhythmic drugs. Late follow-up consisted of visits to the hospital and Holter recordings every 3 months. Any undocumented but suggestive symptoms were attributed to AF.

Results

The same focus was found to produce different types of atrial arrhythmias. Single discharges manifested as isolated extrasystoles, repetitive discharges with long cycle lengths as an automatic rhythm; in a small minority of patients shorter cycles resulted in organized monomorphic tachycardia or a pattern of focal flutter, whereas at even shorter cycle lengths an ECG pattern of AF was produced, i.e. rapid and irregular tachycardia without discrete P waves [8]. Sudden variations (up to 350 ms beat to beat) in the focus discharge rate were responsible for the irregular cycle lengths. In the majority, true intracardiac AF was initiated when the focus abruptly discharged a very rapid train with a cycle length of 182 ± 57 ms (330 beats per minute) leading to chaotic atrial activity. The source of isolated extrasystoles was the same, and initiation was therefore the result of sudden transformation of benign isolated extrasystoles into a malignant train of rapid discharges. Initiation of common atrial flutter, its degeneration into AF or its interruption could also be the result of pulmonary vein (PV) discharges. In Holter recordings, multiple daily bouts of varying duration could be recorded, or at other times only isolated ectopics could be found, or even AF without ectopics, because the focus discharged only in rapid bursts, with every burst inducing AF. The ectopic P waves – whether isolated or initiating AF – were superimposed on the T wave of the previous QRS complex because of a characteristically short coupling interval producing a P-on-T pattern recognizable at first sight.

Of the total of 110 patients who were investigated, none had undergone left atrial ablation. Ninety-six percent of foci triggering AF and producing ectopy originated from the PV. In the veins, focal ectopic activity was marked by a spike (the PV potential, PVP) reflecting atrial muscular bundles extending up to 4 cm from the left atrium into the PV. The PVP was tracked from its source inside the veins to its atrial exit, and the source marked by the earliest PVP was very discrete usually, in contrast to the exit. A lower-amplitude far-field PVP (< 0.1 mV) was also recorded from contiguous branches or the corresponding PV trunk or a neighbouring PV trunk. A local high frequency PVP was recorded simultaneously in other parts of the same vein but with a *later timing*, indicating progression towards the ostium and its left atrial exit or bystander activation. Considerably later, conduction was also recorded in different parts of the same vein, so that recording late activity in one sector of the PV during ectopy did not exclude an origin in another part of the same vein; the same source could also produce ectopy with different *activation* patterns. Conduction time to the left atrium was long – up to 160 ms – and exhibited decremental conduction with increasing prematurity. PVP closely coupled to the previous sinus beat were not conducted to the left atrium (i.e. was sequestered within the vein) and were documented in 70% of patients. In all cases, the PVP was also identified during sinus rhythm or coronary sinus pacing at the end of the multicomponent atrial activity, with this sequence inverting during extrasystoles (or repetitive focal tachycardia) in the vein giving rise to ectopy. In other veins, the activation sequence was not reversed, indicating passive (bystander) activation.

There are significant problems that limit effective mapping of PV foci:

1. Spontaneously occurring ectopy is unpredictable and some recording sessions have to be terminated after hours without ectopy. Different manoeuvres are inconsistent in how well they help to elicit ectopy, though isoproterenol infusion is the most effective.
2. Ectopy could induce AF lasting for minutes or hours, enforcing prolonged periods of waiting for its spontaneous interruption or external or internal electrical cardioversion(s) (sometimes multiple).
3. Mechanically produced beats were often observed, confusing mapping data and requiring comparison of their ECG morphology, coupling interval and intra-atrial sequence with those of spontaneous ectopy.
4. Spontaneous or provoked ectopy mapped and ablated in one ablation session did not exclude the possibility of other foci appearing later from another part of the targeted PV or from different PV, requiring further ablation.

Radiofrequency ablation was performed at the site of earliest spike activity (source) or along its intravenous course or at its ostial exit into the left atrium. In patients with rare ectopy, "disconnection" of the arrhythmogenic PV can be performed by sequential radiofrequency applications on the ostium targeting the PVP during sinus rhythm or left atrial pacing. Successful ablation of the focus was strongly associated with disappearance of the local PV potential(s) in sinus rhythm and produced a concomitant significant decrease in total ectopic number (from 4630 ± 3320 to 76 ± 77 per 24 h) as well as elimination of AF paroxysms. PV stenosis, defined as a diameter reduction of 50% or more, was observed in six veins, but only two patients had symptoms. No patient had pulmonary hypertension. The left inferior PV, a distal ablation site (close to PV branching) and the use of radiofrequency power reaching 45-50 W were predictive factors. When radiofrequency power was limited to below 30 W, no PV stenosis occurred. This power was associated with low achieved temperature in the PV owing to the high blood flow.

In a follow-up period of 8 ± 4 months (including repeated Holter recordings), ablation of the initiating trigger alone produced elimination of AF with a success rate depending on the number of arrhythmogenic PV: 90% success in patients with a single arrhythmogenic PV, 67% in those with two PV and 25% when more PV were involved.

Implications of Findings

Focal ablation targeted at arrhythmogenic triggering sources is therefore an important component of AF ablation. The main caveat with this approach is the unpredictable occurrence of ectopias and the inconsistency with which they may be induced. Ablation of focal triggers is presently made easier by the occurrence of ectopics frequent enough to allow mapping in the PV, and minimization of the number of radiofrequency applications. Complete isolation of the arrhythmogenic PV is an alternative solution that requires further study and technical improvements. The long-term effects of ablation in or around PV also needs to be clarified before widespread application can be envisaged [10, 11].

The decision to offer this procedure to patients depends upon an individualized risk/benefit assessment – particularly the risks of persistent AF versus those of an ablation procedure. In view of the difficulties of linear lesion making [11] and PV ablation, and bearing in mind the as yet unclear long-term consequences of extensive ablation, we offer this procedure only to multidrug-resistant symptomatic patients with paroxysmal AF as an alternative to AV junction ablation. A history of thromboembolic phenomena or tachycardia-mediated heart failure, as evidence of AF morbidity, strengthens the indication for the procedure.

References

1. Lévy S, Breithardt G, Campbell RWF, Camm AJ, Daubert JC, Allessie M, Aliot E, Capucci A, Cosio F, Crijns H, Jordaens L, Hauer RNW, Lombardi F, Lüderitz B (1998) Atrial fibrillation: current knowledge and recommendations for management. Eur Heart J 19:1294-1320
2. Cox JL, Canavan TE, Schuessler RB et al (1991) The surgical treatment of atrial fibrillation II: Intraoperative electrophysiologic mapping and description of the electrophysiologic basis of atrial flutter and fibrillation. J Thorac Cardiovasc Surg 101:406-426
3. Allessie MA, Lammers WJEP, Bonke FIM et al (1985) Experimental evaluation of Moes' multiple wavalet hypothesis of atrial fibrillation. In: Zipes DP, Jalife J (eds) Cardiac electrophysiology and arrhythmias. Grune & Stratton, Orlando, pp 265-276
4. Konings KTS, Kirchhof CJHJ, Smeets JRLM et al (1994) High density mapping of electrically induced atrial fibrillation in humans. Circulation 89:1665-1680
5. Kumagai K, Krestian C, Waldo AL (1997) Simultaneous multisite mapping studies during induced atrial fibrillation in the sterile pericarditis model. Insights into the mechanism of its maintenance. Circulation 95:511-521
6. Wang J, Liu L, Feng J, Nattel S (1996) Regional and functional factors determining induction and maintenance of atrial fibrillation in dogs. Am J Physiol 271:40
7. Haïssaguerre M, Jaïs P, Shah DC et al (1996) Right and left atrial radiofrequency catheter therapy of paroxysmal atrial fibrillation. J Cardiovasc Electrophysiol 12:1132-1144
8. Jaïs P, Haïssaguerre M, Shah DC et al (1997) A focal source of atrial fibrillation treated by discrete radiofrequency ablation. Circulation 95:572-576
9. Haïssaguerre M, Jaïs P, Shah DC, Takahashi A, Hocini M, Quiniou G, Garrigue S, Le Mouroux A, Le Métayer P, Clémenty J (1998) Spontaneous initiation of atrial fibrillation by ectopic beats originating in the pulmonary veins. N Engl J Med 339:659-666
10. Robbins IM, Colvin EV, Doyle TP, Kemp E, Loyd JE, McMahon WS, Kay N (1998) Pulmonary vein stenosis after catheter ablation of atrial fibrillation. Circulation 98:1769-1775
11. Jaïs P, Shah DC, Haïssaguerre M, Takahashi A, Lavergne T, Hocini M, Garrigue S, Barold SS, Le Métayer P, Clémenty J (1999) Septal and left atrial linear ablation for atrial fibrillation. Efficacy and safety. Am J Cardiol (in press)

How Common Is a Genetic Origin of Atrial Fibrillation?

R. Brugada[1], J. Brugada[2] and R. Roberts[1]

Introduction

Few disciplines will have the impact of molecular genetics. Cardiology has benefited from its techniques and, since 1989, with the discovery of the first chromosomal locus for a cardiac disease, multiple disease-causing genes have been discovered. The field is progressing rapidly, and it is certain that in the coming years
genetics will play a role not only in diagnostics, but in prevention and treatment
of these inherited diseases. Arrhythmias, like most diseases, result from an interaction of environmental and genetic factors. In the last few decades we have
acquired extensive knowledge about environmental factors triggering arrhythmias. The role of genetics has been described at all levels of the conduction system of the heart by the documentation of families with several individuals suffering from an inherited form of arrhythmia. However, it has not been until this last
decade, with the introduction of molecular biology and the techniques of genetic
mapping, that we have been able to study these families and identify the genes
that cause their disease.

Atrial Fibrillation

Atrial fibrillation is the most common sustained arrhythmia encountered in clinical practice. It is the most common cause of embolic stroke, accounting for
approximately 75 000 strokes per year in the United States, and leads to more hospital admissions than any other arrhythmia [1]. In addition to causing symptoms
of dizziness and dyspnea, atrial fibrillation may precipitate heart failure, syncope,
angina, and myocardial infarction, and may trigger ventricular arrhythmias in
susceptible individuals. Age is a major determinant of the prevalence of atrial fibrillation. At present there are over 3 million cases of atrial fibrillation in the US.

[1]Department of Cardiology, Baylor College of Medicine, Houston, Texas, USA; [2] Cardiovascular Institute, Hospital Clinic, University of Barcelona, Spain

The overall prevalence of 0.5%-1% rises to about 10% in people over the age of 70. It is claimed that atrial fibrillation accounts for about one-third of strokes in people over the age of 65 [2]. There is no known cure for atrial fibrillation, and therapy is palliative and directed towards heart rate control and prevention of systemic emboli with anticoagulant therapy.

Identification of Families with Atrial Fibrillation

A molecular basis for atrial fibrillation is yet to be determined. The identification of genes causing a familial form of the disease could be an effective method to elucidate the pathogenesis of at least some of the mechanisms that trigger the arrhythmia. It is not generally appreciated that atrial fibrillation may be familial. This was evident from a search in the literature, which showed only a few publications referring to the familial form of the disease. It was first reported as a familial form in 1943 [3], and while it is probably very uncommon, there has been no systematic study to determine the overall prevalence of the disease. The report in the Spanish journal of cardiology helped identify five families in Catalonia, Spain [4] (Fig. 1), with atrial fibrillation who inherited the disease in an autosomal

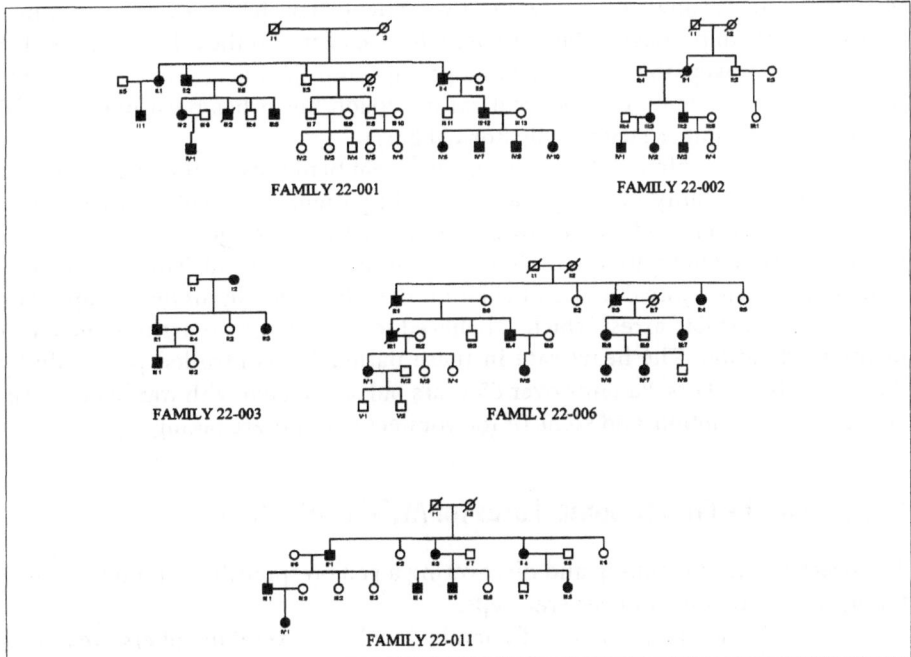

Fig. 1. Pedigree of the families identified in Catalonia, Spain, with a common locus on chromosome 10, segregating with familial atrial fibrillation. Solid blocks represent affected individuals, squares represent males and circles females. Slashed blocks represent deceased individuals

dominant pattern. In these families there were a total of 103 individuals. Forty-two of them presented with atrial fibrillation. The age at diagnosis of the arrhythmia was 1-45 years. The disease (age at presentation of the arrhythmia) occurs early in life and penetrance is very high; in the last generations three individuals were diagnosed in their first month of life. The elderly generations were diagnosed at a later age although the age at presentation of the disease is unknown, mainly due to the lack of symptoms and lack of any routine examinations until recently.

Clinical Data

The majority of the individuals in these five families are asymptomatic. The arrhythmia is very well tolerated in the young population, to the point that some of the individuals were diagnosed in their 20s during family screening. Only six patients presently suffer from palpitations, and otherwise continue a normal life. The disease is chronic in all but two individuals. Both of them have symptoms associated with the paroxysms but are unaware of any triggering factors for the arrhythmia. The echocardiograms were within the normal range when the patients were diagnosed. Some of them have subsequently developed dilatation of the left atrium as shown on follow-up. Two patients have left ventricular dysfunction; one of them probably related to her advanced age and the other possibly due to tachycardiomyopathy secondary to a poorly controlled heart rate. Six patients have undergone attempted electrical cardioversion but it has been unsuccessful in all of them despite a structurally normal heart.

The lack of symptomatology and the apparent benignity of the disease do not exclude the possibility of complications. Eight patients have suffered complications. Seven of them had a cerebrovascular accident before age 70 and it was fatal in five of them. One patient suffered sudden death at age 36. This patient was intolerant to paroxysmal atrial fibrillation despite antiarrhythmic therapy. The patient had a cardiac arrest which is believed to be due to a proarrhythmic effect of the medication. The heart rate in these patients is controlled primarily by digoxin or β-blockers. Patients over 65 years old are treated with warfarin to prevent systematic emboli, and some of the younger patients are taking aspirin.

Mapping of the Chromosomal Locus for Atrial Fibrillation

The overall goal of mapping and discovering a gene responsible for a disease in a family may be divided into several steps.

The first is the identification of a family in which several members are affected with an inherited disease. The initial steps must of necessity be undertaken by the clinician. The diagnosis needs to be made using consistent and objective data. Usually there are three diagnostic categories: affected, normal, and indeterminate. One must also exclude other causes that may simulate the phenotype. For example, in familial atrial fibrillation, it is important to rule out valvular disease, which could by itself cause atrial fibrillation. The initial diagnostic assessment is with a history taking and physical examination, an electrocardiogram, and an echocardiogram. The genetic studies require a blood sample. DNA is obtained from the white cells and the lymphocytes are cultured in the presence of an Epstein Barr virus to generate immortal cell lines for a renewable source of DNA.

The second step is the identification of the chromosomal locus carrying the gene. The technique used is genetic linkage analysis. The genes are spread among the 23 pairs of chromosomes. These chromosomes contain markers that are different among the individuals and make it possible to track how the areas of the chromosomes or *loci* have been transmitted through the generations in a family. It is usual to select 300 evenly distributed markers, which provides a marker for every 10 million base pairs. The identification of an area of a chromosome that has been inherited by all the affected individuals, and by none of the nonaffected, indicates that this area probably contains the gene causing the disease. This is a statistical analysis, and for the result to have enough power a family of a minimal size with enough affected individuals is required.

The third step is to identify the gene. There are two overall approaches: one the candidate gene approach, and the other, positional cloning. The first attempt is always the candidate gene approach, which involves determining whether genes already mapped to the region are responsible for the disease. The candidate genes are sequenced to determine whether a mutation is present that is coinherited with the disease in affected individuals but not in normal subjects. Positional cloning refers to the isolation of the region to identify new genes which could cause the disease.

The final step is the confirmation that it is this mutation that causes the disease, by finding it in all affected person and none of the normal ones. Ultimate proof is induction of the disease in an animal by a mutated transgene or through homologous recombination.

Linkage was performed on family 22-001 [5] using chromosomal markers as previously outlined. The locus responsible for the disease was shown to be on the long arm of chromosome 10q22-q24. The affected members of family 22-001 shared an area of 28 cM (28 million base pairs). With the four additional families several genetic crossovers were identified which narrowed the region containing the gene to less than 0.5 cM. We have sequenced several candidate genes including a β-adrenergic receptor, α-adrenergic receptor, G-protein-coupled receptor kinase, and a potassium channel, none of which contained a mutation and thus were excluded. Positional cloning of the region is ongoing to identify the gene since all candidate genes have been excluded. At this point, the whole region has been isolated in bacterial artificial chromosomes (BAC), and two new genes have been identified that are presently being sequenced.

Screening for Additional Families

Based on clinical experience and the few reports in the literature, familial atrial fibrillation would appear to be rather uncommon. To further ascertain its incidence, we established a toll-free number through the internet. We indicated we were primarily interested in individuals below the age of 50 with a diagnosis of atrial fibrillation on electrocardiogram, with a family history of the disease and without other structural heart disease. All individuals who responded underwent the regular screening for genetic cardiac disease, namely: history, physical, electrocardiogram, echocardiogram, and a blood sample for DNA analysis. We have found that familial atrial fibrillation appears to be much more common than previously anticipated. We have identified more than 100 probands with the familial form of the disease in the United States of America and 15 probands from six other countries [6]. Analysis of four of these families has shown no link with chromosome 10. This means that familial atrial fibrillation is a heterogeneous disease caused by more than one gene. This is not at all surprising given the experience with other cardiac diseases such as congenital long QT or hypertrophic cardiomyopathy, in which several disease-causing genes have been identified.

Conclusions

Familial atrial fibrillation should provide us with some understanding of the development of the arrhythmia in the normal heart. Despite the familial form being very uncommon, no study has been performed to evaluate its real prevalence. We do recommend the screening of family members of individuals affected with so called lone atrial fibrillation to rule out the familial form. The disease is better tolerated if it is developed in early stages of life and it is in general resistant to cardioversion even with normal size atria. The disease is not benign though, and with seven patients with history of stroke, anticoagulation is recommended medication after 65 years of age in all individuals.

Acknowledgements. This work is supported in part by grants from the National Heart, Lung, and Blood Institute, Specialized Centers of Research (P50-HL42267-01), the National Institutes of Health Training Center in Molecular Cardiology (T32-HL07706), the American Heart Association, Bugher Foundation Center for Molecular Biology (86-2216), ACC/Merck Fellowship Awards/International Exchange Committee Award (ID#67567), and the Fundacion MAPFRE MEDICINA, Madrid, Spain.

References

1. Feinberg WM, Blackshear JL, Laupacis A, Kronmal R, Hart RG (1995) Prevalence, age distribution, and gender of patients with atrial fibrillation. Arch Intern Med 155:469-473
2. Albers GW (1994) Atrial fibrillation and stroke: three new studies, three remaining questions. Arch Intern Med 154:1443-1448
3. Wolff L (1943) Familial auricular fibrillation. N Engl J Med 229:396-397
4. Girona J, Domingo A, Albert D, Casaldaliga J, Mont L, Brugada J (1997) Fibrilación auricular familiar. Rev Esp Cardiol 50:548-551

5. Brugada R, Tapscott T, Czernuszewicz GZ, Marian AJ, Iglesias A, Mont L, Brugada J, Girona J, Domingo A, Bachinski LL, Roberts R (1997) Identification of a genetic locus for familial atrial fibrillation. N Engl J Med 336:905-911
6. Brugada R, Bachinski LL, Hill R, Roberts R (1998) Familial atrial fibrillation is a genetically heterogeneous disease. J Am Coll Cardiol 31:349A (abstr)

Lone Atrial Fibrillation: What Is the Anatomical and the Electrophysiological Substrate?

G. Bagliani[1], M. Adam[2], M. Villani[†3], M. Pirrami[2], P. Franciosa[2], G. Carreras[2], R. Apolloni[2], M.G. Bendini[2], M. Ridarelli[2] and A.S. Montenero[2]

Introduction

Atrial fibrillation is commonly associated with a structural heart disease such as valvular disease, coronary artery disease, or dilated cardiomyopathy. Lone atrial fibrillation may be defined as a form of paroxysmal, persistent, or permanent atrial fibrillation with a "pure" electrophysiological substrate. But, does a pure lone atrial fibrillation really exist? To answer this question, it is important to investigate carefully both the anatomic and the electrophysiologic substrates, including all modulating factors that may increase the probability of induction of atrial fibrillation.

Anatomic Consideration

Although the hearts of patients with lone atrial fibrillation are normal in conventional diagnostic procedures, sometimes they show evidence of structural alterations at autopsy or biopsy. Primary atrial cardiomiopathy or significant pathology of the sinus node has been highlighted, and in some cases a dramatic decrease in the nerve endings confirms a purely neurogenic mechanism to be at the base of lone atrial fibrillation. In these cases, the diagnosis of lone atrial fibrillation is incorrect because we are unable to demonstrate the true anatomic substrate of the arrhythmia. In fact, in a group of patients with drug-refractory paroxysmal lone atrial fibrillation, Frustaci et al. [1] demonstrated significant abnormality at the atrial biopsy in the form of:
- Atrial myocarditis in 66% of patients
- Noninflammatory cardiomyopathic process in 17%
- Patchy fibrosis in 17%

Thus, these alterations, absent in patients without atrial fibrillation, may contribute to the arrhythmic process.

[1]Dipartimento di Cardiologia, Ospedali di Foligno, Foligno, Italy; [2]Dipartimento di Cardiologia, Ospedale S. Maria, Terni, Italy; [3]Dipartimento di Cardiologia, Università "La Sapienza", Roma, Italy

Electrophysiologic Substrate

Atrial fibrillation has been demonstrated to be a reentrant arrhythmia. On the basis of the wavelength theory proposed by Alessie [2], for atrial fibrillation to be sustained requires from four to six circuits traveling simultaneously into the atria. The wavelength of a reentry arrhythmia can be obtained as the product of the conduction velocity and the refractory period. In the case of atrial fibrillation, the wavelength of each circuit is short (8 cm) due to a low conduction velocity and short atrial refractory period. Atrial fibrillation happens when zones of slow conduction and zones of heterogeneous refractoriness are simultaneously present in atria with a critical mass able to contain an adequate number of waves (4-6) circulating simultaneously. An exception to the reentrant mechanism is the focal form of atrial fibrillation that has been recently demonstrated [3].

Atrial Conduction Delay

Functional Delay

Delay of conduction of a premature stimulus in a particular site in the atria has been demonstrated to be the critical event which precedes the induction of atrial fibrillation.

In a study of Papageorgiou et al. [4], a premature extrastimulus delivered in the HRA but not in the coronary sinus was able to generate a conduction delay towards the posterior triangle of Koch; this delay was particularly evident and statistically significant in patients with a previous episode of atrial fibrillation, and was independent of age, atrial dimension, intramyocardial fibrosis, or myocyte apoptosis.

Delayed conduction and dispersion of refractoriness appear to be the purely electrophysiologic substrate of lone atrial fibrillation. This substrate is probably based on some spatial characteristics of the membranes [5] – connexin, ion channels, regulatory proteins – that may influence the propagation of the impulse, which may lead to the tissue anisotropism necessary to maintain atrial fibrillation.

The study by Papageorgiou et al. [4] supports the existence of true lone atrial fibrillation on the basis of genetically determined critical areas of conduction in the right atrium.

Stable delay

Patients with a previous episode of atrial fibrillation often show a significant increase in the atrial activation times both at the surface and in intracavitary recording. Conduction over the Bachmann bundle may be the critical point for the interatrial conduction time. Impairment of Bachmann bundle conduction may lead to abnormal activation of the left atrium and facilitate the induction of atrial fibrillation [6].

Multipolar esophageal recordings (Fig. 1) may help to calculate the interatrial

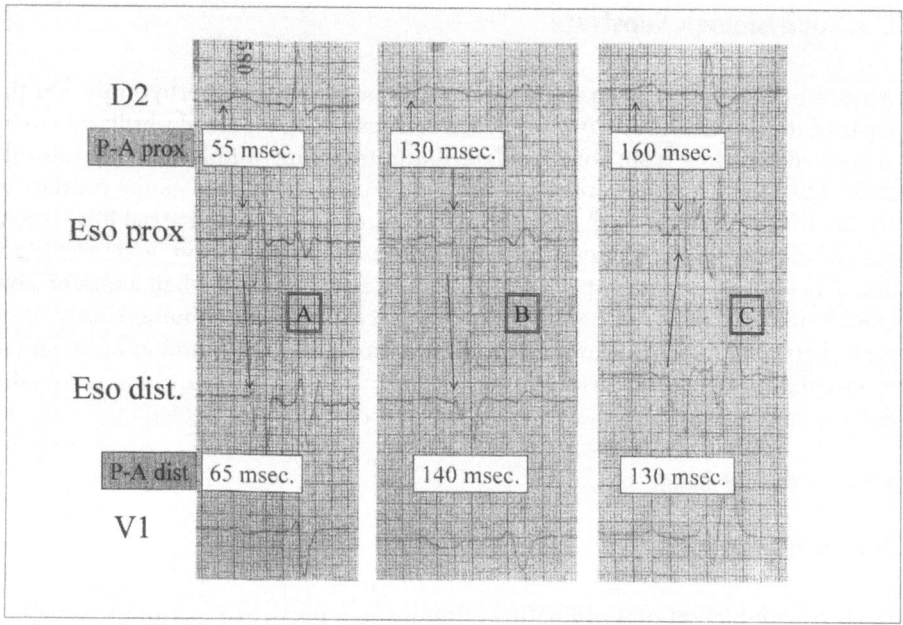

Fig. 1. Patterns of atrial activation using surface ECG and multipolar esophageal lead. A Normal atrial activation is characterized by: normal P wave in D2, normal interatrial conduction time (less than 65 ms), craniocaudal activation of the left atrium (proximal esophageal activation precedes distal). **B** Typical pattern of Bachmann bundle delay: P wave longer than 110 ms in D2 (positive and with a notched apex), prolonged interatrial conduction time (more than 65 ms), craniocaudal activation of the left atrium (proximal esophageal activation precedes distal). **C** Typical pattern of Bachmann bundle block: P wave longer than 110 ms in D2 with a negative terminal component, prolonged interatrial conduction time (more than 65 ms), retrograde activation of the left atrium (distal esophageal activation precedes proximal)

conduction time [7] and the pattern of activation of the left atrium in the longitudinal direction. This method helped us to differentiate three different patterns of activation:

1. Normal activation:
   – Normal P wave in D2
   – Normal interatrial conduction time (< 65 ms)
   – Craniocaudal activation of the left atrium (proximal esophageal activation precedes distal)
2. Bachmann bundle delay:
   – P wave longer than 110 ms in D2, positive and with a notched apex
   – Prolonged interatrial conduction time (> 65 ms)
   – Craniocaudal activation of the left atrium (proximal esophageal activation precedes distal)
3. Bachmann bundle block:
   – P wave longer than 110 ms in D2, with a negative terminal component
   – Prolonged interatrial conduction time (> 65 ms)

– Retrograde activation of the left atrium (distal esophageal activation precedes proximal).

These results support the suggestion of Bayes de Luna [6] that significant disturbance of the interatrial conduction time predicts early recurrence of atrial fibrillation.

Dispersion of Atrial Refractoriness

Atrial refractoriness can be calculated by introducing properly timed extrastimuli in different areas of the atria. The difference between the longer and the shorter refractory period calculated at different atrial sites represents the dispersion of atrial refractoriness.

Patients with lone atrial fibrillation have been demonstrated to have an increased dispersion of atrial refractoriness compared with normal subjects [8, 9]. This may be critical because premature atrial beats may reach some areas of the atria during the recovery time and others during the refractory period, leading to a preferential conduction path and unidirectional block that may facilitate the induction of atrial fibrillation.

Many factors can modify the dispersion of atrial repolarization, generating the substrate for atrial fibrillation. The autonomic nervous system and, in particular, strong vagal stimulation increase the dispersion of refractoriness, and atrial vulnerability [10]. In animals, a sudden stretch of the right atrium produced by increasing the atrial pressure increases the dispersion of atrial refractoriness and the likelihood of developing atrial fibrillation [11]. This mechanism may trigger lone atrial fibrillation due to atrioventricular nodal reciprocating tachycardia or atrioventricular reciprocating tachycardia. In this case, ablation of the primary tachycardia cures the atrial fibrillation.

Atrial Vulnerability

In patients with a potential substrate for atrial fibrillation, a properly timed extrastimulus can induce atrial fibrillation: this identifies patients with high "atrial vulnerability" [12].

Referring to electrophysiologic properties, the concept of atrial vulnerability is consistent with an effective refractory period shorter than the relative refractory period. This difference is the so-called window of vulnerability, which in the normal subject ranges between 20 and 30 ms. An ectopic beat occurring in the window of vulnerability can generate repetitive atrial beats that, in the presence of zones of slow conduction and dispersion of refractoriness, can give rise to atrial fibrillation [13].

Patients with atrial fibrillation have a greater window of vulnerability, in particular at higher heart rates, when the effective refractoy period shortens without a corresponding shortening of the relative refractory period [14].

Focal Mechanism

Atrial fibrillation has been considered exclusively a multiple reentrant arrhythmia for many years. Animal and human studies have confirmed this hypothesis, but Jais and Haïssaguerre recently described a particular form of atrial fibrillation called focal atrial fibrillation [3].

The two superior pulmonary veins appear to be the most important trigger points of focal atrial fibrillation.

These atrial foci exhibited unpredictable firing and delayed conduction to the left atrium. The venous origin of the earliest ectopic activity was demonstrated to be 2-4 cm within the main pulmonary veins and depolarization was marked by a spike preceding the onset of the ectopic P wave by more than 100 ms. Focal atrial fibrillation can be differentiated from the common form of atrial fibrillation by typical patterns both on the surface and in the intracavitary recording.

On the surface ECG focal AF may be suspected in presence of:
– Runs of paroxysmal atrial fibrillation alternating with one or a few sinus beats
– The presence of organized tachycardia at about 400/min in some leads, despite an apparently typical pattern of atrial fibrillation

At endocardial mapping the arrhythmia shows the following characteristics:
– Organized atrial activity with a very short cycle length (up to 130 ms)
– Centrifugal activation of the atria from a single focus (similar to atrial tachycardia)

Focal atrial fibrillation can easily be suppressed by radiofrequency ablation of its site of origin [15].

After ablation of the focus the patients remain free from recurrences and atrial fibrillation does not persist even after artificial desynchronization of the atria by high-rate pacing, further confirming the focal origin of the arrhythmia.

Triggering and Modulating Factors

Ectopic Atrial Beats

The presence of an electrophysiological substrate is not of itself usually able to generate atrial fibrillation. In a recent study [16], Haïssaguerre et al., after detailed mapping of spontaneous-onset, drug-resistent paroxysmal atrial fibrillation, demonstrated that the arrhythmia was initiated by ectopic atrial beats (single or repetitive). Although these may originate in many places in the atria, in 94% of the cases the firing site was very deep in the ostia of the pulmonary veins. The authors concluded that a particular anatomic structure of the pulmonary veins may facilitate the onset of the ectopic beats and trigger drug-refractory atrial fibrillation. It is not clear whether a pulmonary venous origin of ectopic beats can be demonstrated in all patients with atrial fibrillation; this field needs to be investigated further.

Without a doubt, in everyday clinical practice evaluation of the induction sequence of atrial fibrillation by conventional surface ECG or Holter monitoring can be extremely important in understanding the initial mechanism. Suppression of the ectopic beats can itself be the endpoint of antifibrillatory therapy once the ectopic beats have been shown to be responsible for triggering atrial fibrillation (Fig. 2) [17].

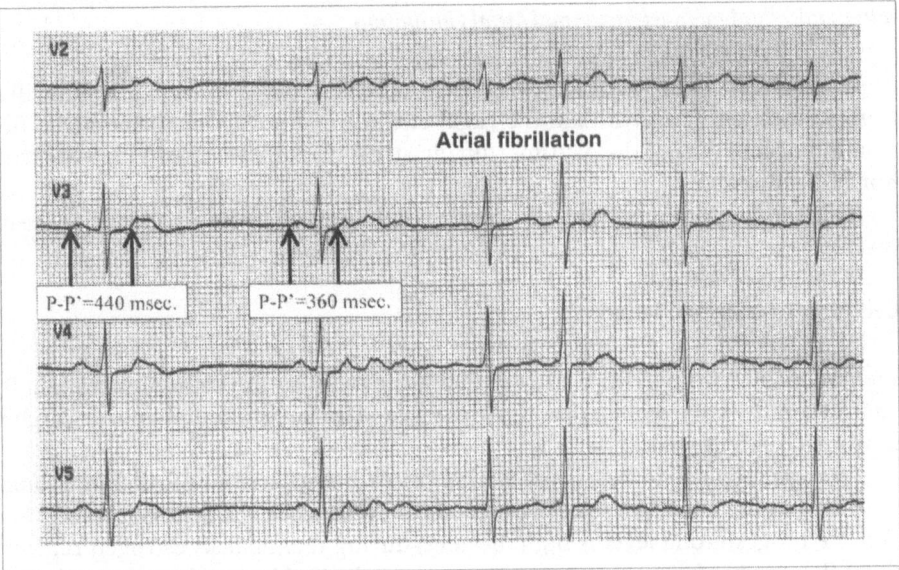

Fig. 2. Induction of atrial fibrillation by a premature atrial beat. A tract of atrial bigeminy has been recorded (both the ectopic beats are blocked at atrioventricular level). The coupling interval of the second ectopic atrial beat is shorter than the first (360 vs 440 ms), thus generating an episode of atrial fibrillation

Autonomic Nervous System

The influence of the autonomic nervous system on the inducibility of atrial fibrillation has been widely described. In humans, both strong vagal stimulation and isoprenaline infusion provoke atrial fibrillation in patients who have previously experienced the arrhythmia [10]. Atrial vulnerability can be greatly changed by vagosympathetic equilibrium. The vagal nerve and the nerves of the sympathetic nervous system have different anatomical distributions, latencies, and durations of their effects [18]. In this context it is easy to understand how an imbalance of the autonomic nervous system may lead to an inhomogeneous substrate.

In the classical definition of Coumel [19], neuromediated paroxysmal atrial fibrillation can be vagally mediated or adrenergically mediated [19].

Vagally Mediated Paroxysmal Atrial Fibrillation

This form of atrial fibrillation occurs most frequently between the ages of 30 and 50 years. No structural heart disease can be demonstrated, and the paroxysms most often develop during the night, at rest, and in the postprandial period. ECG recording before the onset of atrial fibrillation shows a progressive decrease in the heart rate.

Acute alcohol intake increases the risk of atrial fibrillation by both a vagal mechanism and via a direct toxic effect.

Adrenergically Mediated Paroxysmal Atrial Fibrillation

In patients with an apparently normal heart, the adrenergic form of atrial fibrillation is much less frequent than the vagal one. Adrenergically mediated atrial fibrillation occurs during the daytime, during stress or exercise, and in patients with hormonal disease.

This the predominant type of arrhythmia in patients with an identified heart disease.

Gender and Atrial Fibrillation

Premenopausal women have a lower incidence of atrial fibrillation than men. By contrast, in the older population the incidence of atrial fibrillation appears higher in women than in men.

Estrogen appears to be the protecting factor, because atrial fibrillation relapses overall in the luteal phase of the menstrual cycle, when the estrogen level is low and the progesterone level is high; besides, during menopause, estrogen replacement therapy has been demonstrated to reduce the incidence of atrial fibrillation. The mechanism of the protective effect of estrogens is complex and probably multifactorial, involving a direct ionic mechanism at membrane level and an indirect effect mediated by the autonomic nervous system [20].

Conclusions

The word "lone" should be used to refer to a particular form of atrial fibrillation which has a primarily electrophysiologic substrate. Recent studies on the focal mechanisms show that lone atrial fibrillation is probably a real electrophysiological condition. Nonetheless, several factors including myocarditis should be taken into account before a paroxysm of atrial fibrillation is defined as lone atrial fibrillation. Thus, a deep understanding of the electrophysiologic mechanisms is fundamental to any therapeutic decision.

References

1. Frustaci A, Chimenti C, Bellocci F, Morgante E, Russo MA, Maseri A (1997) Histological substrate of atrial biopsies in patients with lone atrial fibrillation. Circulation 96:1180-1184
2. Allessie MA (1995) Reentrant mechanisms underlying atrial fibrillation. In: Zipes DP, Jalife J (eds) Cardiac electrophysiology: from cell to bedside, 2nd edn. Saunders, Toronto, pp 562-566
3. Jais P, Haissaguerre M, Dipen C, Chouairi S, Gencel L, Hocini M, Clementy J (1997) A focal source of atrial fibrillation treated by discrete radiofrequency ablation. Circulation 95:572-576

4. Papageorgiou P, Moahan K, Boyle N, Seifert MJ, Beswick P, Zebeda J, Epstein L, Josephson ME (1996) Site-dependent intra-atrial conduction delay. Relationship to initiation of atrial fibrillation. Circulation 94:384-389
5. Thomas SA, Schussler RB, Saffitz JE (1998) Connexins, conduction and atrial fibrillation. J Cardiovasc Electrophysiol 9:608-1007
6. Bayès de Luna A, Cladellas M, Oter R, Torner P, Guindo J et al (1988) Interatrial conduction block and retrograde activation of the left atrium and paroxysmal supraventricular tachyarrhythmia. Eur Heart J 9:1112-1118
7. Bagliani G, Meniconi L, Raggi F, Corea L (1998) Left origin of the atrial esophageal signal as recorded in the pacing site. Pacing Clin Electrophysiol 21 (I):18-24
8. Michelucci A, Padeletti L, Fradella GA (1982) Atrial refractoriness and spontaneous or induced atrial fibrillation. Acta Cardiol 37:333-341
9. Misier AR, Opthof T, van Hemel NM (1992) Increased dispersion of refractoriness in patients with idiopathic paroxysmal atrial fibrillation. J Am Coll Cardiol 19:1531-1535
10. Zipes DP, Mihalick MJ, Robbins GT (1983) Effect of selective vagal and stellate ganglionic stimulation on atrial refractoriness in man. Am J Cardiol 51:96-100
11. Satoh T, Zipes DP (1996) Unequal atrial stretch in dogs increases dispersion of refractoriness conducive to developing atrial fibrillation. J Cardiovasc Electrophysiol 7:833-842
12. Attuel P, Pellegrin D, Gaston J (1989) Latent atrial vulnerability: new means of electrophysiologic investigations in paroxysmal atrial arrhythmias. In: Attuel P, Coumel P, Janse MJ (eds) The atrium in health and disease. Futura, Mt Kisco, NY, pp 159-200
13. Cosio FG, Palacios J, Vidal JM (1983) Electrophysiologic studies in atrial fibrillation: slow conduction of premature impulses. A possible manifestation of the background for reentry. Am J Cardiol 51:122-130
14. Wyndham CRC, Amat-y-Leon F, Wu D, Denes P, Dhingra R, Simpson R, Rosen KM (1977) Effects of cycle length on atrial vulnerability. Circulation 55:260-271
15. Haïssaguerre M, Markus F, Fischer B, Clementy J (1994) Radiofrequency catheter ablation in unusual mechanisms of atrial fibrillation. J Cardiovasc Electrophysiol 5:743-751
16. Haïssaguerre M, Jaïs P, Shah D, Takahashi A, Hocini M, Quiniou G, Garrigue S, Le Mouroux A, Le Metayer P, Clementy J (1998) Spontaneous initiation of atrial fibrillation by ectopic beats originating in the pulmonary veins. N Engl J Med 339:659-666
17. Capucci A, Santarelli A, Boriani G (1992) Atrial premature beats coupling interval determines lone paroxysmal atrial fibrillation onset. Int J Cardiol 36:87-93
18. Alessi R, Nusynowitz M, Abildskov JA (1958) Nonuniform distribution of vagal effects on the atrial refractory period. Am J Physiol 194:406-410
19. Coumel P (1996) Autonomic influences in atrial tachyarrhythmias. J Cardiovasc Electrophysiol 7:999-1007
20. Rubart M, von der Lohe E (1998) Sex steroids and cardiac arrhythmia: more questions than answers. J Cardiovasc Electrophysiol 9:665-667

Atrial Fibrillation in Apparently Idiopathic Cardiomyopathy: The Chicken or the Egg?

F. Morady

In 1913, Gossage and Hicks reported the case of a previously healthy 23-year-old man who presented with dyspnea and chest pain and was found, on the basis of radial and jugular pulse tracings, to have atrial fibrillation and a rapid ventricular response [1]. On physical examination, there was no evidence of cardiomegaly. He was treated with tincture of digitalis and continued to have atrial fibrillation, and serial physical examinations demonstrated progressive cardiac enlargement. The patient died suddenly approximately 18 months after first presenting with atrial fibrillation. A postmortem examination demonstrated a dilated and hypertrophied left ventricle, with no valvular lesions and normal coronary arteries. Earlier contemporary studies had suggested that dilatation of the heart may be a common cause of atrial fibrillation, but, based on the findings in their patient, Gossage and Hicks concluded that dilatation of the heart may be caused by, rather than being the cause of, atrial fibrillation [1].

The report by Gossage and Hicks demonstrates that the chicken-egg question relating to atrial fibrillation and dilated cardiomyopathy was first posed many years ago. However, several decades elapsed before this important issue was again addressed in the literature. This review will summarize some of the experimental and clinical studies having to do with the phenomenon of atrial-fibrillation-induced dilated cardiomyopathy.

Experimental Studies of Tachycardia-Induced Cardiomyopathy

If dilated cardiomyopathy is caused by atrial fibrillation, it is likely that an important factor is an uncontrolled ventricular rate and prolonged tachycardia. Therefore, experimental studies of tachycardia-induced cardiomyopathy may provide some insight into the clinical syndrome of atrial-fibrillation-induced

Department of Internal Medicine, Division of Cardiology, University of Michigan, Ann Arbor, Michigan, USA

cardiomyopathy. Congestive heart failure has been brought on in dogs and pigs by continuous ventricular pacing at rates of 220-250 beats/min for 1-8 weeks [2-5]. These animals develop ventricular dilatation, a reduced left ventricular ejection fraction, reduced cardiac output, and elevated filling pressures, as are typical of dilated cardiomyopathy.

Perhaps more relevant to the clinical syndrome of atrial-fibrillation-induced cardiomyopathy are the experimental studies that have employed rapid atrial pacing to induce congestive heart failure. Continuous atrial pacing in dogs at a rate of 190 beats/min (with 1:1 atrioventricular conduction) for 12 weeks has been demonstrated to cause ventricular dilatation and a drop in left ventricular ejection fraction from approximately 0.50 to 0.30, with most of the drop occurring in the first 6 weeks of rapid pacing [6]. In pigs, tachycardia-induced cardiomyopathy has been induced by atrial pacing at a rate of 240 beats/min for 3 weeks [7-9]. The hemodynamic profile of this model of congestive heart failure is typical of dilated cardiomyopathy.

Experimental studies have also demonstrated that tachycardia-induced cardiomyopathy is at least partially reversible. In dogs that develop tachycardia-induced cardiomyopathy after 3-8 weeks of ventricular pacing at 220-240 beats/min, wall motion abnormalities resolve within 2-4 days after cessation of rapid pacing [3]. When atrial pacing at a rate of 190 beats/min for 12 weeks induces cardiomyopathy in dogs, the left ventricular ejection fraction returns to normal by 2 weeks after resolution of the tachycardia [6]. In pigs subjected to rapid atrial pacing at 240 beats/min for 3 weeks, all indices of systolic function become abnormal but return to normal during a 4-week recovery period [8].

Although abnormalities of systolic function appear to resolve within a relatively short period of time after cessation of rapid pacing in these experimental models of tachycardia-induced cardiomyopathy, other types of abnormalities may be persistent or may take a longer time to resolve. In dogs and pigs with tachycardia-induced cardiomyopathy who are allowed to recover for 4-12 weeks after cessation of rapid atrial pacing, indices of systolic function return to normal, but there may be persistent left ventricular dilatation, left ventricular hypertrophy, and diastolic dysfunction, reflected in abnormalities in indices of relaxation and filling [6, 8].

Because patients with atrial fibrillation rarely have ventricular rates as high as the rates used to induce cardiomyopathy in experimental studies, the results of these experimental studies are not directly applicable to the clinical arena. The experimental studies demonstrate that sustained tachycardia during a period of several weeks causes a dilated cardiomyopathy, that abnormalities in systolic function resolve within several days to weeks after cessation of tachycardia, and that abnormalities in diastolic function may persist for a longer period of time. However, the experimental studies do not provide information on how long it takes for dilated cardiomyopathy to occur in patients with atrial fibrillation and a rapid ventricular response, who typically have rates varying between 100 and 160 beats/min.

Mechanism of Tachycardia-Induced Cardiomyopathy

Several possible mechanisms of tachycardia-induced cardiomyopathy have been proposed, and it is likely that the mechanism is multifactorial. The possible mechanisms of tachycardia-induced cardiomyopathy include the following: depletion of myocardial energy stores, including creatine, phosphocreatine, and adenosine triphosphate [10]; a decrease in creatine kinase activity [7]; structural and functional abnormalities of mitochondria [10]; a diminished responsiveness of myocytes to an increase in extracellular calcium [9]; abnormalities in cytoarchitecture, with a decrease in the myofibrillar content of myocytes [9]; and biochemical defects in sarcolemmal receptor and transport systems [10].

Deleterious Effect of Irregular Ventricular Rate

In addition to persistent tachycardia, another possible reason for compromised systolic function in patients with chronic atrial fibrillation may be the irregularity of the ventricular rhythm. In a group of 11 patients with atrial fibrillation who had a mean left ventricular ejection fraction of 0.46 ± 0.11 and who underwent catheter ablation of the atrioventricular junction, the cardiac output was found to be significantly lower (by 12%) during irregular ventricular pacing at a mean cycle length of 750 ms than during regular ventricular pacing at a cycle length of 750 ms [11].

Further evidence of a deleterious effect of an irregular ventricular rhythm on left ventricle function is provided by a study in which 14 patients who had chronic atrial fibrillation and a controlled ventricular response (average hourly heart rates of 60-100 beats/min on 24-hour Holter monitor recording) underwent catheter ablation of the atrioventricular junction and implantation of a ventricular pacemaker [12]. Most of the patients had an ischemic or dilated cardiomyopathy. The mean left ventricular ejection fraction before ablation was 0.30 ± 0.11, and rose to 0.39 ± 0.11 by 1 month after ablation. Therefore, it appears that an irregular ventricular rate, even in the absence of tachycardia, may contribute to left ventricular dysfunction that is reversible.

Effect of Cardioversion in Patients with Atrial Fibrillation and Dilated Cardiomyopathy

The first published report of a series of patients with congestive heart failure attributable to idiopathic atrial fibrillation was by Phillips and Levine [13]. They found that 7 of 84 patients (8%) with idiopathic atrial fibrillation had overt congestive heart failure and cardiomegaly. The average duration of atrial fibrillation in the patients with congestive heart failure was 3.7 months, and their average ventricular rate was 146 beats/min at rest (range 122-170 beats/min). In contrast, among the patients who did not have congestive heart failure, the average ventricular rate was 100 beats/min, and only 2 had a ventricular rate greater than 118 beats/min. Of note is that signs and symptoms of congestive heart failure resolved completely among 6 patients with congestive heart failure in whom sinus rhythm was restored after treatment with quinidine. Phillips and Levine concluded that atrial fibrillation may cause a reversible type of heart failure, and emphasized the importance of recognizing that "chronic myocarditis" may be a manifestation rather than a cause of atrial fibrillation.

After a hiatus in the literature of approximately 40 years, the association between atrial fibrillation and dilated cardiomyopathy was again emphasized in a case report by Peters and Kienzle [14]. In a 56-year-old man with a 10-year history of chronic atrial fibrillation, the ventricular rate varied between 120 and 160 beats/min, and the left ventricular ejection fraction was 0.18. Treatment with amiodarone resulted in conversion to sinus rhythm, with an increase in ejection fraction to 0.54.

There have been no large-scale studies of the effect of cardioversion on left ventricular function in patients with idiopathic dilated cardiomyopathy, but there are 3 published studies that have had sample sizes of 10-17 patients [15-17]. In one of these studies, the initial ventricular rate during atrial fibrillation was 120-175 beats/min [16]. The mean baseline left ventricular ejection fractions were in the range of 0.25-0.30. In each of these studies, restoration of sinus rhythm was accompanied by almost a two-fold increase in ejection fraction, with complete normalization of left ventricular function in approximately 50% of patients. These studies suggest that among patients with atrial fibrillation and a dilated cardiomyopathy presumed to be idiopathic, the cardiomyopathy may actually be a result of the atrial fibrillation and reversible in one-half of patients.

Effect of Rate Control on Left Ventricular Function

In patients with a dilated cardiomyopathy and chronic atrial fibrillation, long-term restoration of sinus rhythm may not be possible. Several studies have demonstrated that control of the ventricular rate by atrioventricular node ablation or modification may result in improvement in left ventricular function when rate control cannot be achieved with medications. For example, in a patient who was presumed to have idiopathic dilated cardiomyopathy and who had chronic atrial fibrillation with an uncontrolled ventricular rate, modification of the atrioventricular node resulted in a marked improvement in left ventricular function by echocardiography, with an increase in fractional shortening from 18% to 38% [18].

In four studies, left ventricular function was assessed before and after atrioventricular junction ablation and pacemaker implantation in patients with uncontrolled atrial fibrillation and baseline left ventricular dysfunction [19-22]. The sample sizes in these studies ranged from 5 to 12 patients. There was a consistent improvement in left ventricular function, with fractional shortening or ejection fraction improving by 26-67%. The patients in these studies had various types of heart disease, demonstrating that tachycardia-induced cardiomyopathy may be superimposed on other types of underlying structural heart disease. Thus, even if the patient does not have a completely reversible form of dilated cardiomyopathy caused by atrial fibrillation, it is still important to achieve adequate rate control.

In a study that used radiofrequency modification of the atrioventricular node to control the ventricular rate during atrial fibrillation, there were four patients who had a dilated cardiomyopathy that was presumed to be idiopathic [23]. The baseline left ventricular ejection fraction in these patients ranged from 0.13 to 0.36, and two of the patients had severe congestive heart failure and were awaiting cardiac transplantation. After control of the ventricular rate, the mean left ventricular ejection fraction increased from 0.22 ± 0.10 to 0.48 ± 0.12, and the two patients who had been awaiting transplantation no longer needed a heart transplant. This study demonstrated that even when atrial fibrillation results in tachycardia-induced dilated cardiomyopathy that is severe enough to necessitate cardiac transplantation, the cardiomyopathy may be completely or almost completely reversible with control of the ventricular rate.

Rate Control with Medications vs Atrioventricular Junction Ablation

In a multicenter study, patients with chronic atrial fibrillation, overt congestive heart failure, and a resting ventricular rate greater than 90 beats/min were randomly assigned to atrioventricular junction ablation and pacemaker implantation (32 patients) or pharmacologic treatment for rate control (34 patients) [24]. The most common type of heart disease was coronary artery disease. The baseline mean left ventricular ejection fractions in the two groups were approximately 0.43-0.44, and remained unchanged after 12 months of follow-up. At first glance, the results of this study may seem to contradict the results of the earlier uncontrolled studies that demonstrated a significant improvement in ejection fraction after rate control is achieved. However, the explanation for this apparent discrepancy may be that the entry criterion in this study was a resting rate greater than 90 beats/min, which is lower than in many prior studies [13, 14, 16, 18, 20-23]. In addition, it is possible that a depressed ejection fraction is most likely to improve after treatment of atrial fibrillation when there is an apparently idiopathic dilated cardiomyopathy [16, 17] than when a patient has coronary artery disease or valvular heart disease.

Conclusions

In patients with dilated cardiomyopathy and atrial fibrillation, the atrial fibrillation may be either the chicken or the egg. It is clear that dilated cardiomyopathy of any etiology can be a cause of atrial fibrillation, but there is also ample evidence that atrial fibrillation may be a cause of dilated cardiomyopathy. Therefore, in patients with atrial fibrillation and an apparently idiopathic dilated cardiomyopathy, it is always important to either restore sinus rhythm or ensure that the ventricular rate is adequately controlled.

References

1. Gossage AM, Hicks BJA (1913) On auricular fibrillation. Q J Med 6:435-640
2. Armstrong PW, Stopps TP, Ford SE, de Bold AJ (1986) Rapid ventricular pacing in the dog: pathophysiologic studies of heart failure. Circulation 74:1075-1084
3. Wilson JR, Douglas P, Hickey WF, Lanoce V, Ferraro N, Muhammad A, Reichek N (1987) Experimental congestive heart failure produced by rapid ventricular pacing in the dog: cardiac effects. Circulation 75:857-867
4. Chow E, Woodard JC, Farrar DJ (1990) Rapid ventricular pacing in pigs: an experimental model of congestive heart failure. Am J Physiol 258:H1603-H1605
5. Kajstura J, Zhang X, Liu Y, Szoke E, Cheng W, Olivetti G, Hintze TH, Anversa P (1995) The cellular basis of pacing-induced dilated cardiomyopathy: myocyte cell loss and myocyte cellular reactive hypertrophy. Circulation 92:2306-2317
6. Damiano RJ, Tripp HF, Asano T, Small KW, Jones RH, Lowe JE (1987) Left ventricular dysfunction and dilatation resulting from chronic supraventricular tachycardia. J Thorac Cardiovasc Surg 94:135-143
7. Spinale FG, Hendrick DA, Crawford FA, Smith AC, Hamada Y, Carabello BA (1990) Chronic supraventricular tachycardia causes ventricular dysfunction and subendocardial injury in swine. Am J Physiol 259:H218-H229
8. Tomita M, Spinale FG, Crawford FA, Zile MR (1991) Changes in left ventricular volume, mass, and function during the development and regression of supraventricular tachycardia-induced cardiomyopathy: disparity between recovery of systolic versus diastolic function. Circulation 83:635-644
9. Spinale FG, Fulbright BM, Mukherjee R, Tanaka R, Hu J, Crawford FA, Zile MR (1992) Relation between ventricular and myocyte function with tachycardia-induced cardiomyopathy. Circ Res 71:174-187
10. Shinbane JS, Wood MA, Jensen DN, Ellenbogen KA, Fitzpatrick AP, Scheinman MM (1997) Tachycardia-induced cardiomyopathy: a review of animal models and clinical studies. J Am Coll Cardiol 29:709-715
11. Daoud EG, Weiss R, Bahu M, Knight BP, Bogun F, Goyal R, Harvey M, Strickberger SA, Man KC, Morady F (1996) Effect of an irregular ventricular rhythm on cardiac output. Am J Cardiol 78:1433-1436
12. Natale A, Zimerman L, Tomassoni G, Kearney M, Kent V, Brandon MJ, Newby K (1996) Impact on ventricular function and quality of life of transcatheter ablation of the atrioventricular junction in chronic atrial fibrillation with a normal ventricular response. Am J Cardiol 78:1431-1433
13. Phillips E, Levine SA (1949) Auricular fibrillation without other evidence of heart disease. Am J Med 7:478-489
14. Peters KG, Kienzle MG (1988) Severe cardiomyopathy due to chronic rapidly conducted atrial fibrillation: complete recovery after restoration of sinus rhythm. Am J Med 85:242-244
15. Sacrez A, Kieny JR, Bouheur JB, Komajda M, Bareiss P, Bouilland H, Ferriere M (1990) Effet de la réduction de la fibrillation auriculaire sur la fonction ventriculaire gauche des cardiomyopathies dilatées. Arch Mal Coeur 83:15-21

16. Grogan M, Smith HC, Gersh BJ, Wood DL (1992) Left ventricular dysfunction due to atrial fibrillation in patients initially believed to have idiopathic dilated cardiomyopathy. Am J Cardiol 69:1570-1575

17. Kieny JR, Sacrez A, Facello A, Arbogast R, Bareiss P, Roul G, Demangeat JL, Brunot B, Constantinesco A (1992) Increase in radionuclide left ventricular ejection fraction after cardioversion of chronic atrial fibrillation in idiopathic dilated cardiomyopathy. Eur Heart J 13:1290-1295

18. Lemery R, Brugada P, Chriex E, Wellens HJJ (1987) Reversibility of tachycardia-induced left ventricular dysfunction after closed-chest catheter ablation of the atrioventricular junction for intractable atrial fibrillation. Am J Cardiol 60:1406-1408

19. Rosenqvist M, Lee MA, Moulinier L, Springer MJ, Abbott JA, Wu J, Langberg JJ, Griffin JC, Scheinman MM (1990) Long-term follow-up of patients after transcatheter direct current ablation of the atrioventricular junction. J Am Coll Cardiol 16:1467-1474

20. Heinz G, Siostrzonek P, Kreiner G, Gossinger H (1992) Improvement in left ventricular systolic function after successful radiofrequency His bundle ablation for drug refractory, chronic atrial fibrillation and recurrent atrial flutter. Am J Cardiol 69:489-492

21. Rodriguez LM, Smeets JLRM, Xie B, de Chillou C, Cheriex E, Pieters F, Metzger J, den Dulk K, Wellens HJJ (1993) Improvement in left ventricular function by ablation of atrioventricular nodal conduction in selected patients with lone atrial fibrillation. Am J Cardiol 72:1137-1141

22. Brignole M, Gianfranchi L, Menozzi C, Bottoni N, Bollini R, Lolli G, Oddone D, Gaggioli G (1994) Influence of atrioventricular junction radiofrequency ablation in patients with chronic atrial fibrillation and flutter on quality of life and cardiac performance. Am J Cardiol 74:242-246

23. Morady F, Hasse C, Strickberger SA, Man KC, Daoud E, Bogun F, Goyal R, Harvey M, Knight BP, Weiss R, Bahu M (1997) Long-term follow-up after radiofrequency modification of the atrioventricular node in patients with atrial fibrillation. J Am Coll Cardiol 27:113-121

24. Brignole M, Menozzi C, Gianfranchi L, Musso G, Mureddu R, Bottoni N, Lolli G (1998) Assessment of atrioventricular junction ablation and VVIR pacemaker versus pharmacological treatment in patients with heart failure and chronic atrial fibrillation. Circulation 98:953-960

Cardioversion for Atrial Fibrillation Today: When and Why?

C. Pandozi, G. Gentilucci, M.C. Scianaro and M. Santini

Atrial fibrillation is a common arrhythmia with a high prevalence in the elderly [1]. One Australian study found a prevalence of atrial fibrillation of 11.6% in people over 75 years of age [2]. The arrhythmia has been considered benign until it was demonstrated that atrial fibrillation carries a significant morbidity and mortality. The mortality risk in patients with atrial fibrillation has been reported to be twice as high as that in controls [1].

Stroke is the most important cause of death, occurring in up to 30% of patients aged 80-89 years and in up to 15% of patients aged 50-59 years [3]. Even in the absence of clinically apparent stroke, patients with atrial fibrillation have a high incidence of abnormal findings suggesting silent cerebral infarction on CT scanning of the brain [4]. An increased risk of stroke has been reported in lone atrial fibrillation only in patients older than 60 years [5, 6].

The etiology of atrial fibrillation is various. While some patients have a definite noncardiac etiology, such as thyreotoxicosis or alcohol abuse, the majority have a clear structural heart disease. Valvular heart disease (in the past the foremost cause of atrial fibrillation), hypertension, coronary artery disease, dilated and hypertrophic cardiomyopathy and sick sinus syndrome are the most frequent pathologies in patients with paroxysmal or permanent atrial fibrillation. In a few patients no evident structural heart disease is present and their atrial fibrillation is termed "lone".

Atrial fibrillation may be asymptomatic or, more frequently, symptomatic. The arrhythmia may cause palpitations or symptoms related to hemodynamic dysfunction such as fatigue, shortness of breath on exertion and dizziness. It may precipitate angina, syncope, and left ventricular dysfunction.

Several classifications of atrial fibrillation have been proposed. The most widely accepted is the so-called 3 Ps classification proposed by Gallagher and Camm [7], which subdivides atrial fibrillation in relation to time course into three forms: paroxysmal, persistent, and permanent. Paroxysmal atrial fibrillation is that in which episodes of atrial fibrillation terminate spontaneously within 24-48 h. Persistent atrial fibrillation continues until some measure is taken to termi-

Dipartimento di Cardiologia, Ospedale San Filippo Neri, Rome, Italy

nate it. Atrial fibrillation is permanent when it has resisted all attempts to restore sinus rhythm or when the physician and patient decide that no such attempt should be made. The term "acute atrial fibrillation" may describe an episode of atrial fibrillation related to an acute curable cause [8].

From the above classification it is evident that when atrial fibrillation is termed "permanent" no attempt should be made to restore sinus rhythm. In patients with paroxysmal atrial fibrillation electrical cardioversion should not be used unless the ventricular rate is very high or there is severe hemodynamic dysfunction. In this form of atrial fibrillation pharmacological cardioversion is generally used to reduce the duration of the episode, prevent the development of atrial electrical remodeling, and avoid transition to the persistent form (when this happens in spite of antiarrhythmic drugs therapy, electrical cardioversion should be planned). Moreover, it is noteworthy that when atrial fibrillation exceeds 48 h duration, the current recommendation is to provide anticoagulant therapy for 3 weeks before attempting arrhythmia conversion to prevent embolic events. For all these reasons, the question of when and why to cardiovert atrial fibrillation relates mainly to the persistent form of atrial fibrillation.

Why should a patient with persistent atrial fibrillation undergo cardioversion? At the moment the "rate versus rhythm" debate is still open. This debate relates to the fundamental question of the efficacy, costs, adverse effects, and benefits of attempting to restore and maintain sinus rhythm in patients with persistent atrial fibrillation compared with a strategy of damage limitation by controlling the ventricular rate and preventing thromboembolic events by anticoagulation. Several ongoing trials are examining this issue, but the results of the AFFIRM [9], PIAF [10], and RACE [11] studies will be available only in the next few years. While waiting for the results of these prospective studies, an answer to the present questions can be proposed. First: *why* cardiovert persistent atrial fibrillation?

The goals of treating atrial fibrillation are the following: improving symptoms and quality of life, improving hemodynamics, and reducing the risk of stroke. Pharmacological rate control ameliorates symptoms and may make the patient asymptomatic despite the loss of atrioventricular synchrony, but it achieves incomplete improvement of the hemodynamics because there is no effect on the contribution of atrial systole to the cardiac output. Moreover, there is no effect on the risk of embolism, and anticoagulation is necessary in the vast majority of patients. Sinus rhythm restoration, on the other hand, improves symptoms, restores atrial contraction, and reduces the embolic risk. Moreover, this treatment increases exercise capacity, particularly in patients with heart failure [12], and improves quality of life [13].

For these reasons, in our opinion rate control is not indicated in the majority of patients with persistent atrial fibrillation. In these patients restoration and maintenance of sinus rhythm is the primary therapeutic goal which improves symptoms and hemodynamics and avoids the need for anticoagulation. Moreover, rate control means anticoagulation monitoring and exposes the patients to bleeding complications. Furthermore, in patients with atrial fibrillation embolic risk is reduced by anticoagulation, but it probably is still higher than that in subjects in sinus rhythm, even though, to be honest, it remains conjecture that cardioversion and maintenance of sinus rhythm restore the risk of stroke to that in a control population.

In the future the ongoing trials will establish whether the benefits associated with restoration and maintenance of sinus rhythm also lead to a decrease in mortality and morbidity.

The other question, *when* to cardiovert atrial fibrillation, introduces another important clinical issue. Not to deny subjects with atrial fibrillation the potential benefits of sinus rhythm, should all patients be considered for cardioversion? We think that all patients with persistent atrial fibrillation merit serious consideration for cardioversion before it is accepted that atrial fibrillation is permanent. A crucial issue is the probability of restoring and maintaining sinus rhythm as well as evaluation of any potentially enhanced risk associated with trying to maintain sinus rhythm, such as occurs, for example, with the use of class I agents in patients with ventricular dysfunction and thyroid disease, in whom amiodarone is contraindicated.

The main factors that increase the likelihood of an early recurrence of atrial fibrillation are the following: previous successful cardioversions followed by early recurrences of the arrhythmia, a long duration of the present episode of atrial fibrillation, or the presence of rheumatic mitral valve disease [11].

At the moment the prognostic value of an enlarged left atrium is disputed, as it is well known that left atrial enlargement may be the consequence and not the cause of atrial fibrillation. Therefore, we think that the majority of new patients presenting with persistent atrial fibrillation should undergo at least one attempt at cardioversion. In the other cases, in patients with previous episodes of persistent atrial fibrillation and successful cardioversion, prior to any attempt at cardioversion an assessment of the risk of relapse from sinus rhythm is required, and prophylactic therapy should be instituted before cardioversion, especially if amiodarone is the drug selected to prevent atrial fibrillation recurrence. Clinical practice has shown that early recurrences of persistent atrial fibrillation following successful cardioversion indicate a high risk of future recurrence, and therefore patients who experienced previous early recurrences should not undergo cardioversion unless there is a modification in the clinical strategy (e.g., use of antiarrhythmic therapy in patients previously cardioverted without antiarrhythmic drugs because it was their first episode of persistent atrial fibrillation, switching from class I antiarrhythmic drugs to amiodarone, and so on).

Once it has been decided that a patient with persistent atrial fibrillation should undergo cardioversion because of a high likelihood of maintaining sinus rhythm, every effort should be made to achieve the goal of sinus rhythm restoration. This means that in patients with persistent atrial fibrillation resistant to external cardioversion, or with a low likelihood of cardioversion with trans-thoracic shocks, internal low energy cardioversion should be performed [14-17]. An atrial fibrillation resistant to external defibrillation should not be defined as permanent unless attempts at internal cardioversion have failed. Moreover, when using internal cardioversion, the optimal lead configuration (right atrium-coronary sinus) should be utilized if other lead configurations associated with a higher atrial defibrillation threshold fail (right atrium-left pulmonary artery and right atrium-right ventricle configurations).

Finally, in deciding when to cardiovert a patient with atrial fibrillation, the issue of anticoagulation should be always carefully addressed. It is now well established that in patients with atrial fibrillation lasting 48 h or more, oral anticoagulation for at least 3 weeks before and 4 weeks after cardioversion is recommended. Therefore, patients with persistent atrial fibrillation can undergo cardioversion only if oral anticoagulation has been given and therapeutic international normalized ratio (INR) values (between 2 and 3) have been achieved for at least 3 weeks. An interesting new approach in patients with persistent atrial fibrillation who for various reasons have not yet been anticoagulated combines transesophageal echocardiography and pre-transesophageal echocardiography heparin – a strategy that reduces the duration of hospitalization and may be cost-effective. Whether this approach is a good one is at the moment unknown, but the answer may be given by the ongoing ACUTE (Assessment of Cardioversion Using Transesophageal Echocardiography) study, the pilot of which showed that the transesophageal echocardiographic approach allows identification of patients who can safely undergo cardioversion without prior prolonged anticoagulation [18].

References

1. Kannel WB, Abbott RD, Savage DD, McNamara PM (1982) Epidemiologic features of chronic atrial fibrillation: the Framingham study. N Engl J Med 306:1018-1022
2. Lake FR, Cullen KJ, de Klerk NH, McCall MG, Rosman DL (1989) Atrial fibrillation and mortality in an elderly population. Aust N Z J Med 19:321-326
3. Wolf PA, Dawber TR, Thomas HE Jr, Kannel WB (1978) Epidemiologic assessment of chronic atrial fibrillation and risk of stroke: the Framingham study. Neurology 28:973-977
4. Petersen P, Madsen EB, Brun B, Pedersen F, Gyldensted C, Boysen G (1987) Silent cerebral infarction in chronic atrial fibrillation. Stroke 18:1098-1100
5. Brand FN, Abott RD, Kannel WB, Wolf PA (1985) Characteristics and prognosis of lone atrial fibrillation: 30 years follow-up in the Framingham study. JAMA 254:3449-3453
6. Kopecky SL, Gersh BJ, McGoon MD (1987) The natural history of lone atrial fibrillation. A population-based study over three decades. N Engl J Med 317:669-674
7. Gallagher MM, Camm J (1998) Classification of atrial fibrillation. Am J Cardiol 82:18N-28N
8. Lévy S, Novella P, Ricard P, Paganelli F (1995) Paroxysmal atrial fibrillation: a need for classification. J Cardiovasc Electrophysiol 6:69-74
9. The Planning and Steering Committees of the Affirm Study for the NHLBI Affirm Investigators (1997) Atrial fibrillation follow-up investigation of rhythm management: the AFFIRM study design. Am J Cardiol 79:1198-1202
10. Hohnloser SF, Kuck KH (1997) Atrial fibrillation: maintaining stability of sinus rhythm or ventricular rate control? The need for prospective data: The PIAF trial. Pacing Clin Electrophysiol 20:1989-1992

11. Sopher SM, Camm AJ (1998) New trials in atrial fibrillation. J Cardiovasc Electrophysiol 9:S211-S215

12. Lipkin DP, Frenneaux M, Stewart R, Joshi J, Lowe T, McKenna WJ (1988) Delayed improvement in exercise capacity after cardioversion of atrial fibrillation to sinus rhythm. Br Heart J 59:572-577

13. Jung W, Lüderitz B (1998) Quality of life in patients with atrial fibrillation. J Cardiovasc Electrophysiol 9:S177-S186

14. Levy S, Ricard P, Lau C, Lok N, Camm J, Murgatroyd FD, Jordaens LJ, Kappemberger LJ, Brugada P, Ripley KL (1997) Multicenter low energy transvenous atrial defibrillation (XAD) trial results in different subset of atrial fibrillation. J Am Coll Cardiol 29:750-755

15. Levy S, Ricard P, Gueunoun M, Yapo F, Trigano J, Mansouri C, Paganelli F (1997) Low-energy cardioversion of spontaneous atrial fibrillation. Immediate and long-term results. Circulation 96:253-259

16. Schmitt C, Alt E, Plewan A, Ammer R, Leibig M, Karch M, Schomig A (1996) Low energy intracardiac cardioversion after failed conventional external cardioversion of atrial fibrillation. J Am Coll Cardiol 28:994-999

17. Santini M, Pandozi C, Toscano S, Castro A, Altamura G, Jesi AP, Gentilucci G, Villani M, Scianaro MC (1998) Low energy intracardiac cardioversion of persistent atrial fibrillation. Pacing Clin Electrophysiol 21:2641-2650

18. Klein AL, Grimm RA (1997) Cardioversion guided by transesophageal echocardiography; the ACUTE pilot study: a randomized, controlled trial. Ann Intern Med 126:200-209

Acute Conversion of Recent-Onset Atrial Fibrillation and Flutter: Class IC or Class III Drugs?

R.F. Guaragna, C.H. Chen and D. Bracchetti

General Principles of Treatment of Recent-Onset Atrial Fibrillation and Flutter

How long atrial fibrillation should go on, in order to be considered of recent onset (less than 24 h? 7 days? more?), is a moot point that raises confusion when it comes to evaluating the efficacy of an antiarrhythmic regimen. In any case, the longer the arrhythmia continues, the less likely is its conversion into sinus rhythm, because of the electric remodeling of the atria (shortening of the refractory period) caused by the persistent fibrillation. Similarly, the risk of thromboembolic complications increases with the duration of the arrhythmia, so that any attempt at cardioversion beyond 48 h must be carried out after full anticoagulation therapy [1]. If recent-onset atrial fibrillation or flutter bring about hemodynamic instability, electrical cardioversion is recommended (success rate 75%-95%), otherwise sinus rhythm can be restored using antiarrhythmic drugs.

Atrial fibrillation is thought to be due to multiple (five or six) reentry circuits, simultaneously and randomly activated under the "leadership" of the smallest one in which a short excitable gap exists [2].

Atrial flutter, on the other hand, depends on the activation of a macro-reentry circuit, with a large excitable gap, in the right atrium, around anatomical obstacles represented by the superior vena cava, the inferior vena cava, and the coronary sinus. Therefore, the vulnerable parameter for both arrhythmias is the atrial refractory period, critical increase of which leads to blocking of the circulating wave. Indeed, when refractoriness reaches the value at which the "wave length" (refractory period x conduction velocity) becomes larger than the available tissue mass, reentry stops [3, 4].

Both class IC and class III antiarrhythmic drugs prolong the refractory period by different electrophysiologic mechanisms, the former delaying the recovery from inactivation of the Na^+ channels after repolarization, the latter blocking the

Unità Operativa di Cardiologia, Ospedale Maggiore, Bologna, Italy delayed rectifier K$^+$ current (I_{Kr}), thus prolonging the duration of the action potential. Owing to their action on the Na$^+$ channels, class IC drugs also decrease conduction velocity, while class III drugs have no effect on conduction [3, 5, 6].

Efficacy of Class IC Antiarrhythmic Agents in Recent-Onset Atrial Fibrillation and Flutter

Propafenone

Propafenone has been demonstrated to be effective in cardioverting recent-onset atrial fibrillation both when given intravenously (2 mg/kg in 10 min) and when administered in a single oral loading dose (600 mg). Success rates reported in the literature vary greatly, ranging from 50% to up 90% when the drug is given intravenously, and from 45% to up 80% when given orally [6-11]. This wide disparity depends upon two factors: the time of data collection and the definition of recent-onset atrial fibrillation, which is different in different studies. The later the evaluation of the drug efficacy with respect to the start of its administration, the higher the conversion rate. Propafenone is more effective when atrial fibrillation has gone on for less than 24-48 h. In one study [8], the drug, given intravenously, was successful within 1 h in 71% of the patients whose arrhythmia had lasted less than 48 h, and in only 26% of the patients with longer-lasting atrial fibrillation. Moreover, propafenone is more effective in patients with normal or mildly enlarged atrial dimensions. In one study [9], the mean left atrial dimension (determined echocardiographically) was significantly higher in nonresponders than in responders within 1 h of intravenous administration of the drug (47 mm vs 41 mm).

When given as a single oral loading dose, propafenone has been found superior to the digoxin-quinidine combination, until recently considered the treatment of choice for recent-onset atrial fibrillation. In one randomized, controlled study [10], at 6 h from the start of both treatments the rate of conversion into sinus rhythm was 62% in the propafenone group, compared to 38% in the digoxin-quinidine group, and 17% in the control group.

Very few data are available about the efficacy of propafenone in converting atrial flutter. In one study [7], the drug given intravenously was successful in 40% of patients within 1 h; in another study [8] the success rate was 33%.

Flecainide

Flecainide has also been found to be effective given either intravenously (2 mg/kg in 10 min) or as a single oral loading dose (300 mg). Rates of conversion to sinus rhythm range between 50% and 92% when the drug is given intravenously and between 50% and 90% when it is administered orally [12-17].

Like propafenone, flecainide is more effective in atrial fibrillation of short duration. In one study [13] sinus rhythm was restored (within 30 min of intravenous administration) in 50% of the patients in whom the arrhythmia continued for less than 24 h, compared to none of the patients with longer-lasting atrial fibrillation. Similarly, the success rate with a single oral loading dose (at 5 h) was 71% when the arrhythmia had gone on for less than 24 h and zero for longer-lasting atrial fibrillation.

Flecainide administered intravenously has been proved more effective than procainamide in cardioversion of atrial fibrillation that has lasted less than 24 h. In one controlled, randomized study [15] conversion to sinus rhythm was achieved within 1 h in 92 % of the patients treated with flecainide (1.5 mg/kg in 15 min followed by an infusion of 1.5 mg/kg over 1 h) and in 65% of those receiving procainamide (1 g infused over 30 min followed by an infusion of 2 mg/min over 1 h).

Very few data are available regarding the efficacy of flecainide in the treatment of atrial flutter. One study [7] reports a poor 13% of conversions within 1 h of intravenous administration of the drug.

When compared with each other, propafenone was less effective than flecainide (both given intravenously) in one study [17], where the rate of conversion to sinus rhythm within 1 h was 55% for the former and 86% for the latter. Moreover, the conversion rate in atrial fibrillation of no more than 24 h duration was 96% in the flecainide group and 57% in the propafenone group (in patients with arrhythmia lasting longer than 24 h, the success rate was 67% in the flecainide group and 50% in the propafenone group). It should be noticed that, in this study, a significant difference between responders and nonresponders was found in the plasma level of propafenone at the time of conversion. This means that propafenone might have been more effective if administered differently (i.e. faster infusion or higher doses) in order to obtain higher plasma levels. When given as a single oral loading dose propafenone and flecainide have shown similar efficacy. In a randomized, controlled study [12], flecainide and propafenone were successful in 59% and 51% of patients respectively at 3 h and in 78% and 72% respectively at 8 h, while the spontaneous conversion rate was 18% at 3 hours and 39% at 8 h in the control group.

As for atrial flutter, in the only two studies comparing the two drugs [7, 17], flecainide was found to be less effective than propafenone (13% versus 40% conversion rate within 1 h of intravenous administration).

Similar side effects have been described for propafenone and flecainide. The cardiovascular side effects include sinus standstill at the moment of cardioversion, QRS lengthening, bundle branch block, bradycardia, atrial flutter preceding sinus rhythm (generally with an A/V ratio of 2/1 or 3/1, seldom 1/1, leading to a fast ventricular rate), hypotension, and heart failure. Cardiovascular side effects are more likely to be observed in patients with underlying heart disease and poor left ventricular function and in patients with latent or manifest automatic and/or conductive disturbances. These side effects have been reported more frequently with flecainide than with propafenone (31% versus 8% incidence in one study) [17].

Efficacy of Class III Antiarrhythmic Agents in Recent-Onset Atrial Fibrillation and Flutter

Amiodarone

In uncontrolled studies of the 1980s, amiodarone was effective in converting recent-onset atrial fibrillation when given intravenously (5-7 mg/kg plus up to 1500 mg/24 h). Success rates ranged between 46% and 85%, depending on the study population with regard to the definition of recent-onset atrial fibrillation and on the time interval from the start of the infusion to data collection [18, 19].

However, more recent, controlled studies have questioned the real efficacy of the drug. In one study [20], of 50 patients whose arrhythmia had lasted for less than 7 days, the conversion rates at 2, 6, 12, and 24 h were 30%, 48%, 56%, and 68% respectively in the amiodarone group, compared to 24%, 46%, 50%, and 60% in the control group. Not even at 24 h was the difference between the two groups statistically significant (given the number of patients included in the study it would have had to be at least 25%).

In another controlled study [14] of 32 patients with atrial fibrillation lasting less than 72 h, the conversion rate at 2 h was 34% in the amiodarone group compared to 22% in the control group, and at 8 h the rates were 59% and 56%, respectively. No difference in drug plasma level was found between responders and nonresponders. In the same study, amiodarone was compared with intravenous flecainide: at 2 h the conversion rate was 34% in the amiodarone group and 59% in the flecainide group, while at 8 h it was 59% in the first group and 68% in the second.

In a third randomized, controlled study [16] comparing intravenous amiodarone with flecainide administered as a single oral loading dose, amiodarone turned out to be less effective than flecainide at 2 h and 8 h (16% and 37% conversion rates as compared to 68% and 91%), with no difference between the amiodarone group and the control group, in which conversion rates were 24% and 48% respectively. But at 24 h, sinusalization was 95% in the flecainide group and 89% in the amiodarone group. This suggests that either amiodarone had a delayed high efficacy, due to its slow action, or, as seems more probable, that late conversions to sinus rhythm were spontaneous. This is not surprising considering that acute administration of amiodarone does not substantially increase the duration of the action potential in the way that chronic oral administration does due to its active metabolite desethylamiodarone.

Dofetilide

Dofetilide does not seem as effective as class IC antiarrhythmic agents in patients with recent-onset atrial fibrillation. Two placebo-controlled studies [21, 22] reported success rates of 14% and 26% within 1 h of administration of two different doses of the drug (4 µg/kg or 8 µg/kg and 8 µg/kg or 12 µg/kg in 15 min). No conversion was seen in the control groups. On the other hand, in one uncontrolled study [23] the overall efficacy of dofetilide was 52% in response to three different regimens (2.5, 4, and 8 μg/kg in 15 min). However, the average duration of atrial fibrillation in this study was shorter than in those already quoted (32 days versus 62 and 65 respectively); moreover, in 7 out of 19 patients, atrial fibrillation had continued for less than 24 h (conversion rate 66%), and in 14 out of 19 no underlying heart disease was present.

Higher doses of the drug seem to bring little advantage. One study [21] reported conversion rates of 10.3% with a 4 μg/kg dose and 19% with an 8 μg/kg dose. Similarly, another study [22] reported 22% success using an 8 μg/kg and 33% using a 12 μg/kg dose.

Dofetilide is much more effective in the treatment of atrial flutter, with success rates ranging between 54% and 80%.

In one placebo-controlled study [21] comparing two different drug administration regimens, the conversion rate was higher when dofetilide was given in higher doses (62% with an 8 μg/kg dosage versus 33% with 4 μg/kg), while no conversion was seen in the control group. Similarly, in one uncontrolled study [24], sinus rhythm was restored in 50% of the patients given 2.5 μg/kg and in 100% of the patients given 4 μg/kg. It is noteworthy that sinus rhythm recovery was always sudden, not preceded by any cycle lengthening, in accordance with the electrophysiologic mechanism of class III agents, which increase the refractory period (as a consequence of the lengthening of the action potential) without affecting the conduction velocity.

In a comparison of flecainide and dofetilide, dofetilide was effective in converting atrial flutter in 70% of patients within 1 h of intravenous administration of 4 or 8 μg/kg in 15 min, while flecainide (2 mg/kg) produced only a 9% conversion rate, without a difference between responders and nonresponders in plasma drug levels at the end of the infusion [24]. Dofetilide causes Q-T interval prolongation, which only relates to the S-T interval, without an effect on the QRS duration, as is the case with class IC antiarrhythmic agents.

The most feared among the cardiovascular side effects of the drug is polymorphic sustained or unsustained ventricular tachycardia (torsade de pointes), whose incidence has been found to range between 3.2% and 13% [21], often associated with the highest doses and with the existence of facilitating factors including hypokalemia, impaired left ventricular function, and concomitant administration of other drugs affecting the Q-T interval (e.g., amitriptyline).

Ibutilide

Ibutilide is a new class III antiarrhythmic agent which, besides inhibiting the delayed rectifier K^+ current, increases a slow inward plateau Na^+ current. Like dofetilide, it has been found more effective in converting atrial flutter than atrial fibrillation. In a double-blind, randomized, placebo-controlled, dose-response trial [25] that enrolled 200 patients with atrial fibrillation and atrial flutter lasting from 3 h to 90 days, sinus rhythm was achieved (within 60 min of intravenous administration at three different dosages) in 29% of the patients with atrial fibrillation and in 38% of those with atrial flutter, while the conversion rate in the control group was only 3%. The drug efficacy was found to correlate with the injected dose and with the arrhythmia duration, the overall conversion rate being 42% when atrial fibrillation and flutter had gone on for less than 30 days, and 16% for longer-lasting arrhythmias.

In another controlled study [26] of 266 patients with atrial fibrillation and flutter lasting from 3 h to 45 days, sinus rhythm was recovered within 1 h of intravenous administration of the drug in 31% of the patients with atrial fibrillation and in 63% of those with atrial flutter, while the conversion rate was only 2% in the control group. It has also been shown that, should ibutilide be unsuccessful in converting atrial flutter, previous drug infusion increases the efficacy of subsequent atrial pacing (success rate 87% versus 18% in a control group pretreated with placebo) and reduces the risk of inducing atrial fibrillation [27]. A relation was found between drug efficacy and the duration of atrial fibrillation as well as the left atrial dimension. Such a correlation was not proved for atrial flutter.

The safety of ibutilide has been reported in 586 patients with atrial fibrillation and flutter [28, 29]. The overall incidence of polymorphic ventricular tachycardia diagnosed as torsade de pointes was 4.3%, including 1.7% of patients in whom the arrhythmia was sustained and required cardioversion. In almost all cases this occurred within 40 min of the start of the initial ibutilide infusion, without a clear relationship with the dose or plasma concentration of the drug.

Sotalol

On the whole sotalol is less effective than the other class III antiarrhythmic agents in treating both atrial fibrillation and flutter. In a randomized, controlled study [30] of 48 patients with atrial fibrillation lasting less than 7 days and treated with two different regimens of sotalol (1.0 and 1.5 mg/kg in 10 min i.v.), sinus rhythm was restored in 17% of the patients receiving the lower dose and in 18% of the patients receiving the higher dose (in total 35% versus 19% in the control group).

Sotalol is less effective than flecainide in converting atrial fibrillation. In one study [31] of 106 patients who were randomly given either sotalol or flecainide (1.5 mg/kg in 15 min), sinus rhythm was restored within 2 h in 23% of the patients given sotalol and in 52% of those treated with flecainide. The highest success rate with both drugs was observed in patients whose arrhythmia had continued for less than 24 h (31% in the sotalol group versus 69% in the flecainide group).

In a double-blind, randomized study [32] comparing sotalol (1.5 mg/kg in 10 min) with two different regimens of ibutilide (1 or 2 mg/kg in 10 min), sotalol turned out to be less effective than ibutilide, both in atrial fibrillation and flutter. For atrial fibrillation, the conversion rate within 1 h was 11% in the sotalol group versus 44% in the group receiving the higher dose and 20% in the group receiving the lower dose of ibutilide. With regard to atrial flutter, sinus rhythm was achieved in 19% of the patients receiving sotalol and in 70% and 59% of those treated with ibutilide at the higher and the lower dose respectively.

There were more proarrhythmic side effects in the ibutilide group than in the sotalol group, where torsade de pointes was not observed.

Role of Class IC and Class III Antiarrhythmic Drugs in Recent-Onset Atrial Fibrillation and Flutter

Some important conclusions can be drawn from the literature survey about the pharmacological cardioversion of recent-onset atrial fibrillation and flutter. Both class IC and class III antiarrhythmic agents are effective in converting atrial fibrillation and flutter, although the conversion rate varies greatly from one study to the other. These differences mainly depend on the time interval from administration of the drug to data collection, together with the duration of the arrhythmia in the study population. As to the first point, when data collection is delayed (12 h) the success rate in atrial fibrillation conversion increases, and so does the probability of spontaneous conversion, as shown by controlled studies. It is therefore inaccurate and misleading to assess the efficacy of a drug far from the time of its peak plasma level, particularly in the absence of a control group, because such an evaluation might include a high proportion of patients with spontaneous cardioversion. As to the second point, short-lasting atrial fibrillation is more likely to convert to sinus rhythm either spontaneously or under the effect of the drug. Hence, studies that enroll the greatest proportion of patients with atrial fibrillation that has lasted for less than 24 h show the greatest success rates.

Indeed, the main predictor of the efficacy of all antiarrhythmic agents is arrhythmia duration. For this reason, whatever the chosen drug, pharmacological cardioversion should be carried out within 24-48 h of the onset of arrhythmia, when also the thromboembolic risk is negligible.

On the whole, class IC drugs are more effective than class III agents in converting recent-onset atrial fibrillation. No substantial advantage stems from the use of flecainide rather than propafenone, both of which can be administered either intravenously or as a single oral loading dose. Owing to their negative inotropic effect and their depressing effect on conduction velocity, class IC drugs should be avoided in patients with poor left ventricular function (in whom they can cause heart failure) and those with patent or latent conduction disturbances (in whom they can precipitate severe bradycardia and proarrhythmia). Class III antiarrhythmic drugs are much more effective in converting atrial flutter. This is not surprising because, due to their selective effect on the refractory period without affecting conduction velocity, they most probably allow the "wave length" to reach the critical value at which the arrhythmia stops [24]. An appealing explanation might also be that because ibutilide and dofetilide, like most I_{Kr} blockers, exhibit the property of reverse use-dependency of action on repolarization, they are likely to be more effective in arrhythmias with slower atrial rates, such as atrial flutter, rather than atrial fibrillation. By contrast, the effects of class IC drugs on the atrial refractory period increase as the rate is increased [5]. In the treatment of atrial flutter, class III agents could even replace the more commonly used non-pharmacological techniques (electrical cardioversion, endoatrial or trans-esophageal pacing), with a cost advantage and less discomfort to the patient. Moreover, since they do not impair contractile function, they can safely be used in patients with depressed left ventricular function. Due to the risk of polymorphic ventricular tachycardia, to some extent linked to the dosage, they are not recommended in patients with significant lengthening of the Q-T interval (> 440 ms), particularly in situations where a membrane instability exists, such as electrolyte imbalance (hypokalemia) or recent administration of drugs affecting the Q-T interval duration (e.g., amitriptyline).

In controlled studies, intravenously administered amiodarone did not prove better than placebo in cardioverting atrial fibrillation or flutter. This is probably because its acute effect on lengthening the action potential is limited compared to its chronic effect, which is to some extent attributable to its active metabolite desethylamiodarone [6]. However, amiodarone is useful in the setting of recent-onset atrial fibrillation, particularly when an impairment of the left ventricular function is to be feared (i.e., acute myocardial infarction): the significant slowing of the ventricular rate may improve the hemodynamic pattern, perhaps facilitating recovery of the sinus rhythm.

Finally, the relatively high number of patients in whom recent onset atrial fibrillation spontaneously converts into sinus rhythm, as documented by controlled studies, should make us question the real necessity of always resorting to drugs, whose potential side effects can be severe and life-threatening.

References

1. Levy S, Breithardt G, Campbell RWF et al, on behalf of the working Group on Arrhythmias of the European Society of Cardiology (1998) Atrial fibrillation: current knowledge and recommendations for management. Eur Heart J 19:1294-1320
2. Lindsay BD, Smith JM (1996) Electrophysiologic aspects of human fibrillation. Cardiol Clinics 14:483-505
3. Janse MJ (1992) To prolong refractoriness or to delay conduction (or both)? Eur Heart J 13:14-18
4. Task force of the working group on arrhythmias of the European Society of Cardiology (1991) The Sicilian gambit. A new approach to the classification of antiarrhythmic drugs based on their actions on antiarrythmic mechanisms. Circulation 84:1831-1851
5. Singh BN (1997) Acute conversion of atrial fibrillation and flutter: direct current cardioversion versus intravenously administered pure class III Agents. J Am Clin Cardiol 29:391-393
6. Singh BN, Nademanee K (1985) Control of cardiac arrhythmias by selective lengthening of repolarization: theoretic considerations and clinical observations.Am Heart J 109:421-430
7. Suttorp MJ, Kingma JH, Jessurun ER et al (1990) The value of class IC antiarrhythmic

drugs for acute conversion of paroxysmal atrial fibrillation or flutter to sinus rhythm. J Am Clin Cardiol 16:1722-1727

8. Bianconi L, Boccadamo R, Pappalardo A et al (1989) Effectiveness of intravenous propafenone for cardioversion of atrial fibrillation of recent onset. Am J Cardiol 64:335-338

9. Bellandi F, Cantini F, Pedone T et al (1995) Effectiveness of intravenous propafenone for conversion of recent onset atrial fibrillation: a placebo-controlled study. Clin Cardiol 18:631-634

10. Capucci A, Boriani G, Rubino I et al (1994) A controlled study on oral propafenone versus digoxin plus quinidine in converting recent onset atrial fibrillation to sinus rhythm. Int J Cardiol 43:305-313

11. Boriani G, Biffi M, Capucci A et al (1997) Oral propafenone to convert recent onset atrial fibrillation in patients with and without underlying heart disease. A randomised controlled trial. Ann Intern Med 126:621-625

12. Capucci A, Boriani G, Botto GL et al (1994) Conversion of recent onset atrial fibrillation by a single oral loading dose of propafenone and flecainide. Am J Cardiol 74:503-505

13. Crijns HJGM, Van Wijk LM, Van Gilst WM et al (1988) Acute conversion of atrial fibrillation to sinus rhythm: clinical efficacy of flecainide acetate. Comparaison of two regimens. Eur Heart J 9:634-638

14. Donovan KD, Power BM, Hockings BEF et al (1995) Intravenous flecainide versus amiodarone for recent onset atrial fibrillation. Am J Cardiol 75:693-697

15. Madrid AH, Moro C, Marin-Huerta E et al (1993) Comparaison of flecainide and procainamide on cardioversion of atrial fibrillation. Eur Heart J 14:1127-1131

16. Capucci A, Lenzi T, Boriani G et al (1992) Effectiveness of loading oral flecainide for converting recent onset atrial fibrillation to sinus rhythm in patients without organic heart disease or with only systemic hypertension. Am J Cardiol 70:69-72

17. Kingma JH, Suttorp MJ (1992) Acute pharmacologic conversion of atrial fibrillation and flutter: the role of flecainide, propafenone and verapamil. Am J Cardiol 70:56A-61A

18. Faniel R, Schoenfeld PH (1983) Efficacy of i.v. amiodarone in converting rapid atrial fibrillation and flutter to sinus rhythm in intensive care patients. Eur Heart J 4:180-185

19. Strasberg B, Arditti A, Sclarowsky S et al (1985) Efficacy of intravenous amiodarone in the management of paroxysmal or new atrial fibrillation with fast ventricular response. Int J Cardiol 7:47-55

20. Galve E, Rius T, Ballester R et al (1996) Intravenous amiodarone in treatment of recent onset atrial fibrillation: results of a randomised controlled study. J Am Coll Cardiol 27:1079-1082

21. Falk RH, Pollak A, Singh SN et al for the intravenous dofetilide investigators (1997) Intravenous dofetilide, a class III antiarrhythmic agent, for the termination of sustained atrial fibrillation or flutter. J Am Coll Cardiol 29:385-390

22. Sedgwick ML, Lip G, Rae AP et al (1995) Chemical cardioversion of atrial fibrillation with intravenous dofetilide. Intern J Cardiol 49:159-166

23. Suttorp JM, Polak PE, Van't Hof A et al (1992) Efficacy and safety of a new selective class III antiarrhythmic agent dofetilide in paroxysmal atrial fibrillation and atrial flutter. Am J Cardiol 69:417-419

24. Crijns HJGM, Van Gelder C, Kingma JH et al (1994) Atrial flutter can be terminated by a class III antiarrhythmic drug but not by a class I C drug. Eur Heart J 15:1403-1408

25. Ellenbogen KA, Stambler BS, Wood MA et al, for the ibutilide investigators (1996) Efficacy of intravenous ibutilide for rapid termination of atrial fibrillation and atrial flutter: a dose-response study. J Am Coll Cardiol 28:130-136
26. Stambler BS, Wood MA, Ellenbogen KA et al, for the ibutilide repeat dose study investigators (1996) Efficacy and safety of repeated intravenous doses of ibutilide for rapid conversion of atrial flutter or fibrillation. Circulation 94:1613-1621
27. Stambler BS, Wood MA, Ellenbogen KA et al (1996) Comparative efficacy of intravenous ibutilide versus procainamide for enhancing termination of atrial flutter by atrial overdrive pacing. Am J Cardiol 77:960-966
28. Murray KT (1998) Ibutilide. Circulation 97:493-497
29. Kowey PR, Vanderlungt JT, Luderer JR (1996) Safety and risk/benefit analysis of ibutilide to acute conversion of atrial fibrillation. Am J Cardiol 78:46-52
30. Sung RJ, Tan HL, Karagounis L et al, for the Sotalol Multicenter Study Group (1995) Intravenous sotalol for the termination of supraventricular tachycardia and atrial fibrillation/flutter: a multicenter randomised double blind placebo controlled study. Am Heart J 129:739-748
31. Reisenger J, Gatterer E, Kuen P et al (1977) Flecainide versus sotalol for immediate conversion of atrial fibrillation. J Am Coll Cardiol 29:471A
32. Vos MA, Golitsyn SR, Stangle K et al, for the Ibutilide/Sotalol Comparator Study Group (1998) Superiority of ibutilide (a new class III agent) over DL-sotalol in converting atrial flutter and atrial fibrillation. Heart 79:568-575

Antiarrhythmic Drug Therapy Before Electrical Cardioversion of Atrial Fibrillation: Is It Really Useful?

A. Capucci, F.F. Tarantino, G.Q. Villani, M.F. Piepoli, D. Aschieri and A. Rosi

Electrical cardioversion is actually the more effective way to convert persistent atrial fibrillation to sinus rhythm. The success rate of electric cardioversion is 75%-93% [1, 2]. The efficacy of the procedure mainly depends on atrial fibrillation duration and left atrial size. The success rate is about 90% in patients with atrial fibrillation duration of less than 1 year and 50% in patients with atrial fibrillation of 5 years duration [3]. Also patients with left atrial enlargement have less probability of returning to sinus rhythm or of maintaining sinus rhythm after successful cardioversion.

Pretreatment with an antiarrhythmic drug may be useful since the incidence of recurrent atrial fibrillation is greatest within the first few hours after cardioversion. The risk of recurrence is relatively high in the first minutes after cardioversion and in the first 24 h after cardioversion and is very high in the long term follow-up. Rossi and Lown [4] reported a 30% recurrence of atrial fibrillation 1 min after cardioversion. Van Gelder et al. [5] observed a 7% recurrence of atrial fibrillaton between 0.5 h and 24 h after sinus rhythm restoration. Antiarrhythmic drug pretreatment has been proposed to reduce early recurrence although few prospective studies have been performed.

Early Recurrence: Which Is the Substrate?

The main problem related to atrial fibrillaton treatment is the maintenance of sinus rhythm after cardioversion. After both pharmacological and electric cardioversion the prophylactic antiarrhythmic approach should be considered according to the presence or absence of factors predisposing the patient to recurrences. It is conventionally accepted that the main factors which may favour relapses are: the presence of heart disease, neurohormonal substrate, arrhythmia duration, left atrial size and patient age. Recently a retrospective study on 85 patients with atrial fibrillation analysed the functional and pharmacological vari-

Divisione di Cardiologia, Ospedale Civile, Piacenza, Italy

ables which could possibly influence the long-term outcome after a first electrical cardioversion [6]. Multivariate analysis, with persistence of sinus rhythm at 100 days as the end-point, confirmed the duration of atrial fibrillation episode and age > 75 years as prognostic factors while echocardiographic parameters and the presence of organic heart disease played no role. Treatment with sotalol also contributed to the maintenance of sinus rhythm.

Immediately after electrical cardioversion, the electrophysiological substrate of the atria may also favour early recurrence (atrial remodelling). An electrophysiological remodelling has been demonstrated by Wijffels et al. [7] in conscious goats in which repetitive induction of episodes of atrial fibrillation resulted in chronic atrial fibrillation after a few days. A marked shortening of the atrial refractory period was observed due to the prolonged duration of atrial fibrillation. In these conditions, the physiological normalization of atrial refractoriness after sinus rhythm restoration was lost and it was recovered only after a few days of stable sinus rhythm. If atrial refractoriness requires a few days to revert completely, this could explain the early recurrences seen after cardioversion.

With this hypothesis, some studies have tested the efficacy of antiarrhythmic treatment before cardioversion in preventing atrial fibrillation relapses, reducing atrial refractoriness, or preventing premature supraventricular beats.

Clinical Results

Tielman et al. [8] demonstrated that the use of intracellular calcium-lowering drugs during atrial fibrillation was the only significant variable related to the maintenance of sinus rhythm after cardioversion ($p = 0.03$). The authors conclusions suggest that pretreatment with calcium-antagonist may reduce atrial electrical remodelling during atrial fibrillation, thus reducing the incidence of early atrial fibrillation relapses.

Oral amiodarone is effective for long-term maintenance of sinus rhythm after electrical cardioversion. Crijns et al. [9] noted that only 31% of patients treated with flecainide remained in sinus rhythm after 2 years follow-up. Switching to amiodarone resulted in 63% response rate. However, amiodarone loading requires at least 3-4 weeks to reach therapeutic plasma levels and during the first weeks of treatment patients may be at risk of recurrences of paroxysmal atrial fibrillation.

Recently we randomized 92 patients with persistent atrial fibrillation and organic heart disease to pretreatment with amiodarone 400 mg or placebo [10]. In the amiodarone group, 25% of patients reversed to sinus rhythm before DC cardioversion. Amiodarone pretreatment increased DC cardioversion efficacy and no significant difference in energy requirement was observed. At 2 months follow-up, patients treated with amiodarone had a lower recurrence rate than the placebo group (32% vs 56%; $p < 0.01$). The high percentage of pharmacological conversion obtained pre-DC shock may be considered an interesting result. Although no embolic event was observed, at the time of sinus rhythm conversion patients had still not reached the recommended 3 weeks of anticoagulation treatment, with possible embolic complication.

In a recent work [11] amiodarone was given at 600 mg/day for 4 weeks before cardioversion in patients in whom previous conventional antiarrhythmic treatment had not been successful. After cardioversion, the daily maintenance dose was 204 ± 166 mg. During the loading period 16% of patients converted to sinus rhythm and after electrical cardioversion 90% of all patients had sinus rhythm restored. After 3-years follow-up, 53% of these patients were still in sinus rhythm.

Bianconi et al. [12] tested propafenone in a placebo-controlled study involving 100 patients and comparing two different strategies: pretreatment with oral propafenone or propafenone only after cardioversion. The pharmacological conversion before DC shock was obtained in 6% of the subjects. In the whole population propafenone did not exert any significant effect on the total energy required for cardioversion or on the success rate of the procedure. Indeed propafenone had differential effects requirements for successful cardioversion. It significantly decreased DC shock energy in those patients (22% of the propafenone pretreatment group) in whom atrial fibrillation was transformed into atrial flutter, whereas energy requirements were increased compared to control if atrial fibrillation pattern did not change. Arrhythmia recurrence was significantly reduced within 10 min after cardioversion (0% vs 17% in placebo group) and also within 24 h and 48 h. After cardioversion the incidence of supraventricular ectopic beats was higher in placebo patients, whereas sinus node dysfunction was more common in patients treated with propafenone.

Flecainide has been evaluated by Van Gelder et al. [13] in a randomized study where it was administered intravenously. Although no differences were found in the energy of the effective shocks, attempts with high-energy shocks were more often required in flecainide group than in the placebo-treated patients.

More recently some studies were performed on patients submitted to low-energy internal atrial cardioversion, a procedure that in some patients can even be done without sedation [14].

Although different protocols were adopted, these studies were aimed at evaluating the effects of different agents on the atrial defibrillation threshold; this kind of evaluation seems interesting even in the perspective of an internal atrial defibrillator. Preliminary data have shown a reduction in defibrillating energies with intravenous sotalol [15], pretreatment with amiodarone [16] and intravenous flecainide [17].

Conclusions

Immediately after electrical cardioversion there is a high rate of atrial fibrillation recurrence, due to a complex electrophysiological remodelling, which interacts with modulating factors, such as the autonomic nervous system.

The administration of class IC and class III antiarrhythmic drugs has a favourable effect in reducing early arrhythmia recurrences, which is counterbalanced by the possibility of post-cardioversion bradyarrhythmias and by variable effects on defibrillation energy requirements. In particular amiodarone seems to be the most effective drug in this new approach to electric cardioversion. In clinical practice an adequate period of anticoagulation before starting amiodarone therapy may be an interesting and useful approach to the treatment of permanent atrial fibrillation in patients with organic heart disease.

An alternative approach to oral pretreatment with antiarrhythmic drugs should be considered, that is administering the drug intravenously immediately after cardioversion, thus avoiding potential unfavourable effects on atrial defibrillation threshold and on post-cardioversion bradyarrhythmias. In this view controlled studies analysing the risk-benefit ratio of these different strategies are required.

References

1. Lown B (1967) Electrical reversion of arrhythmias. Br Heart J 29:469-489
2. Resnekow L, Mc Donald L (1971) Electroconversion of lone atrial fibrillation and flutter, including hemodynamic studies at rest and on exercise. Br Heart J 33:339-350
3. Resnekov L (1980) Direct current shock. In: Chung EK (ed) Cardiac emergency care. (2nd edn) Lea & Febiger, Philadelphia pp 189-214
4. Rossi M, Lown B (1967) The use of quinidine in cardioversion. Am J Cardiol 19:234-238
5. Van Gelder IC, Crijns HJ, Van Gilst WH R, Lie KI (1991) Prediction of uneventful cardioversion and maintenance of sinus rhythm from direct-current electrical cardioversion of chronic atrial fibrillation or flutter. Am J Cardiol 68:41-46
6. Daytschaever M, Haerynck F, Tavernier R, Jordaens L (1998) Factors influencing long-term persistence of sinus rhythm after first electrical cardioversion for atrial fibrillation. PACE 21:284-287
7. Wijffels MCEF, Kirchof CJHJ, Dorland R, Allessie MA (1995) Atrial fibrillation begets atrial fibrillation: a study in awake chronically instrumented goats. Circulation 92:1954-1968
8. Tielman RG, Van Gelder IC, Crijns HJ, Kam PJ de, Van de Berg MP, Haaksma J, Van der Woude HJ, Allessie MA (1998) Early recurrences of atrial fibrillation after electrical cardioversion: a result of fibrillation induced electrical remodeling of the atria? J Am Coll Cardiol 31:167-173
9. Crijns HJ, Van Gelder IC, Van Gilst WH, Hillege H, Gosselink AM, Lie KL (1991) Serial antiarrhythmic drug treatment to maintain sinus rhythm after electrical cardioversion for chronic atrial fibrillation or atrial flutter. Am J Cardiol 68:335-341
10. Capucci A, Aschieri D,Villani GQ, Passerini F, Groppi F, Rosi A, Arruzzoli S (1997) Oral amiodarone increases efficacy of DC cardioversion in patients with chronic atrial fibrillation and organic heart disease. J Am Coll Cardiol 29[2 Suppl A]:443A
11. Gosselink AT, Crijns HJ, Van Gelder IC, Hillige H, Wiesfeld AC, Lie KI (1992) Low dose amiodarone for maintenance of sinus rhythm after cardioversion of atrial fibrillation or flutter. JAMA 267:3332-3333
12. Bianconi L, Mennuni M, Lukic V, Castro A, Chieffi M, Santini M (1996) Effects of oral propafenone administration before electrical cardioversion of chronic atrial fibrillation: a placebo controlled study. J Am Coll Cardiol 28:700-706

13. Van Gelder IC, Crijns HJ, Van Gilst WH, De Lagen CD, Van Mijk LM, Lie KI (1989) Effects of flecainide on the atrial defibrillation threshold. Am J Cardiol 63:112-116
14. Boriani G, Biffi M, Capucci A, Bronzetti G, Sabbatani P, Frabetti L, Zannoli R, Branzi A, Magnani B (1996) Fibrillazione atriale: efficacia, sicurezza e tollerabilità della cardioversione elettrica endocavitaria a bassa energia. Cardiologia 41[Suppl 5]:47 (abstr)
15. Lok NS, Lau CP, Way TY, Wah HS (1995) Effect of sotalol on transvenous atrial defibrillation for acute and chronic atrial fibrillation. J Am Coll Cardiol 25:109 A (abstr)
16. Santini M, Pandozi C, Toscano S, Castro A, Altamura G, Jesi AP, Gentilucci G, Villani M (1996) Intracardiac cardioversion of chronic atrial fibrillation. Cardiostimolazione 14:167 (abstr)
17. Boriani G, Biffi M, Capucci A, Sabbatani P, Bronzetti G, Frabetti L, Ayers GM, Magnani B (1997) Favourable effects of flecainide in transvenous low energy internal atrial cardioversion. PACE 20:1440 (abstr)

Low-Energy Internal Defibrillation: How Many Patients Are Still in Sinus Rhythm After 1 Year?

G. Gasparini, A. Bonso, S. Themistoclakis, F. Giada, A. Corrado and A. Raviele

Low-energy internal atrial defibrillation has recently been introduced into clinical practice as an effective and safe method of restoring sinus rhythm in patients with atrial fibrillation [1-5]. The technique has proved to be particularly useful in patients with long-standing atrial fibrillation or a very enlarged left atrium [1, 2, 6]. However, these patients are considered to be at very high risk of early recurrence of atrial fibrillation. Thus, it seems justified to ask the question: how many patients maintain sinus rhythm after successful internal atrial defibrillation, and for how long?

Factors Influencing the Persistence of Sinus Rhythm After Cardioversion

The probability of maintaining sinus rhythm after cardioversion, regardless of the method used (pharmacological or electrical), seems to depend on several variables [7].

The duration of the last atrial fibrillation episode was found by Duytschaever et al. [8] to be the only significant predictor of maintenance of sinus rhythm 100 days after cardioversion. Alt et al. [2] reported that patients with an atrial fibrillation duration > 2 months had a significantly higher risk of relapsing into atrial fibrillation after internal defibrillation than those with an atrial fibrillation duration < 2 months. It is possible that the long duration of atrial fibrillation favors the persistence of atrial fibrillation as a consequence of the electrophysiological changes induced by the arrhythmia itself in atrial cells, consisting of reduction and dispersion of refractoriness (so-called electrical remodeling of the atrium) [9]. On multivariate analysis, Crijns et al. [10] found left atrial size to be the only significant variable that predicted long-term maintenance of sinus rhythm. Moreover, Omran et al. [11] identified the peak emptying velocity of the left atrial appendage before cardioversion as a predictor of recurrence of atrial fibrillation. Finally, a fundamental role in the prevention of

Reparto di Cardiologia, Ospedale Umberto I, Mestre, Venice, Italy

atrial fibrillation recurrences is played by antiarrhythmic drugs [7]. Without drugs, atrial fibrillation relapses are common (44%-85% at 1 year) after cardioversion. With antiarrhythmic therapy, annual recurrence rates decrease to 17%-89% but still remain significant. Moreover, not rarely antiarrhythmic drugs had to be discontinued because of side effects [8, 12]. Although the presence of a severe heart disease, a long duration of atrial fibrillation and large left atrium size are associated with a lower probability of maintenance of sinus rhythm during follow-up, it is in these conditions that restoration and maintenance of sinus rhythm may yield the best results in terms of hemodynamic improvement and reduction in morbidity and mortality.

Literature Data on Clinical Outcome in Patients Treated with Low-energy Internal Defibrillation

Initial literature data on the use of low-energy internal defibrillation in patients with chronic atrial fibrillation are very interesting [1-5]. First of all, internal defibrillation has shown significantly greater efficacy than external cardioversion (93% vs 79%; $p < 0.01$) [2]. A high efficacy rate of low-energy internal defibrillation in restoring sinus rhythm has been reported: from 70% to 100% in different papers, including patients with long-standing atrial fibrillation and/or patients refractory to pharmacological or external electrical cardioversion [1-6]. The clinical outcome of patients after sinus rhythm restoration has been reported in a few studies: generally, all patients were treated with antiarrhythmic drugs, predominantly with sotalol or amiodarone. During a follow-up period ranging from 5.4 ± 1.9 months to 15 ± 12 months persistence of sinus rhythm was found in 38%-63% of patients [1, 2, 4, 12]. Alt and coworkers [2] compared on an intention-to-treat basis the long-term clinical outcome of patients treated with internal or external cardioversion. In just over 1 year mean follow-up, they found a significantly higher percentage of patients in sinus rhythm when treated with internal cardioversion (48% vs 38%, $p < 0.05$) as compared with those treated with external cardioversion. However, this difference was only apparent. In fact, almost all patients were successfully cardioverted with both methods; the probability of a patient being in sinus rhythm after 1 year when treated with internal cardioversion was the same as when treated with external cardioversion (53% vs 51%); the difference lay in the higher number of patients cardioverted with the first method. It must again be underlined that a large number of patients refractory to external cardioversion might be cardioverted with internal defibrillation [1, 2] and that 1 year sinus rhythm maintenance might be too long.

Personal Experience

In our Institution, since February 1997 we have performed low-energy internal atrial defibrillation in 48 consecutive patients with persistent atrial fibrillation

($\geq$ 1 month) who were refractory to at least 2 attempts at anterior-posterior external electrical cardioversion (200 J and 300 J) and who, before the introduction of low-energy internal defibrillation, would have been considered for permanent atrial fibrillation, according to the Gallagher classification [13]. Twenty-eight patients were male and the mean age was 65 ± 10 years (range 40-85). An organic heart disease was present in 43 cases: hypertensive in 23, valvular in 12, ischemic in 6, dilated in 2; 5 patients had atrial fibrillation alone. The mean duration of the last episode of atrial fibrillation was 8.2 ± 9.8 months (range 1-43). Before internal defibrillation, 2.8 ± 1.8 pharmacological and/or external electrical cardioversions per patient were carried out (range 2-14). All patients were treated with warfarin and the mean value of INR at the procedure was 3.2 ± 1.2. Before internal defibrillation, 39 out of 48 patients were on antiarrhythmic drugs (amiodarone in 35, sotalol in 3, propafenone in 1). Through the femoral and jugular veins, we positioned two custom-made catheters, one in the right atrium (lateral wall) and one in the coronary sinus (13 patients) or, more often, in the left pulmonary artery (35 patients); an additional standard tetrapolar catheter was placed in the right ventricular apex to provide R wave synchronization and back-up pacing. We used an external defibrillator capable of delivering biphasic truncated shock (6+6 ms in duration) from 10 V to 400 V with a minimum pre-shock RR interval of 500 ms. In all patients, we used slow intravenous infusion of midazolam during the procedure to improve patient shock tolerance. Shocks were delivered between 250 V and 400 V in 50-V steps until the sinus rhythm or the capacitor's maximum leading-edge voltage was reached.

The results were as follows. Sinus rhythm was restored in 47 patients (98%). The mean value of defibrillating energy was 6.8 ± 2.6 J (318 ± 60 Volts). A total of 133 shocks were delivered (2.8 ± 1.6 per patient). No complications were observed during or after internal defibrillation.

The follow-up duration of the whole population was 13.2 ± 7.2 months (range 1-25). During this period 14 patients (30%) had an early atrial fibrillation recurrence ($\leq$ 1 week); 17 patients (36%) had a late atrial fibrillation recurrence (> 1 week; mean 1.6 ± 2 months, range 0.3-9) (Fig. 1). Sixteen patients (34%) maintained sinus rhythm (the mean follow-up of these 16 patients was 11.1 ± 6.2 months, range 3-22). There were no differences between patients maintaining sinus rhythm and those with atrial fibrillation recurrences in terms of clinical characteristics or arrhythmia features (p = NS) (Table 1).

Conclusions

In conclusion, low-energy internal defibrillation is a useful tool in patients with persistent atrial fibrillation; in particular, its therapeutic power is higher in patients with atrial fibrillation that is long-standing and/or refractory to external cardioversion.

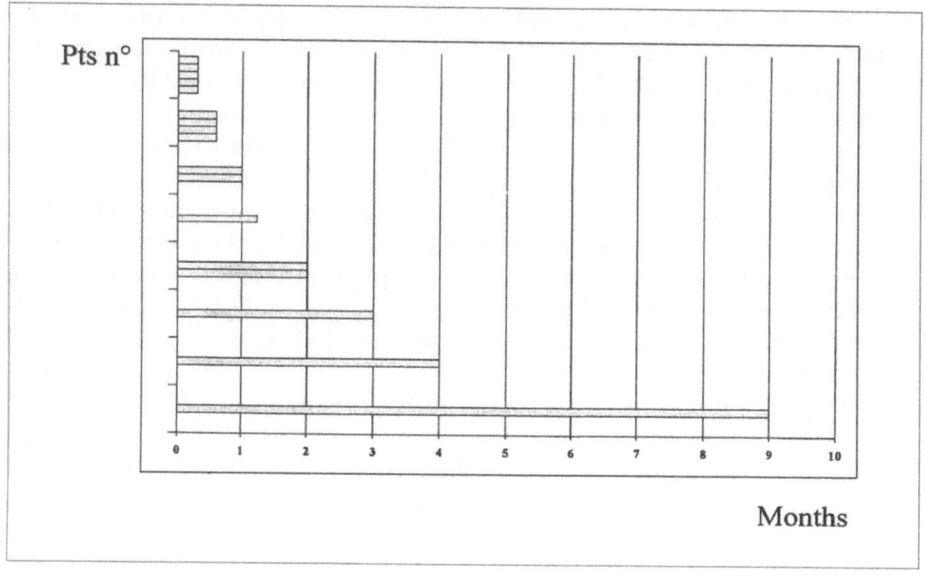

Pts n°

Months

Fig. 1. Late atrial fibrillation recurrences (17 pts: mean 1.6 ± 2 months, range 0.3-9)

Table 1. Clinical characteristics and arrhythmia features in pts with atrial fibrillation (AF) relapse and with maintenance of sinus rhythm

	Pts with AF relapse	Pts in sinus rhythm	p value
Pts number	31	16	
• Sex (male/female)	19/12	8/8	NS
• Age (mean ± SD)	64.7 ± 9.5	65. ± 10.8	NS
• Organic heart disease	29	14	NS
– Hypertensive	16	7	
– Valvular	8	4	
– Ischemic	4	2	
– Dilated	0	1	
• No organic hearth disease	3	2	NS
• LA diameter (mm; mean ± SD)	51 ± 6	50 ± 8	NS
• LVEF (%; mean ± SD)	61 ± 9	54 ± 12	NS
• AF history (years; mean ± SD)	3.7 ± 5.6	4.3 ± 5.1	NS
• Last episode duration (months; mean ± SD)	7.0 ± 8.1	10.6 ± 12.3	NS
• n° previous cardioversion (mean ± SD per pt)	2.9 ± 2.2	2.6 ± 0.6	NS
• n° previous AA drugs used (mean ± SD per pt)	1.3 ± 1.0	1.25 ± 0.7	NS
• Pts on AA drugs at TAD (n°)	25	13	NS

AA, antiarrhythmic; LA, left atrium; LVEF, left ventriculas ejection fraction; NS, not significant

From one-third to a half of patients treated with internal cardioversion maintain sinus rhythm during long-term follow-up (≥ 1 year). It is now thought that no variable can predict maintenance of sinus rhythm after cardioversion. Our data show a longer history of atrial fibrillation, a longer duration of the last episode of atrial fibrillation, and a lower left ventricular ejection fraction (though not statistically significant) in patients whose sinus rhythm is maintained during follow-up as compared with atrial fibrillation relapse patients. In deciding whether to perform internal electrical cardioversion, clinical evaluation of the single case may be more important than consideration of clinical, echocardiographical or pharmacological variables.

In our opinion, moreover, the group of patients with late atrial fibrillation recurrence after low-energy internal defibrillation is very interesting. Indeed, some of these patients could be treated with an implantable atrial defibrillator to resolve their arrhythmia relapses.

References

1. Schmitt C, Alt E, Plewan A et al (1996) Low energy intracardiac cardioversion after failed conventional external cardioversion of atrial fibrillation. J Am Coll Cardiol 28:994-999
2. Alt E, Ammer R, Schmitt C et al (1997) A comparison of treatment of atrial fibrillation with low-energy intracardiac cardioversion and conventional external cardioversion. Eur Heart J 18:1796-1804
3. Levy S, Ricard P, Lau CP et al (1997) Multicenter low energy transvenous atrial defibrillation (XAD) trial results in different subsets of atrial fibrillation. J Am Coll Cardiol 29:750-755
4. Santini M, Pandozi C, Toscano S et al (1998) Low energy intracardiac cardioversion of persistent atrial fibrillation. PACE 21:2641-2650
5. Boriani G, Biffi M, Bronzetti G et al (1998) Efficacy and tolerability in fully conscious patients of transvenous low-energy internal atrial cardioversion for atrial fibrillation. Am J Cardiol 81:241-244
6. Gasparini G, Bonso A, Rigo F, Raviele A (1997) Acute endocavitary atrial cardioversion: what indications and limitations. In: Raviele A (ed) Cardiac arrhythmias 1997. Springer (Satellite Symposia), Milano, pp 15-18
7. Levy S, Breithardt G, Campbell RWF et al (1998) Atrial fibrillation: current knowledge and recommendations for management. Eur Heart J 19:1294-1320
8. Duytschaever M, Haerynck F, Tavernier R, Jordaens L (1998) Factors influencing long-term persistence of sinus rhythm after a first electrical cardioversion for atrial fibrillation. PACE 21:284-287
9. Wijffels MCEF, Kirchhof CJHJ, Dorland R, Allessie MA (1995) Atrial fibrillation begets atrial fibrillation. A study in awake chronically instrumented goats. Circulation 92:1954-1968
10. Crijns HJGM, Van Gelder IC, Tieleman RG et al (1997) Long-term outcome of electrical cardioversion in patients with chronic atrial flutter. Heart 77:56-61
11. Omran H, Jung W, Schimpf R, et al (1997) Echocardiographic parameters for predicting maintenance of sinus rhythm after internal atrial defibrillation. Am J Cardiol 81:1446-1449

12. Lévy S, Ricard P, Gueunoun M et al (1997) Low-energy cardioversion of spontaneous atrial fibrillation. Immediate and long-term results. Circulation 96:253-259
13. Gallagher MM, Camm AJ (1997) Classification of atrial fibrillation.PACE 20:1603-1605

How Useful Is Transoesophageal Echocardiography During Electrical Cardioversion for Predicting Long-Term Sinus Rhythm Maintenance?

B. De Piccoli

Introduction

Both pharmacological and electrical cardioversion are widely used in the management of subjects affected by atrial fibrillation (AF). The tachyarrhythmia recurrence rate after restoration of sinus rhythm (SR) is near 40% [1], and about 57% of cases occur during the first 30 days [2]. This cardiac arrhythmia has a deep impact on patient's haemodynamics and risk of embolic events, so tailored antiarrhythmic and anticoagulant therapy is commonly employed [3] even though it is not free of complications. Many authors have tried to identify predictors of AF reversibility and SR maintenance. Formerly clinical features of the patients affected were focused on [4]. Later, after the introduction of transthoracic echocardiography (TTE), a correlation was established between left atrial (LA) size and AF recurrence [5]. TEE has allowed investigation of the anatomical and functional aspects of the left atrial appendage (LAA) during AF, and it was documented that auricular Doppler flow patterns constitute a predictor of embolic events [6], successful cardioversion [7] and maintenance of SR [8].

Studies performed using TTE have demonstrated that the restoration of mechanical function of LA after cardioversion takes place at a variable time interval after direct shock [9]. Furthermore, a low speed of growth of atrial contractility has proved to be a predictive index for AF recurrence [10]. Later TEE studies [11, 12] concerning LAA function after direct current shock demonstrated auricular stunning following cardioversion which can be fully independent of LA mechanics [11] and constitutes a risk factor for embolic events.

Reports about simultaneous TEE and direct current shock are scarce [11-13] and not addressed to predicting AF recurrence. We may suppose that LAA Doppler flow gives information about arrhythmia relapse after cardioversion as correctly as it does before the procedure. Furthermore, we belive that the use of TEE must be curtailed in these patients because it is a time-consuming and near-invasive tool that cannot be employed for close examinations. After induction of

Unità Operativa di Cardiologia, Ospedale Umberto I, Mestre, Venice, Italy anaesthesia we are able to perform TEE just before and soon after cardioversion without further discomfort for the patient. Thus we adopted this method and a simultaneous TTE investigation in order to obtain indexes of LA, left ventricular (LV) and LAA function as well as of pulmonary venous flow that could correlate better with the persistence of SR 30 days after its restoration.

Patients and Methods

Study Population

Eighteen patients with nonrheumatic AF of a duration ranging from 4 weeks to 6 months were selected to undergo direct current shock and simultaneous TEE examination. Ten were female and eight male; mean age was 56 ± 15 years. Underlying cardiac disease was hypertension in nine patients, ischaemic heart disease in five and lone atrial fibrillation in four. Each subject had received anti-coagulant treatment during the previous 3 weeks in order to achieve an International Normalized Ratio (INR) ≥ 3.

Study Method

Patients had been fasting for at least 12 h prior to the procedure. Sedation was achieved in all cases by propofol 2.5 mg/kg; after its induction an echocardio-graphic transoesophageal single or multiplane probe was inserted into the oesophagus of the subject under the guidance of a laryngoscope. The probe was equipped with a 5-Mhz transducer (HP Sonos 1500) and was left in situ during the direct electrical shock. Imaging was performed both immediately before and soon after (less than 5 min) the shock. LAA was viewed on the basal short axis section or on the longitudinal section; the base of the structure was drawn from the top of the limbus between the left superior pulmonary vein and the nearest point of the aortic wall on the short section or the atrial wall on the longitudinal section. During diastole the widest and the narrowest areas of the cavity area were measured manually using an off-line video analysis system. Spontaneous echo contrast (SEC) was scored according to Fatkin's method [12]. Pulsed Doppler technique was used to measure peak flow velocities at the outlet of both the LAA and the superior pulmonary vein.

Nearly simultaneously to TEE we performed TTE on the same patient utilis-ing a four-chamber apical view in order to outline the LA and LV cavities as well as to measure the transmitral flow by pulsed Doppler technique.

Calculations

Just before administration of the direct current shock, the following parameters were calculated:
By TTE:
1. LV ejection fraction (EF: %)
2. LA area (cm^2)

By TEE:

1. LAA fractional area change (FAC: %)
2. SEC score (+/++++)
3. LAA pulsed Doppler flow (Fig. 1):
    (a) Sum of peak velocities (cm/s) of the outflow (+) and inflow (-) of the maximal fibrillatory wave
    (b) Sum of the duration (ms) of the outflow (+) and inflow (-) of the maximal fibrillatory wave
    (c) Sum of peak velocities (cm/s) of the outflow (+) and inflow (-) of the minimal fibrillatory wave
    (d) Sum of the duration (ms) of the outflow (+) and inflow (-) of the minimal fibrillatory wave
4. Pulmonary vein pulsed Doppler flow (PVF):
    (a) Peak velocity (cm/s) of systolic flow (S)
    (b) Velocity-time integral (cm) of systolic flow (S VTI)
    (c) Peak velocity (cm/s) of diastolic flow (D)
    (d) Velocity-time integral (cm) of diastolic flow (D VTI)
    (e) S peak veocity/D peak velocity
    (f) S VTI/D VTI

Soon after administration of shock the following parameters were calculated:

By TTE:

1. LV EF (%)
2. Transmitral pulsed Doppler flow:
    (a) Peak A-wave velocity (cm/s)
    (b) VTI (cm) of A wave (A VTI)
    (c) Duration (ms) of A-wave
    (d) Ratio between A VTI and VTI of global mitral flow (A VTI/total VTI)

By TEE:

1. LAA FAC (%)
2. SEC score (+/++++)
3. LAA pulsed Doppler flow (Fig. 2)

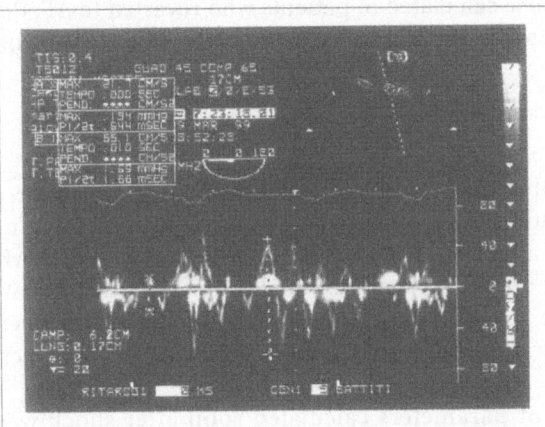

Fig. 1. Pulsed Doppler left atrial appendage flow during AF. Peak velocities of fibrillatory waves were calculated by a line drawn from the top of outflow to the bottom of inflow

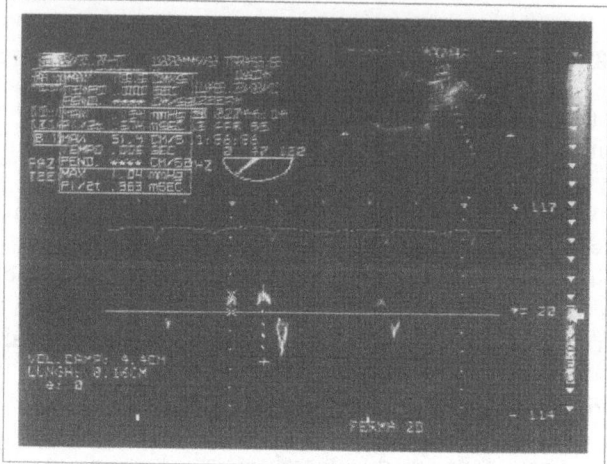

Fig. 2. Pulsed Doppler left atrial appendage flow after SR restoration. Peak velocities of early diastolic (E+E$_1$) and end-diastolic (A+A$_1$) waves were calculated as in Fig. 1. Early diastolic wave in this instance is given only by the outflow component

(a) Sum of peak velocities (cm/s) of end-diastolic contraction (A) and relaxation (A$_1$)

(b) Duration (ms) of A+A$_1$

(c) Sum of peak velocities (cm/s) of early diastolic outflow (E) and inflow (E$_1$)

(d) Duration (ms) of E+E$_1$

4. PVF: the same parameters as were evaluated during AF. We did not analyse the atrial reversal flow because it was well documented in only a few cases (16%) and exhibited a very low velocity.

Follow-Up and Statistical Analysis

Each subject was treated with propafenone 450 mg/day. None took digoxin and only two were treated with β-blockers.

Thirty days after cardioversion, ten patients maintained SR while eight had reverted to AF. The echocardiographic parameters calculated in patients with SR persistence were compared to those calculated in patients who reverted to AF; the Student's unpaired *t* test was adopted. A *p* value < 0.05 was considered significant.

Results

Table 1 summarises the mean values and standard deviation of single parameters calculated before the administration of direct current shock. Subjects who maintained SR showed a smaller LA area ($p = 0.034$) than those who reverted to AF. Peak velocities of maximal (Max.: $p = 0.011$) and minimal (Min.: $p = 0.012$) fibrillatory waves were greater in the former than in the latter group. No other index derived from TTE or TEE exploration exhibited a significant difference between the two groups.

Table 2 contains the values of parameters calculated soon after shock was

Table 1. TTE and TEE results before direct shock treatment

	SR group (n = 10)	AF group (n = 8)	p
Transthoracic echocardiography			
1. LV EF (%)	48.13 ± 7	49.2 ± 3,7	0.760
2. LA Area (cm²)	20.8 ± 4.5	26.4 ± 5.7	**0.034**
Transoesophageal echocardiografy			
1. LAA FAC (%)	22.87 ± 8.36	24.8 ± 15.6	0.775
2. SEC score (+/++++)	0.9 ± 0.7	1.2 ± 0.7	0.32
3. LAA flow			
(a) Peak velocity (cm/s), + and -, of max. wave	87.50 ± 25.56	59.25 ± 11.73	**0.011**
(b) Duration (ms), + and -, of max. wave	168.7 ± 41.3	160 ± 61.9	0.942
(c) Peak velocity (cm/s), + and -, of min. wave	28.7 ± 3.06	23 ± 4.9	**0.012**
(d) Duration (ms), + and -, of min. wave	97.6 ± 27.73	82.5 ± 24.66	0.408
4. PVF			
(a) S peak velocity (cm/s)	40.6 ± 22	24.6 ± 22.81	0.174
(b) S VTI (cm)	7 ± 2.62	4.8 ± 22.81	0.174
(c) D peak velocity (cm/s)	48.87 ± 16.46	43 ± 13.02	0.514
(d) D VTI (cm)	10.5 ± 4	8.2 ± 4.38	0.351
(e) S peak velocity/D peak velocity	0.8 ± 0.4	0.58 ± 0.4	0.431
(f) S VTI/ D VTI	0.68 ± 0.32	0.6 ± 0.38	0.77

See Calculations section for explanations. Significant difference if $p < 0.05$ (in bold face)

Table 2. TTE and TEE results after direct shock treatment

	SR group (n = 10)	AF group (n = 8)	p
Transthoracic echocardiography			
1. LV EF (%)	50.17 ± 6.34	45.06 ± 6,4	0.287
2. Mitral flow			
(a) A peak velocity (cm/s)	30.10 ± 5.24	20.87 ± 7.43	**0.007**
(b) A VTI (cm)	2.80 ± 0.94	1.97 ± 0.41	**0.035**
(c) A Duration (ms)	131.50 ± 33.75	138.75 ± 24.46	0.613
(d) A VTI/ total VTI	0.19 ± 0.05	0.18 ± 0.5	0.7
Transoesophageal echocardiografy			
1. LAA FAC (%)	14 ± 5.87	16.88 ± 7.97	0.391
2. SEC score (+/++++)	2 ± 0.82	2.38 ± 0.52	0.276
3. LAA flow			
(a) A + A₁ peak velocity (cm/s)	57.2 ± 8.8	31.25 ± 9.27	**0.002**
(b) A + A₁ duration (ms)	161.3 ± 28.63	137.6 ± 7.61	**0.03**
(c) E + E₁ peak velocity (cm/s)	23.60 ± 5.87	17 ± 6.21	**0.035**
(d) E + E₁ duration (ms)	93.40 ± 38.59	45 ± 32.29	**0.008**
4. PVF			
(a) S peak velocity (cm/s)	35.3 ± 19	22.1 ± 12	0.25
(b) S VTI (cm)	5.51 ± 3	5.95 ± 3.56	0.78
(c) D peak velocity (cm/s)	40.18 ± 16.46	36 ± 16.02	0.481
(d) D VTI (cm)	11.2 ± 3.1	9.3 ± 3.6	0.331
(e) S peak velocity/D peak velocity	0.87 ± 0.13	0.61 ± 0.4	0.511
(f) S VTI/ D VTI	0.53 ± 0.32	0.65 ± 0.48	0.35

See Calculations section for explanations. Significant difference if $p < 0.05$ (in bold face)

administrated. TTE-derived mitral flow values documented a higher peak velocity ($p = 0.007$) and a larger VTI ($p = 0.035$) of the end-diastolic A-wave in SR patients than in AF ones. Four indexes relating to LAA flow were greater in SR than in AF patients: end-diastolic peak velocities of contraction and relaxation flow (A+A_1: $p = 0.002$), duration of A+A_1 ($p = 0.03$), early diastolic outflow and inflow peak velocities (E+E_1: $p = 0.035$) and duration ($p = 0.008$). The remaining parameters calculated were not statistically different between the two groups.

Discussion

Reversal to AF after cardioversion increases the risk of embolic events; for this reason, identifying indexes predictive of recurrence of the arrhythmia is a challenge that must be met in order to achieve appropriate pharmacological prophylaxis.

Our study, in agreement with previous publications on this subject [5, 14, 15], has established that a larger LA cavity area can constitute a predictor of AF relapse after restoration of SR. Apart from this anatomical aspect, some parameters relating to LA function have proved to correctly predict future arrhythmias: mitral flow A-wave peak velocity and velocity-time integral, which may be considered indexes of the contraction and loading properties of the structure, were smaller in patients who reverted to AF. Thus, in agreement with other reports [10, 15], we can conclude that smaller LA size and quicker restoration of its mechanical function identify subjects with better probabilities of maintaining SR.

Our results relating to LAA Doppler flow during AF also parallel the conclusions of other authors [8, 15]. In the present study we analysed LAA Doppler flow soon after direct current shock by leaving a transoesophageal probe in situ during the electrical shock. Similar investigations have rarely been reported [11-13], and they have not been addressed to predict arrhythmia recurrence. Our study documented that peak velocity as well as duration of both early diastolic (E+E_1) and end-diastolic (A+A_1) auricular outflow and inflow were greater in patients with persistence of SR as a probable consequence of a better auricular contractility and compliance after cardioversion in this group. Thus the present paper emphasises that early restoration of the mechanical properties of both LA and LAA constitutes a good prognostic index for maintenance of SR during the follow-up.

PVF proved not to be involved in this correlation although the pulmonary veins are anatomically related to the LA. Many opposing determinants, such as right ventricular systolic pressure pulse, LA relaxation, pressure and maximal area as well as LV systolic function, are related to LA inflow [16] and consequently to LAA function. Peculiar haemodynamic conditions determined by AF or atrial stunning after cardioversion could functionally disconnect the pulmonary veins from the LA-LAA system and perhaps explain the lack of correlation we found between pulmonary venous flow indexes and FA recurrence.

Hypothetical Influence on Anticoagulation

The parameters we have found to predict AF recurrence are close to those involved in the risk stratification of embolic events related to cardioversion [6, 17]; hence, if we are able to identify these indexes during AF and above all soon after administration of direct current shock, when auricular and atrial stunning are heavy, we could adopt a shorter period of anticoagulation treatment.

Present recommendations about oral anticoagulant treatment provide for its use for 3 weeks before and 4 weeks after cardioversion [18]; the treatment carries the risk of possible haemorrhagic complications and is often problematic in its management.

After the introduction of TEE examination in patients about to undergo direct current shock, a brief period of anticoagulant therapy has been proposed before the cardioversion [19]. Our results could underpin a rational argument for recommending shorter anticoagulation after restoration of SR as well.

Conclusions

In the present study, performed in subjects affected by AF and about to undergo electrical cardioversion, we adopted a single TEE investigation simultaneously with TTE in order to obtain information about cardiac structure and function. We demonstrated that LA size was greater in patients who reverted to AF than in those who still maintained SR 30 days after the procedure; furthermore, in this latter group peak velocities of maximal and minimal LAA fibrillatory waves were higher before shock therapy.

We also demonstrated that soon after cardioversion some indexes of both LA mechanical function, such as mitral flow A-wave peak velocity and velocity-time integral, and indexes of LAA contractility and compliance, such as peak velocity and duration of early diastolic $E+E_1$ waves and end-diastolic $A+A_1$ waves, were greater in subjects who maintained SR.

Thus, by a single echocardiographic evaluation during direct current shock treatment, we were able to identify some useful parameters to predict electrical activity of the heart in the immediate follow-up period in patients subjected to direct current cardioversion. These results could have beneficial consequences for antiarrhythmia and, above all, anticoagulation therapy after restoration of SR.

References

1. The National Heart, Lung and Blood Institute Working Group on Atrial Fibrillation (1993) Atrial fibrillation: current understandings and research imperatives. J Am Coll Cardiol 22:1830-1834
2. Tieleman RG, Van Gelder IC, Crijns HJG et al (1998) Early recurrence of atrial fibrillation after electrical cardioversion: a result of fibrillation-induced electrical remodelling of the atria? J Am Coll Cardiol 31:167-173

3. Cairns JA, Connolly SJ (1991) Nonrheumatic atrial fibrillation. Risk of stroke and role of antithrombotic therapy. Circulation 84:469-481

4. Hall JI, Wood DR (1968) Factors affecting cardioversion of atrial arrhythmias with special reference to quinidine. Br Heart J 30:84-90

5. Hoglund C, Rosenhamer G (1985) Echocardiographic left atrial dimension as a predictor of maintaining sinus rhythm after conversion of atrial fibrillation. Acta Med Scand 217:411-415

6. Mugge A, Kuhn H, Nikuta P et al (1994) Assessment of left atrial appendage function by biplane transesophageal echocardiography in patients with nonrheumatic atrial fibrillation: identification of a subgroup of patients at increased thromboembolic risk. J Am Coll Cardiol 23:599-607

7. Mitusch R, Garbe M, Schmucker G et al (1995) Relation of left atrial appendage function to the duration and reversibility of nonvalvular atrial fibrillation. Am J Cardiol 75:944-947

8. Verhorst PMJ, kamp O, Welling RC et al (1997) Transesophageal echocardiographic predictors for maintenance of sinus rhythm after electrical cardioversion of atrial fibrillation. Am J Cardiol 79:1355-1359

9. Manning WJ, Leeman DE, Gotch PJ, Come PC (1989) Pulsed Doppler evaluation of atrial mechanical function after electrical cardioversion of atrial fibrillation. J Am Coll Cardiol 13:617-623

10. Dethy M, Chassat C, Roy D, Mercier LA (1988) Doppler echocardiographic predictors of recurrence of atrial fibrillation after cardioversion. Am J Cardiol 62:723-726

11. Grimm RA, Stewart WJ, Maloney JD et al (1993) Impact of electrical cardioversion of atrial fibrillation on left atrial appendage function and smoke: characterization by simultaneous transesophageal echocardiography. J Am Coll Cardiol 22:1359-1366

12. Fatkin D, Kuchar DL, Thornburn CW, Feneley MP (1994) Transesophageal echocardiography before and during direct current cardioversion of atrial fibrillation: evidence for "atrial stunning" as a mechanism of thromboembolic complications. J Am Coll Cardiol 23:307-316

13. Rigo F, Raviele A, De Piccoli B et al (1997) Internal atrial defibrillation: what are the effects on mechanical function? In: Raviele A (ed) Cardiac arrhythmias 1997. Proceedings of the 5th International Workshop on Cardiac Arrhythmias. Springer, Berlin Heidelberg New York, pp 89-99

14. Turitto G, Bandarizadeh B, Salciccioli L et al (1998) Risk stratification for recurrent tachyarrhythmias in patients with paroxysmal atrial fibrillation and flutter: role of signal averaged electrocardiogram and echocardiography. Pacing Clin Electrophysiol 21:197-201

15. Mattioli AV, Vivoli D, Bastia E (1997) Doppler echocardiographic parameters predictive of recurrence of atrial fibrillation of different etiologic origins. J Ultrasound Med 16:695-698

16. Barbier P, Alimento M, Salomon S et al (1998) Determinants of pulmonary venous systolic flow. Circulation 98 (suppl I):I-641 (abstr)

17. Garcia-Fernandez MA, Torrecilla EG, San Roman D et al (1992) Left atrial appendage Doppler flow patterns: implications on thrombus formation. Am Heart J 124:955-961

18. Laupacis A, Albers G, Dunn M et al (1992) Antithrombotic therapy in atrial fibrillation. Chest 102 (suppl):426S-433S

19. Grimm RA, Stewart WJ, Black IW et al (1994) Should all patients undergo transesophageal echocardiography before electrical cardioversion of atrial fibrillation? J Am Coll Cardiol 23:533-541

Atrial Stunning Following Sinus Rhythm Restoration: Which Mechanism, Time Course and Implication for Anticoagulation?

F. RIGO, A. RAVIELE, B. DE PICCOLI, F. CAPRIOGLIO, C. ZANELLA AND V. CUTAIA

Introduction

Atrial fibrillation (AF) is one of the most common types of arrhythmia, occurring in up to 4% of patients over 60 years of age [1-3]. Cardioversion is performed in patients with AF in an effort to improve cardiac function, relieve symptoms, and decrease the risk of thrombus formation. Successful cardioversion is associated with a 5%-7% incidence of embolism among patients who have not received adequate anticoagulant therapy [4-9]. In fact, the cardioversion of AF to sinus rhythm is associated with transient mechanical dysfunction of the left atrium (LA) and left atrial appendage (LAA) and the development of spontaneous echocardiographic contrast. This phenomenon has been termed "stunning" and is considered an important factor for thromboembolic stroke following cardioversion of AF to sinus rhythm [10-15].

Mechanism of Atrial Stunning

The exact mechanism by which the conversion of AF results in LA and auricular mechanical dysfunction and predisposes the patient to changes in the grade of spontaneous contrast is not clear [16]. Changes occurring in the atria during AF may have a deleterious effect on the atria once sinus rhythm is restored. The marked increase in the rate of atrial depolarization during AF might result in calcium loading, leading to desensitization or down-regulation of calcium receptors in the atria. Restoration of sinus rhythm and elimination of the calcium-loaded state might then result in a state of relative calcium deficiency and associated decrease in mechanical function, which would be expected to normalize as calcium receptors return to their baseline state [16]. Recently, it has been demonstrated that the LAA shows a divergence in behavior compared with the entire LA and

Unità Operativa di Cardiologia, Ospedale Umberto I, Mestre, Venice, Italy this may be related to intrinsic differences in LAA distensibility and shortening [17]. We are not aware of any studies which examine potential differences in calcium handling by atrial myocytes from the body of the LA and from the LAA during AF. The reduction in LAA contraction velocities has been identified as a risk factor for thrombus formation within the LAA [16, 17].

Time Course

The observation that thromboembolism after cardioversion may more often arise as a consequence of the effects of cardioversion on atrial function than from dislodgement of a preexistent thrombus [18] supports the importance of the magnitude and duration of atrial mechanical impairment of LA. Recovery of atrial contractile function may vary greatly from patient to patient, depending on a number of factors [19, 20], and does not occur immediately after conversion of chronic AF, but proceeds gradually [20].

Mode of Cardioversion

Direct evidence of myocardial injury due to electrical cardioversion has been sustained by the initial evidence of organic damage demonstrated by transient ST changes [21], by CPKmb elevation, by evidence of myocyte necrosis [21] and by presence of free radicals [22]. Fatkin and Kuchar [18] and Grimm and Stewart [23], using transoesophageal echocardiography during electrical cardioversion, demonstrated new or increased spontaneous echo-contrast in a considerable proportion of patients, expression of subsequent LA mechanical dysfunction and specific marker for thromboembolic risk. By contrast, Sparks and Kulkarni [24] recently demonstrated that endocardial and transthoracic DC shocks are not directly responsible for LA and LAA stunning and do not contribute to the stunning that is observed after the cardioversion of AF to sinus rhythm, and that, moreover, this is due to the function of the preceding arrhythmia itself rather than the mode of reversion. Also Abascal and Dubrey [25] found no significant difference in the atrial mechanical recovery between electrically and pharmacologically cardioverted patients and concluded that the degree of LA dysfunction after cardioversion is independent of the mode of cardioversion.

Duration of AF

Harjai and Mobareh [26] and Manning and Silverman [27] demonstrated that immediately after cardioversion and at 24 h and 1 week after cardioversion, atrial mechanical function is better in patients with AF < 2 weeks in duration than in those with atrial fibrillation > 6 weeks in duration. Although there was no difference in the LA diameter between the groups with AF of "brief" (< 2 weeks), "moderate" (2-6 weeks) or "prolonged" (> 6 weeks) duration, other patient characteristics, such as age, LA ejection fraction, underlying cardiac diseases, concomitant antiarrhythmic therapy and mode of cardioversion were not separately reported for the three groups. More recently, always Manning and Silverman [27] concluded that in patients with a clinical duration of AF of < 5 weeks recovery, atrial mechanical function appears to be related to the mode of cardioversion: a more prompt return of atrial mechanical function was seen in patients undergoing successful pharmacological cardioversion than in those undergoing successful electrical cardioversion after unsuccessful pharmacological cardioversion. Duration of AF < 24 h and normal LA size as a result was also associated with early recovery of atrial function [28]. Sparks and Jayaprakash [29] more recently observed that LA stunning was not detected after brief duration of AF in patients with structural heart disease and for this reason concluded that the thromboembolic risk is low after brief duration AF that terminates either spontaneously or with an endocardial DC shock, even in patients with significant structural heart disease. These findings have important implications for recipients of implantable devices that are capable of atrial defibrillation in response to AF.

Other Factors

Various clinical findings have been put forward as risk factors responsible for post-cardioversion atrial dysfunction. Blood hypertension, alcohol abuse, heart rate during the post-conversion, cardiac loading conditions, drugs, the presence of valvular or myocardial diseases, LA size, left ventricular ejection fraction and moreover LAA contraction velocity [28, 30], but the true relationship has not been clear until now.

Clinical Implications

Stroke is the third leading cause of death and long-term disability in the United States. Emboli arising from the heart are estimated to account for 15%-20% of all ischaemic strokes with a high reported prevalence of 34% [26]. It has been well documented that the thromboembolic risk in the pericardioversion period is very high [26-28, 31]. For this reason, the American College of Chest Physicians Consensus Committee on Antithrombotic Therapy Recommendations [31] states that all patients with AF > 2 days in duration should receive warfarin therapy for 3 weeks before and 4 weeks after cardioversion until sinus rhythm has been maintained. There are several practical clinical problems associated with these recommendations, including the complication of bleeding related to warfarin, the requirement of a second hospital admission for cardioversion and the delay in reversion of AF to sinus rhythm. A possible solution can be given by echocardiography which shows a good sensitivity in the screening before cardioversion to look for LA thrombus [18, 26]. The transoesophageal echocardiography has clearly demonstrated superior sensitivity and specificity in detecting pre-thrombotic findings and LAA thrombus [32], and for this reason can be utilized to avoid long-term anticoagulation before cardioversion, especially in those patients with high risk of bleeding. I believe that the transoesophageal echocardiography approach before cardioversion should be reserved for those patients with contraindication to anticoagulation, or who need a short anticoagulation course, or those with inadequate duration or extent of anticoagulation, or with poor documentation of anticoagulation status.

Thromboemboli are known to occur after cardioversion in non-anticoagulated patients despite "negative" transoesophageal echocardiograms immediately before cardioversion [33]. It is most likely that persistent or increased atrial stasis after cardioversion results in the formation of fresh, loosely adherent thrombi, and subsequent embolism and the lack of mechanical activity contributes to stasis in the LA and moreover in the LAA [21-24]. The occurrence of embolism in patients undergoing cardioversion is close to 7% and this finding in a large proportion of patients seems to be due to an increased thrombogenic milieau that happens immediately after cardioversion; this risk is present presumably until such time as "normal" atrial and appendage function resumes [24, 30]. It is unclear how long anticoagulation therapy should be continued after cardioversion; this is because no safe means of demonstration has been found for the recovery of atrial mechanical function and, moreover, LAA persistence of stunning that can have a longer time course in comparison to global atrial restoration [30]. In fact, only the transoesophageal approach allows a clear demonstration of LAA function and subsequent potential thromboembolic risk. This approach has a cost-effective ratio that should be better verified. We have no clinical findings to minimize the cost and potential morbidity associated with anticoagulation. Future research should focus on identifying subsets of patients who do not have prolonged anticoagulation after cardioversion.

References

1. Ostrander LD, Brandt RL (1965) Electrocardiographic findings among the adult population of a total community, Tecumseh, Michigan. Circulation 31:888-898
2. Petersen P (1990) Thromboembolic complications in atrial fibrillation. Stroke 21:4-13
3. Kannel WB, Wolf PA (1992) Epidemiology of atrial fibrillation. In: Falk RH (ed) Atrial fibrillation: mechanism and management. Raven Press, New York, pp 81-92
4. Resnekov L, McDonald L (1967) Complications in 220 patients with cardiac dysrhythmias treated by phased direct current shock, and indications for electrocardioversion. Br Heart J 29:926-936
5. Bjerkelund CJ, Orning OM (1969) The efficacy of anticoagulation therapy in preventing embolism related to D.C. electrical conversion of atrial fibrillation. Am J Cardiol 23:208-216
6. Lown B, Perlroth MG (1963) Cardioversion of atrial fibrillation: a report on treatment of 65 episodes in 50 patients. N Engl J Med 269:325-331
7. Weinberg DM, Mancini GBJ (1989) Anticoagulation for cardioversion of atrial fibrillation. Am J Cardiol 63:745-746
8. Petersen P, Godtfredsen J (1986) Embolic complications in paroxysmal atrial fibrillation. Stroke 17:622-626
9. Rokseth R, Storstein O (1963) Quinidine therapy of chronic auricolar fibrillation: the occurrence and mechanism of syncope. Arch Intern Med 111:184-189

10. Grimm RA, Stewart WJ (1997) Left atrial appendage "stunning"after electrical cardioversion of atrial flutter: an attenuated response compared with atrial fibrillation as the mechanism for lower susceptibility to thromboembolic events. J Am Coll Cardiol 29:582-589

11. Manning WJ, Silverman DI (1994) Impaired left atrial mechanical function after cardioversion: relation to duration of atrial fibrillation. J Am Coll Cardiol 23:1535-1540

12. Omram H, Jung W (1997) Left atrial chamber and appendage function after internal atrial defibrillation: a prospective and serial transesophageal echocardiographic study 29:131-138

13. Irani WN, Grayburn PA (1997) Prevalence of thrombus,spontaneous echo contrast, and atrial stunning in patients undergoing cardioversion of atria flutter. Circulation 95:962-966

14. Santiago D, Warshofsky M (1994) Left atrial appendage function and thrombus formation in atrial fibrillation-flutter: a transesophageal echocardiographic study. J Am Coll Cardiol 24:159-164

15. O'Neill PG, Puleo PR (1990) Return of atrial mechanical function following electrical conversion of atrial dysrhythmias. Am Heart J 120:353-359

16. Falcone RA, Morady F (1996) Transesophageal Echocardiographic evaluation of left atrial appendage function and spontaneous contrast formation after chemical or electrical cardioversion of atrial fibrillation. Am J Cardiol 78:435-439

17. Hoit BD, Shao Y (1994) Influence of acutely altered loading conditions on left atrial appendage flow velocities. J Am Coll Cardiol 24:1117-1123

18. Fatkin D, Kuchar DL (1994) Transesophageal echocardiography before and during direct current cardioversion of atrial fibrillation: evidence for atrial stunning as a mechanism of thromboembolic complications. J Am Coll Cardiol 23:307-316

19. Murgatroyd FF, Camm AJ (1993) Atrial arrhythmias. Lancet 341:1317-1322

20. Jovic A, Troskot R (1997) Recovery of atrial systolic function after pharmacological conversion of chronic atrial fibrillation to sinus rhythm: a Doppler echocardiographic study. Heart 77:46-49

21. Daal CE, Ewy GA (1974) Myocardial necrosis from direct current countershock. Circulation 50:956-961

22. Caterine MR, Spencer KT (1994) Direct current countershocks generate free radicals. Circulation 90:1-5

23. Grimm RA, Stewart WJ (1993) Impact of electrical cardioversion for atrial fibrillation on left atrial appendage function and spontaneous echo contrast: characterization by simultaneous TEE. J Am Coll Cardiol 22:1359-1366

24. Sparks PB, Kulkarni R (1998) Effect of direct current shocks on left atrial mechanical function in patients with structural heart disease. J Am Coll Cardiol 31:1395-1399

25. Abascal VM, Dubrey S (1995) Electrical vs pharmacgological cardioversion on atrial fibrillation:does the atrium really care? Circulation 92[Suppl 1]:I-591

26. Harjai KJ, Mobarek SK (1997) Clinical variables affecting recovery of left atrial mechanical function after cardioversion from atrial fibrillation. J Am Coll Cardiol 30:481-486

27. Manning WJ, Silverman DI (1995) Temporal dependence of the return of atrial mechanical function on the mode of cardioversion of atrial fibrillation to sinus rhythm. Am J Cardiol 75:624-626

28. Mattioli AV, Castellani ET (1996) Restoration of atrial fuction after fibrillation of different etiological origins. Cardiology 87:205-211

29. Sparks PB, Jayaprakash S (1999) Left atrial mechanical function after brief duration atrial fibrillation. J Am Coll Cardiol 33:342-349

30. Louie EK, Liu D (1998) Stunning of the left atrium after spontaneous conversion of atrial fibrillation to sinus rhythm. J Am Coll Cardiol 32:2081-2086
31. Laupacis A, Albers G (1992) Antithrombotic therapy in atrial fibrillation. Third ACCP Conference on antythrombotic therapy. Chest 102 (suppl):S426-S433
32. Pearson AC (1995) Transesophageal echocardiographic screening for atrial fibrillation: when should we look before we leap? J Am Coll Cardiol 25:1362-1364
33. Black IW, Hopkins AP (1993) Evaluation of transesophageal echocardiography before cardioversion of atrial fibrillation and flutter in nonanticoagulated patients. Am Heart J 126:375-381

Drug Prevention of Atrial Fibrillation: Are Novel Agents More Effective Than the Old Ones?

T. Van Noord, I.C. Van Gelder and H.J.G.M. Crijns

Introduction

This report concerns paroxysmal and persistent atrial fibrillation (AF). Paroxysmal AF usually occurs in short episodes which terminate spontaneously. By contrast, persistent AF does not self-terminate and needs electrical cardioversion for restoration of sinus rhythm [1]. Cardioversion for persistent AF is in general successful. However, the Achilles' heel in the treatment of both paroxysmal and persistent AF is arrhythmia recurrence. It should be kept in mind that restoration of sinus rhythm, either chemically or electrically, should only be attempted after adequate treatment of the underlying disease. The present review will deal with prevention of AF, focusing on new antiarrhythmic (Vaughan-Williams class III) drugs, recently discovered beneficial effects of conventional antiarrhythmic drugs, and alternative medical treatment strategies.

Prevention of Paroxysmal and Persistent AF

Conventional Drugs

Paroxysmal and persistent AF are chronic diseases: the first attack will not be the last in over 90% of patients despite antiarrhythmic prophylaxis. As a consequence, the endpoint of treatment is "attack-free rate" or "time to first recurrence". For this reason, when considering drug efficacy it might be more appropriate to focus on quality of life, but firm data concerning this issue are not available. In this respect, however, it is important to note that up to 50% of patients discontinue drug therapy owing to loss of quality of life due to side effects and drug inefficacy.

In patients suffering from frequent attacks of paroxysmal AF, chronic prophy-

Department of Cardiology, Thorax Center, University Hospital Groningen, The Netherlands

laxis can be effective after removal of precipitating factors such as caffeine, alcohol, or stress, and adequate treatment of underlying diseases like myocardial ischemia, thyreotoxicosis, and heart failure. Class IC antiarrhythmic drugs are highly effective but should not be given to individuals with clinical features resembling the CAST (Cardiac Arrhythmia Suppression Trial) individuals, i.e., patients with a previous myocardial infarction [2, 3]. In a placebo-controlled, crossover study Anderson et al. included 53 patients with two or more attacks of AF within a 4-week baseline period [2]. Median dosage of flecainide was 300 mg, which is well above the clinical dosage currently instituted (150-200 mg daily). Compared to placebo, flecainide prolonged the median time to the first recurrence (3 vs 15 days) as well as the time between subsequent attacks (6 vs 27 days). The efficacy of flecainide was maintained during a mean follow-up of 17 months [3]. Compared to quinidine, flecainide seems to be more effective: 46% vs 16% total abolition of supraventricular tachycardia, after dose increase: 50% vs 32% ($p = $ ns). Side effects of flecainide only occurred after dose adjustment, while side effects of quinidine occurred even before dose adjustment [4]. Propafenone is also effective, especially the lower dose (600 mg daily). A higher dose of propafenone is associated with an increased incidence of adverse events [5]. The class IA drug quinidine is as effective as flecainide but is less well tolerated. Naccarelli et al. included 239 patients randomized to receive flecainide (maximum dose 300 mg daily) or quinidine (maximum dose 1500 mg daily) and followed them for 12 months. Inadequate response caused 10% and 12% terminations of the drug, respectively. However, 30% of the patients in the quinidine group stopped taking the drug owing to adverse effects, versus only 18% of the flecainide group [6]. In an open label comparison of sotalol and propafenone in a mixed population with both paroxysmal and persistent AF, 37% and 30% of the patients were attack-free for 1 year [7]. Concerning amiodarone, the evidence available suggests that it is most effective but, unfortunately, its use is associated with a relatively high incidence of side effects [8].

Persistent AF does not disappear spontaneously and is difficult to terminate with drugs. First-choice therapy for restoration of sinus rhythm is direct current electrical cardioversion. However, AF frequently relapses if left untreated. These recurrences are predominantly confined to the first week after electrical cardioversion [9]. Conventional antiarrhythmic drugs are only moderately effective in the prevention of relapses of AF. Even when using a serial cardioversion and antiarrhythmic approach only 30%-50% of patients maintain sinus rhythm for 2 years [10]. Most conventional prophylactic drugs are equally effective, except for amiodarone, which appears to be more efficacious [11]. Quinidine has been studied most frequently. A meta-analysis of six controlled trials showed that quinidine was superior to no treatment (50% vs 25% of the patients respectively remained in sinus rhythm for 1 year). However, the total mortality was significantly higher in the quinidine group (12 of 413 patients (2.9%) versus 3 of 387 patients (0.8%), respectively, $p < 0.05$) [12]. A recent registry also demonstrated a relatively high incidence of sudden death with quinidine [13]. Of 570 patients younger than 65 years, 6 died suddenly, all shortly after restoration of sinus rhythm. These findings make it questionable whether there is still a role for quinidine in the prophylaxis of AF. Only a few trials evaluated the class IC drugs flecainide and propafenone and the class II/III drug sotalol, showing that these drugs are comparable to class IA drugs as far as efficacy is concerned [11]. However, differences may be observed in the adverse event profile, which may guide the choice for one particular drug (see below). In general, class IC drugs and sotalol are better tolerated than class IA drugs and amiodarone. On the other hand, all except amiodarone may cause significant proarrhythmia. Minimal prospective comparative data for amiodarone are available, but a favorable outcome has been reported when amiodarone is instituted as a last resort agent. The drug is particularly useful in AF complicated by heart failure. Unfortunately, its use is limited by potentially severe non-cardiac side effects. However, low dose amiodarone (200 mg daily) is effective and adverse events seem to be limited [14]. Gosselink et al. studied 89 patients with chronic AF who had failed previous treatment aimed at maintenance of sinus rhythm. These patients were treated with a mean dose of amiodarone of 204 ± 66 mg. Actuarially, 53% of these patients were still in sinus rhythm after a follow-up of three years. Adverse events occurred in three patients and were a reason for discontinuation in only one patient [14]. Only limited data on β-blocker therapy for the prevention of AF are available. Theoretically, suppressing adrenergic-dependent premature beats in the early phase after cardioversion may lower the relapse rate. Preliminary data from a large-scale study demonstrate a lower relapse rate in patients treated with metoprolol compared to placebo [15]

Efficacy of New Antiarrhythmic Drugs

Several pure class III agents are currently under investigation. These drugs are specific blockers of the delayed rectifier potassium current, especially its rapidly activating component (I_{KR}). Most drugs show reverse rate-dependency, indicating that prolongation of the action potential duration occurs predominantly at lower heart rates. This also may explain why torsades de pointes usually occur soon after conversion of (rapid) AF into (slow) sinus rhythm. In addition to blockade of I_{KR}, ibutilide acts by augmentation of the inactivated sodium channel. Azimilide blocks both the slow component of the delayed rectifier (I_{KS}) and I_{KR}. As class III agents act by prolongation of repolarization especially at a normal heart rate, these drugs are expected to be effective for the prevention of AF. The Achilles' heel of these drugs, however, is their propensity to induce proarrhythmia, i.e., torsades de pointes, at lower heart rates. This was the reason for stopping the clinical development of, e.g., D-sotalol and almakolant.

The only pure class III antiarrhythmic drug currently available is ibutilide, but this is exclusively for i.v. use, precluding assessment of its long term preventive efficacy. Torsades de pointes may occur (up to 8% of patients), again demonstrating limitations of class III drugs [16, 17]. Dofetilide, another pure class III antiarrhythmic drug, also seems to be effective for the prevention of AF or atrial flutter. In a randomized placebo-controlled study, 70% vs 26% of the dofetilide-treated vs placebo treated patients, respectively, maintained sinus rhythm [18]. In contrast to other pure class III drugs which block only I_{KR}, azimilide blocks both the slowly activating (I_{KS}) and the rapidly activating (I_{KR}) components of the delayed rectifier potassium current. Azimilide's effects on atrial effective refractory period are rate-independent: under conditions of tachycardia and β-adrenergic stimulation, azimilide allegedly prolongs the action potential duration, while pure I_{kr} blockers then lose efficacy [19]. Azimilide seems more effective than dofetilide in acute conversion: in a pacing-induced AF dog model azimilide terminated AF in 13 of 14 dogs (93%), while only 6 of 12 dogs (50%) converted on dofetilide ($p <$ 0.05). Azimilide has been reported to be effective in prolonging the time to recurrences in patients with paroxysmal AF. In a randomized study of placebo vs doses of azimilide, median time to recurrence was 17 days in the placebo group vs 130 days in patients treated with 125 mg azimilide daily [20]. Torsade de pointes was demonstrated in 1 of 270 patients treated with azimilide, which is relatively low, but this may relate to insufficient recording. The suggested safety of azimilide may relate to the absence of reverse use-dependent effects (in contrast to other pure class III antiarrhythmic drugs) [21, 22]. More studies are currently in progress. Dronedarone is another new class III antiarrhythmic drug which resembles amiodarone by having multiple actions (class I, II, III, and IV antiarrhythmic actions), but it lacks amiodarone's iodine subgroup and phospholipase inhibition. At present, this drug is under development. No (preliminary) data are yet available.

Conventional Drugs with New Therapeutic Actions

Recent data on the cellular adaptation processes which occur early after the start of AF [23] suggest calcium overload to be an important pathogenetic trigger [24, 25]. Hypothetically, reduction of electrical remodeling by a calcium-channel blocker may enhance the maintenance of sinus rhythm. This suggests that nondihydropyridine class IV antiarrhythmic drugs contain new therapeutic actions unknown until recently. Evidence for beneficial effects of calcium channel-blockers in patients with AF is still a matter of discussion. Whereas older studies demonstrated proarrhythmic effects of verapamil and diltiazem, i.e., an increase in the number and duration of episodes of paroxysmal AF, recent data seem to be more in accordance with experimental findings on prevention of electrical remodeling. In a post-hoc analysis of 60 patients (not randomized) who underwent electrical cardioversion for persistent AF, maintenance of sinus rhythm was significantly higher in patients using a calcium lowering drug (verapamil, diltiazem, or a β-blocker) before the cardioversion compared to those treated with digoxin. In line with these findings, Tieleman et al. demonstrated that concomitant administration of verapamil during 1 month oral loading with amiodarone was an independent predictor of pharmacological cardioversion of AF [26]. In addition, preliminary data confirm this observation by suggesting higher efficacy of amiodarone in combination with calcium blockers compared to amiodarone alone during serial electrical cardioversion therapy [27].

Tolerability and Safety of Antiarrhythmic Drugs: Old Versus New Drugs

The most important adverse effects of drugs used in AF are ventricular proarrhythmia, heart failure, enhanced atrioventricular nodal conduction, and exacerbation of sick sinus syndrome or atrioventricular conduction disturbances. Sick sinus syndrome may be the basis for AF and can be unmasked by all antiarrhythmic drugs including digitalis.

Ventricular proarrhythmia includes new-onset ventricular fibrillation, ventricular tachycardia, or torsade de pointes. Class IA and (new pure) class III drugs predominantly cause polymorphic ventricular tachycardia, or torsade de pointes [28, 29], whereas class IC drugs may induce incessant monomorphic ventricular tachycardias and ventricular fibrillation [30, 31]. In contrast to the quinidine-like drugs, ventricular proarrhythmia or sudden death due to class IC drugs is virtually absent in patients without overt heart disease. It occurs predominantly late after institution of the drug, and especially during higher heart rates. Patients treated with quinidine or sotalol may experience sudden death especially early after onset of therapy or after dosage increases [32, 29]. Despite the fact that amiodarone prolongs QT_c interval and usually causes bradycardia, it is associated with a low incidence of torsade de pointes and may even be instituted after proarrhythmic events on class IA drugs. This probably relates to its "multichannel" action.

Patients using class IA and IC drugs may experience high ventricular rates during breakthrough AF or atrial flutter. These agents do not suppress and may even augment atrioventricular conduction by anticholinergic stimulation. Atrioventricular conduction is further reinforced by exercise and anxiety. Therefore patients using these drugs prophylactically must be cautioned to avoid exercise during a recurrence of AF. Digoxin, a β-blocker, or a calcium-channel blocker may be added but there are no clinical data to support this approach. New pure class III antiarrhythmic drugs probably do not promote this type of supraventricular proarrhythmia.

Depending on dose and duration of therapy, class IA and IC drugs especially may cause heart failure, mainly through cardiodepression. Disopyramide allegedly has the largest negative inotropic effects and may cause heart failure early but also late (months) after initiation, especially in patients with a history of cardiac insufficiency. The other class IA drugs, as well as β-blockers (including sotalol), calcium-channel blockers, and probably also pure class III antiarrhythmic drugs, rarely cause heart failure in patients with AF. Heart failure induced by amiodarone has not been described.

Future Strategies

Antiarrhythmic therapy is only moderately effective. Amiodarone-like drugs (such as dronedarone and azimilide) may possibly exhibit comparable efficacy but fewer adverse events. In the future, hybrid therapy may be an important tool to improve treatment outcome. One example are patients who develop atrial flutter while receiving class IC antiarrhythmic drugs prophylactically ("class IC atrial flutter"). These patients may benefit from radiofrequency ablation of their atrial flutter with continuation of the class IC drug thereafter [33]. Of the 16 patients who were scheduled for atrial flutter radiofrequency ablation, successful isthmus ablation was achieved in 15 patients. After a follow-up of 4 ± 2 months 13 patients successfully maintained sinus rhythm. In patients with paroxysmal AF a hybrid therapy with both antiarrhythmic drug treatment and (single- or dual-site) atrial pacing may also be effective for the prevention of relapses of AF. Delfaut et al. [34] demonstrated in 30 patients with drug-refractory symptomatic AF (and primary or drug-induced bradycardia) a marked increase in arrhythmia free intervals during both single-site (143 ± 110 days) and dual-site right atrial pacing (195 ± 96 days) combined with antiarrhythmic drug treatment compared to 9 ± 10 days during the control period ($p < 0.0001$). Pretreatment with safe antiarrhythmic drugs in persistent AF is a promising approach enhancing the duration of sinus rhythm after electrical cardioversion [35].

Conclusions

Antiarrhythmic drugs are the mainstay of AF treatment but they are usually only moderately effective. Amiodarone seems to be most effective, and the proarrhythmia risk is low, but its use is restricted by noncardiac adverse events. New (pure) class III antiarrhythmic drugs carry a considerable risk of ventricular proarrhythmia. However, the new class III drugs which not only block I_{kR} but also have other effects, like azimilide which also inhibits I_{kS}, and dronedarone, are promising both in terms of efficacy and safety. Treatment with calcium entry blockers, whether or not combined with class I or III antiarrhythmic drugs, may appear a safe and efficacious alternative.

Hybrid therapy with antiarrhythmic drugs in combination with radiofrequency ablation or atrial pacing may become important tools for the treatment of refractory patients.

References

1. Gallagher MM, Camm J (1998) Classification of atrial fibrillation. Am J Cardiol 82:18N-28N
2. Anderson JL, Gilbert EM, Alpert BL, Hernthorn RW, Waldo AL, Bhandari AK, Hawkinson RW, Pritchett ELC (1989) Prevention of symptomatic recurrences of paroxysmal atrial fibrillation in patients initially tolerating antiarrhythmic therapy. Circulation 80:1557-1570
3. Anderson JL, Platt ML, Guarnieri T, Fox TL, Maser MJ, Pritchett ELC, and the Flecainide Supraventicular Tachycardia Study Group (1994) Flecainide acetate for paroxysmal supraventricular arrhythmias. Am J Cardiol 74:578-584
4. Van Wijk LM, Den Heijer P, Crijns HJGM, Van Gilst WH, Lie KI (1989) Flecainide versus quinidine in the prevention of paroxysms of atrial fibrillation. J Cardiovasc Pharmacol 13:32-36

5. UK Propafenone PSVT Study Group (1995) A randomized, placebo-controlled trial of propafenone in the prophylaxis of paroxysmal supraventricular tachycardia and paroxysmal atrial fibrillation. Circulation 92:2550-2557

6. Naccarelli GV, Dorian P, Hohnloser SH, Coumel P, for the Multicenter Atrial Fibrillation Group (1996) Prospective comparison of flecainide versus quinidine for the treatment of paroxysmal atrial fibrillation/flutter. Am J Cardiol 77:53A-59A

7. Reimold SC, Cantillon CO, Friedman PL, Antman EM (1993) Propafenone versus sotalol for suppression of recurrent symptomatic atrial fibrillation. Am J Cardiol 71:558-563

8. Horowitz LN, Spielman SR, Greenspan AM, Mintz GS, Morganroth J, Brown R, Brady PM, Kay HR (1985) Use of amiodarone in the treatment of persistent and paroxysmal atrial fibrillation resistant to quinidine therapy. J Am Coll Cardiol 66:366-367

9. Tieleman RG, Van Gelder IC, Crijns HJGM, De Kam PJ, Van den Berg MP, Haaksma J, Van der Woude HJ, Allessie MA (1998) Early recurrences of atrial fibrillation after electrical cardioversion: a result of fibrillation-induced electrical remodeling of the atria? J Am Coll Cardiol 31:167-173

10. Van Gelder IC, Crijns HJGM, Tieleman RG, Brügemann J, De Kam PJ, Verheugt FWA, Lie KI (1996) Value and limitation of electrical cardioversion in patients with chronic atrial fibrillation – importance of arrhythmia risk factors and oral anticoagulation. Arch Intern Med 156:2585-2592

11. Crijns HJGM, Gosselink ATM, Van Gelder IC, Wiesfeld ACP, Van den Berg MP, Tuininga YS, Lie KI (1992) Drugs after cardioversion to prevent relapses of chronic atrial fibrillation. In: Kingma JH, van Hemel NM, Lie KI (eds) Atrial fibrillation, a treatable disease? Kluwer Academic, Dorchecht, pp 105-148

12. Coplen SE, Antman EM, Berlin JA, Hewitt P, Chalmers TC (1990) Efficacy and safety of quinidine therapy for maintenance of sinus rhythm. A meta-analysis of randomized control trials. Circulation 82:1106-1116

13. Carlsson J, Tebbe U, Rox J, Harmjanz D, Haerten K, Neuhaus KL, Seidel F, Niederer W, Miketic S, for the ALKK Study group (1996) Cardioversion of atrial fibrillation in the elderly. Am J Cardiol 78:1380-1384

14. Gosselink ATM, Crijns HJ, Van Gelder IC, Hillige H, Wiesfeld ACP, Lie KI (1992) Low-dose amiodarone for maintenance of sinus rhythm after cardioversion of atrial fibrillation or flutter. JAMA 32:3289-3293

15. Kuehlkamp V, Schirdewan A, Stangl K, Homberg M, Ploch M, Beck OA (1998) Use of metoprolol CR to maintain sinus rhythm after conversion from persistent atrial fibrillation. A randomized double-blind placebo-controlled study. Circulation 98:I-633 (abstr)

16. Vos MA, Golitsyn SR, Stangl K, Ruda MY, Van Wijk LV, Harry JD, Perry KT, Touboul P, Steinbeck G, Wellens HJ (1998) Superiority of Ibutilide (a new class III agent) over DL-sotalol in converting atrial flutter and atrial fibrillation. The Ibutilide/Sotalol Comparator Study Group. Heart 79:568-575

17. Stambler BS, Wood MA, Ellenbogen KA, Perry KT, Wakefield LK, Van der Lugt JT (1996) Efficacy and safety of repeated intravenous doses of ibutilide for rapid conversion of atrial flutter or fibrillation. Ibutilide repeat dose study investigators. Circulation 94:1613-1621

18. Singh SN, Berk MR, Yellen LG, Zoble RG, Haley JA, Abrahamson D, Satler CA (1997) Efficacy and safety of oral dofetilide in maintaining normal sinus rhythm in patients with atrial fibrillation/flutter: a multicenter study. Circulation 96:I-383 (abstr)

19. Nattel S, Liu L, St-Georges D (1998) Effects of the novel antiarrhythmic agent azimilide on experimental atrial fibrillation and atrial electrophysiologic properties. Cardiovasc Res 37:627-635

20. Pritchett E, Page R, Conolly S, Marcello S, Schnell D, Wilkinson W (1998) Azimilide treatment of atrial fibrillation. Circulation 98:I-633 (abstr)
21. Karam R, Marcello S, Brooks RP, Corey AE, Moore A (1998). Azimilide dihydrochloride, a novel antiarrhythmic agent. Am J Cardiol 81:40D-46D
22. Singh BN (1999) Current antiarrhythmic drugs: an overview of mechanisms of action and potential clinical utility. J Cardiovasc Electrophysiol 10:283-301
23. Wijffels MCEF, Kirchhof CJHJ, Dorland R, Allessie MA (1995) Atrial fibrillation begets atrial fibrillation. A study in awake chronically instrumented goats. Circulation 92:1954-1968
24. Tieleman RG, De Langen C, Van Gelder IC, De Kam PJ, Grandjean J, Bel KJ, Wijffels MCEF, Allessie MA, CrijnsHJGM (1997) Verapamil reduces tachycardia-induced electrical remodeling of the atria. Circulation 95:1945-1953
25. Daoud EG, Knight BP, Weiss R et al (1997) Effect of verapamil and procainamide on atrial fibrillation-induced electrical remodeling in humans. Circulation 96:1542-1550
26. Tieleman RG, Gosselink AT, Crijns HJGM, Van Gelder IC, Van den Berg MP, De Kam PJ, Van Gilst WH, Lie KI (1997) Efficacy, safety and determinants of conversion of atrial fibrillation and flutter with oral amiodarone. Am J Cardiol 79:53-57
27. Natale A, Tomassoni G, Beheiry S, Zimerman L, Kim YH, Pisano E, Leonelli F, Potenza M, Fanelli R (1998) Prospective randomized evaluation of combined therapy with amiodarone and a calcium antagonist for treatment of refractory atrial fibrillation. Circulation 98:I-103 (abstr)
28. Hohnloser SH, Van de Loo A, Baedeker F (1995) Efficacy and proarrhythmic hazards of pharmacologic cardioversion of atrial fibrillation: prospective comparison of sotalol versus quinidine. J Am Coll Cardiol 26:852-858
29. Jackman WM, Friday KJ, Andersen JL, Alliot EM, Clark M, Lazzaro R (1988) The long QT syndrome: a clinical review, new clinical observations and a unifying hypothesis. Prog Cardiovasc Dis 31:115-172
30. Falk RH (1989) Flecainide-induced ventricular tachycardia and fibrillation in patients treated for atrial fibrillation. Ann Intern Med 111:107-111
31. Flaker GC, Blackshear JL, McBride R, Kronmal RA, Halperin JL, Hart RG, on behalf of the Stroke Prevention in Atrial Fibrillation Investigators (1992) Antiarrhythmic drug therapy and cardiac mortality in atrial fibrillation. J Am Coll Cardiol 20:527-532
32. Carlsson J, Tebbe U Rox J, Harmjanz D, Haerten K, Neuhaus KL, Seidel F, Niederer W, Miketic S, for the ALKK Study group (1996) Cardioversion of atrial fibrillation in the elderly. Am J Cardiol 78:1380-1384
33. Nabar A, Rodriguez LM, Timmermans C, Van de Dool A, Smeets JL, Wellens HJ (1999) Effect of right atrial isthmus ablation on the occurrence of atrial fibrillation: observations in four groups having type I atrial flutter with or without associated atrial fibrillation. Circulation 99:1441-1445
34. Delfaut P, Saksena S, Prakash A, Krol RB (1998) Long-term outcome of patients with drug-refractory atrial flutter and fibrillation after single- and dual-site right atrial pacing for arrhythmia prevention. J Am Coll Cardiol 32:1900-1908
35. Bianconi L, Mennuni M, Lukic V, Castro A, Chieffi M, Santini M (1996) Effect of oral propafenone administration before electrical cardioversion of chronic atrial fibrillation: placebo controlled study. J Am Coll Cardiol 28:700-706

Atrial Pacing for Prevention of Atrial Fibrillation: Where and How to Stimulate?

S. Saksena

Introduction

Nonpharmacologic therapies are now being increasingly used in patients with recurrent and refractory atrial fibrillation (AF). These include direct atrial surgery, catheter-based atrial ablation, internal atrial defibrillation and atrial pacing. In retrospective and prospective studies, atrial pacing has reduced the frequency and incidence of AF in patients with sick sinus syndrome without and with manifest AF [1-3]. Similar observations have been made in populations with bradycardia or vagally mediated AF [4]. More sophisticated pacing algorithms and methods such as continuous atrial pacing and dual-site atrial pacing have been suggested to enhance efficacy of atrial pacing [5, 6]. The application of appropriate atrial pacing methods in specific populations with AF or at risk for AF is examined in this commentary. To comprehend the basis for future recommendations, it is valuable to consider the electrophysiologic basis for antiarrhythmic effects of atrial pacing and the clinical data presently available for making current recommendations.

Electrophysiologic Rationale for AF Prevention with Pacing

Effective prevention of AF may potentially be achieved by suppression of atrial premature complexes (APCs), prevention of the onset arrhythmia for AF or rapid AF termination. One antiarrhythmic mechanism of atrial pacing that has not been widely recognized is its direct effect on the atrial substrate that prevents initiation or sustenance of AF [7]. Increasing the atrial pacing rate can suppress atrial ectopy [8, 9]. In the NIPP-AF study, Lau and coworkers demonstrated a marked reduction in overall APC burden over 3-month treatment periods using device counters [9]. In vagal AF, clinical reports have documented that APCs that initiate

Arrhythmia & Pacemaker Service, Eastern Heart Institute, Passaic; Robert Wood Johnson School of Medicine, New Brunswick; Electrophysiology Research Foundation, Millburn, New Jersey, USA

AF are frequently preceded by bradycardia. Increasing the pacing rate eliminates pause-dependent substrate effects and suppresses atrial ectopy and initiation of AF [10]. One of the most significant effects of pacing, hitherto unappreciated, is a change in the atrial activation sequence and its secondary effect on induced and spontaneous atrial tachyarrhythmias [11]. Activation of both atria and their recovery of excitability is advanced to a modest extent by coronary sinus or septal pacing methods, but more significantly by multisite atrial pacing [11]. We and others have shown that maximal effects are obtained by dual-site right atrial pacing as compared to single-site methods. Using basket catheters for detailed biatrial endocardial mapping, Khoury and coworkers have demonstrated a marked reduction in right atrial, septal and left atrial activation with dual-site right atrial pacing. In contrast, single-site septal pacing advanced left atrial activation but did not impact the right atrium to any appreciable extent. APCs from multiple atrial sites of origin are more likely to encounter an altered coupling interval in the abnormal substrate, preventing the initiation of reentry, after dual-site than after single-site atrial pacing. Another antiarrhythmic mechanism is that change in the atrial pacing rate can reduce the dispersion of refractory periods in animal experiments but has not been as well established in clinical studies.

The effects of different modes of atrial pacing have now been studied [11]. Single-site right atrial pacing, particularly if performed from the appendage or septum, can advance septal and adjoining left atrial activation but may have few effects on the lateral right atrium. Dual-site right atrial pacing advances both right and left atrial activation in most sites, such as the septum, crista, coronary sinus and left atrium. Biatrial pacing produces similar effects. P-wave duration is reduced. Data suggest that dual-site right atrial pacing can attenuate by up to 25% the incremental delay encountered by closely coupled APCs. This results in suppression of induced AF in 56%-67% of patients with reproducibly induced AF from a specific atrial site with programmed atrial stimulation [12, 13]. Dual-site atrial pacing may also improve the hemodynamics and atrial emptying and facilitate a greater antiarrhythmic effect [14]. Preventing initiation and prompt termination of AF can also have a cumulative effect on its sustenance. Studies suggest that when animals with chronic AF are maintained in sinus rhythm, it is much more difficult to sustain AF [15].

Optimal Stimulation Sites for AF Prevention

Stratification of AF subpopulations based on AF burden, coexisting arrhythmias and heart disease is desirable in the decision to select an appropriate stimulation site (or sites) for atrial pacing.

In Sick Sinus Syndrome or Atrioventricular Block, Where There May or May Not Be Manifest AF, And AF Overall Burden Is Likely to Be Low

Several moderate to large clinical trials have now been reported that suggest that single-site atrial pacing in the right atrium may be satisfactory for AF prevention.

Andersen et al. noted a reduction in the development of chronic AF in patients with sick sinus syndrome [16]. In the Pacemaker Selection in the Elderly (PASE) pilot study, a trend toward reduction in AF events was noted [17]. However, the Canadian Trial on Physiologic Pacing (CTOPP) did not demonstrate such benefit [18]. However, all of these studies were focused and powered for survival endpoints with physiologic pacing, had variable methods of physiologic pacing (AAI vs DDD) with or without rate response and used single-site pacing. Thus, no estimate of the extent of atrial pacing achieved is obtainable, and in large measure antiarrhythmic drug therapy was not systematically used. At the current time, attention should be paid to the achievement of effective atrial pacing by programming in these populations. Early data suggest some advantage of mid to high septal pacing over high lateral right atrial pacing, albeit in a different population, discussed below. Inferentially, such benefits may accrue even in this population.

Single-Site Atrial Pacing in Symptomatic AF, with a Significant AF Burden

Single-site pacing in patients with symptomatic AF has been examined in prospective trials such as PAC-A-TACH and PA3, which have noted no overall benefit in AF prevention [19, 20]. Subgroup analysis shows benefit in patients receiving concomitant sotalol or quinidine therapy with atrial pacing. The extent of atrial pacing is not quantifiable from these data. Similarly, PA3, a trial of short-term (3-month) atrial pacing in prevention of chronic AF in patients awaiting atrioventricular junctional ablation, failed to demonstrate any increase in the time to first recurrence [20]. This trial employed high right atrial pacing and achieved 62% atrial pacing. These data suggest a limited role for single-site pacing alone in these populations.

Pilot studies of atrial septal pacing from both the high septum, near Bachmann's bundle, and mid to low septal sites show more encouraging results in AF prevention in patients with recent-onset AF. Padeletti et al. performed septal atrial pacing in 25 patients with very frequent AF, refractory on average to one antiarrhythmic drug, just above the coronary sinus ostium [21]. Rhythm control was achieved during a mean follow-up of 10 months in over 90% of patients, most often on pacing alone. Longer-term data and larger multicenter clinical trials, particularly in drug-refractory AF, are awaited. Initial reports from another trial show only a trend to benefit relative to high right atrial pacing alone [22]. Percent atrial pacing and drug therapy cannot be quantified from available data at the present. Thus, at the present time use of septal pacing may be considered in patients without drug refractory AF, but other data suggest that this is inferior to dual site right atrial pacing [23]. Thus, at the present time, septal pacing should be undertaken only in patients without drug-refractory AF in whom there is inability to institute dual-site atrial pacing.

Dual-Site Atrial Pacing in Symptomatic Refractory AF, with a High AF Burden

Clinical studies have now provided long-term data on dual-site atrial pacing and have been encouraging in AF prevention. Daubert et al. have reported on 86 patients with refractory AF or flutter and interatrial block during long-term follow-up (mean > 40 months) [24]. Sixty-four percent of these patients achieved rhythm control. Our data in patients with highly refractory and symptomatic AF (paroxysmal, 50%; persistent, 30%; chronic, 20%) suggest rhythm control can be achieved in > 80% of patients [23]. In our study, > 80% of continuous overdrive pacing was sought and preoperatively ineffective antiarrhythmic drugs were administered concomitantly in most patients, though usually in a lower dose than previously. Time course of recurrent AF showed a progressive decline over the first 6 months with a suggestion of an "atrial remodeling" process that improved AF control over time [25]. Other reports have substantiated the efficacy of dual-site right atrial pacing in combination with drugs. Vardas and coworkers demonstrated an 80% efficacy rate in a pilot study of 10 patients when combined with β-blocker drug therapy [26]. Boccadamo et al. noted similar success in 19 patients with a variety of pacemaker generators and refractory symptomatic AF [27]. Failure to use drug therapy lowered efficacy rates in the Vardas study. It has been suggested dual-site right atrial pacing or other forms of atrial pacing are efficacious solely in patients with preexisting bradycardias. In our studies, these comprised < 35% of patients, with most having drug-induced bradycardia. While patients without bradycardias have shorter AF-free intervals (approximately 500 vs 1000 days), both were markedly greater than preimplant AF-free intervals (9 days). Lau et al. reported successful suppression of recurrent AF in refractory AF patients without primary bradyarrhythmias with dual-site right atrial pacing in controlled prospective comparison [9]. Experience from other centers suggests a 50%-60% efficacy rate when drug therapy is not used in patients with refractory AF. The safety of the technique has been established for dual-site right atrial pacing with coronary sinus os lead dislodgment rates of < 1%. In contrast, lead dislodgment is > 15% with biatrial pacing, even with newer leads. Thus, dual-site right atrial pacing should be considered the pacing method of choice when multisite atrial pacing is considered for AF prevention in patients with refractory AF.

How to Stimulate for Pacing Prevention

Clinical trials of multisite pacing are providing some insight into this issue. One short-term comparison of biatrial pacing, single-site atrial pacing and support pacing showed only a trend toward benefit without significant increase in time to first AF recurrence, though an overall trend to reduced AF burden was seen in many patients [28]. However, triggered pacing was used, extent of atrial pacing was not established, and drug therapy was not systematically added. Furthermore, the study used 3-month on-treatment periods and these do not allow for a "remodeling process" to improve AF control as seen in the pilot data. In our studies on dual-site right atrial pacing, the AF prevention regimen includes drug therapy, quantifies pacing and has a longer period in the chosen pacing mode to allow for the remodeling process. Adjunctive therapy such as catheter ablation of coexisting or induced atrial flutter, and even right atrial compartmentalization with linear lesions, has been employed to suppress recurrent AF and maintain rhythm control.

Atrial pacing is now being combined with other therapies – electrical, ablative and, as mentioned, drugs – to achieve rhythm control. Antitachycardia pacing, as used in the Medtronic Jewel AF trial currently in progress, and defibrillation provide back-up to reestablish rhythm control and allow preventative therapies to achieve maximal effect. Pilot data on combining atrial ablation and atrial pacing with and without drug therapy are showing promise in rhythm control in refractory AF [29, 30].

Conclusions

Progressive clinical experience is now providing significantly more data on the potential role of atrial pacing in AF prevention. These data support the belief that appropriate stimulation methods and lead placement in combination with adjunctive antiarrhythmic therapies can enhance the efficacy of atrial pacing for establishing rhythm control in recurrent AF and delay the onset of AF in populations at risk.

References

1. Sgarbossa EB, Pinski SL, Maloney JD, Simmons TW, Wilkoff BL, Castle LW, Trohman RG (1993) Chronic atrial fibrillation and stroke in paced patients with sick sinus syndrome. Relevance of clinical characteristics and pacing modalities. Circulation 88:1045-1053
2. Reimold SC, Lamas GA, Cantillon CO, Antman EM (1995) Risk factors for the development of recurrent atrial fibrillation: role of pacing and clinical variables. Am Heart J 129:1127-1132
3. Hesselson AB, Parsonnet V, Bernstein AD, Bonavita G (1992) Deleterious effect of long-term single chamber ventricular pacing in patients with sick sinus syndrome: the hidden benefits of dual chamber pacing. J Am Coll Cardiol 19:1542-1549
4. Coumel P, Friocourt P, Mugica J, Attuel P, LeClercq JF (1983) Long-term prevention of vagal atrial arrhythmias by atrial pacing at 90/minute: experience with 6 cases. PACE 6:552-560
5. Daubert C, Mabo PH, Berder V, Gras D, Leclercq C (1994) Atrial tachyarrhythmias associated with high degree interatrial conduction block: prevention by permanent atrial resynchronisation. Eur J CPE 1:35-44
6. Saksena S, Prakash A, Hill M, Krol RB, Munsif AN, Mathew PP, Mehra R (1996) Prevention of recurrent atrial fibrillation with chronic dual site right atrial pacing. J Am Coll Cardiol 28:687-694
7. Saksena S, Prakash A, Krol RB, Munsif AN, Giorgberidze I, Mathew P, Kaushik RR (1997) Prevention of atrial fibrillation with a single and multisite atrial pacing. In: Murgatroyd FD, Camm AJ (eds) Nonpharmacological management of atrial fibrillation. Futura, Armonk, NY, pp 339-356
8. Murgatroyd F, Slade A, Nitzsche R, Limousin M, Rosset N, Camm AJ, Ritter P (1994) A new pacing algorithm for the suppression of atrial fibrillation. PACE 17:863-867

9.   Lau CP, Tse HF, Yu CM, Teo WS, Ng KH, Huang SK, Leung SK, Tsang V, Hill M (1999)
     Dual site right atrial pacing in paroxysmal atrial fibrillation without bradycardia
     (NIPP-AF Study). PACE 22(II):804 (abstr)
10. Mehra R, Hill MRS (1996) Prevention of atrial fibrillation/flutter by pacing techni-
     ques. In: Saksena S, Luderitz B (eds) Interventional electrophysiology, 2nd edn.
     Futura, Armonk, NY, pp 521-540
11. Prakash A, Delfaut P, Krol RB, Saksena S (1998) Regional right and left atrial activa-
     tion patterns during single- and dual-site atrial pacing in patients with atrial fibrilla-
     tion. Am J Cardiol 82:1197-1204
12. Prakash A, Saksena S, Hill M, Krol RB, Munsif AN, Giorgberidze I, Mathew P, Mehra R
     (1997) Acute effects of dual-site right atrial pacing in patients with spontaneous and
     inducible atrial flutter and fibrillation. J Am Coll Cardiol 29:1007-1014
13. Chen YJ, Chen SA, Tai CT, Yu WC, Feng AN, Ding YA, Chang MS (1998) Electrophy-
     siologic characteristics of a dilated atrium in patients with paroxysmal atrial fibrilla-
     tion and atrial flutter. J Intervent Cardiac Electrophysiol 2:181-186
14. Daubert C, Mabo P, Berder V, De Place C, Kermarrec A, Paillard F (1991) Simulta-
     neous dual atrium pacing in high degree interatrial blocks: hemodynamic results.
     Circulation 84:II-453 (abstr)
15. Wijffels MCEF, Kirchhof CJHJ, Dorland RD, Allessie MA (1995) Atrial fibrillation
     begets atrial fibrillation. A study in awake chronically instrumented goats.
     Circulation 92:1954-1968
16. Andersen HR, Nielsen JC, Thomsen PEB, Thuesen L, Mortensen PT, Vesterlund T,
     Pedersen AK (1997) Long-term follow-up of patients from a randomized trial of
     atrial versus ventricular pacing for sick sinus syndrome. Lancet 305:1210-1216
17. Lamas GA, Ellenbogen KA, Griffin JJ, Wilkoff BL, Sgarbossa E, Huang S, Marinchak
     RA, Mitchell G, Estes M, Venditti FJ, Maloney JD, Rizo-Patron C, Lieberman EH,
     Mangione C, Orav J, Goldman L, for the PASE Investigators (1995) Quality of life and
     clinical events in DDDR versus VVIR paced patients: design and preliminary results
     of a randomized trial. Circulation 92[Suppl]:I-533 (abstr)
18. Connolly S, for CTOPP Investigators (1998) Results of the Canadian Trial of
     Physiologic Pacing. Presented at American Heart Association Scientific Sessions,
     November 1998
19. Wharton JM, Sorrentino RA, Criger D, Shenasa M, Brownstein S, Derring T, Gering L,
     Grill C, Lee KL (1999) Predictors of death in VVI-R and DDD-R paced patients with
     the tachycardia-bradycardia syndrome. ACC 33:153A (abstr)
20. Gillis AM, Connolly SJ, Yee R, Dubuc M, Phillipon F, Lacombe P, Kerr CR, Wyse DG,
     for the PA3 Investigators (1998) atrial pacing peri-ablation for paroxysmal atrial
     fibrillation - Phase I. PACE 21(II):872 (abstr)
21. Padeletti L, Porciani MC, Michelucci A, Colella A, Ticci P, Vena S, Costoli A, Ciapetti C,
     Pieragnoli P, Gensini GF (1999) Interatrial septum pacing: a new approach to prevent
     recurrent atrial fibrillation. J Intervent Cardiac Electrophysiol 3:35-43
22. Bailin SJ, Adler SW, Guidici MC, Hill MRS, Solinger B, Bachmann's Bundle Pacing
     Trial Centers (1999) Bachmann's bundle pacing for the prevention of atrial fibrilla-
     tion: initial trends in a multi-center randomized prospective study. PACE 22(II):727
     (abstr)
23. Delfaut P, Saksena S, Prakash A, Krol RB (1998) Long-term outcome of patients with
     drug-refractory atrial flutter and fibrillation after single and dual site right atrial
     pacing for arrhythmia prevention. J Am Coll Cardiol 32:1900-1908
24. d'Allones GR, Victor F, Pavin D, Mabo P, Daubert C (1999) Long-term effects of bia-
     trial synchronous pacing to prevent drug refractory atrial tachyarrhythmias: a pilot
     study. PACE 22(II):755 (abstr)

25. Saksena S, Prakash A, Krol R, Delfaut P (1999) Time dependence and pattern of atrial fibrillation recurrences after single and dual site right atrial pacing. (abstract) J Am Coll Cardiol 33:140A

26. Vardas PE, Simantirakis EM, Manios EG, Parthenakis FI, Chrysostomakis SI, Zuridakis EG (1996) Acute and chronic hemodynamic effects of bifocal vs. unifocal right atrial pacing. (abstract) J Am Coll Cardiol 27:74A

27. Prakash A, Boccadamo R, Di Belardino N, Mammucari A, Krol RB, Sroczynski H, Mackenzie P, Saksena S (1999) Multicenter experience with dual site atrial pacing using different pacemaker generator systems: long-term results. (abstract) Submitted for presentation at American Heart Association Scientific Sessions, November

28. Mabo P, Daubert C, Bouhour A, on behalf of the SYNBIAPACE Study Group (1999) Biatrial synchronous pacing for atrial arrhythmia prevention: the SYNBIAPACE study. (abstract) PACE 22(II):755

29. Prakash A, Krol RB, Saksena S, Sumar R (1999) Ablation of coexisting atrial flutter elicited using an electrophysiologic strategy in atrial fibrillation improves drug efficacy. (abstract) PACE 22(II):743

30. Krol RB, Prakash A, Saksena S, Sroczynski H, Sumar R, Mackenzie P (1999) Initial experience with an electrophysiologic strategy using a combination of atrial pacing and atrial ablation therapy for management of refractory atrial fibrillation. (abstract) PACE 22(II):A27

Implantable Atrial Defibrillator: What are the Results of Initial Experience?

G. Gasparini, A. Bonso, S. Themistoclakis, F. Giada, A. Corrado and A. Raviele

Atrial fibrillation (AF) is the most common arrhythmia in clinical practice for which patients are hospitalized, engendering high human and economic costs [1, 2]. The limited efficacy and the side effects of drugs used both to maintain sinus rhythm and to control the heart rate have increased interest in the development of non-pharmacological therapy for AF [3]. The implantable atrial defibrillator (IAD) is one such therapeutic tool.

Among other alternative non-pharmacological therapies, AV node ablation with pacemaker implantation and atrium compartmentalization by linear radiofrequency ablation or surgical lesions (the maze operation) are irreversibly destructive procedures that are feasible only in a limited number of selected patients. By contrast, focal radiofrequency ablation, although still experimental, is emerging as an interesting approach which targets, limited lesions in patients with paroxysmal "fire" AF. Finally, multisite atrial pacing, including algorithms of overdrive pacing and/or suppression of post-extrasystolic compensatory pauses, seem to be a promising means for preventing AF.

Both the introduction into clinical practice of low-energy internal atrial defibrillation [4] and the concept that early restoration of sinus rhythm might decrease the recurrence rate of AF (AF begets AF) [5] have led to the development of the IAD. This device was thought to be able to restore sinus rhythm quickly by the use of low-energy shocks and, therefore, by lengthening AF-free intervals, to reduce the complications of AF and its negative effects on cardiac function.

At present, two models of IAD are manufactured by two different companies: the Metrix Atrioverter 3000 or 3020 (Guidant Corporation), which specializes in atrial defibrillation and provides ventricular back-up pacing, and the 7250 Jewel AF (Medtronic Corporation), which is capable of defibrillating and pacing both atria and ventricles. The number of these devices implanted worldwide is still low (less than 400) and preliminary clinical data have only recently been published or presented at international congresses.

Reparto di Cardiologia, Ospedale Umberto I, Mestre, Venice, Italy

Metrix Atrioverter 3000 or 3020

The Metrix system consists of an IAD (model 3000 or 3020) connected to right atrial (Perimeter right atrial model 7205) and coronary sinus (Perimeter coronary sinus model 7109) defibrillation leads and a bipolar endocardial ventricular pacing lead. The device has a volume of 53 cc and weighs 79 g or 82 g (3000 or 3020 respectively). It detects AF by means of specific algorithms and delivers R-wave synchronous defibrillation shocks to convert AF to sinus rhythm; it is also able to pace the ventricle after shock in the event of bradycardia. The 3000 IAD model has an 80-μF capacitor with a maximal shock of 3 J with a biphasic waveform of 3 ms/3 ms. The 3020 IAD model has a 160-μF capacitor with a maximal shock of 6 J with a biphasic waveform of 6 ms/6 ms. The device can be programmed in the monitor mode, in the patient- or physician-activated mode and in the automatic mode.

The Metrix device has been implanted in slightly over 200 patients and new implants have currently been suspended because of a technological improvements to the system. Preliminary data regarding 51 patients from 19 different centers have recently been reported by Wellens and coworkers [6]. All patients had frequent recurrences (> 1 week and < 3 months) of paroxysmal or persistent AF in spite of drug therapy (mean 3.9 drugs tested per patient). These belonged to a larger group of patients screened for defibrillator implantation (119 patients), of whom 44 (36%) were excluded because of a high defibrillation threshold (> 6 J). The majority of the 51 patients treated with IAD were free from organic heart disease, and had normal left ventricular function and a low risk of ventricular tachyarrhythmias. In all patients the device was set to the physician-activated mode. During a mean follow-up of 259 ± 138 days (minimum 3 months) 41 patients (80%) had 227 episodes of AF. Sinus rhythm was restored by the Metrix system in 96% of episodes, with a mean number of three shocks per episode. In ten cases (4%) in 9 different patients (22%) the device was not able to restore sinus rhythm. Early recurrences of AF (within 1 min of sinus rhythm restoration) were observed in 62 episodes (27%) in 21 patients (51%), and 36 of these (58%) were once again shock-treated after pharmacological therapy. The success rate of the device in achieving a stable sinus rhythm was therefore 86%.

With regard to safety, it is mandatory to underline that on a total of 3719 R-wave synchronized shocks delivered (during implantation and follow-up) with a minimum pre-shock RR interval of 500 ms, no ventricular arrhythmias were induced. The defibrillation threshold was substantially the same at the time of implantation and after 3 months. Analysis of the AF detection algorithm performance during observed operations revealed a 92% sensitivity (1178 tests for the detection of AF) and 100% specificity (1062 tests for the recognition of sinus rhythm). Regarding complications, one cardiac tamponade, two subclavian vein thromboses, two lead dislocations and two device and lead explantations (because of infection) were observed. Marked variability in shock tolerance between patients was reported. The number of shocks is important, since discomfort grows as the number of shocks increases.

The Metrix system can be considered an efficacious and safe device, at least in the population studied by Wellens; this has been confirmed in many other patients (about 200) implanted worldwide. Therefore, in some subjects the IAD was programmed in the patient-activated mode and activated out-of-hospital, without inducing proarrhythmic effects. The activation of the IAD within a few minutes of the beginning of AF should be useful in avoiding atrial electrical remodeling, thus favoring sinus rhythm restoration and reducing early and late AF recurrences. Indeed, preliminary data by Timmermans and Wellens [7] would seem to confirm that prompt cardioversion of AF prolongs arrhythmia-free intervals. However, this model of IAD has several limitations: (1) the maximum energy delivery is too low and in many patients the device cannot be implanted because of a high defibrillation threshold; (2) as this atrioverter is a single-chamber non-rate-responsive pacing device, it does not enable single-site or multisite atrial pacing to be carried out to prevent and/or treat AF recurrences; (3) lack of ventricular defibrillation does not allow implantation in patients with organic heart disease and high risk of ventricular arrhythmias; (4) since shock tolerance is low, quality of life would not be improved in patients with a high number of AF relapses, but paradoxically worsened because of the many painful shocks delivered.

7250 Jewel AF

The Jewel 7250 AF is a dual-chamber implantable cardioverter defibrillator capable of pacing and defibrillating both atria and ventricles. It is 55 cc in volume and 93 g in weight and is connected to two or three catheters: two catheters are positioned in the right ventricular apex (Sprint 6932 or 6943 with single spring or Sprint 6942 or 6945 with dual spring) and in the right atrium (Sprint 6932 or 6943 with single spring or Capsure Fix 6940 without spring) respectively; another catheter (Sprint 6932 with single spring) is positioned in the coronary sinus if the atrial defibrillation threshold during implantation is high (about 7% of patients). This device has an important effect on AF prevention, as it provides atrial pacing both during bradycardia periods and with overdrive atrial pacing and/or post-extrasystolic pacing by means of specific algorithms. Moreover, it is possible to treat other supraventricular arrhythmias, such as atrial flutter and atrial tachycardia (AT) by delivering burst pacing, ramp pacing or 50 Hz burst pacing. The device can be set to the monitor mode, patient- or physician-activated mode or automatic mode.

So far, data on patients treated with the Jewel 7250 AF have been presented at international congresses or in abstract form only. Preliminary clinical experience worldwide [8] involves 142 patients with malignant ventricular tachyarrhythmias and paroxysmal AF. During a mean follow-up of 4.5 months, 19 patients had 220 episodes of atrial flutter and 23 patients had 119 episodes of AF. When used, antitachy pacing interrupted atrial flutter in 87% of episodes, 50 Hz burst pacing in 31% and atrial shocks in 75%. In patients with AF recurrence, atrial defibrillation was performed in only a few cases and atrial shocks were successful in 88% of episodes. No proarrhythmic effects were observed. Data from a multicenter study on patients with AT and AF and no prior ventricular tachycardia/ventricular fibrillation (VT/VF) who underwent implantation of the Jewel 7250 AF have recently been presented [9]. Worldwide experience concerns 51 patients (left ventricular ejection fraction: 55 ± 16%, left atrial size: 43 ± 9 mm) of whom 35% were in NYHA class II or III. During a mean follow-up of 3.2 ± 2.5 months, 13 patients had 156 spontaneous AT episodes and 28 patients had 206 spontaneous AF episodes. In the former, antitachy pacing was successful in 33/37 (89%) episodes, 50 Hz burst pacing in 22/95 (23%) and atrial shocks in 24/24 (100%). In the latter, 50 Hz burst pacing was successful in 22/55 (40%) episodes and atrial shocks in 139/151 (92%). Nine patients successfully treated 43/44 spontaneous AF episodes themselves using the patient activator (model 9464). Moreover, 2 patients without prior history of VT/VF received successful shock therapy for a spontaneous VF episode.

Painless successful therapy of 35% of spontaneous AT and 11% of spontaneous AF is an important new exclusive aspect of this IAD. While the efficacy of atrial shock in treating spontaneous recurrences of AF is similar to that of the Metrix system, the opportunity of ventricular defibrillation may be a significant advantage in patients with an organic heart disease.

Conclusions

In conclusion, both IAD systems are efficacious and safe in the treatment of spontaneous recurrences of AF; the prompt restoration of sinus rhythm seems to decrease atrial remodeling and to prolong AF-free intervals (data are still preliminary and concern few patients and a short follow-up period). However, patient shock tolerance is very low and constitutes a major limitation to extending implantation. Indeed, more or less intense discomfort is reported for energies between 1 J and 3 J, and real pain is reported for energies > 3 Joules, which are needed to treat almost all arrhythmia recurrences. This low tolerance and the cost of the devices necessitate selecting which patients to treat with IAD. At present, IAD implantation is usually suggested for patients without heart disease and with a high AF recurrence rate who do not respond to pharmacological treatment. Neverthless, in our opinion, IAD could be more beneficial to heart disease patients for example those with low left ventricular function or with a restrictive pattern, in whom sinus rhythm restoration really determines a hemodynamic advantage that improves quality of life and is likely to decrease in thromboembolic events and mortality [10]. A foreseeable, future development may well involve the integration of a pharmacological reservoir into the IAD to provide pharmacological atrial defibrillation associated with electrical defibrillation [11]. Such a system should be more acceptable to the patient and lead to an extension of IAD indications. Moreover, technological improvements, such as the implementation of rate-responsive atrial pacing, could extend current implant indications to brady-tachy syndrome patients, in whom atrial pacing can represent a useful objective option to prevent or interrupt some arrhythmia recurrences.

References

1. Bialy D, Lehmann MH, Schumacher DN, Steinman RT, Meissner MD (1992) Hospitalization for arrhythmias in the United States: importance of atrial fibrillation. J Am Coll Cardiol 19:41A (abstr)
2. Wolf PA, Mitchell JB, Baker CS, Kannel WB, D'Agostino RB (1995) Mortality and hospital costs associated with atrial fibrillation. Circulation 92:I-140 (abstr)
3. Keane D, Zou L, Ruskin J (1998) Nonpharmacologic therapies for atrial fibrillation. Am J Cardiol 81:C 41-C45
4. Levy S, Ricard P, Lau CP et al (1997) Multicenter low energy transvenous atrial defibrillation. J Am Coll Cardiol 29:750-755
5. Wijffels MCEF, Kirchof CJHJ, Dorland R, Allessie MA (1995) Atrial fibrillation begets atrial fibrillation: a study in awake chronically instrumented goats. Circulation 92:1954-1968
6. Wellens HJJ, Lau CP, Lüderitz B et al (1998) Atrioverter: an implantable device for the treatment of atrial fibrillation. Circulation 98:1651-1656
7. Timmermans C, Wellens HJJ (1998) Effect of device-mediated therapy on symptomatic episodes of atrial fibrillation. J Am Coll Cardiol 31:331A (abstr)
8. Wharton M (1998) Treatment of spontaneous atrial tachyarrhythmias with the Medtronic 7250 Jewel AF: worldwide clinical experience. Circulation 98:I-190 (abstr)
9. Sulke N, Bailin SJ, Swerdlow CD, for the Worldwide 7250 Jewel AF-Only Investigators (1999) Worldwide clinical experience with a dual chamber implantable cardioverter defibrillator in patients with atrial fibrillation and flutter. Eur Heart J (in press) (abstr)
10. Raviele A, Gasparini G, Bonso A et al (1998) Trattamento non farmacologico della fibrillazione atriale parossistica refrattaria ai farmaci: defibrillatore atriale o ablazione + pacemaker? In: Alboni P (ed) Controversies in clinical arrhythmology. Cento (FE), pp 118-120
11. Raviele A, Brignole M, Menozzi C et al (1998) Development of an implantable drug delivery system for the treatment of vasovagal syncope: a dream or a real prospect? In: Raviele A (ed) Cardiac arrhythmias 1997. Springer, Milano, pp 422-427

Implantable Atrial Defibrillator: What Are the Future Perspectives?

W. JUNG, C. WOLPERT, S. HERWIG AND B. LÜDERITZ

Introduction

Atrial fibrillation (AF) is a frequent and costly health care problem, being the most common arrhythmia that leads to hospital admission. The overall prevalence of AF in the United States ranges from less than 1% in young, otherwise healthy individuals up to nearly 9% in elderly patients. AF may cause disabling symptoms and serious adverse effects such as impairment of cardiac function or thromboembolic events. Due to the limited efficacy of antiarrhythmic drugs for AF, several nonpharmacologic options have evolved, including pacemaker therapy, transvenous catheter ablation techniques, surgical procedures, and treatment with an implantable atrial defibrillator (IAD). The high prevalence of AF and its clinical complications, the poor efficacy of medical therapy in preventing recurrences, and dissatisfaction with alternative modes of therapy stimulated interest in an IAD [1]. We report on the worldwide experience with the first IAD, the Metrix system, model 3000 and 3020 (InControl Inc., Redmond, Wash., USA).

The Metrix System

Recently, a standalone IAD, the Metrix system (models 3000 and 3020), has entered clinical investigation [2-6]. The Metrix model 3000 and its successor 3020 differ principally in their maximum energy output, 3 J for the Metrix 3000 and 6 J for the Metrix 3020. Both deliver a biphasic truncated exponential waveform of 3/3 ms and 6/6 ms duration respectively, which accounts for the increased energy output of the model 3020. The device, with a weight of 79 g and a volume of 53 ml, is intended for implantation in the pectoral region like a conventional antibradycardiac pacemaker (Fig. 1). Graded shock therapy is available for up to eight shocks (two at each level) for each episode of AF. Biphasic shocks are programmable in 20-V increments up to 300 V. Atrial defibrillation is accomplished by a shock delivered between electrodes

Department of Medicine-Cardiology, University of Bonn, Germany

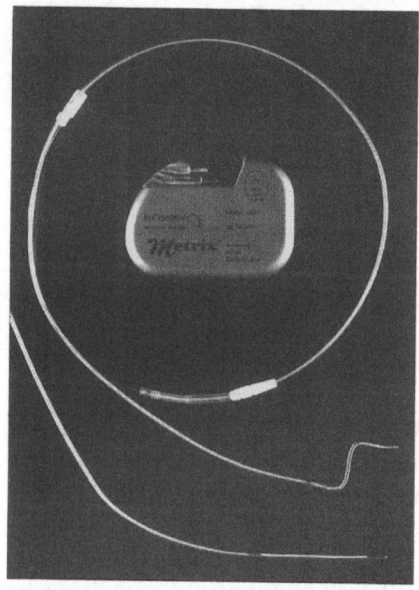

Fig. 1. The Metrix implantable atrial defibrillator and the atrial defibrillation leads. The device has a weight of 79 g and a volume of 53 ml, and is implanted in the pectoral region. The defibrillation coils for the right atrium and the coronary sinus leads are each 6 cm long. The defibrillation lead for the right atrium has a nonretractable screw-in active fixation and the defibrillation lead for the coronary sinus has a spiral configuration at the end, designed to stabilize the lead in the coronary sinus

in the right atrium and the coronary sinus. The right atrium lead has an active fixation in the right atrium. The coronary sinus lead has a natural spiral configuration for retention in the coronary sinus, and can be straightened with a stylet. Both leads are 7 French in diameter and the defibrillation coils are each 6 cm in length. The electrodes may be placed using separate leads, or, very soon, by using a single bipolar lead. A separate bipolar right ventricular lead is used for R wave synchronization and postshock pacing. The Metrix defibrillator can be used to induce AF by using R-wave synchronous shocks and can store intracardiac electrograms for up to 2 min from the most recent six AF episodes. The device can be programmed into one of the following operating modes: fully automatic, patient activated, monitor mode, bradycardia pacing only, and off. As AF is not life-threatening, in the automatic mode the device is only intermittently active in detecting and treating AF, and this "sleep-wake-up" cycle interval is programmable. At the end of the interval it "awakens" and runs its detection algorithm. If AF is not detected it returns to the "sleep" mode for another cycle. The sleep mode significantly reduces energy consumption and prolongs device life. The patient-activated mode differs from the automatic mode in that the device "awakens" only when a magnet is placed briefly over it. This allows the patient to control when the device is able to deliver therapy, yet does not allow the patient to initiate a shock in the absence of AF.

Results

The first Metrix atrial defibrillator was implanted on October 30, 1995, and two further devices were implanted on November 7 and 10, 1995. Initial clinical experience with these three human implants has been recently reported [7].

In April 1996, the phase I Metrix multicenter clinical trial was started [8]. The primary objective of this clinical study is to evaluate the safety of the device in terms of appropriate shock synchronization to avoid shock induced ventricular proarrhythmia. The secondary endpoint is to assess efficacy in detecting and terminating AF. Preimplant testing was performed using designated temporary catheters. The purpose of this testing is to ensure that the atrial defibrillation level obtained is suitable for implantation of the device. Three endocardial catheters were positioned in the coronary sinus, the right atrium, and the apex of the right ventricle. Biphasic shocks were delivered between the catheters placed in the coronary sinus and the right atrium. A separate endocardial lead placed in the right ventricle was used for proper R wave synchronization. As of May 1997, a total of 51 Metrix systems had been implanted as part of the phase I multicenter clinical trial. These 51 patients were selected from 119 patients undergoing a screening test procedure. Figure 2 shows a chest X-ray of a patient with an implanted Metrix system. The results of this phase I clinical trial have been recently published [9]. The findings suggest that both defibrillation thresholds and electrograms are stable over time (implant to 3 months). The device is effective in converting spontaneous episodes of AF. Detection accuracy has been excellent and there have been no errors of R wave selection for synchronization. No proarrhythmias have resulted from over 3500 shocks delivered [8-10].

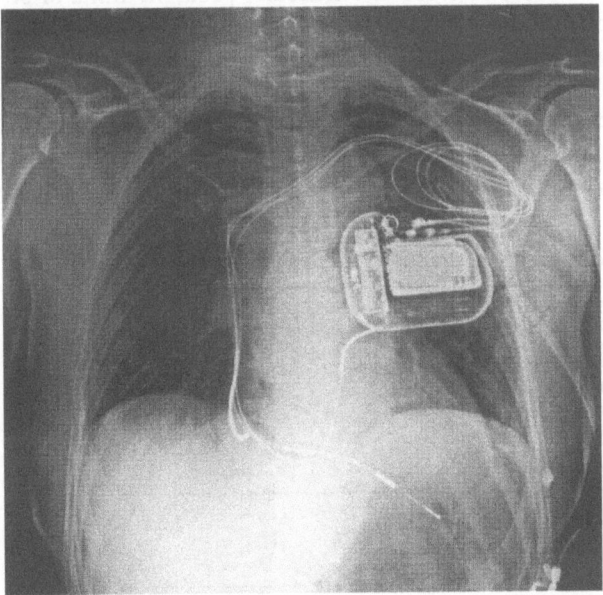

Fig. 2. Chest X-ray (posteroanterior view) of the implanted Metrix system. The pulse generator is implanted subpectorally in the left pectoral region and combined with an active fixation lead placed in the right atrium, a passive fixation lead advanced deep in the coronary sinus, and a conventional bipolar lead positioned in the right ventricle for proper R wave synchronization and postshock VVI pacing

Out-of-Hospital Treatment

As of October 1998, more than 200 Metrix systems have been implanted world-wide [11]. Safety and efficacy data are available for the first 186 implants. To date, most Metrix patients have presented at implant as highly symptomatic and refractory to or intolerant of conventional medical management. In addition, many have experienced external cardioversion one or more times. The majority of patients implanted with the Metrix atrial defibrillator have presented with a relatively healthy cardiovascular history. On average, in this patient population the AF has proven refractory to medical therapy. The presentation of AF has ranged from paroxysmal to long-standing and persistent. In general, the study has excluded patients whose AF episode frequency is greater than once per week or less than once per 3 months. Patient demographics are listed in Table 1. Because AF is not acutely life-threatening, it needs not be treated immediately upon detection. Unlike an implantable ventricular defibrillator, the Metrix system is designed to be highly specific and conservative in its detection and treatment decisions. In over 3300 AF detection tests, the "Mirror" detection algorithm exhibited 100% specificity with a sensitivity of 90.8% using default values (Table 2). To date, no inappropriate shocks have been delivered. Of a total of 336 587 analyzed R waves, about one-third (170 295) have been marked as suitable for potential shock delivery. Out of 8358 shocks delivered, no cases of ventricular proarrhythmia or stroke have been observed (Table 3). There have been no dislodgments of the coronary sinus lead. This lead plays a critical role in enhancing AF detection and lowering conversion energies. The number of shocks delivered per AF episode is 2.4 in the ongoing study versus 3.0 in the phase I clinical study. The conversion to sinus rhythm and the clinical success rate are similar in both studies, with electrical success rates of 93% and 96%, and clinical efficacy rates of 84% and 86%, respectively.

Table 1. Patient demographic characteristics

Number of patients	186
Male/female	138/48
Average age (years)	59
Preimplant drugs failed (mean no.)	3.8
Left atrial size (cm)	2.5-8.0
Ejection fraction (%)	57
Mean follow-up (months)	9.4

Table 2. Mirror detection algorithm

AF detection tests	3313
Specificity	100%
Sensitivity	90.1%
Positive predictive value	100%
Negative predictive value	90.8%
No inappropriate therapy	

Table 3. R wave synchronization

R waves analyzed	336587
R waves marked	170295
Synchronization accuracy	100%
Shocks delivered	8358
No proarrhythmia	

Patient-Activated Mode

The Metrix system provides a programmable, patient-controlled mode. As of August 1998, 57 patients had their Metrix devices programmed to this mode. This treatment option enables these patients to deliver therapy when and where it is appropriate and convenient for them. So far, 267 spontaneous episodes of AF have been treated in this way. Most patients have chosen to deliver with no analgesia or sedation. Most AF episodes treated outside the hospital have been terminated with a single shock, with a mean number of shocks per episode of 1.7. No inappropriate shocks have been discharged. In order to allow patients to cardiovert themselves outside the hospital, implanting centers must complete an observed (in-hospital) therapy phase. Experience to date suggests that clinical success of the Metrix system is not dependent on the setting in which therapy outside the hospital is administered. Patients administering therapy outside the hospital have successfully terminated 81% of spontaneous AF episodes, versus 84% in the hospital.

What Are the Future Perspectives?

For any new therapy, it is imperative to demonstrate safety, efficacy, tolerability with improvement in quality of life, and cost-effectiveness compared to already available therapeutic options. Most importantly, the efficacy and safety rates with a new therapy should be better or at least as good than those observed with previously available means. Maintenance of sinus rhythm or prolonged duration of arrhythmia-free intervals should be clearly demonstrated with an IAD. There is still concern among several physicians that one of the adverse effects of an IAD, shock-induced ventricular proarrhythmia, may in fact have a negative impact on survival. Furthermore, wide experience gained with the implantable ventricular defibrillator has shown that the short- and long-term morbidity and complications associated with such devices are not negligible. Further efforts have to be undertaken to reduce the patient discomfort associated with internal atrial defibrillation in an attempt to make this new therapy acceptable to a larger patient population with AF. Finally, cost-effectiveness and quality-of-life analyses comparing an IAD with alternative therapeutic approaches will be needed.

Many of the future improvements in AF therapy will follow improved patient identification and categorization. There appears to be a subset of patients with recurrent AF who can be treated with atrial defibrillation today. A further subset of the population with bradyarrhythmias will benefit from combined pacing and defibrillation. The subset of patients with a history of ventricular tachyarrhythmias will benefit from a device that has ventricular back-up defibrillation capabilities. Finally, those patients currently labeled as having permanent AF may end up having recurrent AF following either ablation or serial cardioversion [12].

The spectrum of nonpharmacologic therapeutic modalities that are evolving to treat AF will probably require that patients undergo a more detailed evaluation to best characterize their AF so that the most appropriate treatment modalities can be prescribed. Given the complex pathophysiology underlying AF, it is unlikely that one therapeutic modality will adequately treat the majority of AF. Instead, hybrid therapies including ablation and/or electrotherapy in conjunction with pharmacotherapy will probably be required to offer patients the best outcome.

References

1. Lüderitz B, Pfeiffer D, Tebbenjohanns J, Jung W (1966) Nonpharmacologic strategies for treating atrial fibrillation. Am J Cardiol 77:45A-52A
2. Jung W, Lüderitz B (1997) Implantable atrial defibrillator: which results and indications. In: Raviele A (ed) Cardiac arrhythmias. Springer, Berlin Heidelberg New York, pp 100-109
3. Jung W, Wolpert C, Esmailzadeh B et al (1998) Specific considerations with the automatic implantable atrial defibrillator. J Cardiovasc Electrophysiol 9:S193-S201
4. Jung W, Lüderitz B (1997) Implantable atrial defibrillator: quo vadis? (editorial) Pacing Clin Electrophysiol 20:2141-2145
5. Jung W, Tebbenjohanns J, Wolpert C et al (1995) Safety, efficacy, and pain perception of internal atrial defibrillation in humans. Circulation 92:472 (abstr)
6. Jung W, Lüderitz B (1998) Quality of life of patients with atrial fibrillation. J Cardiovasc Electrophysiol 9:S177-S186
7. Lau CP, Tse HF, Lok NS et al (1977) Initial clinical experience with an implantable human atrial defibrillator. Pacing Clin Electrophysiol 20:220-225
8. Jung W, Kirchhoff PG, Lau CP, Tse HF, Lüderitz B, for the Metrix System Clinical Investigational Group (1997) Therapy delivery with the METRIX automatic atrial defibrillation system: threshold stability and shock safety. J Am Coll Cardiol 29:78A (abstr)
9. Wellens HJJ, Lau CP, Lüderitz B et al, for the Metrix Investigators (1998) The atrioverter, an implantable device for treatment of atrial fibrillation. Circulation 98:1651-1656
10. Jung W, Wolpert C, Herwig S et al (1998) Initial experience with the implantable atrial defibrillator. G Ital Cardiol 28 (suppl 1):592-594
11. Jung W, Wolpert C, Spehl S et al, for the Worldwide Metrix Investigators (1998) Worldwide experience with the Metrix implantable atrial defibrillator. In: Adornato E (ed) Rhythm control from cardiac evaluation to treatment. Edizioni Luigi Pozzi, Rome, pp 139-143
12. Reuter D, Ayers GM (1998) Future directions of electrotherapy for atrial fibrillation. J Cardiovasc Electrophysiol 9:S202-S210

Implantable Atrial Defibrillator: Why not a Patient-Activated Drug Delivery System?

A. BONSO, G. GASPARINI, S. THEMISTOCLAKIS, F. GIADA AND A. RAVIELE

Epidemiology of Atrial Fibrillation

Atrial fibrillation is a very frequent and potentially dangerous cardiac arrhythmia, increasing in prevalence with advancing years (from < 0.3% between 25 and 35 years of age to > 5% between 62 and 90 years of age) [1]. The arrhythmia is a source of substantial morbidity and mortality and is associated with increased medical care costs. The risk of systemic embolism and stroke is approximately 3- to 5-fold enhanced in patients with atrial fibrillation and full anticoagulation is frequently recommended in these patients [2]. The loss of atrial contraction and the irregularity of RR intervals reduce cardiac performance and may precipitate heart failure in patients with organic heart disease. It is also possible that a tachycardia-induced cardiomyopathy develops as consequence of a persistently high ventricular rate during atrial fibrillation [3]. Quality of life is frequently compromised by the occurrence of atrial fibrillation and patients often complain of disabling symptoms such as palpitations, fatigue, dyspnea and angina [4]. Finally, the risk of dying is 1.5- to 1.9-fold increased in patients with atrial fibrillation, even after adjustment for other variables [5]. Atrial fibrillation is also the most common cardiac rhythm disorder associated with hospitalization, being responsible for 0.5% of all hospital admissions and for one-third of all arrhythmia principal diagnoses [6]. It has been estimated that hospital costs are 12% to 24% higher in patients with atrial fibrillation compared with those without atrial fibrillation [7].

Rationale for Restoration of Sinus Rhythm

The high prevalence of atrial fibrillation and its clinical and socioeconomic consequences justify the growing interest in this arryhthmia as well as the numerous therapeutical options recently developed in an attempt to restore and mantain sinus rhythm. Restoration of sinus rhythm, indeed, may reduce thromboembolic complications, correct heart failure, eliminate symptoms and most likely improve

Reparto di Cardiologia, Ospedale Umberto I, Mestre, Venice, Italy

survival. Established methods for conversion of atrial fibrillation to sinus rhythm include treatment with antiarrhythmic drugs, external high-energy shocks and internal low-energy defibrillation. This latter method allows to restore sinus rhythm in the majority of patients (77%-100%, 88% as mean) [8], including those that in the past were considered to be poorly responder to external atrial defibrillation such as patients with long-lasting atrial fibrillation (duration > 1-2 years) or very enlarged atria (left atrial diameter > 5-6 cm). Once restoration of sinus rhythm has been achieved, antiarrhythmic drugs are usually prescribed in an attempt to prevent arrhythmia recurrences. However, chronic oral therapy with these drugs is of limited efficacy and not rarely is associated with intolerable side-effects, potential risk for proarrhythmia and aggravation of heart failure, and poor patient compliance. For these reasons, several nonpharmacologic options have evolved in the last years, including pacemaker therapy, transvenous catheter ablation techniques, surgical procedures, and treatment with an implantable atrial defibrillator.

Implantable Electrical Atrial Defibrillator: Results and Limitations

This latter device has been recently introduced into clinical practice with the purpose to keep patients in sinus rhythm by converting atrial fibrillation as soon as it occurs. Indeed, recent studies have suggested that quick interruption of atrial fibrillation is crucial in order to avoid the so-called electrical remodeling of the atria (consisting in a reduction and dispersion of refractoriness) that tends to perpetuate the arrhythmia and to favor early recurrences after successful cardioversion [9]. Up to now two models of electrical atrial defibrillator have entered clinical investigation, the stand-alone device Metrix Atrioverter series 3020 and 3022 (In Control, Redmond, WA) and the combined dual-chamber device Jewel 7250 AF (Medtronic-Minneapolis, MN). Both these models have proven to be either effective (acute success > 90% and clinical success > 80%) and safe (no case of ventricular proarrhythmia in > 3000 shocks delivered) in converting spontaneous episodes of atrial fibrillation [8, 10-12]. However, the current models of electrical atrial defibrillators have a major limitation represented by the poor patient tolerability of the shock and acceptance of the device. Indeed, a mild to moderate discomfort is already felt for shock energy > 1 J and a true pain for shock energy > 3J, that is the energy usually required in clinical practice to interrupt arrhythmic recurrences [13-15].

Rationale for an Implantable Pharmacological Atrial Defibrillator

The problem of shock-related discomfort or pain has stimulated the concept and development of an implantable drug delivery system for treatment of atrial fibrillation, the so-called pharmacological atrial defibrillator [16, 17]. Such a device would allow the automatic, "on demand" intravenous or intracardiac delivery of a bolus of an antiarrhythmic drug able to painlessly terminate most episodes of atrial fibrillation. Ideally, the pharmacological defibrillator should be coupled with an electrical defibrillator to permit shock delivery and electrical cardioversion in case of drug failure. Also, the implementation of additional features, such as dual-chamber rate-responsive pacing and back-up ventricular defibrillation, seem to be desirable in order to increase the efficacy and safety of the system.

Key-issues

The main key-issues to be addressed prior to implementation of a fully automatic pharmacological atrial defibrillator include:
1. The choice of a reliable algorithm to recognize arrhythmia occurrence
2. The search for the most appropriate drug
3. The conception and building of the device.

Algorithms for Detection of Atrial Fibrillation

At present, there are many algorithms to allow detection of atrial fibrillation. Those chosen for the currently available models of electrical implantable atrial defibrillator (Metrix Atrioverter 3022 and Jewel 7250 AF) have shown to be highly sensitive (92%) and specific (100%) [18] and may be also used in an implantable drug pump.

Most Appropriate Drug

Many drugs have been proposed for the chronic oral therapy of atrial fibrillation. However, only few of them have the characteristics that are indispensable for the intermittent use required in an implantable drug delivery system. The ideal drug for this purpose [19] should be highly effective and safe to allow arrhythmia termination in the majority of cases and to avoid unpleasant side effects, proarrhythmia and other serious complications. Moreover, it should be fast-acting and its action duration should be short to permit rapid interruption of atrial fibrillation and repeated drug infusions, if necessary. Finally, it should be stable over time at body temperature for a long period of time (at least several months) and its effective dose should be contained in a small volume to avoid the use of a big reservoir and frequent refilling of the pump.

Among the theoretically potential candidates, procainamide, flecainide and ibutilide have been advocated as possible agents to be used with an implantable pump [17]. However, in literature there is only little information on the effects of these drugs when rapidly and directly injected into the right atrium. This way of administration is believed to allow to temporarily achieve higher plasma and myocardium concentration with a smaller dose. However, conflicting results have been reported to this regard with procainamide [17, 20]. Thus, studies are needed to assess the usefulness of the different antiarrhythmic drugs when centrally delivered into the circulation. A multicenter study with flecainide has recently started in Italy with this goal. The protocol of this study may be summarized as follows. To be included into the study patients must have atrial fibrillation > 2 h in duration, with onset within 48 h. The main exclusion criteria are the following: acute or transient cause of atrial fibrillation; ischemic heart disease or any heart disease with moderate to severe hemodynamic compromising; hypotension; relevant sick sinus syndrome and/or atrioventricular and/or intraventricular conduction disturbances; history of life-threatening ventricular arrhythmias; treatment with class I or III antiarrhythmic drugs. The study has two phases. In phase 1, patients with recent-onset atrial fibrillation are treated with an intravenous infusion of flecainide (2 mg/kg in 10 min). If flecainide restores sinus rhythm and the drug is well tolerated, the patient is advanced to phase 2. In phase 2, an electrophysiologic study is performed. If atrial fibrillation (> 10 min duration) is induced, flecainide is administered directly into the right atrium at progressively increasing doses, starting with a bolus of 0.25 mg/kg in 15 s up to reach the maximum tolerated dose. The primary endpoint of the study is restoration of sinus rhythm either during or by 10 min after the end of flecainide infusion. Secondary endpoints to be evaluated are the proportion of patients converting to sinus rhythm and time to conversion by 24 h after the start of the infusion.

Conception and Building of the Device: Fully Automatic System and Patient-Activated System

Nowadays, a fully automatic implantable drug delivery system for treatment of atrial fibrillation does not exist. However, its realization is not difficult with the formidable technology currently available. Obviously, such a pump should have all the necessary elements, such as drug reservoir, telemetry, electronic controls, and power source. It would be important to incorporate this pump into a more "universal" device capable of stimulating and defibrillating the atria and the ventricles, besides delivering drugs. While waiting for this device, it is already possible to use a modified version of Algomed system (Medtronic, Minneapolis, MN), that has been recently built for treatment of vasovagal syncope, as a manual drug delivery system to be activated by the patient at time of symptom occurrence.

References

1. Kannel WB, Wolf PA (1992) Epidemiology of atrial fibrillation. In: Falk RH, Podrid PJ (eds) Atrial fibrillation. Mechanisms and management. Raven, New York, pp 81-93
2. Atrial fibrillation Investigators (1994) Risk factors for stroke and efficacy of antithrombotic therapy in atrial fibrillation: analysis of pooled data from five randomized controlled trials. Arch Intern Med 154:1449-1457
3. Shinbane JS, Wood MA, Jensen DN et al (1997) Tachycardia-induced cardiomyopathy: a review of animal models and clinical studies. J Am Coll Cardiol 29:709-715
4. Jung W, Herwig S, Newman D et al (1999) Impact of atrial fibrillation on quality of life: a prospective, multicenter study. Circulation 33[Suppl A]:104A (abstr)
5. Benjamin EJ, Wolf PA, D'Agostino RB et al (1998) Impact of atrial fibrillation on the risk of death. The Framingham heart study. Circulation 98:946-952
6. Bialy D, Lehmann MH, Schumacher DN, et al (1992) Hospitalization for arrhythmias in the United States: importance of atrial fibrillation (abstract). J Am Coll Cardiol 19:41A
7. Wolf PA, Mitchell JB, Baker CS et al (1995) Mortality and hospital costs associated with atrial fibrillation. Circulation 92 [Suppl I]:I-140 (abstr)

8. Raviele A, Gasparini G, Bonso A et al (1999) Current role of implantable atrial defibrillator in the treatment of paroxysmal atrial fibrillation. G Ital Aritmol Cardiostim 1 (in press)

9. Wijffels MCEF, Kirchof CJHJ, Dorland R, Allessie MA (1995) Atrial fibrillation begets atrial fibrillation. A study in awake chronically instrumented goats. Circulation 92:1954-1968

10. Wellens HJJ, Lau CP, Luderitz B et al (1998) Atrioverter: an implantable device for the treatment of atrial fibrillation. Circulation 98:1651-1656

11. Lerman B, Stein K, Markowitz S (1998) Worldwide clinical experience with the model 7250 Jewel AF dual chamber arrhythmia management device. PACE 21:872 (abstr)

12. Wharton M (1998) Treatment of spontaneous atrial tachyarrhythmias with the Medtronic 7250 Jewel AF: worldwide clinical experience. Circulation 98[Suppl]:I-190 (abstr)

13. Murgatroyd FD, Slade AKB, Sopher SM et al (1995) Efficacy and tolerability of transvenous low energy cardioversion of paroxysmal atrial fibrillation in humans. J Am Coll Cardiol 25:1347-1353

14. Santini M, Pandozi C (1997) La cardioversione endocavitaria a bassa energia nella fibrillazione atriale: efficacia, sicurezza, tollerabilità, indicazioni e prospettive future. G Ital Cardiol 27:191-196

15. Tomassoni G, Newby KH, Kearney MM et al (1996) Testing different waveforms and capacitances: effect on atrial defibrillation threshold and pain perception. J Am Coll Cardiol 28:695-699

16. Bump T, Yurkonis C, Brown J et al (1989) Automatic implantable drug delivery for conversion of atrial fibrillation. In: Update in drug delivery systems. Futura Mt Kisco NY, pp 303-309

17. Arzbaecher R, Gemperline J, Haklin M et al (1998) Rapid drug infusion for termination of atrial fibrillation in an experimental model. PACE 21:288-291

18. Tse H, Lau C, Sra J et al (1999) Atrial fibrillation detection and R-wave synchronization by Metrix implantable atrial defibrillator. Implications for long-term efficacy and safety. Circulation 99:1446-1451

19. Raviele A, Brignole M, Menozzi C et al (1998) Development of an implantable drug delivery system for the treatment of vasovagal syncope: a dream or a real prospect? In: Raviele A (ed) Cardiac arrhythmias 1997. Springer, Milano, pp 422-427

20. Vereckei A, Arnett CJ, Warman E et al (1999) Comparison of the effects of right atrial and intravenous procainamide delivery on drug levels, electrophysiological parameters and termination of atrial fibrillation in dogs. PACE 22:18 (abstr)

Ablation of Atrial Fibrillation: How Should Patients Be Selected?

F. Gaita, R. Riccardi, L. Calò, L. Garberoglio, M. Scaglione, L. Coda, P. Di Donna, R. Massa, M. Bochiardo, L. Vivalda, S. Miceli and S. Leuzzi

Atrial fibrillation is the most frequent supraventricular arrhythmia, and recently it has become clear that it is not a completely benign arrhythmia, since complications such as thromboembolism or ventricular impairment may sometimes occur. Even in absence of associated cardiac disease, when the incidence of these complications is relatively low, the presence of atrial fibrillation generally causes a worsening of quality of life, due to the irregularity of the rhythm or the high ventricular rate, and therefore generally requires life-long therapy.

Despite the high prevalence of atrial fibrillation in the general population – about 4% in patients older than 60 years – treatment of this arrhythmia is still unsatisfactory because of the relatively low success rate of drugs in preventing recurrences. This may be explained by both the heterogeneity of the term "atrial fibrillation" and our lack of knowledge of the mechanisms underlying this arrhythmia. Atrial fibrillation may be present in very different clinical situations, and as a consequence its electrophysiologic substrate and clinical significance are different, too. The high incidence of atrial fibrillation in patients with hypertensive, dilated and valvular cardiopathy is due to the atrial enlargement present in these conditions; the mechanisms responsible for atrial fibrillation in patients without any organic heart disease, or at least any detectable etiology, are probably different, and in such cases the arrhythmia is generally defined as idiopathic atrial fibrillation. In this latter, various factors have been suggested, ranging from atrial myocarditis or adipose replacement to an imbalance of the autonomic tone.

Some of the lack of knowledge about atrial fibrillation may indeed stem from the fact that few data exist about atrial mapping during atrial fibrillation in the different clinical situations, especially in humans. This lack of knowledge may be the reason why therapy is generally unsatisfactory, and the cardiologists have been studying new non-pharmacological treatments such as cardiac single or multisite atrial stimulation, AV node modulation/ablation and, more recently, atrial endocardial catheter ablation.

However, in many cases, non-pharmacological therapy too has been used without any regard to the type of atrial fibrillation. Moreover, nowadays we know

Divisione di Cardiologia, Ospedale Civile di Asti, Italy

that some differences in atrial electrophysiologic features are present even in patients with idiopathic atrial fibrillation. It has been clearly established that during atrial fibrillation different regions of the atria may show differing electrophysiologic behaviour [1, 2]; some regions may show fast, irregular, disorganised atrial activity while, simultaneously, others may be activated by fast but relatively organised and almost regular electrical wavefronts. These different activation patterns may reflect different characteristics of the different parts of the atria, and it can be assumed that the regions showing the most irregular and disorganised activity may be crucial for the maintenance of the arrhythmia, while other regions with relatively regular activation may only be bystanders, and thus ablation in the latter regions may be useless.

In our experience [2] we have observed that in most cases the posterior, posteroseptal and septal regions of both atria are the sites where the most irregular activation is generally present during atrial fibrillation. Similarly it has been demonstrated that the electrical features of the atria during atrial fibrillation are different between patients with the chronic form and those with the paroxysmal form. The more irregular atrial activation and the increased number of regions involved by the presence of disorganised activity in patients with chronic atrial fibrillation may be an expression of electrical remodelling of the atria, with a shortening of refractory periods and an increase in the number of circulating wavelets. Similarly, although it has not been clearly established, it can be assumed that patients with atrial fibrillation associated with cardiac disease have a different atrial electrophysiologic pattern from patients with idiopathic atrial fibrillation.

Moreover, it has been recently demonstrated, that although the classical concept of the multiple reentrant wavelets (Moe's hypothesis) is accepted and considered to be the basis for the maintenance of atrial fibrillation in most cases, a focal drive has been observed in few patients [3], and a focal trigger has been shown to be important in the initiation of the atrial fibrillation [4].

In view of all this, it is clear how atrial fibrillation is a too "generic" term to define an arrhythmia which is actually a group of different arrhythmias with different clinical and electrophysiologic patterns. These observations lead to the assumption that no single technique exists for ablation of atrial fibrillation, but that in all probability different techniques should be used in different patients to cure this arrhythmia, and therefore precise evaluation of the nature of the arrhythmia should be performed.

Cure of atrial fibrillation may be performed by trying either to modify the anatomical substrate responsible for the arrhythmia or to eliminate the trigger underlying the initiation of the arrhythmia. An effective way to modify the substrate is to reduce the critical mass with linear lesions in both atria, as has been demonstrated by surgical ablations, particularly the Maze procedure proposed by Cox [5]. In this approach multiple incisions are created in both atria close enough to prevent wavelet formation and propagation, also reducing the critical mass that must be present for induction and maintenance of the atrial fibrillation, and thus to control the genesis of the arrhythmia. This technique has shown a high success rate but requires a complex surgical procedure with general anaesthesia, thoracotomy and cardiopulmonary by-pass, with related complications and a perioperative mortality varying from 1.3% to 2.1% [6, 7].

More recently, Sueda et al. [8] developed a simpler surgical procedure to be performed on the posterior wall of the left atrium for the treatment of chronic atrial fibrillation associated with mitral valve disease. These authors reported disappearance of atrial fibrillation in 78% of patients 6 months after operation. Our group (data not published) is testing a new and more selective approach to cure atrial fibrillation in patients with concomitant valve surgery, who undergo cardiovascular surgery creating linear lesions between the pulmonary veins and the mitral annulus using cryoablation. The lesions are created by freezing the tissue at -60° for 120 s at each site. The time required to perform our cryoablation procedure was about 20 min. A follow-up period of 6 ± 1 months (range 1-12 months) showed very good success, with 28 of 32 patients (87%) in stable sinus rhythm and with preserved contractility of both atria.

The atrial linear lesions created by cryoablation, being transmural and located in areas that are critical for the initiation and maintenance of atrial fibrilllation, may obviate the need for extensive atrial incision that characterises the Maze procedure and therefore minimize exsanguination and reduce myocardial ischaemic time. For this reason, we believe that nowadays in patients with mitral and/or aortic valvular disease affected by atrial fibrillation who require valve surgery, this is an acceptable indication for concomitant ablation of this arrhythmia. Nevertheless, long-term follow-up of patients who have undergone valve repair or replacement and concomitant ablation is necessary to obtain information about survival and morbidity.

The high success rate of these surgical procedures has led electrophysiologists to develop a catheter technique that mimics these techniques without the need for open chest surgery and its related complications. Swartz et al. [9] and Haïssaguerre et al. [10] were the first who reproduced this technique in humans, demonstrating the feasibility of atrial compartmentalization. Swartz, using a combined approach in the right and left atrium, had a success rate of 79% in a group of 28 patients. However, in some patients two or more procedures were necessary, procedure and fluoroscopy duration were long and, above all, severe complications such as cerebral stroke, cardiac tamponade, bleeding or respiratory distress occurred in more than 20% of cases.

Haïssaguerre in the same period used a similar technique in a group of patients with atrial fibrillation. The technique was effective in about 33% of patients when the ablation was limited to the right atrium and this increased to 60% when an additional ablation was performed in the left atrium. It is worth noting that, although no thromboembolisms occurred during the procedure, pericardial effusion due to cardiac perforation during anticoagulant therapy did occur.

The risk of complication of extensive ablation in the right and left atrium seems, therefore, to be too high for a relatively benign arrhythmia such as atrial fibrillation; on the basis of this consideration new strategies of ablation limited to the right atrium have been developed. Some data support the hypothesis that an ablation limited to the right atrium might be effective in some cases. Atrial fibrillation may be present in different clinical situations and the electrophysiologic substrate may be different, meaning that the left atrium may not necessarily be involved in all kinds of atrial fibrillation, especially in the absence of associated cardiac disease and when an imbalance of the autonomic tone seems to play an important role in its appearance. Furthermore, some experimental data presented by Tondo et al. [11] and Kumagai et al. [12] showed a high success rate in preventing the induction of atrial fibrillation in dogs by creating linear lesions in the right atrium in the midseptum or anteriorly in the region of Bachmann's bundle.

Therefore, in May 1995 our group [1] began performing catheter ablation limited to the right atrium in patients with idiopathic atrial fibrillation, with success in 56% of patients over a mean follow-up period of 11 months, although in about half the successfully treated patients a previously ineffective drug therapy was still necessary to prevent atrial fibrillation recurrences. It is worth underlining that no complications occurred in any patient. Our strategy was to make three linear lesions in the right atrium. The sites of the lesions were decided on the basis of two observations. First, some anatomic barriers are already present in the right atrium; the septum is delimited by some of these (superior and inferior vena cava, crista terminalis, coronary sinus os, Todaro's tendon) and is characterized by the presence in its centre of a non-homogeneous structure that is the fossa ovalis. Second, in our experience, the septum was the region of the right atrium where a more irregular and disorganized electrical activity was recorded; assuming that this factor might be critical for the maintenance of the atrial fibrillation, our ablation strategy considered a linear lesion in the atrial septum to be the first step. The second lesion was performed in the inferior vena cava-tricuspid valve isthmus, because the creation of a lesion from the superior to the inferior vena cava could facilitate the reentrant circuit of atrial flutter. The third transverse lesion, from the fossa ovalis through the posterior wall to the lateral edge of the tricuspid annulus, was performed only in the first patients in an attempt to compartmentalize the right atrium.

In this group of patients a retrospective analysis of atrial mapping and the results of catheter ablation showed some interesting findings. Patients with successful ablation generally present a peculiar pattern characterized by non-homogeneity of the atrial activation in different regions of the right atrium, while this was less evident in patients with unsuccessful ablation. Considering that in this study radiofrequency was delivered mainly in the septal area, and that catheter ablation was more frequently successful in those patients in whom the septum was the region of the right atrium with the shortest FF interval and with the most irregular activation compared to the lateral wall, we might hypothesize that in these patients the lateral wall might be a bystander. By contrast, in the patients with unsuccessful ablation both the lateral and the septal regions showed similar irregular activations, so in these cases the lateral wall may be directly involved in the perpetuation of the arrhythmia. Possible explanations of the lack of success of ablation in these patients may be the difficulty in creating continuous linear lesions in the lateral wall, due to the anatomy of this area, or the need for either more detailed atrial mapping, with evaluation of more sites, or more extensive radiofrequency lesions that would include the left atrium.

These data suggest that catheter ablation of atrial fibrillation might be guided by the localisation of critical areas necessary for the perpetuation of atrial fibrillation, at least in some patients with idiopathic atrial fibrillation. This is in agreement with the hypothesis recently suggested by Konings et al. [13] that, although the atria participate as a whole in the process of atrial fibrillation, not all parts of the atria contribute equally to the perpetuation of the fibrillatory process, suggesting that selective ablation of the areas characterised by abnormal conduction patterns may be effective in the treatment of atrial fibrillation. Moreover, the importance of the septum in the perpetuation of atrial fibrillation has been recently highlighted by Kumagai et al. [14], who showed in dogs that a reentrant circuit in the septum may be a major factor in the maintenance of this arrhythmia.

The initial aim of this experience was to limit the ablation to the right atrium in order to avoid the risks related to extensive ablation in the left atrium, and the ablation was limited to those patients with idiopathic atrial fibrillation and a normal or only mildly dilated left atrium; therefore the results cannot be extrapolated to patients with associated cardiac disease or significant enlargement of left atrium, in whom ablation limited to the right atrium may not be effective.

In some of our patients catheter ablation in the right atrium was effective in eliminating sustained episodes of atrial fibrillation but unmasked the presence of atrial focal tachycardia localised in pulmonary veins, and the ablation of those foci has been effective in the elimination of those tachycardias.

Based on the data published by Haïssaguerre et al. [4] showing that atrial foci may be found in many patients with paroxysmal atrial fibrillation, and in view of the fact that atrial fibrillation may be abolished by elimination of the trigger even without modifying the substrate, our therapeutic strategy has been modified such that, in patients with paroxysmal recurrent atrial fibrillation, atrial foci in pulmonary veins are searched for as a first step (Fig. 1). In a group of 18 patients these foci were found in 12 and ablation was effective in 7 of these 12.

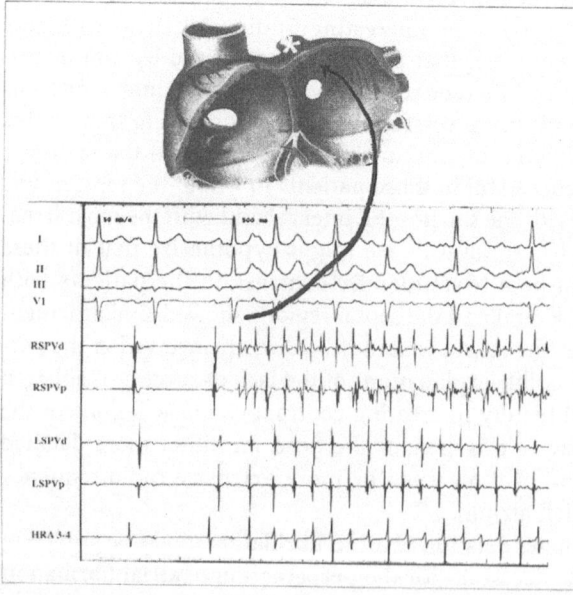

Fig. 1. The figure shows the onset of an episode of atrial fibrillation. The arrhythmia is initiated by a rapid focus on the RSUP. The arrow indicates the first beat of the focus and the site of the successful ablation in the drawing on the top.
RSVP, right superior pulmonary vein; LSPV, left superior pulmonary vein; HRA, right atrium; I, II, III, V1, surface ECG leads

The localisation of these foci allows ablation with selective lesions and a relatively high success rate. However, the technique is more effective in patients with paroxysmal than chronic atrial fibrillation and with many atrial extrasystoles or many non-sustained episodes of atrial fibrillation each day, allowing accurate mapping of these foci that initiate the atrial fibrillation.

Conclusions

Catheter ablation of atrial fibrillation is a new, experimental technique that has shown interesting and promising results, but it cannot be considered as a routine first-choice procedure. Its success in preventing atrial fibrillation recurrences is very variable in the different studies, using different techniques, and so is the incidence of complications.

Two different approaches are nowadays available to cure atrial fibrillation. The first is to modify the substrate responsible for the arrhythmia; this can be performed with linear lesions in the right atrium only – a technique effective only in a small percentage of patients with idiopathic atrial fibrillation – or, in most of the patients with associated heart disease, with linear lesions in the posterior region of left atrium. The second approach consists of eliminating the trigger of the atrial fibrillation, and in these cases ablation of atrial foci generally localised inside pulmonary veins seems to be particularly promising. These two approaches are not in contrast to each other but can be useful in different patients. Improvement in our knowledge of the different electrophysiologic substrates in the different settings of atrial fibrillation, and development of technologies such as catheter cryoablation or ultrasound may influence the development of these techniques to cure atrial fibrillation.

References

1. Gaita F, Riccardi R, Calò L, Scaglione M, Garberoglio L, Antolini R, Kirchner M, Lamberti F, Richiardi E (1998) Atrial mapping and radiofrequency catheter ablation in patients with idiopathic atrial fibrillation. Electrophysiologic findings and ablation results. Circulation 97:2136-2145
2. Gaita F, Calò L, Scaglione M, Riccardi R, Lamberti F, Antolini R, Pecora D, Licciardello G, Kirchner M (1998) Different patterns of atrial activation during paroxysmal and chronic atrial fibrillation. Pacing Clin Electrophysiol 21 (II):937
3. Jais P, Haïssaguerre M, Shah DC, Chouairi S, Gencel L, Hocini M, Clementy J (1997) A focal source of atrial fibrillation treated by discrete radiofrequency ablation. Circulation 95:572-576
4. Haïssaguerre M, Jais P, Shah DC, Takahashi A, Hocini M, Quiniou G, Garrigue S, Le Mouroux A, Le Metayer P, Clementy J (1998) Spontaneous initiation of atrial fibrillation by ectopic beats originating in the pulmonary veins. N Engl J Med 339:659-666
5. Cox JL (1991) The surgical treatment of atrial fibrillation. IV: Surgical technique. J Thorac Cardiovasc Surg 101:584-592

6. Cox JL, Schuessler RB, Lappas DG, Boineau JP (1996) An 8 1/2 year experience with surgery for atrial fibrillation. Ann Surg 224:267-273

7. Kawaguchi AT, Kosakai Y, Isobe F et al (1996) Factors affecting rhythm after the Maze procedure for atrial fibrillation. Circulation 94[Suppl II]:139-142

8. Sueda T, Nagata H, Orihashi K, Morita S, Okada K, Sueshiro M, Hirai S, Matsuura Y (1997) Efficacy of a simple left atrial procedure for chronic atrial fibrillation in mitral valve operations. Ann Thorac Surg 63:1070-1075

9. Swartz JF, Pellersels G, Silvers J, Pattern L, Cervantez D (1994) A catheter-based curative approach to atrial fibrillation in humans. Circulation 90[Suppl I]:I-335 (abstr)

10. Haïssaguerre M, Jais P, Shah DC, Gencel L, Pradeau V, Garrigues S, Chouairi S, Hocini M, Le Métayer P, Roudaut R, Clémenty J (1996) Right and left atrial radiofrequency catheter therapy of paroxysmal atrial fibrillation. J Cardiovasc Electrophysiol 7:1132-1144

11. Tondo C, Scherlag BJ, Otomo K, Antz M, Patterson E, Arruda M, Jackman WM, Lazzara R (1997) Critical atrial site for ablation of pacing-induced atrial fibrillation in the normal dog heart. J Cardiovasc Electrophysiol 8:1255-1265

12. Kumagai K, Uno K, Krestian C, Waldo AL (1996) Single site radiofrequency catheter ablation of atrial fibrillation. J Am Coll Cardiol 27[Suppl A]:4A

13. Konings KTS, Smeets JLRM, Penn OC, Wellens HJJ, Allessie MA (1997) Configuration of unipolar atrial electrograms during electrical induced atrial fibrillation in humans. Circulation 95:1231-1241

14. Kumagai K, Khrestian C, Waldo AL (1997) Simultaneous multisite mapping studies during induced atrial fibrillation in the sterile pericarditis model. Insight into the mechanism of its maintenance. Circulation 95:511-521

An Anatomical Approach to Curing Atrial Fibrillation: Pulmonary Vein Isolation with Through-the-Balloon Ultrasound Ablation

M.D. Lesh, C. Diederich, P. Guerra, Y. Goseki and P.B. Sparks

Introduction

Atrial fibrillation (AF) is the most common sustained arrhythmia in clinical practice. Drug therapy can be associated with a number of untoward effects, such as proarrhythmia, long-term inefficacy and even an increase in mortality. Catheter ablation of the atrioventricular node with pacemaker implantation [1], or modification of the AV node without pacer implantation [2] can facilitate ventricular rate control, but thromboembolic risk is unchanged and atrial systole is not restored. Given these limitations, an approach that cures atrial fibrillation would be highly desirable.

Recently, it has come to be understood that the initiating event in many cases of AF is a "focal trigger" arising in the vast majority of cases from within one of the pulmonary veins [3, 4]. The purpose of the present paper is to briefly describe the development of a novel technology addressing this particular class of AF mechanism.

The "Dual Substrate" for AF

As shown in Fig. 1, our current understanding is that AF has not one but two distinct mechanisms or substrates: the substrate for initiation of AF, and the substrate for maintenance supported by multiple wandering reentrant circuits. The pulmonary vein on the left in Fig. 1 shows sparse, anisotropic atrial fibers extending well onto the body of the vein. It is possible that stretch-induced depolarizations from such fibers may give rise to focal AF triggers.

Can We Ablate AF Triggers?

Of course, even if AF is triggered or driven from a focal source, there is little chance in successfully ablating this source if there are a large number of foci

Department of Medicine and the Cardiovascular Research Institute, University of California, San Francisco, USA

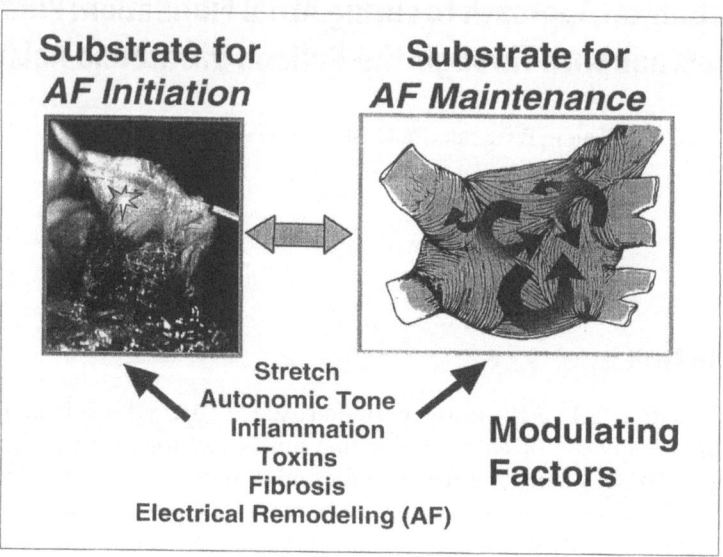

Fig. 1. Concept of dual substrates for atrial fibrillation (AF): that for initiation, and that for maintenance. A dissection of a human upper pulmonary vein is shown on the left. Note sparse, spindly fibers extending well onto the body of the vein. The highly anisotropic fiber pattern in the back of the left atrium is shown on the right. See text for further discussion. Dissection performed with kind assistance of A.E. Becker

throughout the atrium. The work of Haissaguerre, Jais and colleagues, also confirmed now in a number of laboratories, supports this notion of focal triggers. Careful mapping studies have shown that many patients have either a focal trigger or a focal driver [3-5] from the ostium or within one of more pulmonary vein. The more patients are studied, the more it has come to be recognized that this mechanism is common even in those with structural heart disease.

Because these tachycardias have a focal mechanism, they may be abolished using standard radiofrequency (RF) ablation electrode catheters [3, 4]. In a recent report on 55 patients, 78 of 83 focal triggers (94%) arose from the pulmonary veins. In 12 patients, 2 foci were present, in 6 there were 3 foci, and in 1 there were 4 foci. Despite the convincing evidence of pulmonary vein triggers in this important body of work, the recurrence rate was high and many patients required multiple procedures.

Limitations of Traditional Mapping and Ablation of Focal AF Triggers

The pulmonary veins appear to be a crucial source of triggers initiating AF, and mapping and ablation of these triggers appears to be curative in most patients with paroxysmal and even persistent AF. However, there are a number of significant limitations to treating patients with possible focal triggers using the technique of mapping the earliest site of activation and ablating with a "point" lesion – the method that is used, for example, for ablation of ectopic focal atrial tachycar-

Table 1. Limitations of "point" mapping and ablation of focal AF triggers

---

Complex, three-dimensional branching structure of pulmonary veins
No consistent method of trigger induction
No predictability of spontaneous firing
On-going atrial fibrillation masks focal trigger
Endpoint in electrophysiology laboratory poorly defined; high "recurrence" rate
Multiple pulmonary vein foci

---

dias. These limitations are listed in Table 1. First, the pulmonary veins are large, branching, complex structures with atrial tissue extending well onto the veins [6] which makes detailed mapping difficult. Second, it is difficult to induce focal sources in the electrophysiology laboratory which do not respond predictably to alterations in autonomic tone or pacing maneuvers. Ongoing AF will mask any potential focal trigger, requiring multiple electrical cardioversions to map triggers in patients with persistent AF or those in whom sustained AF occurs repeatedly in the electrophysiology laboratory. Because of the difficulty in inducing focal triggers, the endpoint of ablation is poorly defined. Finally, patients with focal triggers may have more than one focus, either two in the same pulmonary vein, or in multiple veins.

A New Approach to AF Ablation: Anatomic Isolation of the Pulmonary Veins

One way to circumvent theses limitations would be use of an anatomically guided ablative approach. If the pulmonary veins are the origin of focal triggers in well over 90% of patients with paroxysmal AF, then targeting this anatomic substrate is possible. If one or more pulmonary veins from the left atrium were electrically isolated with a circumferential lesion, firing from within those veins would be unable to reach the body of the atrium, and thus could not trigger AF (Fig. 2). The advantage of this anatomically guided approach is that it could be done quite rapidly and no detailed mapping would be required. Indeed, one would not even require spontaneous triggers during electrophysiological testing.

The technical requirements of such a circumferential lesion include the following: (a) assurance that the lesion is anatomically positioned at the left atrial/pulmonary vein junction; (b) a morphology that is 2-3 mm in width, but up to 7-8 cm in "length" (circumference); (c) transmural and continuous; (d) lesion is not acutely thrombotic; and (e) minimal long-term vein stenosis present. While RF energy is a convenient source of ablation for focal lesions, it is more difficult to produce the lesion required here.

We have developed a novel over-the-wire catheter design which integrates a cylindrical ultrasound transducer within a saline filled balloon, termed TTB-USA (through-the-balloon ultrasound ablation) in order to produce narrow circumferential zones of hyperthermic tissue death at the pulmonary vein ostia (Figs. 2-4). Ultrasound has been used in the past for ablation of cardiac tissue [7, 8], though

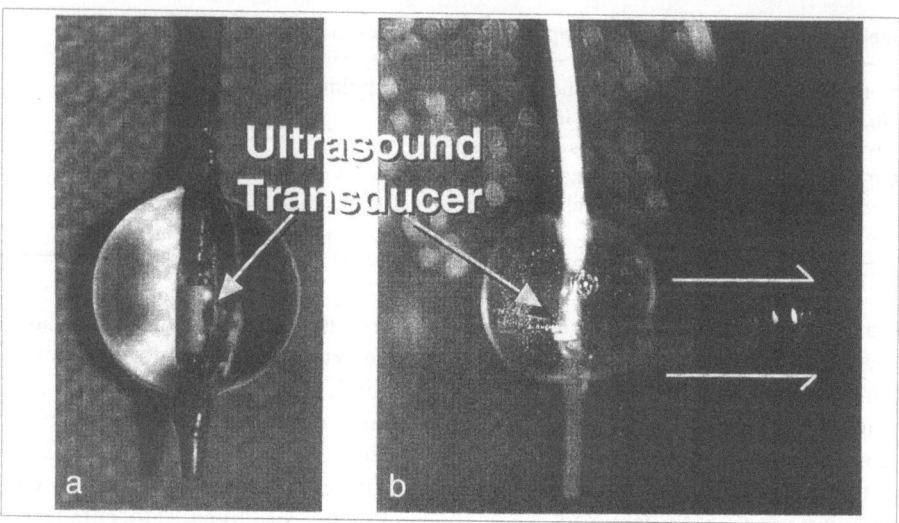

Fig. 2a,b. Novel circumferential ablation device employing a cylindrical ultrasound transducer within a water-filled balloon (**a**). When the transducer is activated (**b**) on the surface of a water bath, a sharp highly collimated wake is noted, indicating that ablation would occur perpendicular to the axis of the transducer (*arrows*)

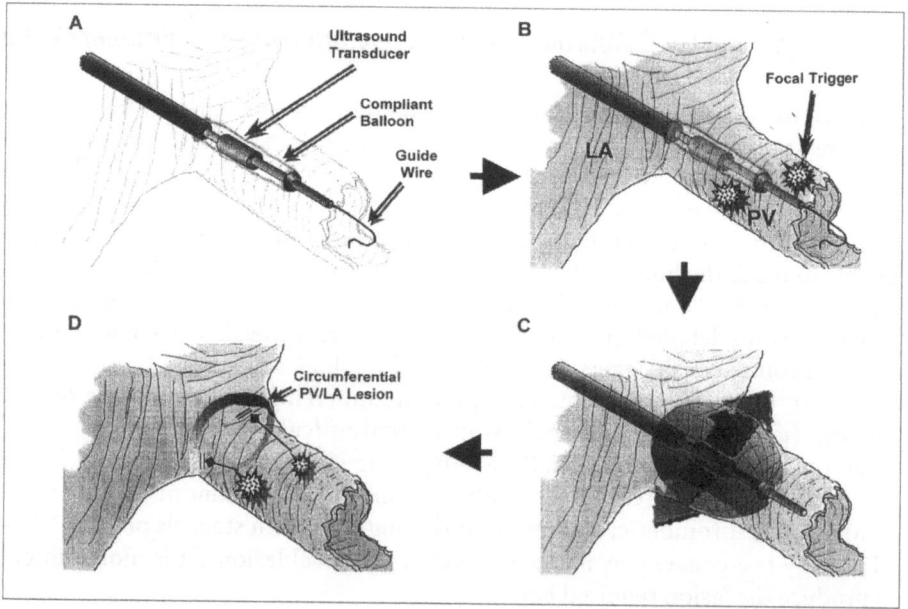

Fig. 3a-d. The concept of through-the-balloon ultrasound ablation (TTB-USA) is demonstrated. **a** A cylindrical ultrasound transducer is mounted to a catheter shaft and **b** deployed over a guide-wire into a pulmonary vein (PV) from which focal triggers emerge. **c** The balloon is inflated, and ultrasound energy is delivered and radiates into the tissue producing **d** a complete circumferential lesion blocking the egress of focal triggers

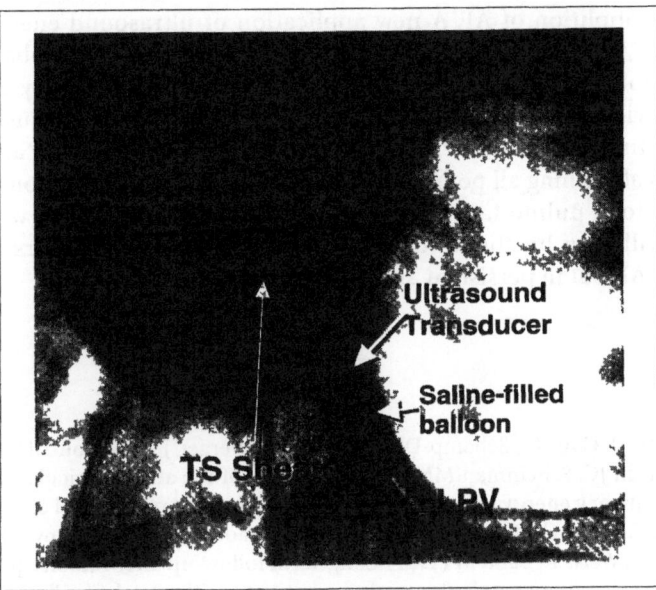

Fig. 4. Circumferential ablation device employing a cylindrical ultrasound transducer within a saline-filled balloon deployed over a guide-wire in the left lower pulmonary vein (LLPV) of a dog. With the balloon inflated with saline plus radiocontrast, an angiogram has been performed in the vein (TS transseptal)

not in the configuration developed here [9]. When a current is passed through the ultrasound transducer at its resonant frequency, it vibrates and sound energy radiates out perpendicularly to the axis of the transducer. When the energy hits cardiac tissue it is absorbed and the molecules vibrate. Molecular friction causes heating. One does not rely on extensive heating of the vein surface and conduction of heat into the cardiac tissue, as is required with RF ablation. Furthermore, heating uniformly at lower temperatures (50°C, for example) with ultrasound does not denude the endothelium and therefore thrombosis and stenosis are unlikely to occur. The balloon in the TTB-USA device serves multiple purposes, including precise positioning and anchoring the applicator, providing a standoff from the targeted tissue, allowing non-attenuating acoustic coupling, and insulating the lesion from cooling by the pulmonary venous blood flow and the blood from the heated cardiac surface. Preliminary efforts have indicated that circumferential ablation of cardiac tissue using TTB-USA catheters is quite feasible, and devices with balloon diameters of up to 2 cm are capable of producing uniform zones of hyperthermic necrosis more than 5 mm in depth.

Summary

The recognition that many cases of paroxysmal AF are initiated by a trigger from one of the pulmonary veins has allowed us to propose an anatomical approach towards the abolition of AF. A new application of ultrasound energy will, it is hypothesized, prevent AF initiation via a TTB-USA (through-the-balloon ultrasound ablation). Further studies are needed for evaluation of safety and efficacy, but if the device can be used with a high degree of safety, avoiding such complications as pulmonary vein stenosis [10], then one can envisage an empirical approach to abolishing all potential AF triggers by electrical isolation of one, two, or even all four pulmonary veins at their ostia. Clinical trials with such an approach will then be able to determine the role of focal triggers not only in paroxysmal AF, but in persistent and even chronic AF as well.

References

1. Langberg JJ, Chin M, Schamp DJ, Lee MA, Goldberger J, Pederson DN, Oeff M, Lesh MD, Griffin JC, Scheinman MM (1991) Ablation of the atrioventricular junction with radiofrequency energy using a new electrode catheter. Am J Cardiol 67:142-147
2. Morady F, Hasse C, Strickberger SA, Man KC, Daoud E, Bogun F, Goyal R, Harvey M, Knight BP, Weiss R, Bahu M (1997) Long-term follow-up after radiofrequency modification of the atrioventricular node in patients with atrial fibrillation. J Am Coll Cardiol 29:113-121
3. Haissaguerre M, Jais P, Shah DC, Takahashi A, Hocini M, Quiniou G, Garrigue S, Le Mouroux A, Le Metayer P, Clementy J (1998) Spontaneous initiation of atrial fibrillation by ectopic beats originating in the pulmonary veins. N Engl J Med 339:659-666
4. Jais P, Haissaguerre M, Shah D, Chouairi S, Gancel L, Hocini M, Clememty J (1997) A focal source of atrial fibrillation treated by discrete radiofrequency ablation. Circulation 95:572-576
5. Haissaguerre M, Jais P, Shah D, Lavergne T, Takahashi A, Barold S, Clememty J (1997) Predominant origin of atrial arrhythmia triggers in the pulmonary veins: a distinct electrophysiologic entity. PACE 20(II):1065
6. Nathan H,Eliakim M (1996) The junction between the left atrium and the pulmonary veins. An anatomic study of human hearts. Circulation 34:412-422
7. Zimmer JE, Hynynen K, He DS, Marcus F (1995) The feasibility of using ultrasound for cardiac ablation. IEEE Trans Biomed Eng 42:891-897
8. He DS, Zimmer JE, Hynynen K, Marcus FI, Caruso AC, Lampe LF, Aguirre ML (1995) Application of ultrasound energy for intracardiac ablation of arrhythmias. Eur Heart J 16:961-966
9. Hynynen K, Dennie J, Zimmer JE, Simmons WN, He DS, Marcus FI, Aguirre M (1997) Cylindrical ultrasonic transducers for cardiac catheter ablation. IEEE Trans Biomed Eng 44:144-151
10. Robbins IM, Colvin EV, Doyle TP, Kemp WE, Loyd JE, McMahon WS, Kay GN (1998) Pulmonary vein stenosis after catheter ablation of atrial fibrillation. Circulation 98:1769-1775

Ablate and Pace Therapy or AV Junction Modification for Medically Refractory Atrial Fibrillation?

P. Della Bella[1], C. Tondo[1], C. Carbucicchio[1], S. Riva[1], A. Proclemer[2], D. Facchin[2] and P. Fioretti[2]

Currently available nonpharmacological techniques for ventricular rate control in patients with drug refractory atrial fibrillation (AF) include radiofrequency ablation of the atrioventricular (AV) junction with pacemaker implantation [1-4] and modulation of AV node conduction [5-8]. The former is an already established approach with a high success rate and predictable long-term effects; it also has limitations that include a nonphysiological pattern of ventricular activation and possible risk of late sudden death [9, 10]. Modulation of the AV node conduction has been introduced more recently into clinical practice, and, although it eliminates lifetime pacemaker dependence, it is less widely accepted because of a lower acute success rate, risk of inadvertent AV block, and persistence of irregular heartbeat. Since recent randomized studies [10, 11] comparing acute and medium term outcomes of the two techniques have given contrasting results, at the present time the relative merits of the two techniques are not well defined.

Accordingly, the acute results and long-term follow-up data of two large patient populations with drug-refractory AF, treated by either technique, were compared in our dual-center nonrandomized prospective study. The first group consisted of 60 consecutive patients treated by ablation of the AV junction and pacemaker implantation in one hospital, the second group of 60 consecutive patients in whom modulation of the AV node was attempted as a first-line approach in the other hospital.

Methods

Ablation of the AV Junction and Pacemaker Implantation

Sixty consecutive patients (30 male) with a mean age of 64 ± 11 years were admitted to the Institute of Cardiology of Udine (Italy) because of symptomatic

[1]Istituto di Cardiologia, Centro Cardiologico, Fondazione Monzino, Milan, Italy; [2]Istituto di Cardiologia, Ospedale S. Maria della Misericordia, Udine, Italy

episodes of paroxysmal (24 patients, 40%) or chronic AF (36 patients, 60%). Forty-three (72%) of them had organic heart disease; the mean left ventricular ejection fraction (assessed by echocardiography) was 50 ± 15% and in 12 patients it was less than 40%. The mean number of hospital/emergency room admissions was 3.2 ± 1.5 per patient in the previous year. A mean number of 4.3 ± 1.3 drugs had failed to preventing arrhythmia recurrences or adequately control the ventricular rate.

AV block was obtained by positioning a 7 French 4-mm tip steerable catheter across the tricuspid valve to record a His bundle electrogram that was hence withdrawn to obtain the smallest His bundle deflection. Radiofrequency energy was delivered by the impedance control (first 30 patients) or temperature control mode (following 30 patients). The goal of the procedure was the appearance of a complete AV block; if failure persisted after seven attempts, a left-sided retrograde approach was effected. During the same session the pacemaker implantation was performed using a rate-responsive single-chamber unit in patients with chronic AF, or a rate-responsive dual-chamber unit with mode switch in patients with paroxysmal AF. Both accelerometric and activity sensors were used.

Modulation of AV Node Conduction

Sixty consecutive patients (32 male) with a mean age of 58 ± 12 years were admitted to the Institute of Cardiology of Milan (Italy) because of paroxysmal (43 patients, 72%) or chronic AF (17 patients, 28%). A mean of 5 ± 2 antiarrhythmic drugs had proven ineffective in preventing severe clinical symptoms, causing an average of 4.2 ± 2.0 hospital admissions per patient in the year preceding the procedure. Fifty patients (83%) had structural heart disease; the mean left ventricular ejection fraction was 54 ± 12%.

Thus, the incidence of underlying heart disease and impaired heart function, as well as the occurrence of severe clinical symptoms, were similar in both groups, but patients treated by ablation of the AV node were older and had an higher rate of chronic AF than the other group. Modulation of AV node conduction was performed by positioning a 4-mm tip steerable catheter over the tricuspid annulus to perform mapping of Koch's triangle and to deliver radiofrequency energy. When the modulation was carried out during sinus rhythm, the AH interval, the anterograde effective refractory period, and the Wenckebach cycle length of the AV node were assessed before and after ablation. When the procedure was performed during AF, the average ventricular rate over 30 min was evaluated. The ablation was performed during sinus rhythm in 30 patients, targeting the so-called "slow AV node pathway potential". An accelerated junctional rhythm (60-100 bpm) with 1:1 ventriculo-atrial conduction was considered a marker of success. Radiofrequency current applications were performed at closely spaced target sites, with the purpose of achieving prolongation of the Wenckebach circle length as near as possible to a target value of 500 ms (complete success); intermediate values (430-500 ms) were considered partial results, while persistence of a value less than 430 ms was defined as an acute failure.

When the modulation of the AV node was attempted during AF (30 patients), the ablation catheter was initially positioned approximately 1 cm inferior to the His bundle, in order to record an A/V ratio of 0.5 to 1; a persistent slowing of the heart rate to below100 bpm was considered a success, while values above 100 bpm defined an acute failure.

Isoproterenol (up to 4 µg/min) was administered in a minority of patients (21 patients, 13 with sinus rhythm, 8 with AF) to confirm whether the procedure had been effective; modification of Wenckebach cycle length and heart rate were acutely evaluated, but a systematic analysis of the predictive value of isoproterenol infusion was not performed.

An echocardiogram was performed after the procedure and before discharge. Oral anticoagulants or antiaggregants were administered according to clinical needs.

Treatment with β-blockers or calcium-antagonists, digoxin, and antiarrhythmic drugs was continued in patients who had undergone modulation when complete acute success was not achieved or when recurrences of rapid AF were observed.

Follow-Up

The follow-up was organized according to the same protocol for all patients. Only patients with a minimum of 12 months follow-up are included. Outpatient visits and standard electrocardiograms were planned at 1, 3, and 6 months after discharge, and then at regular 6-month intervals. Patients with a pacemaker had the device regularly checked, with particular reference to the mode switch and the activity sensor operation, and to the onset of spontaneous rhythm during transient pacemaker inhibition. Among patients who had undergone modulation, a Holter recording was required at each visit; furthermore, patients were asked to obtain an electrocardiogram if relevant symptoms occurred. Treatment with antiarrhythmic drugs was instituted according to clinical indications.

Endpoints

Clinical endpoints in both groups were: occurrence and cause of death, number of hospital admissions by the end of the first year of follow-up, occurrence of syncope or acute heart failure, and recurrence of severe palpitations or hypotension. A favorable long-term follow-up was defined by absence of recurrence of the presenting clinical symptoms. Life quality parameters were evaluated in all patients by means of a semiquantitative questionnaire [12], comparing the scores (0-10 according to severity of symptoms) obtained before and 1 year after the procedure and relating to the following: palpitations, rest dyspnea, effort dyspnea, exercise intolerance, and weakness. Lost to quality-of-life follow-up were patients who died before 1-year evaluation, as well as patients who had undergone unsuccessful modulation with pacemaker implantation, who were excluded from the symptom score analysis.

Results

Acute Findings

Ablation of the AV junction. Acute success (complete AV block) was obtained in all cases (100%), with a right-sided approach in 53 (90%) and a sequential right-and left-sided approach in the remaining 7 (10%), with a mean number of 3.4 ± 3 pulses. No complications occurred after the procedure. A VVIR pacemaker was implanted in 36 patients and a DDDR pacemaker in 24 patients without any complications or infections.

Modulation of AV node conduction. Among 30 patients in sinus rhythm the anterograde AV Wenckebach cycle length was prolonged, after 12 ± 8 pulses, from 328 ± 85 to 466 ± 80 ms ($p < 0.01$). Full or partial success was obtained in 11 (37%) and 6 (20%) of the patients, respectively; in the remaining 13 patients (43%) the procedure was considered an acute failure. In the 30 patients in whom the procedure was attempted during AF, the heart rate decreased from 178 ± 35 to 96 ± 35 bpm ($p < 0.01$) after 10 ± 6 radiofrequency pulses: acute success was achieved in 17 patients (57%). Complete AV block was deliberately induced in two patients during sinus rhythm and in seven patients during AF because of ineffectiveness of the procedure; the overall rate of acutely induced AV block was therefore 15% (9/60 patients). In the case of remaining failures the patients were treated by antiarrhythmic drugs. Isoproterenol infusion (13 patients with sinus rhythm, 8 patients with AF) showed a reduction in Wenckebach cycle length from 476 ± 55 to 381 ± 60 ms and an increase in heart rate from 54 ± 36 to 86 ± 32 bpm.

Mean procedure and fluoroscopy time was significantly lower for patients treated by ablation and pacemaker than for those treated by modulation (75 ± 15 vs 135 ± 45 min, $p < 0.05$, and 9 ± 5 vs 39 ± 9 min, $p < 0.05$, respectively). The following long-term antiarrhythmic treatment was maintained in patients after ablation and modulation, respectively: digoxin (27 and 10 patients), β-blockers (4 and 4 patients), verapamil or diltiazem (6 and 0 patients), class I or III antiarrhythmics (12 and 4 patients).

Long-Term Outcome: Comparison of Clinical Events in the Study Groups

After a similar follow-up period for both groups (27 ± 7 vs 26 ± 6 months), there were one cardiac death among patients treated by ablation and pacemaker, and one cardiac death among patients who had undergone modulation. Both patients who died had severe cardiac disease (one had severe valvular heart disease, left ventricular ejection fraction 40%, and an escape rhythm of 40 bpm; the other had combined mitral and aortic disease and a baseline left ventricular ejection fraction of 20%).

The mean number of hospital admissions decreased significantly to 0.2 patients per year in both treatment groups. Similarly, the incidence of acute heart failure episodes was markedly diminished in both groups: 3.3% (2 cases) in the group treated by ablation, and 1.6% (1 case) in the group treated by modulation.

There has been no recurrence of syncope or tachycardia-related severe hypotension in both groups.

Late failures, defined by recurrence of palpitations and documented AF with high ventricular rate, were documented in 4 of 60 (6%) patients 3 ± 2 months after ablation of the AV junction, and in 7 of 60 (12%) patients 4 ± 2 months following a modulation; a second procedure causing permanent AV block was performed in all patients with a pacemaker and in two of those who had undergone modulation. Early pacemaker dysfunction (no sensor activity) requiring replacement of the unit was detected in 1 of 60 (2%) patients following ablation of the AV node. Three patients with paroxysmal AF and a DDDR unit complained of mild palpitations related to the onset of AF, as documented by the pacemaker memory function.

Subjective Symptom Score

The analysis of the modification of the scores after 1 year was performed separately in patients with chronic and in those with paroxysmal AF. Subjective score analysis comprised 58 patients with ablation of the AV junction and 51 patients with modulation of AV node conduction (97% and 85% of the respective study group).

The decrease in the score for weakness and rest dyspnea was significant and occurred to a similar extent after either ablation or modulation in both groups of patients (chronic AF and paroxysmal AF). Effort dyspnea and exercise intolerance after modulation in both paroxysmal and chronic AF patients decreased slightly more than in those treated by ablation and subsequent pacemaker implantation. In patients with chronic AF, the decrease in palpitation score at 1 year was far less evident in those who had undergone modulation (from 8.4 to 4.5, p n.s.) than in those who underwent AV junction ablation and pacemaker implant (8.0 to 1.7, p < 0.001). On the other hand, in patients with paroxysmal AF the decrease in palpitation score was similar among those who had ablation of the AV junction and those treated by modulation of the AV node conduction.

Conclusions

The data presented in this dual-center, nonrandomized, prospective study provide a comparison of the acute and long-term results of two ablative techniques aimed at controlling ventricular rate in patients with drug-refractory AF, either chronic or paroxysmal. The endpoint of the procedure (complete AV block) was consistently obtained with ablation of the AV junction in all cases; on the other hand, the acute success rate of AV node conduction modulation, although defined upon arbitrary values, was markedly lower (ranging from 57% to 63% of the underlying atrial rhythm) but in accordance with the mean values reported in previous studies [7, 9]. Ablation of the AV junction is conceptually easier, as supported by the shorter procedure and fluoroscopy time and by the smaller number of radiofrequency pulses. By contrast, the persisting uncertainties concerning the mechanism of modulation underline the more complex electrophysiological substrate involved in this approach. Moreover, the occurrence of complete AV block during a modulation procedure has to be considered an acute failure of this approach and although in this series there were no cases of accidental AV block, AV block was intentionally induced in 15% of our patients, because of poor modification of the AV node conduction parameters. Other authors have reported a similar incidence of complete AV block, ranging from 10% to 16% [7, 13].

Both procedures appear very effective over the long term. There were no further complaints of major symptoms in any of the patients in either treatment group. As a consequence, the need for hospital admissions decreased dramatically to a similar extent after modulation and after ablation of the AV node, thus confirming the primary role of heart rate control in AF [14-16]. In our series the beneficial effects of decreasing the heart rate by modulation have extended over the long term and the electrocardiographic documentation revealed that in most patients the mean rate during AF was far lower than would be expected on the basis of the acute results.

An improvement in quality-of-life indexes was achieved in both study groups, as assessed through a semiquantitative questionnaire already used in similar studies [4, 12]. The reduction in perceived weakness and rest dyspnea was similar after both ablation and modulation, and might be related to a reduction in the mean heart rate per se, to regularization of the rhythm, or to an increase in left ventricular function [12, 17]. The improvement in effort dyspnea and exercise intolerance in patients with paroxysmal AF was significant after both ablation and modulation. The palpitation score was also greatly diminished in both treatment groups, although it was a persistent complaint in some patients, particularly those treated by modulation, due to the persistence of irregular heart beat.

In conclusion, both modulation of AV node conduction and ablation of the AV junction and pacemaker implantation can be offered as an effective means to achieve ventricular rate control in patients with drug-refractory AF. Acute success appears to be higher after ablation and pacemaker implantation. Given acute success of the procedures, however, both approaches are similarly effective in achieving long-term ventricular rate control and symptom score improvement.

References

1. Jackman WM, Wang X, Friday KJ et al (1991) Catheter ablation of atrioventricular junction using radiofrequency current in 17 patients: comparison of standard and large-tip catheter electrodes. Circulation 83:1562-1576
2. Yeung-Lai-Wah J, Alison J, Lonergan L et al (1991) High success rate of atrioventricular node ablation with radiofrequency energy. J Am Coll Cardiol 18:1753-1758
3. Rodriguez LM, Smeets JLRM, Xie B et al (1993) Improvement in left ventricular function by ablation of atrioventricular nodal conduction in select patients with lone atrial fibrillation. Am J Cardiol 72:1137-1141
4. Brignole M, Gianfranchi L, Menozzi C et al (1997) Assessment of atrioventricular junction ablation and DDDR mode-switching pacemaker versus pharmacological

treatment in patients with severely symptomatic paroxysmal atrial fibrillation. Circulation 96:2617-2624

5. Feld GK, Fleck RP, Fujimura O et al (1994) Control of rapid ventricular response by radiofrequency catheter modification of the atrioventricular node in patients with medically refractory atrial fibrillation. Circulation 90:2299-2307

6. Della Bella P, Carbucicchio C, Tondo C et al (1995) Modulation of atrioventricular conduction by ablation of the "slow" atrioventricular node pathway in patients with drug-refractory atrial fibrillation or flutter. J Am Coll Cardiol 25:39-46

7. Morady F, Hasse C, Strickberger SA et al (1997) Long-term follow-up after radiofrequency modification of the atrioventricular node in patients with atrial fibrillation. J Am Coll Cardiol 27:113-121

8. Carbucicchio C, Tondo C, Fassini G, Riva S, Agostoni PG, Galli C, Della Bella P (1999) Modulation of the atrio-ventricular node conduction to achieve rate control in patients with atrial fibrillation: long-term results. PACE 22:442-452

9. Vanderheyden M, Goethals M, Anguera I et al (1997) Hemodynamic deterioration following radiofrequency ablation of the atrioventricolar conduction system. Pacing Clin Electrophysiol 20:2422-2428

10. Geelen P, Brugada J, Andries E et al (1997) Ventricular fibrillation and sudden death after radiofrequency catheter ablation of the atrioventricular junction. Pacing Clin Electrophysiol 20:343-348

11. Lee S, Chen S, Tai C et al (1998) Comparison of quality of life and cardiac performance after complete atrioventricular junction ablation and atrioventricular junction modification in patients with medically refractory atrial fibrillation. J Am Coll Cardiol 31:637-644

12. Twidale N, McDonald T, Nave K Seal A (1998) Comparison of the effects of AV nodal ablation versus AV nodal modification in patients with congestive heart failure and uncontrolled atrial fibrillation. Pacing Clin Electrophysiol 21(Pt I):641-651

13. Brignole M, Gianfranchi L, Menozzi C et al (1994) Influence of atrioventricular junction radiofrequency ablation in patients with chronic atrial fibrillation and flutter on quality of life and cardiac performance. Am J Cardiol 74:242-246

14. Chen SA, Lee SH, Chiang CE et al (1996) Electrophysiological mechanisms in successful radiofrequency catheter modification of atrioventricular junction for patients with medically refractory paroxysmal atrial fibrillation. Circulation 93:1690-1701

15. Kreiner G, Heinz G, Siostrzonek P et al (1996) Effect of slow pathway ablation on ventricular rate during atrial fibrillation. Circulation 93:277-283

16. Markowitz SM, Stein KM, Lerman BB (1996) Mechanism of ventricular rate control following radiofrequency modification of atrioventricular conduction in patients with atrial fibrillation. Circulation 94:2856-2864

17. Fitzpatrick AP, Kourouyan HD et al (1996) Quality of life and outcomes after radiofrequency His-bundle catheter ablation and permanent pacemaker implantation: impact of treatment in paroxysmal and established atrial fibrillation. Am Heart J 131:499-507

18. Heinz G, Siostrzonek P, Kreiner G et al (1992) Improvement in left ventricular systolic function after successful radiofrequency His bundle ablation for drug refractory, chronic atrial fibrillation and recurrent atrial flutter. Am J Cardiol 69:489-492

Atrial Fibrillation After Heart Surgery: How to Identify and Protect Predisposed Patients?

C. Zussa and E. Polesel

Introduction

Supraventricular arrhythmias (SVA), mostly atrial fibrillation (AF), are the most frequent complications after cardiac surgery. In patients undergone coronary artery bypass grafting (CABG), the incidence of postoperative AF (pAF) ranges from 20% to 40% [1-10]. The figure rises to 50% after valvular surgery [11, 12].

Although the consequences of this arrhythmia are usually not life-threatening, AF aggravates the risk of stroke, hemodynamic impairment, heart - failure and prolonged hospital stay, with consequent increased costs [7, 13-15]. For these reasons, several studies have been performed to try to identify and provide prophylactic treatment for predisposed patients [16-19]. Many factors have been tested by several authors as independent variables predictive of pAF, from systemic hypertension to postoperative bleeding, withdrawal of β-blockers, atrial manipulation, myocardial protection, cross-clamping time, respiratory or renal parameters, and others [4, 7, 17, 20, 21], but most proved to be poorly correlated with the onset of pAF.

From the meta-analysis of these clinical reports, age and occurrence of preoperative AF episodes have been found to be the only independent factors mildly correlated with an increased risk of pAF [4, 7, 18, 20, 22]. This lack of significant correlations may be related to the probably multifactorial mechanisms responsible for pAF development, such as pericardial inflammation or effusion, autonomic nervous system imbalance, etc. [1, 5, 7, 11].

Based on previous results, some authors have tried to identify subgroups of patients, possibly more predisposed to pAF, and prophylactically treated them with various pharmacological agents such as β-blockers, verapamil, digoxin, procainamide, etc. [23-27]. Not surprisingly, again, the results showed only a mild, not statistically significant, reduction in the incidence of pAF [7]. Indeed, the treatments had been not specifically aimed at modifying the causes of pAF, which are still unknown.

Reparto di Cardiochirurgia, Ospedale Umberto I, Mestre, Venice, Italy

Interesting results were obtained with prophylactic utilization of amiodarone. Two studies were published in 1991 and 1993 [28, 29] about short-term (24-h) prophylaxis with this drug given intravenously, but, despite promising results, the side effects meent that infusion was discontinued in about 20% of cases. In 1997 prophylaxis with amiodarone given orally was reported to produce positive results with good tolerance [30].

Taking a different approach, recently the utilization of temporary large-surface epicardial wire electrodes was tested to treat pAF, with immediate successful conversion to sinus rhythm in most of the cases, but with significant early recurrence [31, 32].

The lack of securely determined factors predisposing patients to pAF, the resulting still controversial pharmacological prophylaxis, and the insufficiently proven nonpharmacological early treatment of pAF constituted the starting point of our study. Our aim was to find a more effective and convenient approach to pAF.

Patients and Methods

From 1 July 1998 to 28 February 1999, 60 consecutive patients scheduled to undergo cardiac surgery were included in the study. The exclusion criteria were current AF, previous episodes of paroxysmal AF, treatment with anti-arrhythmic agents during the year before operation, contraindications to the use of amiodarone (i.e., thyroid disease), and atrial dimensions > 50 mm on echocardiography. The five patients scheduled for beating-heart myocardial revascularization during this period were included as well, to evaluate possible differences in pAF incidence and treatment.

The patients were randomly divided in three groups. Group A consisted of 20 patients prophylactically treated with amiodarone, one 200-mg tablet three times a day for 7 days before operation, then one tablet daily, only while hospitalized (7.3 ± 0.8 days). Group B consisted of 20 patients in whom two dedicated temporary large-surface (60 mm^2) wire electrodes (TADpole 7950, InControl, Inc., Redmond, Wash., USA) were positioned in contact with the epicardium of the atria (Fig. 1), while a traditional temporary wire electrode was positioned on the anterior surface of the right ventricle. Group C was the control group and consisted of 20 patients in whom neither prophylaxis nor dedicated electrodes were utilized (Table 1). Informed consent was obtained from each patient included in groups A and B. In the case of pAF in group B patients, the electrodes were utilized to defibrillate the atria through an interface module (InControl, Inc.) connected to an external defibrillator (Hewlett-Packard, Geneva, Switzerland). The first shock delivered was always 0.7 J, followed, if unsuccessful, by stepwise increasing energy of 1, 2, 2.3, or 3 J. In these patients amiodarone was utilized if pAF recurred more than once during hospitalization (200 mg, one tablet three times a day for 2 weeks, then one tablet a day for 1 month). In group C amiodarone was infused to restore sinus rhythm with an intravenous bolus of 5 mg/kg followed by continuous infusion of 900 mg during a 24-h period and oral admin-

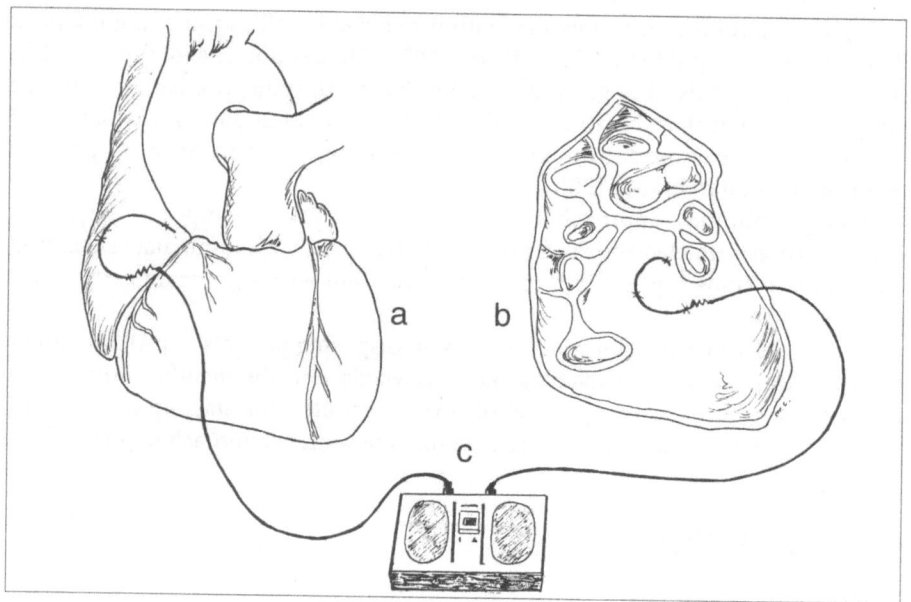

Fig. 1. Positioning of the temporary large-surface wire electrodes for atrial defibrillation. They are placed on the anterolateral surface of the right atrium (**a**) and on the posterior pericardium close to the surface of the left atrium (**b**). They will be connected to the interface module (**c**) to defibrillate

Table 1. Demographic and clinical characteristics of the patient groups

	Group A (n = 20)	Group B (n = 20)	Group C (n = 20)
Age (years; mean ± SD)	59.6 ± 8.4	62.8 ± 8.1	66.1 ± 10
Male sex (n)	13	12	13
NYHA class (mean ± SD)	2.6 ± 0.8	2.7 ± 0.7	2.6 ± 0.9
Mitral regurgitation (n)	6	7	6
Previous myocardial infarction (n)	4	5	6
Systemic hypertension (n)	9	8	10
LVEF (mean ± SD)	0.51 ± 0.14	0.49 ± 0.12	0.48 ± 0.16
Surgery (n)			
CABG, CPB	9	12	8
CABG, beating heart	2	1	2
Mitral valve	4	2	4
Aortic valve	3	2	4
Combined valve + CABG	2	3	2
CPB time (min; mean ± SD)	136 ± 42	148 ± 51	140 ± 52
Aortic c-c time (min; mean ± SD)	96 ± 32	103 ± 36	101 ± 32

CABG, coronary artery bypass grafting; CPB, cardiopulmonary bypass; c-c, cross-clamp

istration of one 200-mg tablet a day for 1 month thereafter. A total of 55 patients underwent cardiac surgery in moderate hypothermic cardiopulmonary bypass and blood cardioplegic arrest. Five patients underwent myocardial revascularization under beating-heart conditions, utilizing a Medtronic Octopus (Medtronic, Inc., Minneapolis, Minn., USA) or a Baxter CAB SuperSlide (Baxter Healthcare Corporation, Irvine, Calif., USA) stabilizer. After surgery each patient was admitted to intensive care and subsequently transferred to the floor, where three-lead telemetry monitoring was utilized until discharge from the hospital. Patients were followed for cardiac rhythm on out-patient basis once a week for 1 month after operation.

Statistical analysis was performed by the χ^2 test or analysis of variance, as appropriate.

Results

Clinical results are summarized in Table 2. No significant differences in 30-day mortality and morbidity were found among the groups.

A significantly smaller incidence of pAF was found in group A than in either of the others, while no difference was found between group B and group C (Table 3). Regarding the type of surgery, pAF occurred at a higher rate in patients who had undergone any kind of valve procedure, compared with a CABG-alone operation, in all groups. The differences within each group and among the groups were not statistically significant, due to the small number of events. Two patients (one in group B and one in group C), among those operated in beating-heart conditions without cardiopulmonary by-pass, experienced pAF as well.

Amiodarone prophylaxis resulted in a lower ventricular rate at pAF onset. The only patient in group A in whom pAF occurred was subsequently treated according to the amiodarone protocol, as described for group C patients.

The characteristics of atrial defibrillation in group B patients are described in Table 3. In five patients of this group with early recurrence of pAF, the second-defibrillation protocol started with a shock of 1 J followed by subsequent shocks up to 2.3 J, if necessary. Three of these last patients had a second recurrence of pAF, which was treated with the amiodarone therapeutic protocol described above. In two of them sinus rhythm was restored, and one was discharged in AF. This patient, like those discharged in AF from among the group C patients, was successfully converted to sinus rhythm 1 month later by means of external DC shock. None of the patients discharged in sinus rhythm showed AF during the month of follow-up after discharge. No adverse effects were observed related to the positioning and extraction of the defibrillating temporary epicardial wires.

A protective effect of amiodarone prophylaxis resulted also from the absence of early recurrence of pAF in group A, although the differences among the three groups are not statistically significant due to the small number of pAF recurrences.

Hospital stay was significantly longer for group C patients, compared with both group A and B patients, while the difference was mildly significant between groups A and B.

Table 2. Clinical results

	Group A	Group B	Group C
30-Day mortality	0	0	0
Perioperative myocardial infarction (n)	0	0	1
Bleeding	0	0	0
Ventricular arrhythmias (n)	0	1	1
Low output syndrome (n)	0	1	0
Prolonged intubation (n)	0	0	1

Table 3. Postoperative atrial fibrillation data

	Group A	Group B	Group C	p
No. of patients with pAF	1	8	9	0.011
Surgery				
No. of patients with pAF/valve ± CABG group	1/9	4/7	5/10	ns
No. of patients with pAF/CABG alone group	0/11	4/13	4/10	ns
pAF onset (days after surgery)	2.9 ± 1.4	2.4 ± 1.7	2.7 ± 1.9	ns
Vr mean ± SD	108 ± 0	130.5 ± 8.3	135.3 ± 11.4	0.004
Time from pAF to shock (min, mean ± SD)		19.5 ± 7.0		
Time from pAF to shock (min, minimum-maximum)		10 - 30		
No. of shocks (mean ± SD)		2.0 ± 0.76		
No. of shocks (minimum-maximim)		1 - 3		
Energy per shock (J, mean ± SD)		1.3 ± 0.7		
Energy per shock (J, minimum-maximum)		0.7 - 3		
Early pAF recurrence	0	5	3	ns
No. of shocks (mean ± SD)		1.6 ± 0.6		
No. of shocks (minimim-maximum)		1 - 2		
Energy per shock (J, mean ± SD)		1.7 ± 0.6		
Energy per shock (J, minimum-maximum)		1 - 2.3		
AF at discharge	0	1	2	ns
Hospital stay (days, mean ± SD)	7.3 ± 0.8	7.9 ± 1.1	9.3 ± 1.9	*
Hospital stay (days, minimum-maximum)	6 - 10	6 - 10	6 - 14	

Vr, ventricular rate
*, $p = 0.03$ between A and B, $p = 0.01$ between B and C, $p = 0.001$ between A and C

No side effects were observed related to the amiodarone protocols, either prophylactic or therapeutic.

Discussion

Postoperative AF represents the most frequent, although rarely life-threatening, complication after cardiac surgery, with clinical and economic implications [1-10, 13-15]. Prophylactic treatment with many pharmacological agents, both before and early after surgery, has failed to demonstrate efficacy in most cases [7, 30, 31]. However, β-blockers (sotalol) and amiodarone seem to produce some positive results.

Sotalol, administered twice a day for 3 months, starting 2 h before operation, provided a significant reduction in occurrence of pAF compared to placebo [27]. However, in this study pAF still occurred in 26% of the patients treated with sotalol – an incidence also reported in patients without any prophylaxis [7, 9, 14, 19, 31]. Moreover, β-blockers may be contraindicated in patients with severe LV dysfunction, chronic obstructive pulmonary disease, and peripheral vascular disease, which seems to represent the population most prone to developing pAF [14, 19, 30, 31].

Amiodarone was tested with positive results in preventing pAF, but with some drawback. Hohnloser et al. [28] and Butler et al. [29] reported a significant reduction in pAF incidence with intravenous infusion of amiodarone during the perioperative period, but the side effects, mostly severe bradycardia, warranted discontinuation of treatment in 10%-20% of cases. In a more recent study, oral administration of amiodarone allowed good prevention of pAF to be achieved without significat side effects [30].

Our experience in the group of patients prophylactically treated with amiodarone confirmed the efficacy of this approach. The reduction in pAF occurrence in these patients was significant ($p = 0.01$) compared with the other groups and no adverse effects were observed. The only patient with pAF in this group maintained sinus rhythm after therapeutic administration of amiodarone following the group C protocol.

Obviously, group B patients showed a similar incidence of pAF as control patients. The low-energy epicardial atrial defibrillation procedure proved to be safe and effective, but was associated with a significant number of pAF early recurrences. These required repeated defibrillation and suggested adding the amiodarone therapeutic protocol after the second recurrence. Therefore, at discharge, amiodarone was prescribed to 1, 3, and 9 patients in groups A, B, and C, respectively.

On the basis of our experience we could not find any statistically significant difference in demographic and clinical characteristics between patients who experienced pAF and those who maintained sinus rhythm, either within each group or in the entire study population as a whole.

Our results confirmed that the incidence of pAF is higher in patients treated with any valve procedure than in those who undergo CABG alone [11, 12], although the difference was not significant, probably due to the small number of events. In our study, the occurrence of pAF even in patients who had undergone CABG alone, under beating-heart conditions, without cardiopulmonary bypass, confirms a multi-etiological origin of pAF, beyond cardiopulmonary bypass-related factors [7, 17, 21].

From our experience, it is still impossible effectively to identify groups of patients who are more predisposed to pAF, and consequently it seems to be a better strategy to focus on the best method of prophylaxis of pAF and the most safe and effective treatment of this event when it occurs. Amiodarone short-term prophylaxis appeared a safe and adequate method to reduce the incidence of pAF, without adverse effects. On the other hand, although defibrillation via temporary large-surface wire electrodes was effective in restoring sinus rhythm, it was associated with a significant incidence of pAF recurrences that in some patients required the addition of short-term amiodarone therapy.

It has been suggested that pAF produces a significant increase in hospital stay and consequent costs. Our experience confirmed this. Both amiodarone prophylaxis and the application of temporary defibrillating electrodes reduced the duration of hospitalization compared with the control group; moreover, amiodarone prophylaxis was associated with a mildly significantly shorter hospital stay than was the treatment with electrodes.

While we await the results of more extensive ongoing prospective studies, we suggest the adoption of a short-term oral prophylaxis with amiodarone, chiefly in patients scheduled to undergo valve procedures, although it seems effective also in CABG-alone procedures. In the case of urgent or emergent operation, or amiodarone intolerance that precludes prophylaxis, we suggest the placement of temporary large-surface electrodes to restore sinus rhythm if pAF occurs. If amiodarone is not contraindicated, after more than one recurrence of pAF, successful defibrillation by the temporary electrodes should be followed by oral administration of amiodarone for 1 month. In the case of ineffective defibrillation, amiodarone should also be prescribed for an adequate period of time before restoring sinus rhythm by a traditional external DC shock. Following the protocols described, our results showed that, at discharge, treatment with amiodarone was indicated in none, 15%, and 45% of group A, B, and C patients, respectively ($p = 0.006$).

More extensive studies are necessary to identify the best prophylaxis for pAF, given that it remains impossible at present to identify patients who are predisposed to this significant postoperative complication.

Acknowledgements. The authors thank Mrs. Marta Casella for her valuable assistance with preparation of the manuscript and the drawing of the figure.

References

1. Ormerod OJM, McGregor CGA, Stone DL, Wisbey C, Petch MC (1984) Arrhythmias after coronary by-pass surgery. Br Heart J 51:618-621
2. Rubin DA, Nieminski KE, Reed GE, Herman MV (1987) Predictors, prevention, and

long-term prognosis of atrial fibrillation after coronary artery by-pass graft operation. J Thorac Cardiovasc Surg 94:331-335

3. Lauer MS, Eagle KA, Buckley MJ, DeSanctis RW (1989) Atrial fibrillation following coronary bypass surgery. Prog Cardiovasc Dis 31:367-378

·4. Fuller JA, Adams GG, Buxton B (1989) Atrial fibrillation after coronary artery grafting: is it a disease of elderly? J Thorac Cardiovasc Surg 97:821-825

5. Yousif H, Davies G, Oakley CM (1990) Peri-operative supraventricular arrhythmias in coronary artery bypass surgery. Int J Cardiol 26:313-318

6. Crosby LH, Woll KR, Wood KL, Pifalo WB (1990) Effect of activity on supraventricular tachyarrhythmias after coronary bypass surgery. Heart Lung 19:666-670

7. Frost L, Molgaard H, Christiansen EH, Hjortholm K, Paulsen PK, Thomsen PEB (1992) Atrial fibrillation and flutter after coronary artery bypass surgery: epidemiology, risk factors and preventive trials. Int J Cardiol 36:253-261

8. Cox JL (1993) A perspective of postoperative atrial fibrillation in cardiac operations. Ann Thorac Surg 56:405-409

9. Pires LA, Wagshal AB, Lancey R, Huang S (1995) Arrhythmias and conduction disturbances after coronary artery bypass graft surgery: epidemiology, management, and prognosis. Am Heart J 129:799-808

10. Gaylard E (1996) Changing incidence of atrial fibrillation following coronary artery bypass grafting: a retrospective analysis. Br J Clin Pract 50:164-165

11. Ommen SR, Odell JA, Stanton MS (1997) Atrial arrhythmias after cardiothoracic surgery. N Engl J Med 336:1429-1434

12. Asher CR, Miller DP, Grimm RA, Cosgrove DM, Chung MK (1998) Analysis of risk factors for development of atrial fibrillation early after cardiac valvular surgery. Am J Cardiol 87:892-895

13. Creswell LL, Schuessler RB, Rosenbloom M (1993) Hazards of postoperative atrial arrhythmias. Ann Thorac Surg 56:539-549

14. Aranki SF, Shaw DP, Adams DH, Rizzo RJ, Couper GS, VanderVliet M, Collins JJ, Cohn LH, Burstin HR (1996) Predictors of atrial fibrillation after coronary artery surgery: current trends and impact on hospital resources. Circulation 94:390-397

15. Borzak S, Tisdale JE, Amin NB, Goldberg AD, Frank D, Padhi D, Higgins RSD (1998) Atrial fibrillation after bypass surgery: does the arrhythmia or the characteristics of the patients prolong hospital stay? Chest 113:1489-1491

16. Parker FB, Greiner-Hayes L, Bove EL, Marvasti MA, Johnson LW, Eich RH (1983) Supraventricular arrhythmias following coronary artery bypass. J Thorac Cardiovasc Surg 86:594-600

17. Crosby LH, Pifalo WB, Woll KR, Burkholder JA (1990) Risk factor for atrial fibrillation after coronary artery bypass grafting. Am J Cardiol 66:1520-1522

18. Andrews TC, Reimold SC, Berlin JA, Antman EM (1991) Prevention of supraventricular arrhythmias after coronary bypass surgery: a meta-analysis of randomized control trials. Circulation 84[Suppl III]:236-244

19. Mathew JP, Parks R, Savino JS (1996) Atrial fibrillation following coronary artery bypass graft surgery: predictors, outcomes, and resources utilization. JAMA 276:300-306

20. Leitch JW, Thomson D, Baird DK, Harris PJ (1990) The importance of age as a predictor of atrial fibrillation and flutter after coronary bypass grafting. J Thorac Cardiovasc Surg 100:338-342

21. Caretta Q, Mercanti CA, De Nardo D, Chiarotti F, Scibilia G, Reale A, Marino B (1991) Ventricular conduction defects and atrial fibrillation after coronary bypass grafting. Multivariate analysis of preoperative, intraoperative and postoperative variables. Eur Heart J 12:1107-1111

22. Kowey PR, Taylor JE, Rials SJ, Marinchak RA (1992) Meta-analysis of effectiveness drug therapy in preventing supraventricular arrhythmia early after coronary artery bypass grafting. Am J Cardiol 69:963-965

23. Davison R, Hartz R, Kaplan K, Parker M, Feiereisel P, Michaelis L (1985) Prophylaxis of supraventricular tachyarrhythmia after coronary artery bypass surgery with oral verapamil: a randomized, double-blind trial. Ann Thorac Surg 39:336-339

24. Weiner B, Rheinlander HF, Decker EL, Cleveland RJ (1986) Digoxin prophylaxis following coronary artery bypass surgery. Clin Pharm 5:55-58

25. Martinussen HJ, Lolk A, Szezepanski C, Alstrup P (1988) Supraventricular tachyarrhythmias after coronary artery bypass surgery: a double blind randomized trial of prophylactic low dose propranolol. Thorac Cardiovasc Surg 36:206-207

26. Gold MR, Ungaro MA, Ory DS, O'Gara PT, Buckley MJ (1991) Procainamide prevents arrhythmia following coronary bypass surgery. Circulation 4[Suppl II]:285

27. Pfisterer ME, Kloter-Weber UCD, Huber M, Osswald S, Buser PT, Skarvan K, Stulz PM (1997) Prevention of supraventricular tachyarrhythmias after open heart operation by low-dose sotalol: a prospective, double blind, randomized, placebo-controlled study. Ann Thorac Surg 64:1113-1119

28. Hohnloser SH, Meinertz T, Dammbacher T (1991) Electrocardiographic and antiarrhythmic effects of intravenous amiodarone: results of a prospective, placebo-controlled study. Am Heart J 121:89-95

29. Butler J, Harris DR, Sinclair M, Westby S (1993) Amiodarone prophylaxis for tachycardias after coronary bypass surgery: a randomized, double blind, placebo controlled trial. Br Heart J 1993:56-60

30. Daud EG, Strickberger SA, Man KC, Goyal R, Deeb GM, Bolling SF, Pagani FD, Bitar C, Meissner MD, Morady F (1997) Preoperative amiodarone as prophylaxis against atrial fibrillation after heart surgery. N Engl J Med 337:1785-1791

31. Liebold A, Wahba A, Birnbaum DE (1998) Low-energy cardioversion with epicardial wire electrodes: new treatment of atrial fibrillation after open heart surgery. Circulation 98:883-886

32. Mehmanesh H, Lange R, Hagl S (1998) Temporary atrial electrode for the treatment of supraventricular tachycardia after cardiac operations. Ann Thorac Surg 65:632-636

OTHER SUPRAVENTRICULAR TACHYCARDIAS

Clinically Documented but Not Inducible Atrioventricular Nodal Reentrant Tachycardia: To Ablate or Not To Ablate?

S.-A. CHEN

Several studies have shown that most sustained supraventricular tachycardia can be induced during electrophysiological studies. However, some documented tachyarrhythmias could not be induced during such studies despite infusion of isoproterenol and atropine [1-10]. It is important to study the electrophysiological mechanisms and characteristics of these patients, because the correct diagnosis and target site selected for ablation may be overlooked.

This laboratory found that patients with inducible AV node reentrant tachycardia after isoproterenol and atropine, and patients with noninducible AV node reentrant tachycardia, had a lower incidence of sustained anterograde slow pathway 1:1 conduction, a lower incidence of anterograde dual pathway physiology, and shorter AHmax after isoproterenol and atropine [11]. The possible mechanisms of noninducibility after administering drugs included: (1) isoproterenol and atropine facilitated anterograde fast AV node conduction more than anterograde slow pathway conduction and prevented achievement of slow pathway conduction, and (2) marked shortening of the AH interval over the slow pathway during atrial stimulation, preventing retrograde activation of the fast pathway and initiation of reentrant movement.

Similar to our results, Bogun et al. [12] reported successful slow pathway ablation in six patients with clinically documented but noninducible AV node reentrant tachycardia, and recurrence of tachycardia occurred in one patient during a follow-up period of 8 ± 8 months. However, patients with noninducible AV node reentrant tachycardia needed longer procedure time and longer radiation exposure time because of the strict criteria of endpoints.

Our study had some limitations. First, the presumed mechanism of the noninducible tachyarrhythmia may be incorrect in a small percentage of patients. Second, the number of patients with noninducible tachyarrhythmia is too small to give a good estimate of the complication rates of radiofrequency ablation.

Although a small percentage of patients (2.7%) with presumed diagnosis of AV node reentrant tachycardia and orthodromic AV reciprocating tachycardia

National Yang-Ming University, and Veterans General Hospital-Taipei, Taiwan, R.O.C.

had noninducible tachycardia in the electrophysiological laboratory, application of radiofrequency energy to the presumed arrhythmogenic sites could achieve a high success rate, with a low recurrence rate in these patients.

References

1. Wellens HJJ, Durrer D (1975) The role of an accessory atrioventricular pathway in reciprocal tachycardia: observation in patients with and without the Wolff-Parkinsons-White syndrome. Circulation 52:58-72
2. Josephson ME, Kastor JA (1977) Paroxysmal supraventricular tachycardia: mechanisms and management. Ann Intern Med 87:346-359
3. Farshidi A, Josephson ME, Horowitz LN (1978) Electrophysiologic characteristics of concealed bypass tracts: clinical and electrophysiologic correlates. Am J Cardiol 41:1052-1060
4. Akhtar M, Damato AN, Batsford WP, Caracta AR, Ruskin JN, Weisfogel GM, Lau SH (1975) Induction of atrioventricular nodal reentrant tachycardia after atropine: report of five cases. Am J Cardiol 36:286-291
5. Wu D, Denes P, Bauernfeind R, Dhingra RC, Wyndham C, Rosen KM (1979) Effects of atropine on induction and maintenance of atrioventricular nodal reentrant tachycardia. Circulation 59:779-788
6. Brownstein SL, Hopson RC, Martins JB, Aschoff AM, Llshansky B, Constatin L, Kienzle MG (1988) Usefulness of isoproterenol in facilitating atrioventricular nodal reentry tachycardia during electrophysiologic testing. Am J Cardiol 61:1037-1041
7. Toda I, Kawahara T, Murakawa Y, Nozaki A, Kawakubo K, Inoque H, Sugimoto T (1989) Electrophysiological study of young patients with exercise related paroxysms of palpitation: role of atropine and isoprenaline for initiation of supraventricular tachycardia. Br Heart J 61:268-273
8. Huycke EC, Lai WT, Nguyen NX, Keung EC, Sung RJ (1989) Role of intravenous isoproterenol in the electrophysiologic induction of atrioventricular node reentrant tachycardia in patients with dual atrioventricular node pathways. Am J Cardiol 64:1131-1137
9. Neuss H, Schlepper M, Spies HF (1975) Effects of heart rate and atropine on dual AV conduction. Br Heart J 37:1216-1227
10. Hariman RJ, Pasquariello JL, Gomes JAC, Holtzman R, El-Sherif N (1985) Autonomic dependence of ventriculoatrial conduction. Am J Cardiol 56:285-291
11. Lee SH, Chen SA, Chiang CE, Tai CT, Wen ZC, Ueng KC, Chiou CW, Chen YJ, Yu WC, Huang JL, Cheng JJ, Chang MS (1997) Results of radiofrequency ablation in patients with clinically documented, but noninducible, atrioventricular node reentrant tachycardia and orthodromic atrioventricular reciprocating tachycardia. Am J Cardiol 79:974-978
12. Bogun F, Castellani M, Chan KK, Harvey M, Goyal R, Daoud E, Niebauer M, Man KC, Morady F (1996) Slow pathway ablation in patients with documented but not inducible paroxysmal supraventricular tachycardia. J Am Coll Cardiol 28:1000-1004

Permanent Junctional Reentry Tachycardia: When to Ablate, Where and With Which Results?

M. Lunati[1], G. Magenta[1], G. Cattafi[1], R. Vecchi[1], M. Paolucci[1] and G. Vignati[2]

Introduction

The permanent junctional reentry tachycardia (PJRT) is a rare form of reentrant supraventricular tachycardia (SVT), accounting for 1% of all SVTs, originally described by Coumel et al. in 1967 [1].

PJRT is characterized by an incessant SVT with a long RP interval, narrow QRS complex, generally inverted P waves in inferior leads, at a rate ranging from 110 to 200 bpm.

During SVT antegrade conduction occurs through the AV node and His-Purkinje system, whereas retrograde conduction returns through a slowly conducting accessory pathway (AP) which, like AV nodal tissue, has decremental properties and is generaly located in the posteroseptal zone.

The arrhythmia is characterized by an onset at birth or early childhood, has a wide clinical spectrum (probably the use of the term "persistent" should be preferred to "permanent"), may induce a form of "tachycardiomyopathy" reversible with control of SVT, and is generally refractory to antiarrhythmic drug therapy.

Radiofrequency catheter ablation (RFCA) has become the treatment of choice for this arrhythmia because of its effectiveness and safety. The objective of our work will be to review old and new concepts of the clinical course of the arrhythmia, of the electrophysiological characteristics, and of the results of RFCA derived from recent studies and our own experience [1-9].

When To Ablate

According to the most recent data [4, 5, 8, 9], even if the clinical course of PJRT is incompletely characterized, some considerations can be made in this regard.

There is an equal distribution between male and female (10 M and 11 F in the

[1]Aritmologia Clinica ed Interventistica, Dipartimento Cardiologico "A. De Gasperis";
[2]Cardiologia Pediatrica, Ospedale Ca' Granda, Niguarda, Milan, Italy

study of Dorostkar et al. [9], 9 M and 15 F in the study of Aguinaga et al. [8], 20 M and 12 F in the study of Gaita el al. [5], 2 M and 3 F in the study of Shih et al. [4]).

In approximately 50% of the patients the diagnosis is made at birth, or soon after; in the others the arrhythmia is recognized during infancy, adolescence or adulthood and the prior duration of PJRT is largely unknown.

In about one-fourth of the patients there is an impaired ventricular function tachycardia-related and occasionally symptoms of congestive heart failure (11/21 in the series of Dorostkar et al. [9], 6/24 in the series of Aguinaga et al. [8], 7/32 in the series of Gaita et al. [5]).

Dorostkar et al. [9] demonstrated that the mean PJRT cycle length tends to increase with age (from a mean value of 308 ± 64 ms in the patient < 2 years to 414 ± 57 ms in the patient > 2 years and < 5 years, to 445 ± 57 ms in the patient > 5 years) and this is due to slowing of retrograde conduction in the AP. Probably the spontaneous improvement in ventricular function, which is documented, can be partly related to modifications of the characteristics of the arrhythmia (from incessant to paroxismal SVT).

Up to now RFCA of PJRT was generally performed in adults (mean age at RFCA: in the study of Gaita et al. [5] 29 ± 15 years, in the study of Aguinaga et al. [8] 42 ± 22 years). More recently some authors tend to anticipate the cure of arrhythmia (mean age at RFCA in the study of Dorostkar et al. [9]: 12.8 years).

At our institution, 13 patients with documented PJRT were seen between 1991 and 1998 and successfully treated with RFCA. The clinical characteristics of the study patients were the following: 7 F, 6 M; mean age 22.7 years (range 7-70); in 7/13 the diagnosis was made at birth; 11/13 had incessant SVT which provoked palpitations; 3/13 had evidence of mild decreased left ventricular function (EF 50%); 5/13 had received antiarrhythmic medications (more than one drug) without consistent effects.

Where to Ablate

The explanation for the occurrence of the retrograde conduction only and the decremental properties of the AP associated with PJRT are not completely known: decremental conduction may be due to AP geometry or fiber orientation, the AP may have a tortuous course and impedance mismatch between atrium and ventricle has also been suggested. The frequent location of the pathways in the posteroseptal region raises the possibility that the AP has an AV node-like structure [6, 7, 9].

The methods for an effective RFCA in this arrhythmia are standardized [5, 8, 9].

After the diagnosis of PJRT has been clinically made, the presence of reentry is shown, and the peculiar properties of AP are characterized, the aim of the ablative procedure is to identify the location of the AP recording the shortest VA interval during SVT or ventricular pacing over or under the AV rings. More than 85% of the AP are located at or near the ostium of the coronary sinus and/or in the posteroseptal region (17/21 in Dorostkar's series [9], 25/32 in Gaita's series

[5], 22/24 in Aguinaga's series [8]), thus, RFCA can be successfully performed with a right approach around the coronary sinus ostium (outside or inside the first segment).

A preliminary study of P-wave configuration can be extremely useful in this regard: a negative retrograde P wave in leads II, III, aVF is always present except in patients with an AP with decremetal properties in the left lateral region (positive P wave). A positive P wave in lead I suggests that RFCA can be performed from the right side; a negative P wave does not rule out this possibility [5].

Occasionally, but not exceptionally, PJRT is caused by AP in the free wall (right or left) or by multiple APs [4], (Figs. 1-4). APs located outside the coronary sinus region were 4/21 in Dorostkar's series [9], 8/32 in Gaita's series [5], 2/22 in Aguinaga's series [8].

The success of the procedure is indicated by the immediate stop of SVT during RF delivery (60°-70°), by the impossibility of reinducing SVT, by the evidence of block of retrograde conduction through the extranodal AP 30' after the procedure.

In our series all the patients, except one, had a single AP. The location of AP and the site of effective RFCA were the coronary sinus ostium or posteroseptal region in 11/13, the left lateral region in 1/13; one patient had two AP (one at the ostium of coronary sinus, one in midseptal region).

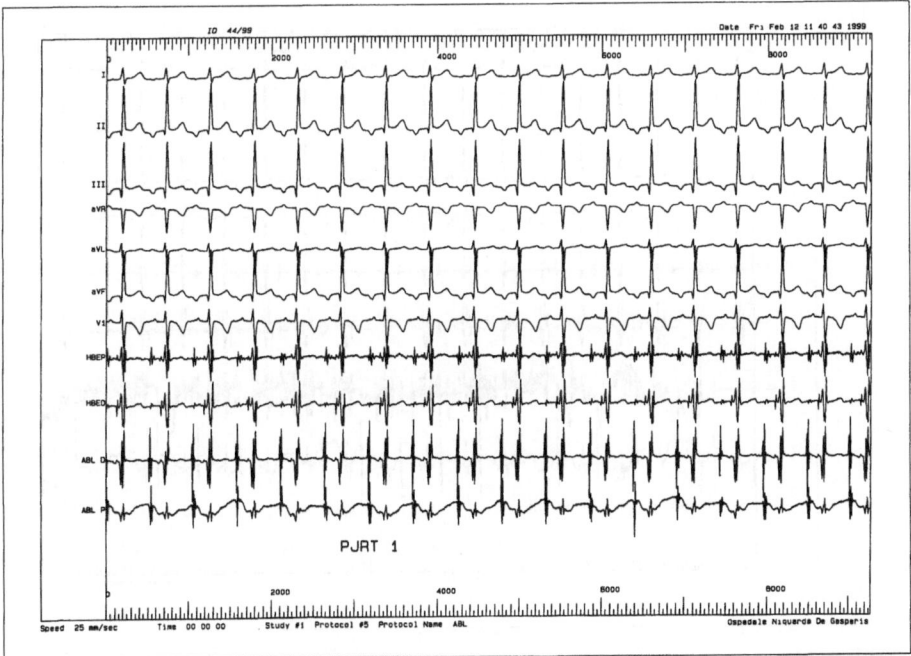

Fig. 1. ECG and intracardiac electrograms of clinical arrhythmia in a patient, 7 years old, with permanent junctional reentry tachycardia (PJRT 1)

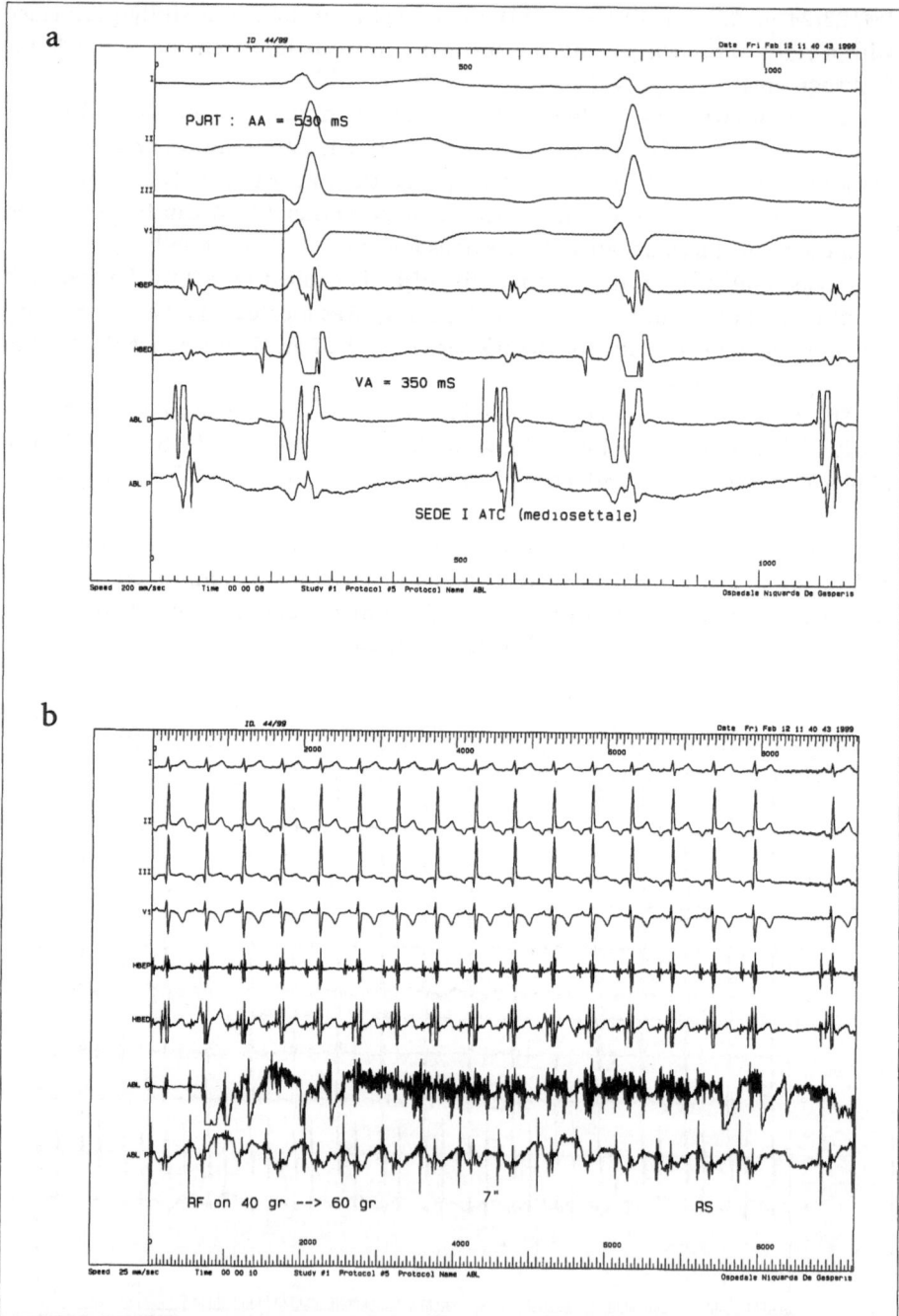

Fig. 2 a,b. Cycle length of the first PJRT (PJRT 1) was 530 ms; earliest atrial activation was recorded from midseptal region (mediosettale, ABL D) (a). PJRT 1 terminated 7 s after onset of radiofrequency (*RF ON*) pulse (b)

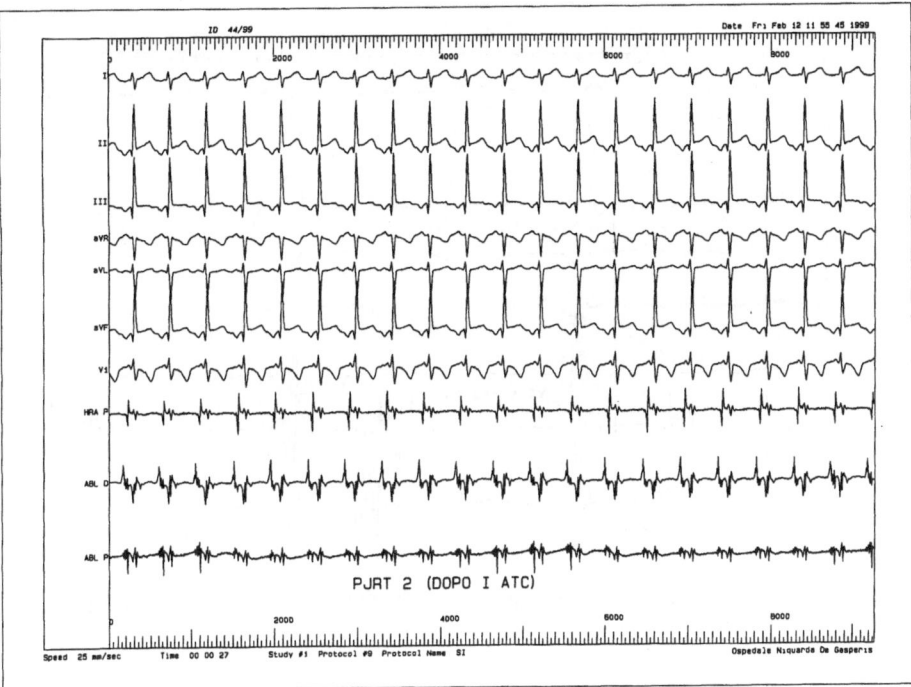

Fig 3. ECG and intracardiac electrograms of a second form of PJRT (PJRT 2) inducible after effective ablation of PJRT 1. Note difference in morphology of retrograde P waves and PR interval between PJRT 1 and PJRT 2

With Which Results

RFCA is extremely effective and safe in this arrhythmia. In Dorostkar's series [9] RFCA was effective in 19/21 patients in a long-term follow-up (range from 2.9 to 8 years) with disappearance of symptoms and improvement of ventricular function in all. In Aguinaga's study AP was successfully ablated in 23/24 patients. All the patients with left ventricular dysfunction experienced an improvement, and after a mean follow-up period of 21 ± 16 months all the patients remain asymptomatic. In Gaita's study [5] 31/32 patients were successfully treated with RFCA, and at a mean follow-up of 18 ± 12 months 31 patients were asymptomatic.

Recurrences are rare (< 10%) and a repeat RFCA is generally completely effective.

Complications are exceptional and not serious: 1 transient AV block in Gaita's and Dorostkar's series [5, 9].

At our institution RFCA was effective in 13/13 patients (in 10/13 with a single session and in 3/13 with a second procedure after a transient success and recurrence of SVT). We did not observe any complications.

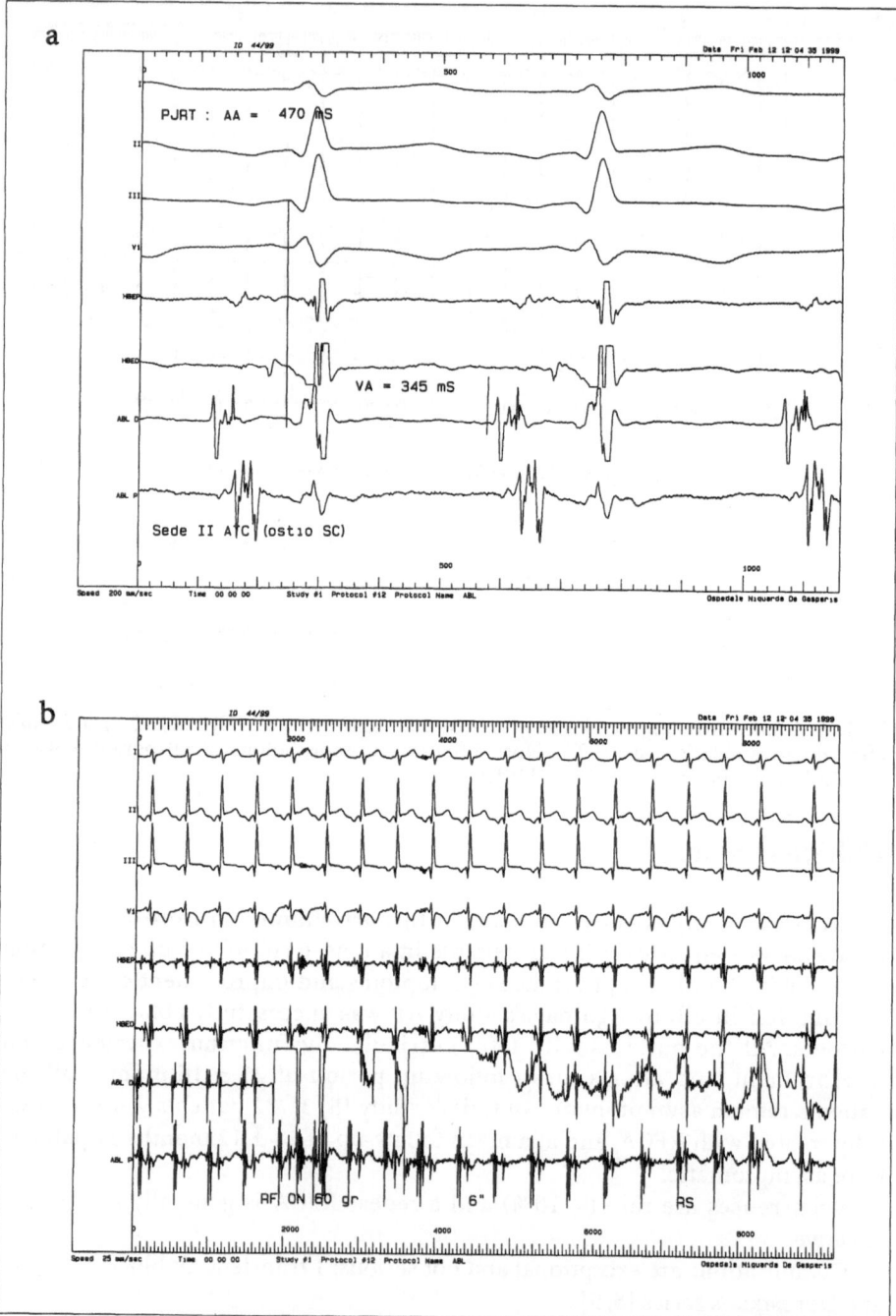

Fig. 4 a,b. Cycle lenght of the second PJRT was 470 ms; earliest atrial activation was recorded from the ostium of the coronary sinus (ostio SC, ABL D) (a). PJRT 2 terminated 6 s after onset of radiofrequency pulse (RF ON) (b)

Conclusions

According to the data presented some conclusions can be drawn.

PJRT has a very wide clinical spectrum with an onset more often in early childhood. The age-related prolongation of the SVT cycle length, due primarily to conduction delay in the concealed AP, explains why clinically asymptomatic adults are not uncommon, why SVT may be incessant or paroxysmal with periods of remission (but exceptionally spontaneous resolution), and why patients with tachycardiomyopathy may improve spontaneously.

Because of unsatisfactory antiarrhythmic treatment of PJRT and the extremely effective cure with RFCA, this option should be considered as the treatment of choice and the indications should be extended to most patients.

In the presence of significant symptoms (intractable SVT, exercise intolerance, etc) and suitable patient size for ablation ($\geq$ 20 kg), RFCA, which provides definite and safe treatment of PJRT, should be applied.

References

1. Coumel P, Cabrol C, Fabiato A et al (1967) Tachycardie permanent par rhythm reciproque. Arch Mal Coeur 60:1830-1864
2. Critelli G, Gallagher JJ, Monda V et al (1984) Anatomic and electrophysiologic substrate of the permanent form of junctional reciprocating tachycardia. J Am Coll Cardiol 4:601-610
3. Chien WW, Cohen TJ, Lee MA et al (1992) Electrophysiological findings and long-term follow-up of patients with the permanent form of junctional reciprocating tachycardia treated by catheter ablation. Circulation 85:1329-1336
4. Shih HT, Miles WM, Klein LS et al (1994) Multiple accessory pathways in the permanent form of junctional reciprocating tachycardia. Am J Cardiol 73:361-367
5. Gaita F, Haissaguerre M, Giustetto C et al (1995) Catheter ablation of permanent junctional reciprocating tachycardia with radiofrequency current. J Am Coll Cardiol 25:648-654
6. Yagi T, Ito M, Odakura H et al (1996) Electrophysiologic comparison between incessant and paroxysmal tachycardia in patients with permanent form of junctional reciprocating tachycardia. Am J Cardiol 78:697-700
7. Chen SA, Tai CT, Chiang CE et al (1996) Electrophysiologic characteristics, electropharmacologic responses and radiofrequency catheter ablation in patients with decremetal accessory pathway. J Am Coll Cardiol 28:732-737
8. Aguinaga L, Brugada J, Anguera I et al (1998) Seguimiento a largo plazo de pacientes con la forma permanente de taquicardia reciproca de la union tipo Coumel tratados mediante ablación con radiofrequencia. Rev Esp Cardiol 51:218-223
9. Dorostkar PC, Silka MJ, Morady F et al (1999) Clinical course of persistent junctional reciprocating tachycardia. J Am Coll Cardiol 33:366-375

How to Predict and Avoid Complete AV Block Complicating Radiofrequency Ablation of AV Nodal Slow Pathway

P. Delise[1], A. Bonso[2], L. Coro[1], M. Fantine[1], A. Raviele[2], G. Gasparini[2] and S. Themistoclakis[2]

Slow pathway ablation is currently used to cure common and uncommon A-V node reentrant tachycardia (AVN RT). The technique has a success rate of about 100% and a 0.5%-2% risk of inadvertent complete AV block [1-4]. Although the risk of block is low, it is difficult to tolerate in patients with a benign arrhythmia, especially when they are young.

Thakur et al. [5] reported that a relatively fast rate of junctional tachycardia (JT) caused by radiofrequency (RF)associated with loss of V-A conduction is related to increased risk of AV block. However, these markers of impending heart block do not allow the risk of AV block to be determined before RF energy delivery. Indeed AV block may occur concurrently with the development of retrograde fast pathway block during JT induced by RF. Hintringer et al. [6] suggested that a useful electrophysiological marker to assess the risk of block is the interval between the atrial component of the His bundle electrogram and the atrial signal of the distal mapping catheter [A(H)-A(Md) interval]. Indeed these authors suggest that a short A(H)-A(Md) interval (17 ± 8 ms) should be associated with a high risk of inadvertent AV block. According to the authors the longer the interval, the greater the distance between the mapping catheter and the compact AV node should be.

The explanation of inadvertent AV block during slow pathway ablation suggested by Hintringer et al., however, is not completely convincing nor is their method of avoiding AV block completely satisfactory. Indeed, the causes of inadvertent AV block during slow pathway ablation vary and may not involve a lesion of the compact AV node. In some cases, the block may be due to intentional damage to the AVN-His junction due to delivery of the energy to the anterior aspect of the triangle of Koch in the junction between the His bundle and compact AV node. In other cases, the block is related to the injury of both fast and slow pathways during serial attempts at ablation of both pathways [4]. In yet other cases, however, the cause of block is unclear because the energy is delivered to the posterior aspect of the triangle of Koch, far from the usual site of the anterograde

[1]Unità Operativa di Cardiologia, Ospedale di Feltre, Belluno, Italy; [2]Unità Operativa di Cardiologia, Ospedale di Mestre, Venice, Italy

fast pathway and far from the compact AV node. A possible explanation in the latter case is an atypical location of the fast pathway or the absence of its anterograde conduction.

Anatomical studies [7] have demonstrated that AV node morphology is quite variable in man and reproduces the electrophysiological model of the duality in only few cases. Electrophysiological studies [8] have confirmed that the AV node is á complex and variable structure. For example, multisite simultaneous catheter mapping of Koch's triangle had demonstrated that retrograde conduction of the AV node both during ventricular pacing and AVN RT is heterogeneous, indicating that in most patients multiple retrograde fast pathways are often present, even if not all are used during AVN RT. Indeed, in about two out of three patients, early retrograde breakthrough is observed in multiple sites of the Koch's triangle or in a large area of a broad wave front activation. Furthermore, it has been suggested that the site of the anteriorly conducting fast pathway is not always coincident with the posteriorly conducting fast pathway (which is retrogradely utilized during AVN RT). For example, in some cases, the anterograde fast pathway is located in the anterior aspect of the Koch's triangle, while the retrograde fast pathway is located in the posterior aspect. It has also been suggested that in some cases the fast pathway is able to conduct only retrogradely, while its anterograde conduction is absent [9]. Such variability explains why in selected cases unexpected AV block can occur during radiofrequency ablation of AVN RT. Indeed, the lesion of the slow pathway can also damage the anterograde fast pathway if the latter is located close to the slow pathway itself. AV block can also follow slow pathway ablation in cases in which the anterograde conduction of the fast pathway is absent and when AVN RT has as the retrograde limb a fast pathway which is capable of retrograde conduction only. Some authors suggest that the absence of anterograde conduction of the fast pathway correlates with a long PR interval and have found a high percentage of AV block during slow pathway ablation in these cases [10]. Other authors, however, have not confirmed this finding [11].

If the mechanism of AV block is an abnormally located or a non-conducting fast pathway, such risk should be reduced by localizing the site of the anterogradely conducting fast pathway. With this purpose, we suggested localizing the site of the anterogradely conducting fast pathway in patients with AVN RT by the pacemapping of Koch's triangle.

Pacemapping of Koch's Triangle

The rationale of the pacemapping of the Koch's triangle is to localize the site of the anterogradely conducting fast pathway on the basis of the shortest St-H interval. Indeed, on stimulating the site where the fast pathway is present, a short St-H interval is recorded and, conversely, the greater the distance between the mapping catheter and the anterograde conducting fast pathway, the longer the St-H interval. The triangle of Koch can be easily identified by using the apex of its virtual three angles as reference points: the catheter positioned on the His bundle (which represents the apex of the triangle), the proximal electrodes of the catheter inserted into the coronary sinus (which represents the apex of the second angle of the triangle), and the atrial insertion of the tricuspid valve in the area surrounding the ostium of the coronary sinus (identified on the basis of the electrophysiological recordings by the mapping catheter). At least three main regions of the Koch's triangle should be mapped: anteroseptal (AS), midseptal (MS) and posteroseptal (PS). Pacemapping is performed by stimulating at a rate slightly faster than the sinus rate (generally 100/min) with an output twice that of the diastolic threshold. The stimulation of the AS aspect of the triangle of Koch is obtained by first placing the catheter where the highest His deflection is recorded. By stimulating at this site, the right ventricle or His bundle is generally captured. During continuous stimulation, the catheter is then slowly withdrawn until the atrium is captured. The first 2-3 beats are used for calculations. During this maneuvre particular attention must be paid in order to avoid stimulating the right septum posteriorly to the tendon of Todaro. Consequently, when necessary, the maneuvre must be repeated more than once and the shortest St-H should be chosen. Stimulation of the posterior aspect of the triangle of Koch is obtained by placing the catheter in front of the ostium of the coronary sinus. Finally, the MS aspect of the triangle of Koch is stimulated by placing the catheter in an intermediate position between the AS and PS regions.

When stimulating from the AS, MS and PS regions, the St-H and AH intervals are calculated in the catheter positioned on the His bundle.

Radiofrequency Ablation Guided by the Pacemapping of Koch's Triangle

We studied 55 patients with common AVN RT (19 M, 36 F, mean age 52 ± 16 years). In all cases a complete electrophysiological study was performed, followed, in the same session, by radiofrequency ablation. In all cases AVN RT tachycardia was inducible (mean RR 410 ± 50 ms).

By pacemapping Koch's triangle in 49/55 patients (Gr.A, 89%) the shortest St-H interval was recorded on stimulating the AS region (Fig. 1a-c). In such cases, the longer St-H intervals obtained by stimulating in the MS and PS regions were related to longer St-A intervals, while AH intervals remained unchanged (Table 1). In 4 patients (Gr.B, 7%) the shortest St-H was recorded in the MS region (Fig. 2 a-c and Table 1). Finally, in two patients (Gr.C, 4%) the shortest St-H was recored in the PS region (Table 1). AH interval was significantly longer in patients of Gr.C than in those of Gr.A and B (200 ± 99 ms vs 64 ± 18 and 62 ± 3 ms respectively). In Gr.A, on stimulation in the AS, MS and PS regions, AH interval remained constant in all cases (AS 64 ± 18, MS 65 ± 19, PS 65 ± 17 ms respectively). In contrast, both in Gr.B and Gr.C, on stimulation in the MS and PS regions, AH shortened (in Gr.B from 62 ± 3 to 32 ± 3 and to 57 ± 3 ms respectively; in Gr.C from 200 ± 99 to 170 ± 100 and to 137 ± 109 ms respectively).

At the end of the electrophysiological study, ablation of the slow or fast pathway was performed. The choice of ablating slow or fast pathway was guided by

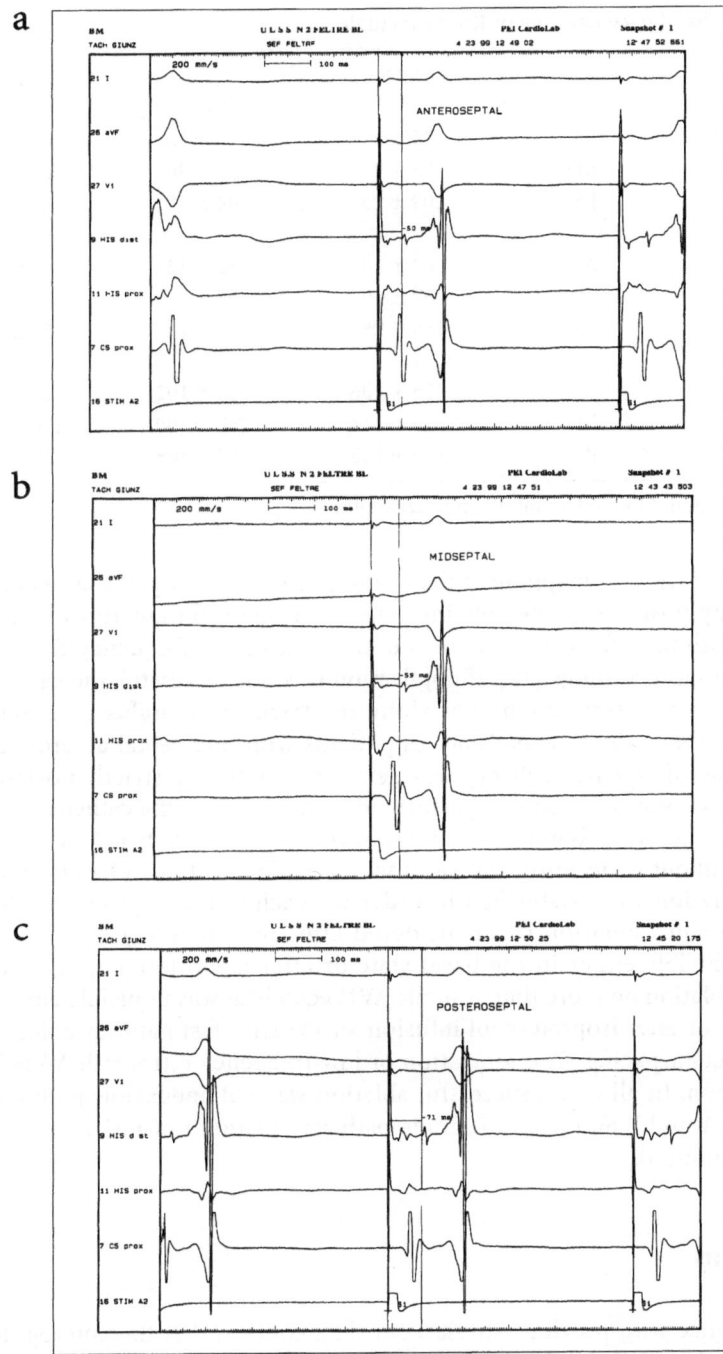

Fig. 1a-c. Pacemapping of Koch's triangle. St-H interval is calculated stimulating in anteroseptal (**a**), midseptal (**b**) and posteroseptal (**c**) areas. The shortest St-H interval is recorded stimulating in anteroseptal area, where the anterogradly conducting fast pathway is located

Table 1. Results of pacemapping of Koch's triangle

		St-H	St-A	AH
Gr.A (*n.* 49)	AS	79 ± 21	15 ± 16	64 ± 18
	MS	95 ± 20	31 ± 20	65 ± 19
	PS	109 ± 23	44 ± 18	64 ± 18
Gr.B (*n.* 4)	AS	80 ± 14	18 ± 12	62 ± 3
	MS	67 ± 10	35 ± 8	32 ± 3
	PS	110 ± 28	53 ± 18	57 ± 3
Gr.C (*n.* 2)	AS	215 ± 106	15 ± 102	200 ± 99
	MS	200 ± 113	30 ± 100	170 ± 100
	PS	190 ± 120	53 ± 108	137 ± 109

AS, anteroseptal; MS, midseptal; PS, posteroseptal

the results of the pacemapping of the triangle of Koch. Slow pathway ablation was obtained by positioning the ablating catheter in the right anterior oblique view near the ostium of the coronary sinus in the zone of low-frequency, fractionated, slow potential recordings [12]. If application was not successful, the catheter was repositioned progressively higher along the tricuspid annulus in a continued attempt to ablate the slow pathway. In patients with mid-septal anterograde fast pathway radiofrequency delivery was performed only in a strictly posteroseptal area. Fast pathway ablation was performed by first placing the catheter in the site where the highest His bundle potential was recorded. The catheter was then withdrawn by about 1 cm until A/V ratio was > 1. The protocol of radiofrequency energy ablation was established in order to reach at least 50°-60° for 20"-30". Radiofrequency ablation was considered effective when: (1) AVN RT was no longer inducible either in the basal state or after isoproterenol, (2) after slow pathway ablation no more than a single AVN echo beat was inducible either in the basal state or after isoproterenol infusion, or (3) after fast pathway ablation during ventricular pacing VA dissociation or low-frequency retrograde Wenchebach phenomenon. In all cases, successful ablation was obtained: slow pathway ablation in Gr.A and B and fast retrograde pathway ablation in Gr. C. In no case was AV block induced.

Conclusions

In accordance with previous studies, our data confirm that the anterograde fast pathway is localized in the anterior aspect of the triangle of Koch in the vast majority of patients. Indeed, in such cases, the shortest St-H interval is recorded on stimulating the AS region, while on stimulating the MS and PS regions, St-H

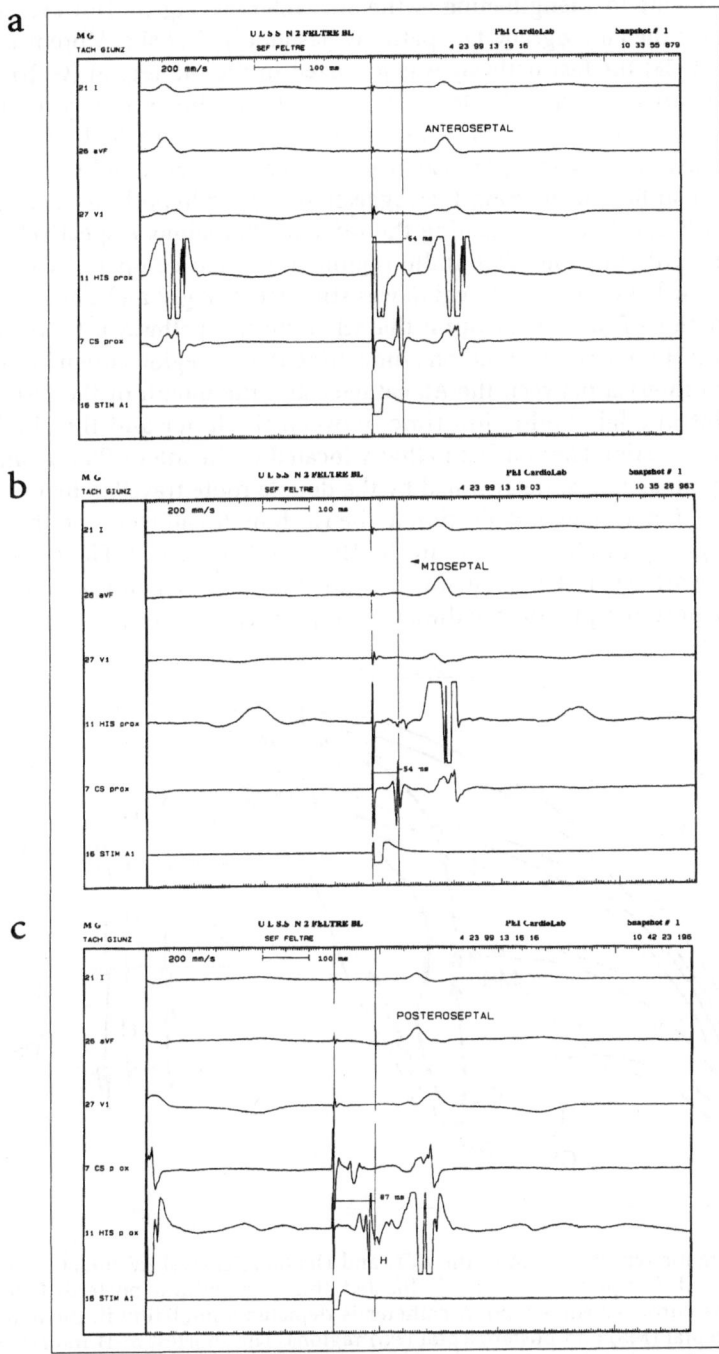

Fig. 2a-c. Pacemapping of Koch's triangle. The shortest St-H interval is recorded stimulating in the midseptal area where the fast pathway is located lengthens owing to a lengthening of the St-A interval (Fig. 3). However, in about 10% of cases the anterograde fast pathway has an atypical site. More precisely, in 4/55 cases (7%) the fast pathway was localized in the MS region (Gr.B) while in 2/55 (3%) cases, which had a long PR interval, the shortest St-H interval was recorded on stimulating the PS region (Gr.C). It is not clear whether, in the latter cases, the fast pathway was posteriorly located or whether it had no anterograde conduction, although the long PR suggests the latter hypothesis. Interestingly, both in Gr.B and C, on stimulating the MS and PS regions respectively, the AH interval recorded in the His bundle region shortened compared with the AH interval recorded when the AS region was stimulated (Fig. 2 a-c).The most probable explanation of such behaviour is that when the fast pathway is far from the AS region the AH interval recorded on stimulating the AS region comprises both the intra-atrial interval between the AS catheter and the mouth of the fast pathway and the intranodal conduction time between the latter and the His bundle. Conversely, on stimulating a fast pathway located in the MS or PS region, the AH interval is a fusion beat determined by the double route travelled by the impulse along the atrium (giving A deflection in the His bundle catheter) and the compact AV node (giving the H deflection in the His bundle catheter). The same mechanism is at work when the fast pathway is not capable of anterograde conduction and only a posteroseptal slow pathway anterogradely conducts (Fig. 4).

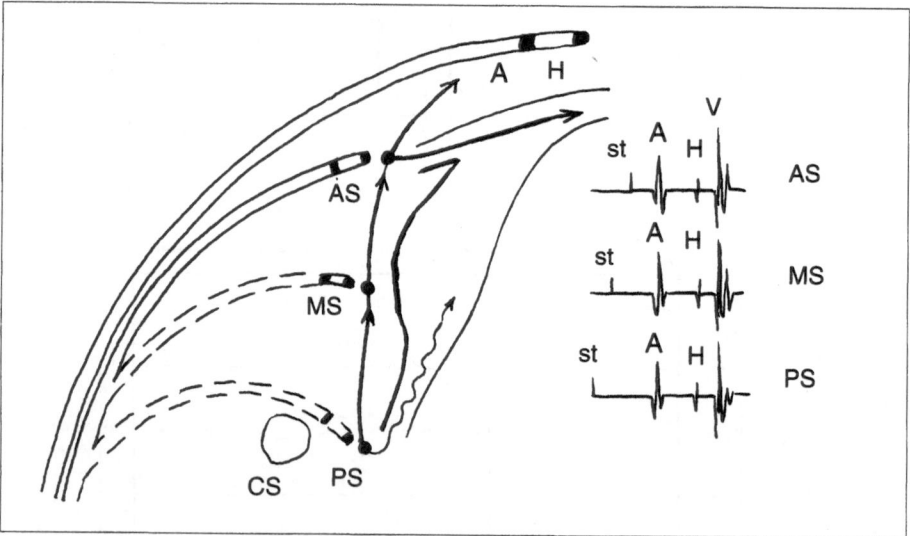

Fig. 3. Schematic representation of the AVN and His bundle. Dual AV nodal pathways can be recognized: fast pathway anteriorly located and slow pathway posteriorly located in front of the coronary sinus (CS). A catheter is depicted stimulating in the anteroseptal (AS), midseptal (MS) and posteroseptal (PS) regions. The shortest St-H interval is recorded in the AS region where fast pathway is located. The greater the distance between the mapping catheter and the anterograde conducting fast pathway, the longer the St-H interval. The longer St-H intervals obtained stimulating in MS and PS regions are related to longer St-A intervals, while AH intervals are constant

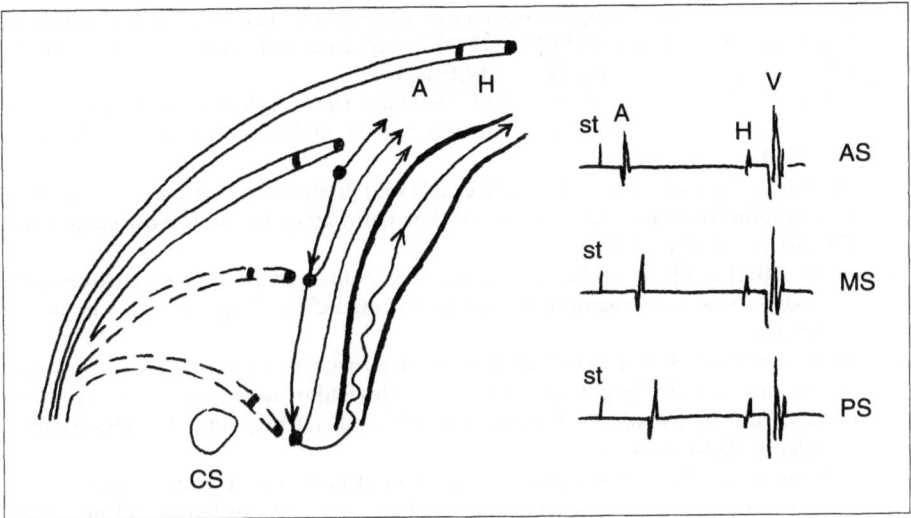

Fig. 4. Schematic representation of the AVN and His bundle. Anterograde fast pathway is absent. Slow pathway is posteriorly located in front of the coronary sinus (CS). A catheter is depicted stimulating in the anteroseptal (AS), midseptal (MS) and posteroseptal (PS) regions. The shortest St-H interval is recorded in the PS region. When compared with the stimulation of AS region, during stimulation of PS region St-A lengthens and AH shortens. For explanations see text

Our data confirm that the risk of AV block related to an atypical location of the fast pathway or to the absence of its conduction is low. In most cases, in fact, the fast and slow pathways are far enough apart to render the simultaneous damage of both pathways by RF energy unlikely. The pacemapping of Koch's triangle, however, demonstrates that, in selected cases this risk does exist, either because the two pathways are closely located or because only the slow pathway anterogradely conducts. In these cases, the risk can be reduced by performing slow pathway ablation in a site sufficiently far from the site of the anterograde fast pathway or ablating the retrogradely conducting fast pathway.

References

1. Haissaguerre M, Gaita F, Fischer B et al (1992) Elimination of atrioventricular nodal reentrant tachycardia using discrete slow potentials to guide application of radiofrequency energy. Circulation 85:2162-2175
2. Jackman WM, Beckman KJ, McClelland JH et al (1992) Treatment of supraventricular tachycardia due to atrioventricular nodal reentry by radiofrequency catheter ablation of slow-pathway conduction. N Engl J Med 327:313-318
3. Wu D, Yeh S-J, Wang C-C, Wen M-S, Lin F-C (1993) A simple technique for selective radiofrequency ablation of the slow pathway in atrioventricular node reentrant tachycardia. J Am Coll Cardiol 21:1612-1621
4. Hindricks G, on behalf of the MERFS investigators of the Working Group on

Arrhythmias of the European Society of Cardiology: The Multicenter European Radiofrequency Survey (MERFS) (1993) Complication of radiofrequency catheter ablation of arrhythmias. Eur Heart J 14:1644-1653

5. Thakur RK, Klein GJ, Yee R, Stites HW (1993) Junctional tachycardia: a useful marker during radiofrequency ablation for atrioventricular node reentrant tachycardia. J Am Coll Cardiol 22:1706-1710

6. Hintringer F, Hartikainen J, Davies W et al (1995) Prediction of atrioventricular block during radiofrequency ablation of the slow pathway of the atrioventricular node. Circulation 92:3490-3496

7. Inoue S, Becker AE (1998) Posterior extensions of the human compact atrioventricular node. A neglected anatomic feature of potential clinical significance. Circulation 97:188-193

8. Anselme F, Hook B, Monahan K et al (1996) Heterogeneity of retrograde fast-pathway conduction pattern in patients with atrioventricular nodal reentry tachycardia. Observations by use of simultaneous multisite catheter mapping of Koch's triangle. Circulation 93:960-968

9. Reithmann C, Hoffmann E, Grunewald A et al (1998) Fast pathway ablation in patients with common atrioventricular nodal reentrant tachycardia and prolonged PR interval during sinus rhythm. Eur Heart J 19:929-935

10. Ridgen LB, Klein LS, Mitrani RD et al (1995) Increased risk of heart block following slow pathway ablation for AV nodal reentrant tachycardia in patients with marked PR interval prolongation during sinus rhythm. PACE 18:II-918

11. Sra JS, Jazayeri MR, Blank Z et al (1994) Slow pathway ablation in patients with atrioventricular node reentrant tachycardia and a prolonged PR interval. J Am Coll Cardiol 24:1064-1068

12. Delise P, Themistoclakis S, Corò L et al (1996) Radiofrequency ablation of atrioventricular node reentrant tachycardias: which results and predictors of success and recurrence? In: Raviele A (ed) Cardiac arrhythmia. Springer, Berlin Heidelberg New York, pp 177-180

Ablation of Antero-Septal and Intermediate Septal Accessory Pathways: How Safe Is It? How Can One Minimize the Risk of AV Block?

R. De Ponti[1], C. Storti[2], M. Zardini[1], M. Tritto[1], M. Longobardi[2], P. Fang[1] and J.A. Salerno-Uriarte[1]

Introduction

The current goal of radiofrequency catheter ablation of supraventricular tachycardias is to cure a large cohort of patients with a primary success rate close to 100% and a complication and recurrence rate close to 0%. In this setting, the ablation of the atrioventricular (A-V) accessory pathway in the triangle of Koch may still represent a grey area, since the strict anatomical relationship between the bypass tract and the A-V node-His bundle may affect the feasibility and safety of the procedure. Consequently, the only rationale for successful ablation with no complication in this area relies on the assumption that the accessory pathway is more sensitive to radiofrequency energy delivery than the normal A-V conduction system [1]. The risk of damaging the normal A-V conduction pathway and of inducing a complete A-V block requiring a permanent pacemaker has been pointed out by both early [2, 3] and recent [4-6] reports, although successful and safe ablation has been described in limited series of cases [7, 8], even with "para-hissian" accessory pathways [1]. Moreover, in the risk/benefit ratio of ablation of by-pass tracts in the Koch's triangle one must consider not only failure and the risk of permanent complete A-V block, but also the theoretical possibility of creating an incessant reentrant circuit by partially damaging both the accessory pathway and the A-V node conduction.

According to our experience, catheter ablation of antero-septal and intermediate septal accessory pathways can be highly successful and safe, the only complication being persistent right bundle branch block in a limited group of patients. On the basis of the previous experience in mapping and ablation of the fast A-V node pathway in patients with A-V nodal reentrant tachycardia [9], we developed and refined a method of ablating these accessory pathways. This paper sets out to answer the questions proposed in the title by describing this method and reporting the results achieved in our series of patients.

[1]Istituto di Cardiologia "Mater Domini", Università degli Studi dell'Insubria, Sede di Varese, Castellanza (VA); [2]Divisione di Cardiologia, Istituto "Città di Pavia", Pavia, Italy

Preliminary Anatomical and Electrophysiological Considerations

From the anatomical point of view, the accessory pathways located in the triangle of Koch can be classified as follows. Among "antero-septal" accessory pathways, the "para-hissian" should be distinguished from the "anterior (or superior) para-septal" by-pass tracts. The para-hissian accessory pathways are those adjacent to the His bundle [1]. Consequently: (1) a His bundle electrogram is recorded at the site of successful ablation; (2) there is practically no distance on fluoroscopy between the ablation catheter and the His bundle catheter; (3) in the His bundle electrogram, the delta wave-V interval is negative. These accessory pathways should be distinguished from the anterior para-septal Kent bundles. In fact, although (1) the anterior para-septal accessory pathways have a close anatomical relationship with the His bundle area, (2) they are usually located antero-superiorly to where the best His bundle electrogram is recorded and (3) the potential risk of damaging the normal conduction pathway during ablation is not consistently decreased, the above-mentioned criteria for para-hissian accessory pathways are not met. Finally, the "intermediate septal" accessory pathways, less commonly observed, are those located in the "true septum", primarily on the right side, in close anatomical proximity to the posterior input of the A-V node [10]. Although they are less close to the His bundle area and the risk of inducing a distal A-V block is less likely, the possibility of damaging the A-V nodal conduction, requiring permanent pacing, should not be underestimated.

Population and Method

Population

Among 1054 patients who underwent radiofrequency catheter ablation of accessory pathways between May 1991 and December 1998, 83 (7.8%) showed an antero-septal or intermediate septal accessory pathway. Demographic data and the location of the accessory pathways, according to the above-mentioned criteria, are shown in Table 1. The four asymptomatic subjects were athletes in whom electro-

Table 1. Demographic data and accessory pathway characteristics in patients with antero-septal and intermediate septal Kent bundles

Number of patients	83
Sex (M/F)	71/12
Age (years ± SD)	29 ± 13 (range 10-71)
Asymptomatic subjects	4 (5%)
Concomitant organic heart disease	5 patients (6%)
Manifest preexcitation	69 patients (83%)
Para-hissian accessory pathway	38 patients (4%)
Anterior para-septal accessory pathway	28 patients (34%)
Intermediate septal accessory pathway	17 patients (20%)
Multiple accessory pathway	5 patients (6%)

physiological testing revealed good conduction properties of the accessory pathway and inducibility of sustained A-V reentrant tachycardia and/or preexcited atrial fibrillation with very fast ventricular response. In the first 41 of these 83 patients the radiofrequency energy was delivered in power control mode, while in the remaining 42 patients temperature control mode was used.

Mapping and Localization of the Accessory Pathway

Since the triangle of Koch is an anatomically complex structure, prior to the mapping/ablation phase one should familiarize oneself with this area by placing multipolar catheters in the His bundle area and coronary sinus and precisely identifying the orientation of the Koch's triangle, together with the limits and extension of essential anatomical landmarks, such as the His bundle, A-V node and coronary sinus os. In order to localize and subclassify (para-hissian, para-septal or intermediate septal) the accessory pathway, a careful mapping is performed on sinus rhythm, searching for optimal A-V and delta wave-V intervals as well as a putative Kent bundle potential. The ratio between the atrial and ventricular deflection should not be inferior to 1; this prevents energy delivery at the ventricular insertion of the accessory pathway, minimizing the risk of inducing permanent right bundle branch block. Particularly, in cases with a manifest para-hissian accessory pathway, the identification of the His bundle location in sinus rhythm may be difficult. In some patients preexcitation hampers a distinct recording of the His bundle electrogram, whereas in other cases a His bundle potential follows the ventricular deflection (see Fig. 1). In these cases additional mapping in orthodromic atrioventricular reentrant tachycardia is required.

Catheter Manipulation and Contact

Since the antero-septal accessory pathways are particularly sensitive to mechanical injury resulting in conduction block [11], the mapping/ablation catheter should be gently manipulated in this area. In our series, a persistent traumatic accessory pathway conduction block occurred in four patients and a second postponed ablation procedure was required in all. For this reason, we never use a long sheath to stabilize the catheter in the antero-septal region in case poor catheter contact is obtained by using the inferior vena cava approach. As shown in Fig. 1, it is useful in these cases to approach the antero-septal (para-hissian and anterior para-septal) area from the superior vena cava with a long curve (diameter > 55 mm) catheter.

Preset Values for Radiofrequency Energy Delivery

Titration of radiofrequency energy delivery together with a stable catheter contact are the key issues for a successful and safe ablation of the accessory pathways in the Koch's triangle. Since power output of radiofrequency energy does not predict temperature during ablation [12], temperature control mode is essential in

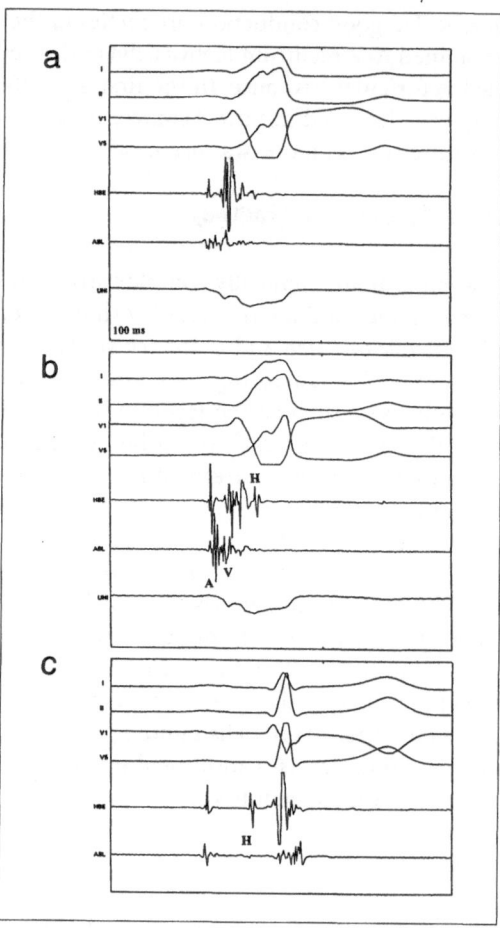

Fig. 1a-c. Fourteen-year-old patient with a para-hissian accessory pathway. In this patient, the change from inferior to superior vena cava approach dramatically improved catheter contact and allowed safe and successful ablation by a single radiofrequency energy pulse. **a** The delta wave-V interval in the His bundle electrogram (HBE) is negative (-10 ms), but no distinct His bundle potential can be recorded. The bipolar signal from the ablation catheter (ABL), positioned through the inferior vena cava, is unsuitable for ablation, due to poor contact. **b** When the catheter is re-positioned through the superior vena cava in the same area, as assessed on fluoroscopy and by the identical morphology of the unipolar signal recorded from the tip of the ablation catheter (UNI), the contact is consistently improved. The amplitude of the bipolar signal has greatly increased and it is now stable, the A-V and delta wave-V intervals are 20 ms and -16 ms, respectively, and a high-frequency potential (putative Kent bundle potential) can be observed between the atrial and the ventricular deflection. Although the ventricular deflection in the unipolar lead has multiple components, the initial component is negative. Moreover, also the His bundle catheter contact is improved and now a distinct high-frequency potential in the HBE can be recorded after the ventricular deflection. The chronology and the polarity of this potential, compared with that recorded postablation, suggest that this is an antegradely activated His bundle potential. **c** After a single radiofrequency energy pulse (55 °C, 15 s, 360 J), conduction through the accessory pathway is permanently abolished; a small His bundle potential can also be recorded at the site of successful ablation the subset of patients with antero-septal and intermediate accessory pathways. In our series of patients, the use of power control mode was limited to the initial phase (1991-1994). The power output of the first radiofrequency pulse was preset at 5 W for 10-15 s; in the subsequent pulses the power was increased to as much as 20 W with the same duration. With the temperature control mode, the cut-off temperature is preset at 55°C. In our experience, this seems to be the optimal value to avoid damage of the normal conduction pathway and to minimize the occurrence of partial ablation of the accessory pathway, which could result in late resumption of conduction. Accordingly, the maximum power is preset at 30 W and the duration at 15 s; radiofrequency generators with a smooth power delivery curve at the beginning of the application are preferable. Only when the applications are unsuccessful due to a low tip temperature or the conduction resumes after a successful application may the power be increased to 50 W and the duration to 30 s, provided that none of the events mentioned in the following paragraph occurs.

Radiofrequency Energy Delivery

Radiofrequency energy should be delivered during a stable cardiac rhythm, preferably in sinus rhythm. In cases with a concealed accessory pathway, in order to monitor the response to the radiofrequency pulse, the energy is delivered on A-V reentrant tachycardia, but the catheter position is carefully and continuously checked, since termination of tachycardia may displace the ablation catheter. Energy delivery during ventricular pacing is to be avoided, since interruption of conduction through the normal pathway cannot be detected during the application. The radiofrequency pulse is promptly interrupted in case the ablation catheter displaces (its position is continuously checked on fluoroscopy), junctional rhythm appears or an increase in the degree of preexcitation is observed. In the latter two situations, the cut-off temperature value must be reduced and the duration of the application shortened. Finally, during radiofrequency energy delivery, once ventricular preexcitation has disappeared, the A-H interval should be carefully monitored, since its prolongation could be a sign of initial damage to the A-V node conduction due to heat propagation in Koch's triangle. When A-H interval prolongation is noted, the radiofrequency application must be discontinued.

Follow-up and Treatment of Recurrence

After successful ablation, the patient undergoes 1 h of observation, during which time a postablation electrophysiological study is carried out. The patient is discharged 48 h after the procedure and followed up for 5 weeks. During this period, a 12-lead electrocardiogram is recorded weekly. If conduction through the accessory pathway resumes, an electrophysiological session is rescheduled; a second ablation is performed only if the accessory pathway is responsible for reentrant tachycardia and/or preexcited atrial fibrillation. Patients with a concealed accessory pathway routinely undergo a follow-up electrophysiological study.

Results

The results of catheter ablation in the overall population and in each subgroup of patients are reported in Table 2. Interruption of conduction through the accessory pathway was achieved in every patient; in 12 patients more than one procedure was necessary to obtain successful ablation. The superior vena cava approach was used in some patients with an antero-septal accessory pathway, predominantly in those with a para-hissian location. As for complications, no A-V block was induced in any case; a persistent postablation right bundle branch block was induced in five patients, all with a para-hissian accessory pathway. No other complications were observed. Fourteen patients had a recurrence within 1 month after the procedure; all were successfully retreated by catheter ablation. The overall recurrence rate was 17%, but as high as 26% when only para-hissian accessory pathways were considered. This rate was significantly higher than in the patients with other accessory pathways, in whom recurrences were observed in 6.4% of cases ($p < 0.05$).

Table 3 shows that, in patients with a para-hissian accessory pathway, the results mainly depend on the operators' experience, although a postprocedure persistent right bundle branch block or an increased recurrence rate can never be excluded in this subset of patients. In any case, experience significantly decreases radiation exposure and increases primary success rate. Yet, the role of mechanically induced accessory pathway block during mapping must be underlined. Among the last 19 cases with a para-hissian accessory pathway, in both patients with an unsuccessful first ablation procedure the failure was due to a traumatic block of the accessory pathway during catheter positioning. The block lasted for several hours and therefore a second procedure was necessary.

Finally, as shown in Table 1, multiple accessory pathways may be present in patients with antero-septal and intermediate septal Kent bundles. These cases show neither higher prevalence nor a preferential location of the associated accessory pathway compared with other patients with Wolff-Parkinson-White syndrome.

Table 2. Success, recurrence and complication rates according to the location of the accessory pathway

	Para-hissian	Para-septal	Intermediate	Overall
Number of patients	38	28	17	83
Success[a]	38 (100%)	28 (100%)	17 (100%)	83 (100%)
Recurrences	10 (26%)	2 (7%)	2 (12%)	14 (17%)
Success after recurrence	10 (100%)	2 (100%)	2 (100%)	14 (100%)
Complications				
A-V block	-	-	-	-
persistent right bundle				
branch block	5 (13%)	-	-	5 (6%)
Number of procedures per patient[b]	1.55	1.17	1.23	1.30
Change from inferior to superior				
vena cava approach	7 (18%)	3 (11%)	-	10 (12%)

[a]Including concomitant accessory pathways in patients with multiple by-pass tracts
[b]Including re-treatment after recurrence

Table 3. Comparison between the first and the second half of the thirty-eight patients undergoing catheter ablation of a para-hissian accessory pathway

	First 19 patients	Second 19 patients
Primary success	12 (63%)	17 (90%)
Recurrence	6 (31%)	4 (21%)
Persistent right bundle branch block	3 (16%)	2 (10%)
Mean fluoroscopy time per patient (min)	57	27

Conclusions

Like other arrhythmogenic substrates [13], the accessory pathways located in the triangle of Koch are a weak substrate or, at least, they are more sensitive to heating than the normal A-V conduction pathway. Therefore, catheter ablation of these Kent bundles is highly successful and safe, provided that a careful and minimally aggressive approach is used. In the method we have described in this paper, the key points are accurate mapping, stable catheter positioning and a low cut-off temperature (only temperature control mode should be used). The main drawback of this approach is an increased incidence of recurrence, which, however, can be successfully retreated and is in accordance with data from the literature [14, 15]. It is likely that the increased recurrence rate in patients with an accessory pathway located in the Koch's triangle is strictly related to the lower amount of radiofrequency energy used in these (especially para-hissian) cases, which may result in partial ablation of the Kent bundle, as suggested by previous histological data [16]. Therefore, every patient undergoing catheter ablation of an accessory pathway located in the triangle of Koch should be followed up for 1-2 months after the procedure and follow-up electrophysiological testing should be scheduled whenever deemed necessary.

Although our experience as well as that of other authors demonstrates the feasibility and safety of ablation of accessory pathways in the Koch's triangle, a careful approach is always to be recommended. One must bear in mind that the ablation results in this area depend mainly on the operator's experience.

Acknowledgements. We are deeply grateful to Dr. Alfredo Vicentini from Electrophysiology Laboratory, C.C. "Pederzoli", Peschiera del Garda (VR), for his kind cooperation.

References

1. Haïssaguerre M, Marcus F, Poquet F, Gencel L, Le Metayer P, Clementy J (1994) Electrocardiographic characteristics and catheter ablation of para-hissian accessory pathways. Circulation 90:1124-1128
2. Yeh SJ, Wang CC, Wen MS, Lin FC, Koo CC, Lo YS, Wu D (1994) Characteristics and radiofrequency ablation therapy of intermediate septal accessory pathway. Am J Cardiol 73:50-56

3. Xie B, Heald SC, Bashir Y, Camm AJ, Ward DE (1994) Radiofrequency catheter ablation of septal accessory atrioventricular pathways. Br Heart J 72:281-284

4. Schaffer MS, Silka MJ, Ross BA, Kugler JD (1996) Inadverted atrioventricular block during radiofrequency catheter ablation. Results of the Pediatric Radiofrequency Ablation Registry. Pediatric Electrophysiology Society. Circulation 94:3214-3220

5. Brugada J, Puigfel M, Mont L, Garcia-Bolao I, Figueiredo M, Matas M, Navarro-Lopez F (1998) Radiofrequency ablation of anteroseptal, para-Hisian, and mid-septal accessory pathways using a simplified femoral approach. Pacing Clin Electrophysiol 21:735-741

6. Lin JL, Huang SK, Lai LP, Cheng TF, Tseng YZ, Lien WP (1998) Radiofrequency catheter ablation of septal accessory pathways within the triangle of Koch: importance of energy titration testing other than local electrogram characteristics for identifying the successful target site. Pacing Clin Electrophysiol 21:1909-1917

7. Kuck KH, Schluter M, Gursoy S (1992) Preservation of atrioventricular nodal conduction during radiofrequency current ablation of midseptal accessory pathways. Circulation 86:1743-1752

8. Schluter M, Kuck KH (1992) Catheter ablation from right atrium of antero-septal accessory pathways using radiofrequency current. J Am Coll Cardiol 19:663-670

9. Storti C, Salerno JA, Stanke A, De Ponti R, Ferrari A, Longobardi M (1994) Junctional area mapping for radiofrequency catheter ablation of the fast pathway in patients with AV nodal reentrant tachycardia. Pacing Clin Electrophysiol 17:846

10. Ho SY, Anderson RH (1998) Anatomy of the accessory pathways: are there lessons relevant to radiofrequency catheter ablation? In: Farrè J, Moro C (eds) Ten years of radiofrequency catheter ablation. Futura, Armonk, NY, pp 149-163

11. Belhassen B, Viskin S, Fish R, Glick A, Glikson M, Eldar M (1999) Catheter induced mechanical trauma to accessory pathways during radiofrequency ablation: incidence predictors and clinical implications. J Am Coll Cardiol 33:767-774

12. Langberg JJ, Calkins H, El-Atassi R, Borganelli M, Leon A, Kalbfleisch SJ, Morady F (1992) Temperature monitoring during radiofrequency catheter ablation of accessory pathways. Circulation 86:1469-1474

13. Salerno JA, De Ponti R, Storti C, Zardini M, Tritto M, Longobardi M (1999) Focal atrial tachycardia originating from the apex of the Koch's triangle: a weak arrhythmogenic substrate in a risky site? Pacing Clin Electrophysiol 22:845

14. Twidale N, Wang XZ, Beckman KJ, McClelland JH, Moulton KP, Prior MI, Hazlitt HA, Lazzara R, Jackman WM (1991) Factors associated with recurrence of accessory pathway conduction after radiofrequency catheter ablation. Pacing Clin Electrophysiol 14:2042-2048

15. Calkins H, Prystowsky E, Berger RD, Saul JP, Klein LS, Liem LB, Huang SK, Gillette P, Yong P, Carlson M (1996) Recurrence of conduction following radiofrequency catheter ablation procedures: relationship to ablation target and electrode temperature. The Atakr Multicenter Investigators Group. J Cardiovasc Electrophysiol 7:704-712

16. Vassilikos VP, Ho, SY, Wong CY, Nathan AW (1997) Recurrence of accessory pathway conduction after successful radiofrequency ablation: histological findings. J Interv Card Electrophysiol 1:311-315

Acute Treatment of Atrial Flutter: Ibutilide, Transesophageal Pacing, or DC Shock?

M. Disertori

Introduction

Drug therapy with class IA and IC antiarrhythmic agents has proven relatively disappointing for the termination of atrial flutter. Unike all other agents, ibutilide, a new pure class III agent, is more effective in patients with atrial flutter than in patients with atrial fibrillation.

Transesophageal atrial pacing (TAP) is an effective, minimally invasive, simple and cheap method of treating atrial flutter; unfortunately, TAP is effective only in typical (type I) atrial flutter and is only minimally effective in atypical (type II) atrial flutter.

DC shock is a safe and highly effective way of terminating atrial flutter, but it needs general anesthesia and can be dangerous in patients with underlying sick sinus syndrome.

In this paper we shall analyze the pros and cons of these three different approaches in the acute treatment of atrial flutter.

Ibutilide

Ibutilide was the first pure class III agent to become clinically available and was developed to rapidly terminate atrial fibrillation and flutter by acutely prolonging the duration of the atrial action potential and effective refractory period (ERP). The clinical data show that the agent is effective in terminating recent onset atrial fibrillation and flutter.

A dose-ranging, randomized, blinded study was performed comparing placebo to four different doses of ibutilide (0.005, 0.010, 0.015, or 0.025 mg/kg administered intravenously over 10 min) in 200 patients, a significant proportion of patients having underlying heart disease [1]. Overall, ibutilide converted 34% of drug-treated patients within 1 h of administration, compared to 3% of patients

Divisione di Cardiologia, Ospedale S. Chiara, Trento, Italy

receiving placebo, and the two higher doses of ibutilide converted 45%-46% of the patients ($p < 0.001$).

The second major placebo-controlled, blinded randomized trial of ibutilide [2] examined 266 patients with atrial fibrillation and flutter lasting from 3 h to 45 days: patients were randomized to receive placebo or up to two 10-min ibutilide infusions (1.0 mg followed by either 0.5 or 1.0 mg) separated by a 10 minute observation period. The patient population was notable for a significant degree of underlying heart disease. The overall conversion efficacy of ibutilide was 47% as compared to 2% for placebo ($p < 0.001$). The conversion rate for atrial flutter (63%) was significantly greater than that for atrial fibrillation (31%; $p < 0.001$).

Ibutilide has also shown to be effective in treating patients who have recently undergone cardiac surgery [3].

There is a definite risk of torsades de pointes secondary to the class III action of the drug, demonstrating the need for careful selection and monitoring of patients receiving ibutilide.

In a randomized study ibutilide (1.0 or 2.0 mg iv) has been compared to intravenous D,L-sotalol (1.5 mg/kg) [4]. In this study, 2.0 mg ibutilide was more effective than 1.0 mg ibutilide, which was more efficacious than intravenous sotalol. Ibutilide, at the higher dose, converted 49% of patients to sinus rhythm as compared to 13% in the sotalol group ($p < 0.01$). Ibutilide converted 70% of patients with atrial flutter and 43% with atrial fibrillation compared to D,L-sotalol induced conversion rates of 19% and 11% respectively ($p < 0.01$).

While it might be hypothesized that ibutilide and D,L-sotalol work through the same mechanism (increasing the action potential duration) and thus should have a similar efficacy in converting atrial fibrillation and atrial flutter to sinus rhythm, it is possible that the observed differences in efficacy are related to their different frequency-dependent effects. At short pacing cycle lengths, D,L-sotalol induced atrial ERP prolongation is significantly attenuated (reverse frequency dependence), while ibutilide exerts a similar ability to prolong ERP independent of atrial cycle length.

Volgman et al. [5] compared intravenous ibutilide (1.0 mg followed by a second 1.0 mg dose if the patients failed to convert) to intravenous procainamide (400 mg iv x three doses). Ibutilide was significantly more efficacious than procainamide, converting 58% of patients to sinus rhythm as compared to 18% ($p < 0.01$). Subgroup analyses demonstrated that ibutilide converted 77% of patients with atrial flutter and 51% with atrial fibrillation as compared to 14% and 21% respectively in the procainamide group.

Ibutilide in the Treatment of Atrial Flutter

Unlike all other antiarrhythmic agents, ibutilide is more effective in patients with atrial flutter than in patients with atrial fibrillation, as reported above.

Atrial flutter is due to a macro reentrant circuit, usually contained within the right atrium and crucially involving an area of slowed conduction around the area of the mouth of the coronary sinus and the inferior vena cava. The nature of the electrical components in this circuit is such that termination of the arrhythmia by class IA and IC drugs requires either creation of conduction block or, at least, marked conduction delay. Perhaps for this reason, class IA and IC drugs have proven relatively disappointing for termination of the arrhythmia.

Termination of experimental atrial flutter has been achieved with some success following the administration of class III agents. Some experimental observations based on a prominent effect on the refractory period led to the hypothesis that abolition of the excitable gap could be the mechanism for atrial flutter termination [6]; this could be the mechanism of the very high clinical efficacy of ibutilide in the treatment of atrial flutter (60%-80% sinus rhythm resumption).

At the moment, ibutilide seems to be the most effective drug in atrial flutter treatment.

Transesophageal Atrial Pacing

TAP is a very effective, minimally invasive, simple and cheap method for treating atrial flutter; the results are only slight poorer than those of the endocavitary technique. TAP avoids the use of fluoroscopy and the sterile precautions and potential complications associated with the transvenous catheter (and also the possible complications of general anesthesia and DC countershock). Serious arrhythmias induced by TAP are very rare and generally related to the use of very high stimulation current (> 20mA) with unwanted ventricular pacing [7].

We have used TAP in the treatment of typical atrial flutter during the last 16 years (more than 600 patients treated). In our experience [8, 9], TAP was effective in terminating atrial flutter in 90% of the episodes. In 20% of patients sinus rhythm followed immediately after TAP was stopped; in 35% of patients sinus rhythm resumed after a short period of atrial fibrillation. Finally, in 35% stable atrial fibrillation was obtained.

Generally patients have no noteworthy side effects during TAP, except for a mild retrosternal burning sensation or chest pain, related to the current output. These discomforts vanish immediately when pacing is interrupted.

Pretreatment with class IC antiarrhythmic agents can favor TAP results in the management of typical atrial flutter [10]. There are no data about ibutilide and TAP, only a demonstration that ibutilide signficantly enhances ($p < 0.001$) endocavitary pacing-induced termination of atrial flutter compared with placebo [11].

DC Shock

Cardioversion of atrial flutter, when used properly, is safe and effective. The energy and current required to cardiovert atrial flutter are less than the energy and current required to cardiovert atrial fibrillation. Excessive current reduces the success of shock treatment.

In an elective situation, 50 J is successful in over 70% of patients as a first shock for typical atrial flutter, and is an appropiate initial shock. If this is ineffective, repeated shocks should be delivered incrementally at 100, 200, 300, and then 360 J. With this approach, a success rate of over 90% should be expected for atrial flutter.

In atypical atrial flutter, or in an emergency, the first shock should be 100 J.

DC shock has comparable efficacy to endocardial and epicardial atrial pacing, but is more effective than TAP. However, it is important to emphasize some advantages of pacing in comparison to DC shock: (1) general anesthesia is not needed, (2) it can treat recurrent episodes of atrial flutter, (3) it can provide backup pacing if bradycardia follows cardioversion.

On the other hand, the disadvantage of pacing is that TAP can be uncomfortable and less effective than shock.

Cost-Effectivenes of Ibutilide Vs Electrical Cardioversion

Recently the cost-effectiveness of ibutilide vs electrical cardioversion in the treatment of atrial fibrillation and flutter was analyzed. Although ibutilide therapy was less expensive than electrical cardioversion, it was also less successful at converting the arrhythmias. However, a stepped treatment regimen of ibutilide as first-line treatment followed by electrical cardioversion for patients who failed to respond was less expensive and more effective than treatment with electrical cardioversion as first-line. This was true also for atrial flutter: ibutilide followed by electrical cardioversion was more successful (96% vs 86% sinus rhythm resumption) and less expensive ($1333 vs $1725) than electrical cardioversion alone [13].

At the moment there are no data comparing the cost-effectiveness of ibutilide to that of TAP.

Conclusions

Pharmacological treatment with ibutilide and electrical treatment with transesophageal pacing or DC shock can each be the best choice for treatment of atrial flutter in different clinical situations.
1. In an emergency, patients should be treated with DC shock, as it is effective and can be performed immediately.
2. In nonemergencies and in situations where the drug is contraindicated (e.g., previous drug treatment, Q-T prolongation) transesophageal pacing could be the first-line treatment, followed, if ineffective, by DC shock.
3. In nonemergencies and in the absence of drug contraindications the choice is affected by the following variables: (1) ibutilide is highly effective but needs at least 4 h monitoring; (2) some patients complain about the electrical techniques; (3) the transesophageal technique is not available in all emergency rooms; and (4) the kind of treatment used as first-line depends on the experience and the preference of the doctor, seeing that the three treatments are quite similar in efficacy.

References

1. Ellenbogen KA, Stambler BS, Wodd MA et al (1996) Efficacy of intravenous ibutilide for rapid termination of atrial fibrillation and flutter: a dose-response study. J Am Coll Cardiol 28:130-136
2. Stambler BS, Wodd MA, Ellenbogen KA et al (1996) Efficacy and safety of repeated intravenous doses of ibutilide for rapid conversion of atrial flutter or fibrillation. Circulation 94:1613-1621
3. Murray KT (1998) Ibutilide. Circulation 97:493-497
4. Sotalol Comparator Study (1996) (protocol 0019) Corvert injection (ibutilide fumarate) Comprehensive review. Appendix I. Pharmacia and Upjohn, Kalamazoo
5. Volgman AS, Stambler BS, Kappagoda C (1996) Comparative efficacy of intravenous Ibutilide versus Procainamide for rapid termination of atrial fibrillation or flutter. Pacing Clin Electrophysiol 9(II):608 (abstr)
6. Inoue H, Yamashita T, Nozaki A et al (1991) Effects of antiarrhythmic drugs on canine atrial flutter due to reentry: role of prolongation of refractory period and depression of conduction to excitable gap. J Am Coll Cardiol 18:1098-1104
7. Disertori M (1993) La stimolazione atriale transesofagea nel trattamento del flutter atriale: utilità e limiti. G Ital Cardiol 23:281-283
8. Disertori M, Inama G, Vergara G et al (1984) Impiego della stimolazione atriale transesofagea nel trattamento del flutter atriale. G Ital Cardiol 14:153-159
9. Guarnerio M, Furlanello F, Del Greco M et al (1989) Transesophageal atrial pacing: a first-choice technique in atrial flutter therapy. Am Heart J 117:1241-1252
10. Doni F, Della Bella P, Kheir A et al (1995) Atrial flutter termination by overdrive transesophageal pacing and the facilitating effect of oral propafenone. Am J Cardiol 76:1243-1246
11. Stambler BS, Wood MA, Ellenbogen KA (1996) Comparative efficacy of intravenous ibutilide versus procainamide for enhancing termination of atrial flutter by overdrive pacing. Am J Cardiol 77:960-966
12. Olshansky B, Kerber RE (1996) Cardioversion of atrial flutter. In: Waldo AL, Touboul P (eds) Atrial flutter: advances in mechanisms and management. Futura, Armonk NY, pp 366-409
13. Zarkin GA, Bala MV, Calingaert B et al (1998) The cost-effectiveness of Ibutilide versus electrical cardioversion in the treatment of atrial fibrillation and flutter. Am J Managed Care 22:211-224

Chronic Atrial Flutter: What Is the Risk of Thromboembolism?

N. Baldi, V.A. Russo, V. Morrone, L. Liconso and G. Polimeni

In a review about atrial flutter, published in 1992, in the section concerning anti-coagulant therapy, Olshansky et al. [1] concluded as follows: "A consensus has not yet been reached about the need for anticoagulation in patients with atrial flutter. It is not possible to make a rational judgement about the need for anticoagulation for patients with atrial flutter based on present data".

Subsequently, due to the contribution of many authors [2-5], cardiologists have once more focused their attention on this issue, since the need for anticoagulation has been underlined, even in patients with atrial flutter as well as those with atrial fibrillation.

In our short presentation we will consider: (a) the incidence of thromboembolism in patients with atrial flutter, whether it is spontaneous or cardioversion-related, (b) the complex problem of the alternation between atrial flutter and fibrillation in the same patient, and (c) the limitations of studies underlining the need for anticoagulation in patients affected by chronic atrial flutter. Finally, we will try to give at least a partial explanation for the possible pathogenesis of thromboembolism in this arrhythmia.

Spontaneous Thromboembolism in Chronic Atrial Flutter

It is difficult to accurately define the incidence of embolism in this condition, since in many studies it is often associated with cardioversion-related cases. However, taking into consideration only the cases of embolism which are not cardioversion-related, percentages resulting from the main studies range between 5% [5], 8.6% [3] and 14% [4] within a period of observation ranging from 26 ± 18 months [5], to 4.5 years [4]. The incidence, therefore, is not negligible, even though these studies have many limitations, the most important of which, in our opinion, are the following. These studies are prevalently retrospective and thus they do not aim at clearly defining an endpoint [3, 4]. Patients studied are often

Unità Operativa di Cardiologia, Azienda Ospedale S.S. Annunziata, Taranto, Italy

referred to a University Hospital to undergo cardioversion or transcatheter ablation. This is reflected in the high frequency of cardiac diseases, history of hypertension and diabetes observed in these groups. It is possible that referral bias may have resulted in a patient group at greater risk of thromboembolic complications than the ordinary patient group with atrial flutter. Subjects studied are often dishomogeneous [3]. Therapeutical behaviors have sometimes changed during the period of observation [5]. The effectiveness of anticoagulant therapy is sometimes determined by a general physician rather than by a reference structure [3]. Finally, we must also consider the possible lack of accuracy in defining embolism, which is not always objectively demonstrated in the patient, but is often derived from the patient's clinical history.

Cardioversion-Related Thromboembolism

The incidence of embolism in this patient group is reported to occur either in association with a non-cardioversion-related embolism or in patients in which both atrial flutter and atrial fibrillation are present.

Recently, Demsen [6] examined eight studies [2, 3, 5, 7-11], including 457 patients bound to elective cardioversion, who had not been suitably anticoagulated (INR < 2.0). He found out that collectively 2.2% of patients had presented with a cardioversion-related thromboembolism. Significantly, no events occurred in the only two cardioversion studies in which 94 patients had been anticoagulated [2, 3], according to fibrillation guidelines. Considering that the incidence of cardioversion-related thromboembolism in atrial fibrillation ranges from 0% to 1.6% in patients who have been anticoagulated and up to 7% in patients who have not been anticoagulated, the percentage of thromboembolism in atrial flutter in patients not treated is about one-third of that found in atrial fibrillation. It must be strongly underlined, however, that these observations too, concerning both atrial flutter and above all atrial fibrillation – including a far greater number of studies – have been derived from non-controlled, almost always retrospective clinical studies with absolutely dishomogeneous casuistics.

Alternation Between Atrial Flutter and Atrial Fibrillation

A basic problem in evaluating the incidence of thromboembolism in patients with atrial flutter is represented by the alternation between atrial flutter and fibrillation.

It is commonly known that atrial flutter rather often changes into atrial fibrillation, and vice versa, both spontaneously and due to the action of some drugs, particularly class IA and IC antiarrhythmic drugs. There are few systematic studies in which the incidence of this alternating process has been analyzed: the study of Murdock et al. [12] analyzed the incidence of flutter in patients with atrial fibrillation treated with propafenone, and in a study by Tunick et al. [13] this phenomenon was observed more organically. Such authors have examined 992 consecutive patients who have undergone ambulatory ECG (Holter) recording. In 96 of them (10%) recording showed atrial fibrillation and/or atrial flutter with or without additional sinus rhythm. There were 24 patients with alternation between fibrillation and flutter, which included 20 patients with paroxysmal combined fibrillation and flutter with alternation between fibrillation, flutter and sinus rhythm and 4 with combined fibrillation and flutter and no sinus rhythm present. In two recent studies [4, 5], the phenomenon of alternation between atrial fibrillation and flutter was observed in about one-third of the groups examined: respectively 30% in the casuistics of Wood et al. [4], and 34% in that of Seidl et al. [5]. In our opinion, the phenomenon of alternation may theoretically account for the incidence of thromboembolism in patients with atrial flutter. Considering again the casuistics of Wood et al. [4], including an overall rate of embolic events in 12 out of 86 patients with atrial flutter (14%), a comparison can be made, as the authors themselves did, with the incidence of thromboembolism in non-valvular atrial fibrillation. Patients with transient ischemic attacks or pulmonary emboli have been excluded in the major trials examining thromboembolic risks in atrial fibrillation. When these patients are excluded from the results of the study of Wood et al. [4], the overall risk in patients with atrial flutter becomes 7% over a mean follow-up period of 4.5 years. Therefore, the annual percentage of risk is about 1.6%. This percentage appears to be approximately one-third of the reported 4.5% annual risk for patients with non-valvular atrial fibrillation. As we observed in about one-third of patients with atrial flutter, an alternation with atrial fibrillation has resulted. Does this subgroup of patients develop thromboembolic phenomena? That is, does the alternation between atrial fibrillation and flutter determine thromboembolism? This is just an assumption that, however, seems to be supported by recent studies carried out by Biblo et al. [14]. These authors analyzed a retrospective cohort study, Medicare patients, hospitalized in 1984, with atrial fibrillation ($n = 396,012$), atrial flutter ($n = 20,209$) and a random sample of other diagnoses ($n = 395,147$). These patients were followed for 8 years. Of the 20,209 patients with atrial flutter, 6599 patients developed atrial fibrillation. The overall risk of stroke in patients with atrial flutter was significantly higher than in the control group (1.303, $p < 0.0001$); however, in the subgroup of patients with atrial flutter who did not develop atrial fibrillation (lone atrial flutter) the relative risk for stroke was 1.112, $p < 0.0005$, while in the subset of patients who did develop atrial fibrillation the relative risk for stroke was 1.564, $p < 0.0001$. Therefore, in patients with atrial flutter the majority of embolic events occurred in those who subsequently developed atrial fibrillation rather than in those with lone atrial flutter. The development of atrial fibrillation in these patients seems to be a strong predictive factor of thromboembolism. Is it possible to identify this subgroup of patients? We know that between atrial flutter and atrial fibrillation there is an intermediate form of arrhythmia, the fibrillo-flutter or impure flutter [15]. In fibrillo-flutter there are F waves, which are not regular regarding their morphology and duration. F-F intervals present a variation which is longer than 0.03 s. Is it possible that these patients are bound to develop atrial fibrillation, thus being more likely to undergo thromboembolism? It is just an assumption, but the need to define whether there are forms of flutter which are more dangerous than others is also felt by Dunn [16], when he asserts in a recently published comment: "In future studies it may be of interest to determine if different focus of atrial flutter carries different risk for thromboembolism".

References

1. Olshansky B, Wilber DJ, Hariman RJ (1992) Atrial flutter. Update on the mechanism and treatment. PACE 15:2308-2335
2. Pagadala P, Gummadi SS, Olshansky B (1994) Thromboembolic risk of chronic atrial flutter: is the risk underestimated? Circulation 90[Suppl]:I-398 (abstr)
3. Lanzarotti C, Olshansky B (1997) Thromboembolic risk of chronic atrial flutter: is the risk underestimated? J Am Coll Cardiol 30:1506-1511
4. Wood KA, Eisemberg SJ, Kalman JM, Drew BJ, Saxon LA, Lee RJ, Lesh MD, Scheinman MM (1997) Risk of thromboembolism in chronic atrial flutter. Am J Cardiol 79:1043-1047
5. Seidl K, Hauer B, Schwick NG, Zellner D, Zahn R, Senges J (1998) Risk of thromboembolism events in patients with atrial flutter. Am J Cardiol 82:580-583
6. Demsen CG (1999) Patients undergoing cardioversion of atrial flutter should be routinely anticoagulated. Am J Cardiol 83:140-141
7. Arnold AZ, Mick MJ, Mazurek RP, Loop FD, Trohman RG (1992) Role of prophylactic anticoagulation for direct current cardioversion in patients with atrial fibrillation or flutter. J Am Coll Cardiol 19:851-855
8. Black IW, Hopkins AP, Lee LC, Walsh WF (1993) Evaluation of transesophageal echocardiography before cardioversion of atrial fibrillation and flutter in non-anticoagulated patients. Am Heart J 126:375-381
9. Moreyra E, Finkelhor RS, Cebul RD (1995) Limitations of transesophageal echocardiography in the risk assessment of patients before non-anticoagulated cardioversion from atrial fibrillation and flutter: an analysis of pooled results. Am Heart J 129:71-75
10. Metha D, Baruch L (1996) Thromboembolism following cardioversion of "common" atrial flutter. Risk factors and limitations of transesophageal echocardiography. Chest 110:1001-1003
11. Klein AL, Grimm RA, Black IW, Leung DY, Chung MK, Vaughn SE, Murray D, Miller DP, Arheart KL, for the ACUTE Investigators (1997) Cardioversion guided by transesophageal echocardiography: the ACUTE pilot study: a randomized, controlled trial. Ann Intern Med 126:200-209
12. Murdock CJ, Kyles AF, Yeung-Lai-Wah JA, Anzehn Q, Vorderbrugge S, Kerr GR (1990) Atrial flutter in patients treated for atrial fibrillation with propafenone. Am J Cardiol 66:755-757
13. Tunick PA, Mc Elhinney L, Mitchell T, Kronzon I (1992) The alternation between atrial flutter and atrial fibrillation. Chest 101:34-36
14. Biblo LA, Chong Y, Kaufman ES, Lewis WR, Mackall JA, Rimm AA (1998) "Lone" atrial flutter, insights to embolic risk. PACE 21:515 (abstr)
15. Oreto G, Luzza F, Satullo G, Donato A (1997) I disordini del ritmo cardiaco. Centro Scientifico, Torino, pp 42-53
16. Dunn MI (1998) Thromboembolism with atrial flutter. Am J Cardiol 82:638

Common and Uncommon Atrial Flutter: What Are the Long-Term Results and Complications of Radiofrequency Ablation?

S. González, J. Almendral, M. Ortiz, J.P. Villacastin, A. Arenal, J. García, N. Pérez Castellano and J.L. Delcan

The availability of nonpharmacological therapeutic options has been a major breakthrough in the treatment of most cardiac arrhythmias. In the case of atrial flutter, radiofrequency catheter ablation has not only increased the therapeutic efficacy of this typically drug-resistant arrhythmia, but has enhanced our knowledge about its mechanisms. The identification of the mechanisms of atrial flutter has been a challenge for several decades [1], but only recently has our understanding about the existence of different types of atrial flutter with different mechanisms allowed the development of a curative approach to some types of atrial flutter.

In this chapter we will describe the different types of atrial flutter with their implications for catheter ablation. We will also discuss the rationale of the two endpoints used for success of catheter ablation of common atrial flutter, and differences in the short and long-term success related to each endpoint.

Classification and Definitions

Atrial flutter has been classically classified into typical and atypical according to its ECG appearance [2] and into type I and type II according to its rate and response to programmed electrical stimulation [3]. It is also conventional to distinguish between atrial flutter and atrial tachycardia based on the slower rate and presence of isoelectric line in the latter.

Although these concepts are constantly repeated in the medical literature, they are probably insufficient, even inadequate, to evaluate the results of catheter ablation in the light of our present knowledge about the mechanisms of regular atrial arrhythmias. For example, the mechanism of common atrial flutter can display a rate that overlaps with that of atrial tachycardia (particularly in patients treated with antiarrhythmic agents), incisional "tachycardias" are considered variously as "flutter" or "tachycardia" although the same arrhythmia is being referred to [4, 5],

Clinical Electrophysiology Laboratory, Departamento de Cardiologia, Hospital General Universitario Gregorio Marañón, Madrid, Spain

and flutter using the same circuit as common flutter but rotating in a clockwise fashion is classified as "typical" or "atypical" depending upon the investigator [6, 7].

Without denying the importance of ECG in planning a particular therapeutic approach for a given patient, we feel that a mechanistically oriented classification is more meaningful at least to compare results of catheter ablation.

Common atrial flutter. The ECG morphology is that of what is usually considered "typical atrial flutter" (although exceptions exist). Pathophysiologically it is presently clear that its mechanism is a macroreentry confined to the right atrium (with passive activation of the left atrium), limited by anatomic and functional barriers around the tricuspid annulus, with caudocranial activation of the septum and craniocaudal activation of the lateral wall (so-called counterclockwise flutter).

Reversed common atrial flutter, also known as clockwise flutter. It has been described as displaying a specific ECG pattern [4, 6, 8], but it is known to display a variety of morphologies [7]. Given that its anatomic substrate is identical to that of the more common counterclockwise form, that its therapeutic ablation approach is also similar, and that the two forms frequently coexist in the same patient, it can be suggested that it should more appropriately be included with the "common" flutter [6].

Incisional Flutter. Atrial arrhythmias not unusually appear after surgical correction of certain forms of congenital heart disease. These arrhythmias are sometimes reentrant, the circuit rotating totally or partially around the surgical scar. They do not have a specific ECG pattern and their existence should be suspected on the basis of the preceding surgery.

"Class I C flutter". It has been recently reported that certain patients with atrial fibrillation treated with class I C antiarrhythmic drugs spontaneously develop atrial flutter [9, 10]. In the majority of cases the flutter observed is of the common type. It is believed to be due to the effect on the critical atrial mass of the electrophysiologic changes produced by class I C drugs.

Atypical or uncommon atrial flutter. There are some cases in which the mechanism of atrial flutter is either unknown or extremely unusual. Rare cases such as those appearing after extensive ablation procedures involving atrial tissue, or using anatomical structures around the coronary sinus [11], or what was previously called type II flutter, would belong into this category.

Results of Ablation of Atrial Flutter

Common Atrial Flutter

Studies in animal models and in humans have demonstrated that the mechanism of common atrial flutter is a macroreentry [12-17]. Several reports using activation mapping techniques [18, 19] and entrainment mapping [20-22] have delineated the circuit as rotating counterclockwise around the tricuspid annulus, with the orifices of the venae cavae, the coronary sinus ostium, the crista terminalis and the eustachian ridge acting as posterior anatomical or functional barriers and the tricuspid annulus itself as anterior barrier.

The above information has led to a variety of procedural approaches. They have been guided by electrophysiologic parameters such as the presence of fragmented electrograms (in a fashion similar to but less justified than in ventricular tachycardia) or entrainment techniques [26, 27]. Cosio et al. [28] and others [29] proposed an anatomical approach based on the anatomical observation that, if the circuit rotates around the tricuspid annulus, the area between the inferior vena cava orifice and the tricuspid ring is a necessary isthmus for the propagating waveform. Blocking conduction in this isthmus was expected to make common atrial flutter impossible. Other groups attempted to guide ablation by a combination of electrophysiologic and anatomic parameters [30-32]. It is interesting to note that difference in acute results does not seem to be significant in comparing reported series, although the anatomic approach resulted in shorter procedures [33].

Suppression of Inducibility as the Endpoint of the Ablation Procedure

In earlier series, the endpoint of the procedure was the termination of flutter by radiofrequency followed by suppression of inducibility by programmed electrical stimulation. The recurrence rate with this endpoint was ≥ 20% (Table 1) [24-29, 32, 34-37].

Although it was realized that some non-electrophysiologic parameters such as

Table 1. Results of ablation of common atrial flutter: endpoint flutter interruption and subsequent noninducibility

Authors	Patients (n)	Success (%)	Recurrences (%)		Previous AF (%)	Follow-up and complications
			AFl	AF		
Cosío et al. [28]	9	78	42	28	11	2-18 Months, no complications
Calkins et al. [26]	16	81	15	8	-	10 ± 4 Months, no complications
Kirkorian et al. [29]	22	86	14	18	23	8 ± 13 Months, no complications
Philippon et al. [34]	59	90	9	26	20	13 ± 6 Months
Nath et al. [35]	22	97	23	23	27	9 ± 5 Months, no complications
Movsowitz et al. [36]	32	97	15	38	56	8.6 ± 5 Months, 1 DVT
Fischer et al. [30]	200	95	15	5.5	5.5	24 ± 9 Months
Saxon et al. [27]	51	88	22	12	45	14 ± 10 Months
Cosío et al. [39]	28	96	58	25	-	40 ± 24 Months
Tai Tai et al. [38]	50	-	16	21	-	17 ± 13 Months

AFl, atrial flutter; AF, atrial fibrillation; DVT, deep venous thrombosis

left atrial dilatation, preexistent atrial fibrillation, or inducibility of atrial fibrilla-tion predicted a worse result [27, 34, 35, 38-40], and that some of the recurrences were arrhythmias other than common atrial flutter, the recurrence rate of flutter was too high.

Conduction Blook in the Cavotricuspid Isthmus as the Endpoint of the Ablation Procedure

It was then proposed that conduction through the cavotricuspid isthmus could be directly evaluated by pacing techniques in the absence of flutter [27, 28, 41], and that this endpoint was a better predictor of absence of recurrences than suppres-sion of inducibility. Subsequent series using this approach have observed that the recurrence rate with conduction block as an endpoint is lower (in the 10% range, Table 2), and that patients who suffered recurrence were those in whom conduction block at the end of the procedure was absent, unidirectional, or rate-dependent, or patients in whom the cavotricuspid isthmus had recovered conduction [42-44].

Cavotricuspid isthmus block is recognized by changes in right atrial activa-tion sequence as compared to the baseline, with lack of atrial fusion when pacing at each side of the line of block [41-46]. It can even be recognized in the surface ECG by a change in P wave morphology or PR duration during low right atrial stmulation [46].

However, evaluation of conduction along the cavotricuspid isthmus may sometimes be difficult. One of the potentially confusing factors is the presence of rate-dependent conduction along the inferior portion of the crista terminalis as recently showed by Arenal et al. [45]. This can simulate conduction through the cavotricuspid isthmus when it is truly blocked, and may explain some cases of clinical success without apparent achievement of the endpoint.

Another source of difficulty arises when radiofrequency applications result in

Table 2. Results of ablation of common atrial flutter: endpoint cavotricuspid isthmus block

Authors	Patients (n)	Success (%)	Recurrences (%)		Previous AF (%)	Follow-up and complications
			AFl	AF		
Cauchemez et al. [42]	20	95	20[a]	-	20	8 ± 2 Months
Poty et al. [43]	44	948	9[b]	7	-	12 ± 5 Months, no complications
Schwartzman et al. [44]	35	97	8[b]	-	-	10 Months
Tai Tai et al. [38]	94		6	21	-	17 ± 13 Months
Cosío et al. [39]	38	100	13	21	-	16 ± 9.5 Months

[a] Recurrence occurred in 43% of patients without cavotricuspid isthmus block vs 8% of patients with cavotricuspid isthmus block
[b] None of these patients had cavotricuspid isthmus block

slowing (but not block) of conduction in the cavotricuspid isthmus. Recently, Villacastin et al. have observed that unipolar recordings obtained close to the ablation line are useful to detect cavotricuspid isthmus block and to distinguish it from slow conduction [47]. Yamabe et al. have reported that bipolar recordings along the line of block can identify gaps of conduction within the line of block in early and late recurrences [48].

In summary, cavotricuspid isthmus block is at the present time the best endpoint for the ablation procedure, but is sometimes difficult to evaluate.

Reversed Common Atrial Flutter

Since both types of common atrial flutter share the same anatomical substrate, they can be equally approached with an anatomically guided line of block in the cavotricuspid isthmus [49]. The acute and long-term success rates are similar to those for the common counterclockwise type [8, 50].

Incisional Flutter

In patients who have undergone surgical atriotomy, the presence of low voltage and fragmented potentials at the level of the surgical scar can be documented [5], suggesting differences in activation times on the two sides. Entrainment studies showed that this type of arrhythmia was reentrant and identified appropriate targets for ablation [5]. The ablation strategy involves the creation of a line of conduction block between one end of the scar and a close anatomic barrier such as the tricuspid annulus. The number of such cases reported is too small to provide an accurate idea of the success rate. The short-term success rate is not higher than 80%, but the long-term success is unclear yet.

"Class I C Flutter"

From the therapeutic standpoint the ablation approach for class I C flutter is identical to that of common flutter. What is interesting in this group of patients, beyond the results of the ablation procedure, is the low recurrence rate of atrial fibrillation when cavotricuspid isthmus block is combined with a continuation of therapy with class I C agents (70%-80% of patients improve or remain free of atrial fibrillation recurrences) [9-11]. However, since the published series are recent, there is no long-term follow-up as yet.

Atypical or Uncommon Atrial Flutter

At the present time there is no definite approach to these arrhythmias using radiofrequency catheter ablation, since the site of origin and mechanisms involved differ among them, and ablation results have not been reported.

Problem of Atrial Fibrillation in Patients with Atrial Flutter

It has been reported that ablation of atrial flutter has a beneficial effect on the incidence of atrial fibrillation in patients with previous documentation of this arrhythmia [30, 34, 36, 51]. Explanations of this include a compartimentalization effect of the cavotricuspid isthmus ablation, a triggering effect of flutter on fibrillation, and facilitation of remodeling due to flutter on the development of fibrillation.

On the other hand, in patients without atrial fibrillation before ablation, a 5%-20% incidence of atrial fibrillation has been reported during follow-up even if the ablation procedure was successful [17, 29, 30, 34, 36, 38, 39]. Although an arrhythmogenic effect of the ablation procedure cannot be excluded, there is no evidence for this, and it is more likely that factors such as the underlying structural heart disease or inducibility of sustained atrial fibrillation play a role, as has been recently demonstrated [38].

Complications of Atrial Flutter Ablation

Risk of Embolism

Sparks et al showed that 80% of patients with atrial flutter had spontaneous echo contrast in the left atrial appendage after conversion to sinus rhythm, and that this phenomenon disappeared after 3 weeks [52]. In a series of 23 patients undergoing elective electrical cardioversion, it was observed that 3 patients had atrial thrombi and another 5 patients had spontaneous echo contrast [53].

In view of these observations it seems reasonable that antithrombotic therapy should at least be considered when a flutter ablation procedure is contemplated.

Atrioventricular Block

Atrioventricular block has been occasionally reported in relation to ablation on the septal aspect in the cavotricuspid isthmus. This was observed in one of 16 patients of one the earlier series of atrial flutter ablation [54].

Experience of Our Group

In our center 71 patients underwent radiofrequency catheter ablation of atrial flutter between 1996 and 1999 with the endpoint of cavotricuspid isthmus. Table 3 summarizes our results. The mechanism of the arrhythmias that were characterized during the procedure common atrial flutter in 50 patients and its reversed form in 16 (most patients with the reversed form also had common flutter). In 10 patients no arrhythmia was induced, in most because the ECG was considered so characteristic of common flutter that no attempt was made to induce flutter. In 10 additional patients atypical flutter was observed without attempting further ablation in most of them.

Acute success was obtained in 64 patients (90%). Peripheral vascular complications were observed in 2 patients. No instances of pericardial, embolic, or bradiarrhythmic complications were detected. During a mean follow-up of 14 ± 9 months sustained atrial tachyarrhythmias were noted in 10 patients (14%). Six

Table 3. The experience of our group ($n = 71$)

Types of atrial flutter studied:	Common: 50 patients Reversed common: 16 patients Incisional: 2 patients Atypical: 10 patients Noninduced: 10 patients
Acute success: Recurrences: Complications:	64 patients (90%) 10 patients (14%) Vascular: 2 patients (3%) Other: 0 patients

patients were restudied: in 4 conduction along the cavotricuspid isthmus had recovered, and common atrial flutter was inducible; in the remaining 2 block along the cavotricuspid isthmus was present, with the origin of flutter documented to be adjacent to the line of block in one patient and in the left atrium in the remaining case.

Long-term mortality was 10% in our series (7 cases). Causes of death included respiratory insufficiency (2 cases), cardiac failure (2 cases), lung carcinoma (1 case), postoperative state after heart transplant (1 case), and cerebrovascular accident (1 case).

Final Considerations

At the present time radiofrequency catheter ablation offers a high success rate with a low incidence of complications in patients with common atrial flutter. The success rate seems to be also high for incisional flutter and the so called class I C flutter. With conduction block in the cavotricuspid isthmus as endpoint for the procedure, the long-term recurrence rate is in the 10% range, although some additional patients (particularly those with a history of atrial fibrillation) may develop atrial fibrillation. Long-term mortality can be significant given the serious underlying disease present in some of these patients. Ablation is still investigational for patients with atypical flutter.

References

1. Jolly WA, Ritchie WJ (1910) Auricular flutter and fibrillation. Heart 2:177-221
2. Puech P, Latour H, Grolleau R (1970) Le flutter et ses limites. Arch Mal Coeur 63:116-144
3. Wells JL, Maclean WAH, James TN, Waldo AL (1979) Characterization of atrial flutter studies in man after open heart surgery using fixed atrial electrodes. Circulation 60: 665-673
4. Cosio FG, Arribas F, Lopez-Gil M, Palacios J (1996) Atrial flutter mapping and ablation I. Studying atrial flutter mechanism by mapping and entrainment. Pacing Clin Electrophysiol 19:841-853

5. Kalman J, Van Hare G, Olgin J,Saxon L, Stark S, Lesh M (1996) Ablation of "incisional" reentrant atrial tachycardia complicating surgery for congenital heart disease. Circulation 93:502-512

6. Kalman J, Olgin J, Sxon L, Lee R, Scheinman M, Lesh M (1997) Electrocardiographic and electrophysiologic characterization of atypical atrial flutter in man: use of activation and entrainment mapping and implications for catheter ablation. J Cardiovasc Electrophysiol 8:121-144

7. Cosio FG, Nuñez A, Arribas F, Lopez-Gil M, Palacios J (1998) Old and new classifications of atrial flutter. In: Saudi N, Schoels W, El-Sherif N (eds) Atrial flutter and fibrillation: from basic to clinical applications. Futura, Armonk, NY

8. Saoudi N, Nair M, Abdelazziz a, Poty H, Daou A, Anselme F, Letac B (1996) Electrocardiographic patterns and results of radiofrequency catheter ablation of clockwise type atrial flutter. J Cardiovasc Electrophysiol 7:931-942

9. Huang DT, Monahan KM, Zimetbaum P, Papageorgiou P, Epstein LM, Josephson ME (1998) Hybrid pharmacological and ablative therapy: a novel and effective approach for the management of atrial fibrillation. J Cardiovasc Electrophysiol 9:462-469

10. Schumacher B, Jung W, Lewalter T, Vahlhaus Ch, Wolpert Ch, Lüderitz B (1999) Radiofrequency ablation of atrial flutter due to administration of class IC antiarrhythmic drugs for atrial fibrillation. Am J Cardiol 83:710-713

11. Nabar A, Rodriguez LM, Timmermans C, Smeets J, Wellens HJJ (1999) Radiofrequency ablation of "class IC atrial flutter" in patients with resistant atrial fibrillation. Am J Cardiol 83:785-787

12. Olgin JE, Jayachandran JV, Engesstein E, Groh W, Zipes DP (1998) Atrial macroreentry involving the myocardium of the coronary sinus: a unique mechanism for atypical flutter. J Cardiovasc Electrophysiol 10:1094-1099

13. Rosenbleuth A, García-Ramos J (1947) Studies on flutter and fibrillation II. The influence of artificial obstacles on experimental auricular flutter. Am Heart J 33:677-684

14. Frame I, Page RL, Hoffman B (1986) Atrial reentry around an anatomic barrier with a partially refractory excitable gap: a canine model of atrial flutter. Circ Res 58:495-511

15. Feld GK, Shahandeh RF (1992) Mechanism of double potentials recorded during sustained atrial flutter in the canine right atrial crush-injury model. Circulation 86:628-641

16. Waldo AL, McLean WAH, Karp RB et al (1977) Entrainment and interruption of atrial flutter with atrial pacing: studies in man following open heart surgery. Circulation 56:737-745

17. IInoue H, Matsuo H, Takayanagi K, Murao S (1981) Clinical and experimental studies of the effects of extrastimulation and rapid pacing on atrial flutter: evidence of macroreentry with an excitable gap. Am J Cardiol 48:623-631

18. Cosio FG, Arribas F, Palacios J, Tascón J, Lopez-Gil M (1986) Fragmented electrogrames and continuous electrical activitiy in atrial flutter. Am J Cardiol 57:1309-1314

19. Olshansky B, Okumura K, Hess PG, Waldo AL (1990) Demonstration of an area of slow conduction in human atrial flutter. J Am Coll Cardiol 16:1639-1648

20. Almendral JM, Arenal A, Abeytua M, San Roman D, Soriano J, Josephson ME (1987) Incidence and patterns of resetting during atrial flutter: role in identifying chamber of origin. J Am Coll Cardiol 9:153 (abstr)

21. Arenal A, Almendral J, San Roman D, Delcan JL, Josephson ME (1992) Frequency and implications of resetting and entrainment with right atrial stimulation in atrial flutter. Am J Cardiol 70:1292-1298

22. Almendral JM, Arenal A (1993) Electrophysiology of human atrial flutter. In:

Josephson ME, Wellens HJJ (eds) Tachycardias; mechanisms and management. Futura, Mount Kisko, NY

23. Olgin J, Kalman J, Lesh M (1996) Conduction barriers in human atrial flutter: correlation of electrophysiology and anatomy. J Cardiovasc Electrophysiol 7:1112-1126

24. Cosio FG, Arribas F, Barbero J et al (1988) Validation of double spike electrograms as markers of conduction delay or block in atrial flutter. Am J Cardiol 61:775-780

25. Olshansky B, Okumuira K, Henthorn RW et al (1990) Characterization of double potentials in human atrial flutter: studies during transient entrainment. J Am Coll Cardiol 15:833-841

26. Calkins H, Leon A, Deam G, Kalbfleisch S, Langberb J, Morady F (1994) Catheter ablation of atrial flutter using radiofrequency energy. Am J Cardiol 73:353-356

27. Saxon L, Kalman J, Olgin J, Scheinman M, Lee R, Lesh M (1996) Results of radiofrequency catheter ablation for atrial flutter. Am J Cardiol 77:1014-1016

28. Cosio FG, Lopez-Gil M, Goicolea A, Arribas F, Barroso JL (1993) Radiofrequency ablation of the inferior vena cava-tricuspid valve isthmus in common atrial flutter. Am J Cardiol 71:705-709

29. Kirkorian G, Moncada E, Chevelier PH, Guillaume C, Vlaudel JP, Bellon CH, Lyon L, Touboul P (1994) Radiofrequency ablation of atrial flutter. Efficacy of an anatomically guided approach. Circulation 90:2804-2814

30. Fischer B, Jaïs P, Shah D, Chouairi S, Haïsaguerre M, Garrigues S, Poquet F, Gencel L et al (1996) Radiofrequency catheter ablation of common atrial flutter in 200 patients. J Cardiovasc Electrophysiol 7:1225-1233

31. Feld GK, Fleck P, Peng-Shen C et al (1992) Radiofrequency catheter ablation for the treatment of atrial flutter. Identification of the critical zone in the reentrant circuit by endocardial mapping techniques. Circulation 86:1233-1240

32. Lesh MD, Van Hare GF, Epstein LM et al (1994) Radiofrequency catheter ablation of atrial arrythmias: results and mechanisms. Circulation 89:1074-1089

33. Chen SA, Chiang CE, Wu TJ et al (1996) Radiofrequency ablation of common atrial flutter: comparison of electrophysiologically guided focal ablation technique and linear ablation technique. J Am Coll Cardiol 27:860-868

34. Philippon F, Plumb V, Epstein A, Kay N (1995) The risk of atrial fibrillation following radiofrequency catheter ablation of atrial flutter. Circulation 92:430-435

35. Nath S, Mounsey P, Haines D, Dimarco JP (1995) Predictors of acute and long-term succes after radiofrequency catheter ablation of type 1 atrial flutter. Am J Cardiol 76:604-606

36. Movzowitz C, Callans D, Schwartzman D, Gottlieb CH, Marchlinski F (1996) The results of atrial flutter ablation in patients with and without a history of atrial fibrillation. Am J Cardiol 78:93-96

37. Poty H, Saoudi N, Aziz A, Nair M, Letac B (1995) Radiofrequency catheter ablation of type 1 atrial flutter. Prediction of late success by electrophysiological criteria. Circulation 1389-1392

38. Tai Tai CH, Chen SA, Chiang CE, Lee SH, Wen Z et al (1998) Long term outcome of radiofrequency catheter ablation for typical atrial flutter: Risk prediction of recurrent arrhythmias. J Cardiovasc Electrophysiol 9:115-121

39. Cosio FG, Lopez-Gil M, Arribas F, Goicolea A, Pastor A, Nuñez A (1998) Radiofrequency ablation of atrial flutter. Long term results after 8 years of experience. Rev Esp Cardiol 51:832-839

40. Frey B, Kreiner G, Binder TH, Heinz G, Baumgartner H, Gössinger H (1997) Relation between left atrial size and secondary atrial arrhythmias after successful catheter ablation of common atrial flutter. Pacing Clin Electrophysiol 20(I):2936-2942

41. Schumacher B, Pfeiffer D, Tebbenjohanns S, Lewalter T, Jung W, Lüderitz B (1998) Acute and long-term effects of consecutive radiofrequency applications on conduction properties of the subeustachian isthmus in type I atrial flutter. J Cardiovasc Electrophysiol 9:152-163

42. Cauchemez B, Haïssaguerre M, Fischer B, Thomas O, Clementy J, Coumel P (1996) Electrophysiological effects of catheter ablation of inferior vena cava-tricuspid annulus isthmus in common atrial flutter. Circulation 93:284-294

43. Poty H, Saoudi N, Nair M, Anselme F, Letac B (1996) Radiofrequency catheter ablation of atrial flutter, further insights into the various types of isthmus block: applications to ablation during sinus rhythm. Circulation 94:3204-3213

44. Schwartzman D, Callans D, Gottlieb C, Dillon S, Movsowitz C, Marchlinski F (1996) Conduction block in the inferior vena cava-tricuspid valve isthmus: association with outcome of radiofrequency ablation of type I atrial flutter. J Am Coll Cardiol 28:1519-1531

45. Arenal A, Almendral J, Alday JM, Villacastin J, Ormaetxe J, Sande JLM, Perez-Castellano N, Gonzalez S, Ortiz M, Delcan JL (1999) Rate-dependent conduction block of the crista terminalis in patients with typical atrial flutter. Influence on evaluation of cavotricuspid isthmus conduction block. Circulation 99:2771-2778

46. Saoudi N, Poty H, Anselme F, Nair M, Abdelazziz A, Letac B (1998) Evolution of concepts and techniques in radiofrequency catheter ablation for the common atrial flutter. In: Saudi N, Schoels W, El-Sherif N (eds) Atrial flutter and fibrillation: from basic to clinical applications. Futura, Armonk, NY

47. Villacastin J, Almendral J, Arenal A, Ortiz M, Perez-Castellano N, Gonzalez S,Velasco D, Valbona B, Delcan JL (1999) Usefulness of unipolar electrograms to confirm isthmus block after radiofrequency ablation of typical atrial flutter. J Am Coll Cardiol 33:117A (abstr)

48. Yamabe H, Okumura K, Misumi I, Fukushima H, Ueno K, Kimura Y, Hokamura Y (1999) Role of bipolar electrogram polarity in localizing recurrent conduction in the isthmus early and late after ablation of atrial flutter. J Am Coll Cardiol 33:39-45

49. Cosio FG, Arribas F, Lopez-Gil M, Gonzalez HD (1996) Radiofrequency ablation of atrial flutter. J Cardiovasc Electrophysiol 7:60-70

50. Tai C, Chen S, Chiang C, Lee S, Ueng K, Wen Z, Chen Y, Yu W, Huang J, Chiou C, Chang M (1997) Electrophysiologic characteristics and radiofrequency catheter ablation in patients with clockwise atrial flutter. J Cardiovasc Electrophysiol 8:24-34

51. Katritsis D, Iliodromitis E, Fragakis N, Adamopoulos S, Kremastinos D (1996) Ablation therapy of type I atrial flutter may eradicate paroxysmal atrial fibrillation. Am J Cardiol 78:345-346

52. Sparks PB, Jayaprakash S, Vohra JK, Mond HG, Yapanis AG, Grigg L Kalman JM (1998) Left atrial "stunning" following radiofrequency catheter ablation of chronic atrial flutter. J Am Coll Cardiol 32:468-475

53. Irani WN, Willett DL, Grayburn PA et al (1995) Prevalence of atrial thrombi and spontaneous echo contrast in atrial flutter: a prospective study using transesophageal echocardiography. Circulation 92(I):537-538

54. Steinberg J, Prasher S, Zelenkofske S, Ehlert F (1995) Radiofrequency catheter ablation of atrial flutter: procedural success and long-term outcome. Am Heart J 130:85-92

Atrial Tachycardia Originating from Crista Terminalis

C. Pappone[1], G. Oreto[2], M.L. Loricchio[1], S. Bianchi[1] and C.D. Dicandia[1]

Atrial tachycardia may be caused by abnormal automaticity, re-entry, or triggered activity. Regardless of the underlying mechanism, it has been observed that, although tachycardia may theoretically arise from any atrial zone, the origin of the arrhythmia is not random, but the ectopic focus or re-entry circuit is frequently located in certain specific areas of the atria [1-4]. It has been suggested that the majority of right atrial tachycardias originate from the crista terminalis (CT) and, accordingly, the term "cristal tachycardia" has been introduced [1-3].

The CT is a vertically oriented prominent band that separates the smooth walled part of the right atrium from the region of the pectinate muscles, which branch out from the crista at right angles. Superiorly, the CT reaches the orifice of the superior caval vein, and inferiorly it approaches the inferior vena cava and the coronary sinus os. The CT plays an important role in atrial flutter, where it works as a barrier preventing the circulating impulse from depolarizing the atrial tissue surrounded by the circuit, thereby contributing to perpetuation of re-entry [5]. This particular CT behavior is dependent on the orientation of its muscle fibers, which ultimately leads to preferentially longitudinal rather than transverse impulse transmission.

Cristal Tachycardia: Electrocardiographic Pattern

The first problem in definition of cristal tachycardia is that in most cases it has a P-wave configuration and axis exactly identical to those observed in normal sinus rhythm [2]. This is not surprising, since: (1) the sinus node is located in the upper part of the CT, in such a way that atrial activation of sinus origin may be indistinguishable from that arising from CT [1]; (2) the sinus pacemaker is not a small structure, but may extend over several centimeters [6]; (3) during sinus rhythm, the atrial site of earliest activation and P wave axis may change under the influ-

[1]Dipartimento di Cardiologia, Ospedale S. Raffaele, Milan, Italy; [2]Dipartimento di Cardiologia, Università di Messina, Italy

ence of autonomic tone variations; in other words, the pacemaker may shift along the CT [1]. Accordingly, distinguishing inappropriate sinus tachycardia from CT tachycardia may often be impossible. Furthermore, the so-called sinus node re-entry tachycardia is likely to represent, at least in some cases, a CT re-entry tachycardia; this is because no direct proof of sustained re-entry in the human or animal sinus node has been provided, but a re-entrant tachycardia has been assumed as arising from the sinus node only on the basis of the P-wave axis, a feature that does not represent a reliable key to determine the precise origin of an impulse.

An important contribution to our understanding of cristal tachycardia was given by Kalman et al. [3], who used intracardiac echocardiography to identify the CT and guide the placement of a 20-pole mapping catheter in close apposition to it. Twenty-seven patients with atrial tachycardia were selected on the basis of a surface electrocardiogram that suggested a right origin of the arrhythmia. Eighteen out of the 27 (67%) had a cristal tachycardia, as defined by intracardiac echocardiography, which, following successful ablation of the arrhythmia, identified the ablation catheter tip in immediate relation to the CT. It is worth noting that four patients showing electrocardiographic features typical of right atrial tachycardia had, in fact, a left atrial tachycardia originating from the right upper pulmonary vein. Recognition of the CT as a common site of origin of atrial tachycardia has been reported by several authors [7-10], but the study by Kalman et al. is the first to validate this assumption by means of intracardiac echocardiography; in previous clinical investigations the relationship between CT and atrial tachycardia was assessed using fluoroscopy alone.

The electrocardiographic pattern of cristal tachycardia was described by Tada et al. [4], based on the observation of 32 patients who underwent successful catheter ablation for right atrial tachycardia. According to the authors, a negative P wave in lead aVR identifies cristal tachycardia with 100% sensitivity and 93% specificity; tachycardias arising from the tricuspid annulus or from the atrial septum, by contrast, show positive P waves in lead aVR, apart from a few exceptions. A further diagnostic clue for cristal tachycardia is provided by lead II: the P wave was positive in 16/17 cases reported by Tada et al. [4], as well as in 13/18 cases in the study of Kalman et al. [3], who also observed in lead II biphasic or isoelectric P waves in 3 cases, and negative P waves in 2 patients whose site of origin of the tachycardia was in the low CT. On the basis of this information, it is reasonable to assume that an atrial tachycardia showing a P wave that is positive in lead II and negative in lead aVR arises from the CT.

Endocardial Activation Mapping in Cristal Tachycardia

Assessment of the atrial activation sequence in cristal tachycardia is facilitated by using a multipolar catheter that provides simultaneous recordings from several endocardial points. Tachycardias arising from the high CT show a high-to-low sequence, a pattern that is identical to that of sinus rhythm; in contrast, a low-to-high impulse progression suggests a low cristal origin of tachycardia, and simultaneous diffusion of the electrical activity towards the high and the low right atrium is typical of tachycardias located in the mid CT [3]. The precise site of the crista from which the arrhythmia arises is revealed by the earliest endocardial activation, which in some cases precedes the surface ECG P wave by a time that usually ranges from 30 to 60 ms. This also identifies the target for ablation; it is worth noting that in atrial tachycardia the mechanical trauma exerted by the catheter may result in sudden and transient disappearance of the arrhythmia, thereby indicating the site for successful ablation [11]. In addition, in cristal tachycardia a fractionated electrogram has been observed at the site of successful ablation [3]; this is likely to express the marked anisotropy that characterizes CT (see below).

Why Does Atrial Tachycardia Frequently Originate from the Crista Terminalis?

Cristal tachycardia appears to be the most common sustained right atrial tachycardia apart from atrial flutter. The reason why cristal tachycardia has a higher incidence than tachycardias arising from other sites is dependent on the particular anatomy of the CT, which contains cells that display automaticity, as well as cells with very few transverse gap junctions [12]. This results in relatively poor cell-to-cell coupling, a phenomenon that forms the basis for anisotropic conduction: CT is, thus, a region of slow conduction, particularly in the transverse direction, and this explains its role as a barrier in atrial flutter [5]. The slow conduction within the CT is a possible explanation for the fragmentation of endocardial potentials recorded at the site of successful ablation [3]. The particular anatomic and physiologic characteristics of CT may lead to tachycardia for more than one reason: (1) the slow conduction is the ideal milieu for re-entry; and (2) poor cell-to-cell coupling may facilitate the expression of atrial ectopic automaticity because of the absence or near-absence of electrotonic inhibitory influence exerted on the focus by the surrounding myocardium [13].

Conclusions

Several studies have pointed out that atrial tachycardia mainly arises from certain preferential regions: the CT is the most common site of origin for right atrial tachycardia [3, 4, 7-10], so that a new term, "cristal tachycardia," has been introduced [3]. When cristal tachycardia originates from the upper part of CT it is indistinguishable from sinus tachycardia, being characterized by a P-wave axis directed inferiorly and to the left. Unfortunately, distinguishing between cristal tachycardia and left atrial tachycardia arising from the right superior pulmonary vein is impossible, so that some left atrial tachycardias may be misclassified as originating in the right atrium. The anatomical basis for cristal tachycardia is the peculiar structure of the CT, the cells of which are characterized by very few transverse gap junctions. This results in poor cell-to-cell coupling, leading to anisotropic conduction. Although the basic mechanism of cristal tachycardia is not absolutely clear, automaticity appears more likely than re-entry in most cases. Cristal tachycardia is usually curable by radiofrequency catheter ablation: in successful ablation sites a fragmented potential may be often recorded, which may be a manifestation of anisotropic conduction within the CT.

References

1. Lesh MD, Kalman JM (1996) To fumble flutter or tackle "tach"? Toward updated classifiers for atrial tachyarrhythmias. J Cardiovasc Electrophysiol 7:460-466
2. Lesh MD, Kalman JM, Olgin JE (1997) An electrophysiologic approach to catheter ablation of atrial flutter and tachycardia: from mechanism to practice. In: Singer I (ed) Interventional electrophysiology. Williams and Wilkins, Baltimore, pp 347-382
3. Kalman JM, Olgin JE, Karch MR, Hamdan M, Lee RJ, Lesh MD (1998) "Cristal tachycardias": origin of right atrial tachycardia from the crista terminalis identified by intracardiac echocardiography. J Am Coll Cardiol 31:451-459
4. Tada H, Nogami A, Naito S, Suguta M, Nakatsugawa M, Horie Y, Tomita T, Hoshizaki H, Oshima S, Taniguchi K (1998) Simple electrocardiographic criteria for identifying the site of origin of focal right atrial tachycardia. Pacing Clin Electrophysiol 21:2431-2439
5. Olgin JE, Kalman JM, Fitzpatrick AP et al (1995) The role of right endocardial structures as barriers to conduction during human type 1 atrial flutter: activation and entrainment mapping guided by intracardiac echocardiography. Circulation 92:1839-1848
6. Boineau JP, Canavan TE, Schuessler RB et al (1988) Demonstration of a widely distributed pacemaker complex in the human heart. Circulation 77:1221-1237
7. Kay GN, Chong F, Epstein AE et al (1993) Radiofrequency ablation for treatment of primary atrial tachycardia. J Am Coll Cardiol 21:901-909
8. Walsh EP, Saul JP, Huise JE et al (1992) Transcatheter ablation of ectopic atrial tachycardia in young patients using radiofrequency current. Circulation 86:1138-1146
9. Shenasa H, Merril JJ, Hamer ME, Wharton JM (1993) Distribution of ectopic atrial tachycardias along the crista terminalis: an atrial ring of fire? Circulation 88 [Suppl I]:I-29 (abstr)
10. Sanders WE Jr, Sorrentino RA, Greenfield RA et al (1994) Catheter ablation of sinus node reentrant tachycardia. J Am Coll Cardiol 23:926-934
11. Pappone C, Stabile G, De Simone A et al (1996) Role of catheter-induced mechanical trauma in localizing of target sites of radiofrequency ablation in automatic atrial tachycardia. J Am Coll Cardiol 27:1090-1097
12. Saffitz JE, Kanter HL, Green KG et al (1994) Tissue-specific determinants of anisotropic conduction velocity in canine atrial and ventricular myocardium. Circ Res 74:1065-1070
13. Joyner R, Van Capelle F (1986) Propagation through electrically coupled cells: how a small SA node drives a large atrium. Biophys J 50:1157-1164

"Incisional" Reentrant Atrial Tachycardia: How to Prevent and Treat It?

J.A. Salerno-Uriarte[1], M. Tritto[1], M. Zardini[1], R. De Ponti[1], P. Fang[1], C. Storti[2] and M. Longobardi[2]

Patients submitted to cardiac surgery for correction of congenital or acquired heart diseases may subsequently experience several types of atrial tachyarrhythmias [1-4]. Most of these are macroreentrant atrial tachycardias strictly related to the presence of scars, prosthetic materials, or conduits and have therefore been named "incisional" or "scar-related" atrial tachycardias. Although their electrocardiographic characteristics may resemble those of atrial flutter, slight differences in P wave morphology and tachycardia cycle length are present and should be identified in order to formulate the correct diagnosis. "Incisional" atrial tachycardia may occur at widely variable times after the operation, most frequently in patients submitted to septal atrial defect repair and Fontan or Mustard procedures for tricuspid atresia or great vessel transposition correction, respectively. The true prevalence of these arrhythmias is unknown; small retrospective series reported a prevalence of 32-57% after the Fontan procedure [4, 6, 7] and about 15% after the Mustard operation [3, 8].

"Incisional" atrial tachycardias often represent a clinically relevant problem. In fact, in patients with reduced ventricular function, their occurrence is frequently associated with hemodynamic deterioration and/or syncope. An increased risk of thromboembolism and death has also been reported [1, 2, 8, 9]. Finally, permanent atrial tachycardias may lead to congestive heart failure in asymptomatic patients.

Pathophysiological Considerations

Several experimental and clinical studies have clearly demonstrated the macroreentrant nature of "incisional" atrial tachycardias [5, 10]. The primary role of natural anatomical (i.e. crista terminalis, eustachian ridge, tricuspid annulus, etc.) or surgically created (scars, prosthetic patches, conduits, etc.) barriers has been pointed out. In fact, such complex obstacles may constrain the electrical impulse propa-

[1]Istituto di Cardiologia "Mater Domini", Università degli Studi dell'Insubria, Sede di Varese, Castellanza (VA; [2]Divisione di Cardiologia, Istituto "Città di Pavia", Pavia, Italy

gation into preferential pathways and represent an ideal substrate for reentry. At least two barriers are required to stabilize reentry [10]. Nevertheless, it has to be considered that the mere presence of a reentrant pathway does not imply that a reentry tachycardia invariably occurs. In fact, according to the wavelength hypothesis, slowing of impulse conduction and/or a proper length of the reentrant pathway are necessary for reentry initiation and perpetuation [11]. However, both these conditions, sooner or later, will take place in enlarged and fibrotic atria such as those of patients submitted to congenital heart disease surgery, but they could account for the wide differences observed in tachycardia time presentation. Finally, slowing of conduction generally occurs at a narrow isthmus bounded by two anatomical or surgical barriers involved in reentry.

Treatment of "Incisional" Atrial Tachycardia

Treatment of "incisional" atrial tachycardia is a challenging problem. Antiar-rhythmic drug therapy has proved to be ineffective in most cases [2, 12, 13]. In addition, its use may be limited in these patients by the frequent association with sinus node dysfunction and impaired ventricular contractility. Serious adverse effects have been reported during antiarrhythmic drug treatment.

Radiofrequency catheter ablation is a recently introduced method to cure patients with various cardiac arrhythmias, including those related to "incisional" reentry [5, 14-19].

Methodological Considerations

Careful and extensive anatomical and electrophysiological cardiac mapping is mandatory in order to elucidate the arrhythmia mechanism and identify the critical components of the reentry circuit to target the radiofrequency current applications. An initial attempt to localize areas of anatomical or functional conduction block, usually characterized by split atrial electrograms, has to be performed during sinus rhythm and induced atrial tachycardia. Subsequently, the endocardial atrial activation sequence has to be reconstructed, by means of several multielectrode catheters, in order to define the path of activation of the atrial chamber during tachycardia. In addition, fragmented, low-amplitude, mid-diastolic or pre-systolic atrial potentials, possibly related to a critical slow-conducting isthmus of the reentrant circuit, have to be identified (Fig. 1). Participation of these areas in the reentrant circuit has to be demonstrated afterwards by pacing maneuvers [20]. Since tachycardia is reentrant in nature, it may be transiently entrained by fixed rate, overdrive atrial stimulation. If stimulation is performed from a non-protected area inside or close to the reentry circuit, an acceleration of the tachycardia to the pacing rate will occur associated with overt P waves and electrogram fusion on surface ECG and intracardiac recordings, respectively. ECG and intracardiac electrogram fusion results from collision of the tachycardia wavefront emerging from the exit site of the reentry circuit with the paced atrial activation. The last paced beat is entrained but not fused. On the other hand, if pacing is performed from a protected area inside the reentrant circuit (such as that bounded by anatomical or

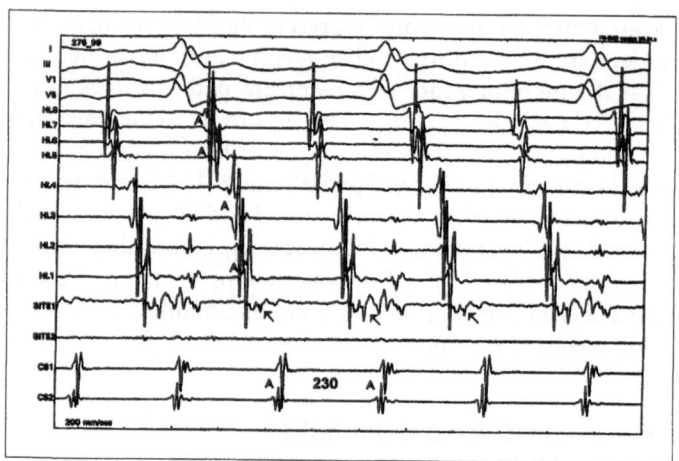

Fig. 1. Fragmented, low-amplitude, pre-systolic potentials recorded during "incisional" atrial tachycardia in a patient previously submitted to atrial septal defect repair. From top to bottom are shown leads 1, Ill, V1 and V5 and the bipolar intracardiac electrograms recorded from the 20-pole "halo" catheter positioned along the tricuspid annulus (HL8-1), the coronary sinus catheter (CS1-2) and the mapping catheter located in the area between the atrial septal patch and the coronary sinus ostium (SITE1-2). An atrial tachycardia with a cycle length of 230 ms and 2:1 AV conduction ratio is present. The lateral atrial wall is activated in a cranio-caudal direction. The bipolar electrogram recorded by the last pair of "halo" electrodes is followed by a fragmented, low-amplitude potential recorded from the mapping catheter (*arrows*) which, in turn, precedes the proximal coronary sinus activation. This signal, which has a 70 ms duration and precedes the surface P wave onset by 70 ms, is possibly related to the slow conduction occurring at the isthmus between the atrial septal patch and the coronary sinus ostium. A, Atrial electrogram. All values given in milliseconds

functional lines of conduction block), the paced rhythm orthodromically propagates to the exit site of the reentry circuit in the same manner as during tachycardia. Therefore, no surface ECG or intracardiac recording fusion will occur (entrainment with concealed fusion) and tachycardia resumes at the end of stimulation with the first post-pacing interval (measured at the site of stimulation) exactly matching the tachycardia cycle length duration (< 30 ms variations). In addition, the interval between the stimulus artifact and the P wave onset is variably prolonged, depending on the site of stimulation inside the protected isthmus (entrance, middle or exit) and the conduction properties of the activated tissues. This interval should also be equal to that measured from the local electrogram to the P wave onset during tachycardia. If all these criteria are met, the critical role of the identified area to the reentrant circuit is demonstrated (Fig. 2). Finally, entrainment with concealed fusion associated with wide differences in post-pacing interval with respect to tachycardia cycle length (> 30 ms) indicates pacing from bystander areas inside the protected isthmus.

Several protected areas may be present and possibly involved in the reentry circuit in patients previously submitted to cardiac surgery for congenital or acquired heart disease repair. They include the areas between the lateral atriotomy and the superior or inferior vena cava, the isthmus between the atrial septal defect closure

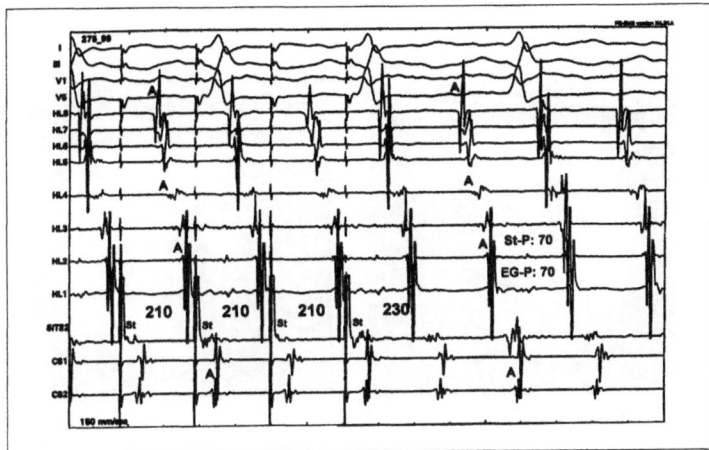

Fig. 2. Concealed entrainment of "incisional" atrial tachycardia in a patient previously submitted to atrial septal defect repair. The surface ECG and intracardiac recordings are arranged as in Fig. 1. In the left part of the panel continuous overdrive pacing at a 210 ms cycle length is performed from the mapping catheter located in the isthmus between the atrial septal patch and the coronary sinus ostium. All the bipolar intracardiac recordings and the surface ECG P waves are accelerated to the pacing rate but no changes in the endocardial activation sequence and surface P wave morphology, as compared to tachycardia, occur (entrainment with concealed fusion). At the end of stimulation tachycardia resumes with the first post-pacing interval measured at the pacing site exactly matching the tachycardia cycle length duration (230 ms). In addition, the interval between the stimulus artifact and the P wave onset is prolonged (70 ms) and equals that measured from the local electrogram and the P wave onset during tachycardia. These findings demonstrate that pacing is being performed from a critical, protected isthmus inside the reentry circuit. St, Stimulus artifact; A, Atrial electrogram; St-P, interval between stimulus artifact and P wave onset at surface ECG; EG-P, interval between onset of bipolar eletrogram recorded by mapping catheter and onset of P wave on surface ECG. Other abbreviations as in Fig. 1. All values given in milliseconds

and the coronary sinus ostium, the area between the Fontan conduit and the lateral atriotomy or the tricuspid annulus, etc. All these zones must be carefully mapped to assess or exclude their critical participation to the reentry circuit.

When a critical, protected isthmus is identified, radiofrequency current should therefore be sequentially delivered across it to create a complete line of block at that level. Complete acute success is obtained when tachycardia terminates during radiofrequency current application and is no longer inducible with subsequent programmed electrical stimulation (Fig. 3). The number of radiofrequency applications necessary to terminate the tachycardia is usually variable, but sometimes success can be obtained just with one or two pulses.

Results of Radiofrequency Catheter Ablation

A few small retrospective studies have been published to date in patients with "incisional" atrial tachycardia submitted to radiofrequency catheter ablation therapy [5, 14-19]. Overall success rates range between 50% and 80%. Follow-up

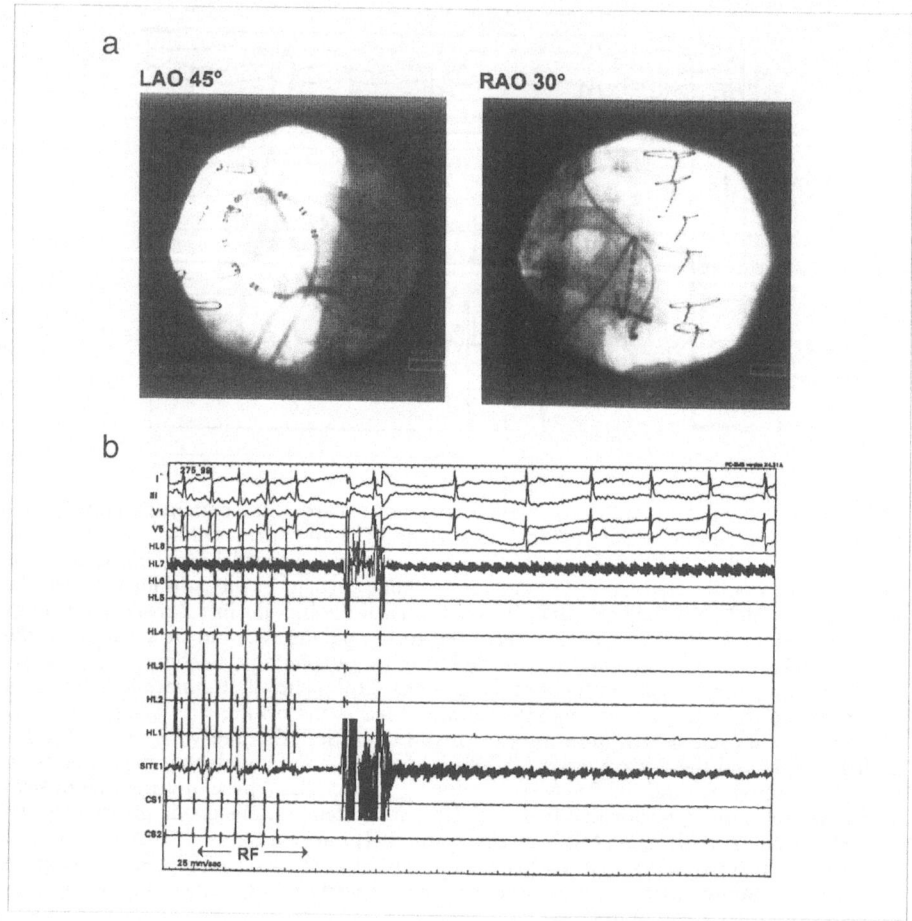

Fig. 3a,b. Tachycardia termination during radiofrequency current application in the area between the atrial septal patch and the coronary sinus ostium in the same patient as in Figs. 1 and 2. **a** 45° left anterior oblique and 30° right anterior oblique views of the "halo", coronary sinus and ablation catheters. **b** the 8-mm tip ablation catheter is positioned at the superior rim of the coronary sinus ostium where radiofrequency current delivery terminates the tachycardia. Note the marked sinus node depression at the end of tachycardia with escape junctional rhythm emergence. Surface ECG and intracardiac recordings in **b** are arranged as in previous figures. RF, Radiofrequency current application. Other abbreviations as in Figs. 1 and 2

studies are lacking, but a 53% recurrence rate at 18 months has been reported [18]. We treated 21 consecutive patients (9 males and 12 females; mean age 42 ± 12 years), with symptomatic "incisional" atrial tachycardia not controlled by several antiarrhythmic drug regimens. The associated cardiac diseases are reported in Table 1. As a whole, 30 different atrial tachycardias were clinically documented and/or induced during the electrophysiological evaluation. Complete success was obtained in 21/30 tachycardias (70%) in 14 patients. One

Table 1. Associated cardiac abnormalities in patients with "incisional" atrial tachycardia submitted to radiofrequency catheter ablation

Type	Number
Atrial septal defect	10
Valve disease	2
Endocardial cushion defect	2
Coronary artery disease	1
Atrio-ventricular nodal reentry	1
Transposition of great arteries	2
Tetralogy of Fallot	2
Interatrial myxoma	1

successfully treated patient experienced a clinical recurrence which was cured during a second procedure. Differences in patient population, with few patients submitted to Fontan or Mustard procedures in our series, may account for the low recurrence rate in comparison to other studies [18]. In addition, in 4 patients a partial modification of the reentry circuit was obtained by radiofrequency current delivery as demonstrated by a consistent prolongation of the tachycardia cycle length. In these patients tachycardia control has been obtained by a previously ineffective antiarrhythmic drug regimen. Globally, a clinical success was therefore observed in 18/21 patients (85%).

From analysis of the published data, it seems clear that radiofrequency catheter ablation results in this subset of patients are not as satisfactory as those reported in subjects with Wolff-Parkinson-White syndrome or atrio-ventricular nodal reentrant tachycardia [21]. However, it should be considered that patients presenting with "incisional" atrial tachycardia often have an extremely distorted anatomy which sometimes renders exceedingly difficult even the recognition of simple anatomical landmarks. In addition, many patients have been submitted to several palliative surgical procedures prior to the final congenital heart disease correction. Thus, as demonstrated by the large number of observed or induced tachycardias in a single patient, multiple reentrant circuits may be present due to distinct anatomical substrates or to an extremely diffuse myocardial atrial disease. It is obvious that under these conditions the results of ablative therapy are less than optimal.

Some improvement in the results of catheter ablation therapy may result from either a better understanding of the tachycardia mechanisms and an improvement in mapping techniques. In fact, new mapping systems including multielectrode "basket" catheters, non-contact unipolar mapping and non-fluoroscopic mapping are under investigation or have been recently introduced in clinical practice [22, 23]. Generally, they allow a complete reconstruction of the atrial endocardial activation sequence during tachycardia (Fig. 4) and may visualize the circulating wavefront. These systems seem quite promising, but further investigations are required.

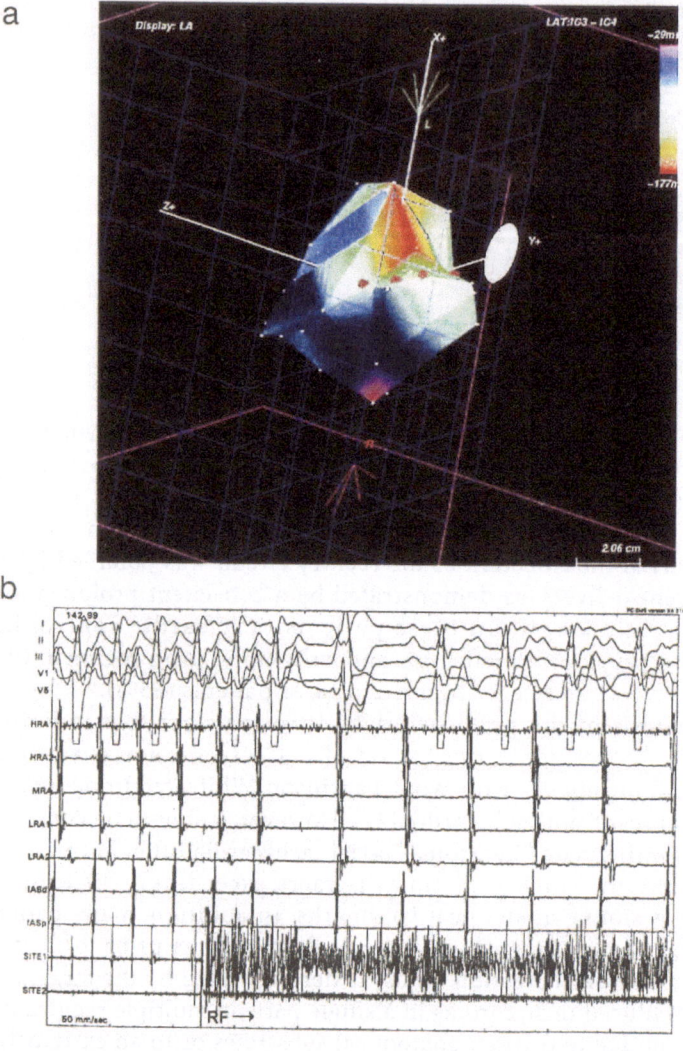

Fig. 4a,b. Atrial endocardial activation map reconstructed by means of a three dimensional, nonfluoroscopic, electroanatomical mapping system (CARTO, Biosense) in a patient with surgically corrected great vessel transposition and "incisional" atrial tachycardia. The point-by-point right atrial map is displayed on a color-code basis (**a**). The red and purple colors indicate the earliest and the latest activated areas, respectively. The red tags indicate the sequentially radiofrequency current pulses which resulted in tachycardia termination (**b**). The target site was identified according to the reconstructed endocardial atrial activation sequence and the response to pacing maneuvers. From top to bottom in panel **b** are shown leads I, III, V1 and V5 and the bipolar intracardiac electrograms recorded by the catheter placed in high (HRA), mid (MRA) and low (LRA) right atrium, the interatrial septum (IAS) and the ablation catheter (SITE). RF, Radiofrequency application

Prevention of "Incisional" Atrial Tachycardia

Due to the less than optimal results of catheter ablation therapy and the sometimes dramatic consequences of these tachyarrhythmias, many efforts have to be made to prevent their occurrence after heart disease repair. Improvements in percutaneous transcatheter techniques for atrial septal defect closure will reduce the number of surgical repairs and, thus, their proarrhythmic consequences. In patients with more complex congenital heart disease, close cooperation between the surgeon and the electrophysiologist is needed. Modification of the surgical techniques may lead, for example, to the creation of a complete intercaval right atriotomy, avoiding electrical impulse transmission at the upper and lower border of the scar. In addition, lines of conduction block may be intentionally created by means of cryoablation or direct radiofrequency current application at narrow, barrier-bounded areas of impulse propagation like those between the inferior vena cava and the tricuspid annulus and between the atrial septal patch and the coronary sinus ostium. Promising results at two-year follow-up have been recently published in a limited series of patients with "incisional" atrial tachycardia after Fontan procedure, submitted to surgical revision associated with cryoablation at areas selected anatomically or on the basis of the results of intraoperatory mapping [24]. In addition, in patients requiring Fontan procedures, an extracardiac cavo-pulmonary connection or a lateral-tunnel technique should be preferred since they may decrease the incidence of late atrial arrhythmias [4, 24]. Finally, since atrial enlargement plays a significant role in arrhythmia development, a better hemodynamic status obtained by means of optimal medical therapy or a new surgical procedure may be helpful in reducing tachycardia recurrences.

Conclusions

"Incisional" atrial tachycardia in patients previously submitted to cardiac surgery is a serious complication with clinical and prognostic implications. Tachycardia management is difficult and antiarrhythmic drug therapy results are disappointing. Radiofrequency catheter ablation is feasible and safe in this subset of patients. Although large prospective studies have never been performed, acute success rates of this technique seem to be good and might be furtherly improved by a better knowledge of tachycardia mechanisms and new mapping systems. Atrial disease progression may account for the high recurrence rate reported in some series. Of crucial relevance is prevention of atrial arrhythmias, which could result from modification of the surgical techniques combined with a closer cooperation between surgeons and electrophysiologists.

References

1. Flinn CJ, Wolff GS, Dick MI et al (1984) Cardiac rhythm after the Mustard operation for complete transposition of the great arteries. N Engl J Med 310:1635-1638

2. Garson A, Bink-Boelkens M, Hesslein PS et al (1985) Atrial flutter in the young: a collaborative study of 380 cases. J Am Coll Cardiol 6:871-878
3. Gelatt M, Hamilton RM, McCrindle BW et al (1997) Arrhythmia and mortality after the Mustard procedure: a 30-year single-center experience. J Am Coll Cardiol 29:194-201
4. Gates RN, Laks H, Drinkwater DC, Jr et al (1997) The Fontan procedure in adults. Ann Thorac Surg 63:1085-1090
5. Lesh MD, Van Hare GF, Epstein LM et al (1994) Radiofrequency catheter ablation of atrial arrhythmias: results and mechanisms. Circulation 89:1074-1089
6. Peters N, Somerville J (1992) Arrhythmias after the Fontan procedure. Br Heart J 68:199-204
7. Cromme-Dijkhuis AG, Hess J, Hahlen K et al (1993) Specific sequela after Fontan operation at mid- and long-term follow-up. J Thorac Cardiovasc Surg 106:1126-1132
8. Gewillig M, Cullen S, Mertens B et al (1991) Risk factors for arrhythmia and death after Mustard operation for simple transposition of the great arteries. Circulation 84:187-192
9. Fernandes SM, Mayer JE Jr, Burnett JT, Sloss LJ, Landzberg MJ (1996) Thrombosis and thromboembolism in the adult after Fontan surgery. J Am Coll Cardiol 27[Suppl A]:44A
10. Frame L, Page R, Boyden P et al (1987) Circus movement in the canine atrium around the tricuspid ring during experimental atrial flutter and during reentry in vitro. Circulation 76:1155-1175
11. Prystowsky EN, Klein JG (1994) Mechanisms of tachycardia. In: Prystowsky EN, Klein GJ (eds) Cardiac arrhythmias. McGraw Hill, New York, pp 81-95
12. Balaji S, Johnson TB, Sade RM, Case CL, Gillette PC (1994) Management of atrial flutter after the Fontan procedure. J Am Coll Cardiol 23:1209-1215
13. Weindling SN, Saul JP, Triedman JK, Walsh EP (1995) Recurrent intra-atrial reentrant tachycardia following congenital heart disease surgery: the search for an optimum therapy. Circulation 92[Suppl I]:I-765
14. Van Hare GF, Lesh MD, Stanger P (1993) Radiofrequency catheter ablation of supraventricular arrhythmias in patients with congenital heart disease: results and technical considerations. J Am Coll Cardiol 22:883-890
15. Triedman JK, Saul JP, Weindling SN, Walsh EP (1995) Radiofrequency ablation of intra-atrial reentrant tachycardia after surgical palliation of congenital heart disease. Circulation 91:707-714
16. Kalman JM, Van Hare GF, Olgin JE, Saxon LA, Stark SI, Lesh MD (1996) Ablation of "incisional" reentrant atrial tachycardia complicating surgery for congenital heart disease. Use of entrainment to define a critical isthmus of conduction. Circulation 93:502-512
17. Baker BM, Lindsay BD, Bromberg B, Frazier DW, Cain ME, Smith JM (1996) Catheter ablation of intraatrial reentrant tachycardias resulting from previous atrial surgery: locating and transecting the critical isthmus. J Am Coll Cardiol 28:411-417
18. Triedman JK, Bergau DM, Saul JP, Epstein MR, Walsh EP (1997) Efficacy of radiofrequency ablation for control of intraatrial reentrant tachycardia in patients with congenital heart disease. J Am Coll Cardiol 30:1032-1038
19. Salerno JA, De Ponti R, Zardini M, Storti C, Chioffi M, Tritto M (1997) Cure of right-sided postsurgical atrial tachycardia treated by direct radiofrequency catheter ablation. Eur Heart J 18[Suppl]:150 (abstr)
20. Stevenson WG, Sager PT, Friedman PL (1995) Entrainment techniques for mapping atrial and ventricular arrhythmias. J Cardiovasc Electrophysiol 6:201-216

21. Stevenson WG, Ellison KE, Lefroy DC, Friedman PL (1997) Ablation therapy for cardiac arrhythmias. Am J Cardiol 80:56G-66G
22. Liu ZW, Jia P, Ershler PR et al (1997) Noncontact endocardial mapping: reconstruction of electrograms and isochrones from intracavitary probe potentials. J Cardiovasc Electrophysiol 8:415-431
23. Dorostkar PC, Cheng J, Scheinman MM (1998) Electroanatomical mapping and ablation of the substrate supporting intraatrial reentrant tachycardia after palliation for complex congenital heart disease. Pacing Clin Electrophysiol 21:1810-1819
24. Deal BJ, Mavroudis C, Backer CL, Johnsrude CL, Rocchini AP (1999) Impact of arrhythmia circuit cryoablation during Fontan conversion for refractory atrial tachycardia. Am J Cardiol 83:563-568

Treatment of Tachyarrhythmias Using Cryothermal Energy

D.L. Lustgarten, D. Keane and J. Ruskin

Introduction

There are several energy sources available for the ablation of abnormally conducting cardiac tissue, with radiofrequency currently in clinical use for the treatment of numerous cardiac arrhythmias. There is a great deal of interest in developing alternative energy sources that could allow the creation of longer lesions with less thrombogenicity than are currently possible using radiofrequency. Some modalities that are under investigation are laser and microwave, which, like radiofrequency, rely on hyperthermy to cause tissue destruction. Another alternative is cryoablation, in which tissue destruction is effected through application of freezing temperatures. As will be discussed below, the cryolesion is quite distinct from lesions created by burning, preserving the basic underlying tissue structure which results in lesions that are less thrombogenic and have greater tensile strength. There is extensive clinical experience in the use of cryothermy in the surgical treatment of tachyarrhythmias where it has proven to be a safe and effective means of ablating electrically abnormal cardiac tissue. With the recent advent of percutaneous cryocatheters, there is now wider potential for the application of cryothermy in a variety of clinical settings. The following discussion contrasts potential advantages of using cryothermy versus modalities relying on hyperthermy and reviews the literature of the use of cryothermy in the surgical management of clinically important arrhythmias.

Mechanisms of Tissue Injury During Cryothermia

Sufficient exposure to cryothermy, typically −50 to −70°C for greater than 30 s, results in destruction of local tissue has been well characterized as occurring in

Massachusetts General Hospital, Boston, Massachusetts, USA

three phases; a freeze/thaw phase, a hemorrhagic phase, and finally a replacement fibrosis phase. In the first phase, intra- and extracellular ice crystals cause compression of local cellular structures and distortion of cytoplasmic components and nuclei. It has been demonstrated that the histologic presence of ice crystals is required for cell death to occur at the site of exposure: whether the presence of ice crystals is causative or merely associated with tissue destruction remains a matter of debate that goes beyond the focus of this discussion. Immediately upon thawing, acute changes in myofilaments and mitochondria occur that are the result of increased membrane permeability during the thawing phase [1]. Loss of mitochondrial membrane integrity results in oxidation of endogenous pyridine nucleotides and subsequent membrane lipid peroxidation and enzyme hydrolysis. The latter result in disruption of the electron transport chain such that, despite evidence of late membrane repair, mitochondria become irreversibly de-energized [2]. During this acute phase of cyrothermal exposure, blood vessels within the cryolesion demonstrate endothelial cell damage, platelet aggregation, flow stasis, and occlusion. Recanalization takes place over the course of the hours-to-days following the acute injury [3]. Additionally, however, endothelial cell damage resulting in smooth cell proliferation has been observed as early as 1 week following exposure to cryothermy. Coagulation necrosis becomes apparent within 48 h of thawing, which characterizes the hemorrhagic phase of tissue destruction induced by cryothermy.

The size of the lesion created by cryothermy is determined by a variety of factors, including temperature, the size of the probe employed, and the duration and number of freeze/thaw cycles to which the tissue is subjected. For a given duration of exposure, lower temperatures generate progressively larger lesions. Within 5 min at a given temperature, however, the lesion size plateaus [4-6]. Repetitive freeze/thaw cycles enlarge cryolesions beyond those obtained with prolonged freezing at a given temperature [7-9]. The rate of conduction of the cold front increases with repetitive exposure, suggesting a progressive increase in thermal conductivity of tissue. Although the basis for this is not well understood, it may relate to a change in basic cellular structure and/or changes in the local microperfusion environment during the thaw cycle [4].

Markovitz et al. [10] demonstrated that varying the tank pressure when utilizing nitrous oxide-cooled cryoprobes directly correlated with lesion size, with maximal lesion sizes being obtained at tank pressures greater than 700 psi. They also demonstrated that cold potassium cardioplegia allowed for the formation of larger lesions at a given temperature and duration of cryothermia. The subsequent use of cryoprobes cooled by liquid nitrogen allowed for significantly lower temperatures and hence the generation of larger lesions for a given duration of exposure [11].

A variety of animal studied have been performed analyzing the effect of cryothermy on the histology and function of conduction tissue, demonstrating irreversible loss of conduction following cryothermy [12-15]. Holman et al. evaluated local electrical potentials generated prior to and immediately following the creation of ventricular cryolesions [16]. Unipolar electrical potentials were measured from points spanning the ventricular myocardium using plunge electrodes. Cryolesions were generated by the application of a cryoprobe cooled to -60°C with expanding nitrous oxide for 2 min. There was a proportionate decrease in local electrogram amplitude the closer the measuring electrode was to the developing cryolesion. The observed decrease in amplitude could reflect epicardial ice insulation or functional inhibition of myocardial electrical potential, a point that was not distinguished by the authors. A greater than 70% decrease in absolute amplitude from control unipolar potentials was predictive of cell death, as determined by subsequent histologic analysis 48 h or 2 weeks following the experiment.

In contradistinction to lesions created by coronary occlusion [17], cryolesions exhibit low arrhythmogenic potential [16, 18, 19]. Using a canine model, Klein et al. found that epicardial electrograms recorded directly above acute epicardial or intramural cryolesions showed amplitude loss, while those adjacent to the lesions were unaffected [18]. This observation persisted 4 weeks after the acute lesion formation, clearly demonstrating sustained loss of myocardial potential following cryothermy. Plunge electrode sites in or surrounding cryolesions revealed normal electrical activation in histologically preserved tissue immediately adjacent to the cryothermal scar, with complete loss of conduction within the cryolesions per se. All dogs studied had frequent ventricular premature beats with variable coupling intervals immediately and for four days following the freeze procedure. With the exception of one animal that had frequent ventricular ectopy prior to study, all ventricular ectopic activity had resolved by seven days following cryothermy. None of the animals were inducible for ventricular tachycardia during programmed electrical stimulation. The absence of inducible ventricular tachycardia and the observation of variable ventricular ectopic coupling times suggested to these authors that the observed ectopy represented enhanced automaticity that was benign and short-lived. A similar study performed on eight dogs by Hunt et al. corroborated these results [19].

A useful property of cryothermal energy is its ability to reversibly block electrical conduction at less severe temperatures, a phenomenon referred to as cryotermination [20] or, more commonly, cryomapping. Analysis of canine ventricular myocardium exposed to temperatures decreasing from 37°C to 30°C demonstrated progressive slowing of conduction to the point of complete block [21]. Cooling prolongs the local effective refractory period causing conduction delay and block [22]. These reversible effects of cryothermy on cardiac conduction has allowed the mapping of focal tachycardias and tachycardia circuits, as will be discussed below.

The completed cryolesion consists of physiologically inert fibrosed tissue. Human autopsy studies are consistent with the changes described above. For example, one patient with dilated cardiomyopathy who died suddenly 8 days following AV nodal surgical cryoablation had fibrinoid necrosis within the cryo-ablated AV node [15]. The AV nodal artery had intramural fibrinoid necrosis. The conduction tissue itself showed necrosis and hemorrhage. The cryolesions from another patient who had undergone AV nodal cryoablation two months before death demonstrated discrete fibrosis and intimal narrowing of the AV nodal artery. At autopsy one year after cryotherapy in a third patient, the penetrating and branching portions of the His bundle showed marked fibrotic changes. In each case, the observed lesions were discrete and sharply delimited. None of the deaths were thought to be related to cryosurgery [15].

The ability of cryothermal energy to create discrete, structurally intact, electrically inert foci in ventricular myocardium makes it a potentially useful therapeutic modality in the treatment of a variety of tachyarrhythmias. Cryothermy has been applied to numerous clinical arrythmias, initially in open surgical procedures and, subsequently, in percutaneous approaches using intravascular cryocatheters. The results of these studies, and the technologies as they have evolved, are the subject of the remainder of this chapter.

Clinical Applications

AV Nodal and His Bundle Ablation

AV nodal and/or His ablation for recurrent drug-refractory supraventricular tachycardias and subsequent permanent pacemaker placement has been employed since 1967 [13, 23-25]. Harrison et al. [13] were the first to evaluate cryosurgery as an alternative to surgical dissection, using a cryoprobe to first map and subsequently ablate the AV node. Patients with drug-refractory, life-threatening supraventricular tachyarrhythmias underwent open-heart surgery with cardiopulmonary bypass, and the His bundle identified using intra-operative mapping techniques through the exposed right atrium. Hand-held nitrous oxide-cooled cryoprobes were used to identify the AV node by cooling within the triangle of Koch at 0°C for 30 s, thereby producing reversible complete heart block with junctional escape in each case. Freezing at –60°C for two consecutive 90-s periods caused irreversible complete heart block. In some cases, a third freeze was applied to the area between the first lesion and the coronary sinus. Complete heart block with a subsidiary junctional escape was observed in each patient which remained the case at up to 3 years of follow-up [16]. One patient had complete retrograde and antegrade heart block confirmed at electrophysiology testing 9 days following cryoablation. In a subsequent study, complete heart block was achieved in 17 of 22 patients who had a variety of recalcitrant supraventricular tachycardias (77%). Subsequent electrophysiology evaluation in 16 of these patients 7 to 10 days after the procedure demonstrated complete disruption of AV nodal tissue and preservation of junctional tissue. Two patients developed incomplete right bundle branch block and one patient had new precordial Q waves – the latter had also received ventriculotomy for attempted simultaneous treatment of ventricular tachycardia. This patient died

12 months following the procedure of an unrelated cause at which time autopsy confirmed discrete fibrosis of the common His bundle and the upper right ventricular aspect of the muscular interventricular septum. Post-operative His bundle electrograms were obtained from 3 patients which demonstrated AV block with His deflections preceding each QRS. The results of these studies suggested that cryoablation provided a safe and effective alternative to mechanical disruption of the AV node for patients with drug-refractory supraventricular tachycardia.

Subsequent to these studies, attempts to minimize morbidity and mortality associated with cardiopulmonary bypass have been examined. For instance, Gillette et al. developed an 11 French transvenous cryocatheter that was fluoroscopically guided to the region of the AV node/His bundle in swine [14]. The cryocatheter was cooled to –60°C using pressurized nitrous oxide. Complete AV block during cryothermia was produced in all 5 animals studied. Complete heart block persisted in 4 of the 5 pigs, whereas the 5th animal developed 2:1 AV block at 1 h. The animals were all sacrificed at one hour allowing gross confirmation of localization of the cryolesions to the apex of the triangle of Koch [14].

Using a steerable 8 French Halocarbon cooled cryocatheter with a bipolar electrode tip, M. Dubuc (personal communication, May 1998) has demonstrated the ability to both reversibly and irreversibly block the AV node in dogs via femoral venous cannulation. Reversible block was achieved by progressively lowering the catheter tip temperature until high degree AV block or lengthening of the PR interval by greater than 50% developed. Typically this occurred at temperatures ranging from –20°C to –50°C. Histologic study of the AV node from an animal in which reversible 2:1 block had been achieved showed no evidence of a lesion. Complete irreversible AV block was obtained in another dog by cryoapplication for 5 min at –50°C. Histologic analysis at 6 weeks demonstrated the AV node to be replaced by scar tissue.

Modified surgical approaches have also been explored. Bredikis and coworkers in Lithuania have published a series of patients in which His bundle cryoablation was effected through two atriotomy incisions, one for the cryoprobe and the other for passage of the surgeon's finger into the atrium to allow digital identification of the anatomic landmarks surrounding the AV node and His bundle [27]. The latter were confirmed by recording His bundle potentials, cryothermal mapping, pressure-induced AV block, or by anatomic definition alone. The success rate in this series of 34 patients was 85% (see Table 1). In a less detailed ensuing report by these authors, they performed the procedure in 72 patients with a success rate of 92% with only one complete failure [28]. They reported a single mortality for which details were not given. Another alternative approach avoiding the need for bypass was reported by Louagie et al. who performed epicardial His bundle cryoablation by application of the cryoprobe to the right coronary fossa [29]. The presence of the His bundle was confirmed by cryomapping and subsequent ablation.

Table 1. Summary of the reported use of cryosurgical ablation for treatment of supraventricular tachycardias. (Reprinted with permission from [85])

Ref., Year	Procedure	No. of patients	Age range	Types of arrhythmias	Follow-up (months)	Succes rate	Morbidity	Mortality
[13], 1977	His bundle cryoablation (HBCA) OHS/CB	3	26-52	AT, SSS, SVT	2-6	100%	none	none
[26], 1980	HBCA-OHS/CB	22 (19 new)	24-70	AT, AP, SSS, SVT AF, AFL, EAR	2-37	77° (17/22)	incRBBB-2/17 septalQ-1/17*	2 deaths at one year - unrelated to procedure
[66], 1980	HBCA(8), APCA(4)	12 (15 arrhythmias)	35-63	WPW, PAF, AF, AT	6-20	HB ablation: 62% (5/8) AP ablation: 100% (4/4)	Re-emergent nodal conduction in 1/8 HBCA** VF 6° post-op	none
[27], 1985	HBCA - thoracotomy (off bypass) HBCA-OHS/CB	34 / 77	18-71 / 12-66	AF, AFL, SVT, AT, ST	Mean: 34	85% (29/34)[T] / 100%	Right atriotomy hemorrhage PM poket wound infection	none
[33], 1987	AVNRT ablation-OHS/CB	8	16-46	AVNRT	1-60	100%	RBBB in 3 patients	none
[34], 1988	AVNRT ablation-OHS/CB	5	3-67	AVNRT	6-24	100%	none	none
[67], 1990	AVNRT ablation-OHS/CB	23 (15 new)	12-56	AVNRT	2-70	100%	none	none
[29], 1991	HBCA-epicardial (off bypass)	6	24-73	AF, AFL, AT	14-43	100%	none	none

Cont.

Cont. Table 1.

Ref., Year	Procedure	Number of patients	Age range	Types of arrhythmias	Follow up (months)	Succes rate	Morbidity	Mortality
[38], 1977	APCA-OHS/CB	2	23, 25	WPW	2-3	100%	none	none
[42], 1985	APCA-OHS/CB	21	17-64	WPW	NA	90% (19/21)	Coronary sinus perforation in 2 patients	none
[68], 1988	APCA-OHS/CB	20	21-58	WPW (21)	12-120	77% (17/20)	Reoperation needed in 4 patients-successful in each	none
[40], 1986	APCA-epicardial with and without CB	105	6-66	WPW (108)	2-42	99% (104/105)	4 recurrences, all successfully reoperated 3 CS tears-repaired	none
[41], 1989	APCA-off bypass except 3 patients requiring endocardial ablation	28	13-67	WPW (31)	2-48	100%	CHB requiring permanent pacemaker. Reoperation for early recurrence in 3 patients	none
[43], 1989	Septal CA-OHS/CB	18	1-31	Septal bypass tracts	Mean: 17	89% (16/18)	Transient post-op pancreatitis	none

AF, atrial fibrillation; AFL, atrial flutters; AP, accessory pathway; AT, atrial tachycardia; AVNRT, AV nodal reentrant tachycardia; CA, cryoablation; CPB, cardiopulmonary bypass; CS, coronary sinus; EAR, ectopic atrial rhythm; HB, his bundle; OHS, open heart surgery; PM, pacemaker; SSS, sick sinus syndrome; SVT, supraventricular tachycardia; WPW, Wolff-Parkinson-White syndrome

*Patient had ventriculotomy for simultaneous ventricular tachycardia ablation

**Successfully reoperated on using cryoablation of the AV node

τ 2 patients failed to achieve stable complete heart block but were cured of arrhythmia

Cryoablation for AV Node Reentry Tachycardia

Cryothermal mapping played a central role in our current understanding of AV nodal anatomy, and was the first experimental modality used to ablate AV nodal reentrant tachycardia while preserving normal antegrade AV nodal conduction. The serendipitous surgical cure of AV nodal reentrant tachycardia with preservation of antegrade AV nodal conduction in a single patient by Pritchett et al. in 1979 [30] during routine dissection of the His bundle region prompted Holman and Cox to evaluate the area of the triangle of Koch using hand-held cryoprobes in dogs [31, 32, Cox, 1987 #256]. Cryolesions were placed encircling the triangle of Koch. If AV nodal block occurred during the application of cryothermal energy, the probe was immediately shut off and the area warmed with saline. Antegrade and retrograde conduction studies were performed acutely and chronically: AV nodal conduction delay and refractory period prolongation were present acutely, but had resolved by 14 weeks. AV nodal echo beats present prior to ablation were no longer inducible, suggesting that the anatomical substrate for AV nodal reentrant tachycardia had been ablated. Consistent with this observation, dual AV nodal physiology that had been noted in three dogs at baseline EP testing was uniformly eliminated by the procedure [32].

In light of these findings, Cox et al. [33] and other investigators [34] went on to perform similar procedures in patients with drug-refractory AV nodal reentrant tachycardia (see Table 1). The procedure proved to be 100% effective with no patient requiring permanent pacemaker placement or continued drug therapy. Right bundle branch block was reported in 3 of the first 8 patients studied [33]. This was presumed on the basis of histologic studies in the canine model [35] to represent extension of the cryolesion either into the right bundle itself, or to fibers in the His bundle destined to feed the right bundle.

Accessory Atrioventicular Pathway Ablation

The application of cryothermy to accessory pathway ablation was initially explored as an alternative to surgical treatment, in view of the considerable mortality rate (3.6%-5.4%) associated with conventional surgery [36, 37]. The potential for the formation of a more stable lesion and, with the advent of hand-held probes, a relatively less invasive procedure requiring less cardiopulmonary bypass time made cryosurgery an appealing alternative. Several clinical series and case reports of cryosurgery for accesory pathways have been published and are summarized in Table 1. The earliest report of cryosurgical accessory pathway ablation was a pilot evaluation of two patients, one with a left posterior accessory pathway, the other with an anterior septal pathway [38]. Confirmation of the former was done by direct electrical recording of the accessory pathway and resolution of the delta wave by applying pressure to the putative accessory pathway. In the latter, the presence of a septal pathway capable of only retrograde conduction was confirmed by cryomapping which demonstrated reversible block across the accessory pathway. The pathways identified in both cases were then ablated endocardially with the patients on cardiopulmonary bypass, using a hand-held cry-oprobe freezing the tissue to −60°C for 90 s with two sequential applications. Both patients remained free of arrhythmia at follow-up (see Table 1).

To further minimize surgical morbidity and mortality, an epicardial approach was employed by Guiraudon and colleagues [39] who reported a series of 105 patients with left lateral (74), postero-septal (23), and right ventricular free wall (11) accessory pathways [40]. Depending on the accessory pathway locale and mapping results, some patients had procedures performed off of cardiopul-monary bypass. Generally, cardiopulmonary bypass was utilized in patients with left sided accessory pathways. Efficacy was excellent, with only four patients requiring reoperation, one of whom required a third procedure. There was a sin-gle failure but the patient's arrhythmia became easily controlled with pro-cainamide. Morbidity was minimal − the patient requiring three procedures developed a post-surgical coagulopathy which resolved. There were no deaths.

Using epicardial cryoablation, Watanabe et al. avoided the use of cardiopul-monary bypass in a series of 28 patients who had a total of 31 accessory path-ways [41]. Only three patients had to be converted to an endocardial procedure, two because of failure to achieve ablation epicardially, and one because of a sur-gical atrial wall tear unrelated to the cryosurgical technique. Morbidity was oth-erwise limited to conversion to an open heart procedure in one patient, and effi-cacy was 100%.

The epicardial approach to left lateral and left posterior accessory pathways is limited anatomically during open chest procedures. Bredikis and Bredikis obviat-ed this limitation by introducing a specially designed cryoprobe into the coro-nary sinus. In this manner, the operators were able to perform cryoablation of left sided accessory pathways without the need for cardiopulmonary bypass. Nineteen of 21 patients were successfully managed by this approach. In two cases, the coronary sinus was torn and required surgical ligation [42]. There were no reports of left circumflex coronary artery complications.

Patients with septal accessory pathways have also been successfully treated with cryoablation: Lee et al. described a series of 18 patients, 11 with classic Wolff-Parkinson-White syndrome and 7 with permanent junctional reciprocating tachycardia who underwent surgical endocardial cryoablation [43]. After tricus-pid valve annulus endocardial mapping, lesions were produced at the site of earli-est activation. Overlapping endocardial lesions were subsequently applied toward the AV node and across the septum opposite the initial lesion. Using this method, 16 definitive cures were obtained. One patient who had both an anteroseptal and a posteroseptal pathway was noted to have recurrence of a delta wave on surface electrogram at 10 months, but had no recurrence of tachycardia off medication. Another patient who did not have return of his delta wave did have recurrences of poorly documented tachycardias requiring medical treatment. Morbidity was limited to one case of postoperative pancreatitis. There were no deaths. Five patients had depressed left ventricular ejection fractions preoperatively, all of which normalized post-operatively, consistent with a diagnosis of resolved tachy-cardiomyopathy [43].

Bundle Branch Reentry

Cryoablation has been used successfully to treat a patient with bundle branch reentry with tachycardia recalcitrant to medical treatment, radiofrequency and direct current ablation [44]. The patient was a 30-year-old woman with Ebstein's anomaly who presented with a sustained left bundle branch block morphology tachycardia and who was found to have inducible bidirectional bundle branch reentry on electrophysiology testing. Despite receiving 23 radiofrequency applications, and four 200-300 J direct current shocks to her right bundle branch, the patient returned to her baseline incomplete right bundle branch pattern, and bundle branch reentry was still inducible 48 h following her procedure. Subsequently, the patient had open-heart surgery and received extensive cryoablation over the entire length of her right interventricular septum. Postoperatively she developed stable right bundle branch block and ventricular tachycardia was no longer inducible. The patient remained symptom free over 10 months of follow-up [44].

Ventricular Tachycardia

There is extensive experience with cryosurgery for the treatment of ventricular tachycardia, usually as an adjunct to other surgical modalities such as aneurysmectomy, subendocardial resection, encircling endocardial ventriculotomy, coronary artery bypass grafting, and/or valvular replacement (Table 2). Each of these procedures has been used to either isolate, remove, or destroy arrhythmogenic ventricular myocardium. Although effective in reducing recurrent ventricular tachycardia, subendocardial resection and encircling endocardial ventriculotomy have been associated with progressive deterioration in left ventricular function [45]. Cryosurgery, on the other hand, has minimal untoward effects on cardiac function and preserves the integrity of the fibrous stroma at the site of the cryolesion [46, 47]. Successful application of cryosurgery to drug-resistant ventricular tachycardia associated with a variant of scleroderma [48] and to idiopathic right ventricular tachycardia [49], suggested that this modality could be an effective alternative to established surgical approaches for drug-refractory ventricular tachycardia, or could be used adjunctively. It was anticipated that cryosurgery would limit the extent of resection required in surgical approaches, and would also allow electrical isolation without disrupting functional structures such as the mitral valve apparatus.

There are currently no prospective studies comparing these various treatment modalities with respect to safety or efficacy, however, numerous studies have been generated and can be compared against historical controls. Prior to the addition of cryosurgery, surgical cure rates for drug-refractory (predominantly ischemic) ventricular tachycardia were reported between 60% and 65%, with an additional 25% gleaned from post-operative antiarrhythmic drugs [50, 51]. Analysis of the pooled data from eleven studies of surgically treated ischemic ventricular tachycardia (Table 2) in which cryosurgery was used adjunctively yields a surgical cure rate of 78% and a clinical cure rate of 92%. Whether this can

Table 2. Summary of the reported use of cryosurgical ablation for the treatment ventricular tachycardia. (Reprinted with permission from [85])

Ref., Year	Procedure	Mapping procedure	No. of patients	Age range	Associated disease process	Follow up (months)	Success rate surgical success* clinical success**	Morbidity	Mortality	Pre-op vs Post-op EF
[48], 1978	CS alone	Endocardial and epicardial mapping	1	37	CREST syndrome	12	see text	none	none	na
[49], 1979	CS alone	Endocardial and epicardial mapping	1	46	Idiopathic septal VT-NOS	6	no recurrent VT - off medication	none	none	na
[45], 1982	CS w/ ERP, EEV	na	5	na	IVT	na	no recurrent VT - off medication	none	none	na
[69], 1985	CS ± aneurysmectomy, ERP, and/or CABG	Endocardial and epicardial mapping	12	na	IVT	1-6	-10/11 (91%) -11/11 (100%)	na	1 operative death (9%) - ↓ C.O.	31 ± 12 vs. 27 ± 8 (NS)
[70], 1986	CS ± aneurysmectomy, ERP, and/or CABG	Endocardial and epicardial mapping	5	15-60	ICM (1) WPW w/ idioVT (1) IVT (3)	3-15	all remained free of VT off meds	Post-op recurrent VT w/ successful reoperation	1 late death - CHF	Either no effect or a trend toward improvement
[53], 1986	ERP + CS vs ERP ± CS	Endocardial mapping	15	48-72	IVT	3-17	-13/14 (93%) -14/14 (100%)	na	1 operative death (7%) CHF	NSC
			22	54-68	IVT	28-76	-15/27 (54%) p < .01 -25/27 (93%)		4 operative deaths (13%) CHF	NSC
[71], 1986	CS ± aneurysmectomy, ERP, and/or CABG	Endocardial and epicardial mapping	39	44-75	IVT	1-59	-31/35 (88.6%) -34/35 (97%)	na	4/39 (10.2%)	Not map-guided: 37 ± 8 vs. 39 ± 10 (NS) Map-guided: 32 ± 12 vs. 37 ± 12 (NS)

Cont.

Cont. Table 2.

Ref, Year	Procedure	Mapping procedure	No. of patients	Age range	Associated disease process	Follow up (months)	Success rate surgical success* clinical success**	Morbidity	Mortality	Pre-op vs. Post-op EF
[72], 1987	Excisional biopsy &/or CS	Endocardial and epicardial mapping	14	1.1 mean	myocardial hamartoma	2-74	-13/13 (100%)	none	1 operative death (7%) - ↓ C.O.	na
[73], 1988	CS alone - epi and endocardial	Endocardial and epicardial mapping	3	13-25	monomorphic ventricular bigeminy w/ ass. VT	5-30	-1/3 (33.3%) -2/3 (67%)	na	1 sudden death @ 5 mos	NSC
[52], 1988	CS alone	Endocardial and epicardial mapping	15	64 ± 9	IVT-all IMI's	19 ±7	-11/14 (79%) -13/14 (93%)	1/14 required ACID	No operative death No sudden death	39 ± 11 vs. 42 ± 9 (NS)
[74], 1989	CS alone	Endocardial and epicardial mapping	33	58 ± 10	IVT	3-57	-27/31 (84%) -28/31 (90%)	1/31 required AICD 2/31 required PPM	2 operative deaths 1 late sudden death	26 ± 7 vs. 40±9 (p < 0.01)
[75], 1989	CS ± ERP∞	Endocardial and epicardial mapping	39	61 ± 9	IVT	18 ±12	-28/37 (76%) -34/37 (92%) (63/71 induced VT's were ablated)	No VT recurrence	1 operative death 1 post-operative death	33 ±13 vs. 39±11 (p < 0.01)
[76], 1989	CS s/ ventriculotomy ± CABG	Endocardial and epicardial mapping	7	15-80	IVT ICM	na	-4/7 (57%) -6/7 (86%)	none	1 death @ 8 mos. CHF/VT	na
[77], 1994	CS ± aneurysmectomy, ERP	Endocardial mapping intraoperatively	4	51-70	IVT ICM	na	-3/4 (75%) -3/4 (75%)	none	1 death @ 26 days	na

Cont.

Cont. Table 2.

Ref., Year	Procedure	Mapping procedure	No. of patients	Age range	Associated disease process	Follow up (months)	Success rate surgical success* clinical success**	Morbidity	Mortality	Pre-op vs. Post-op EF
[78], 1994	CS + aneurysectomy	Endocardial and epicardial mapping	2	13,52	Congenital ventricular septal aneurysm	66,88	-2/2	post-op PAF in 1/2	none	na
[79], 1994	CS + ERP	Endocardial and epicardial mapping	3	19-26	RVOT VT s/p Tet repair	mean 40	-2/3 (66%) -3/3 (100%)	none	none	na
[80], 1994	CS ± aneurysmectomy, ERP, and/or CABG	Endocardial and epicardial mapping	48	43-76	IVT	3-96	-25/44 (57%) -37/44 (84%)	4 late VT recurrence 1 required AICD	4 operative deaths 5 late deaths - none sudden	na
[81], 1994	CS + ERP	Endocardial and epicardial mapping	2	1	myocardial hamartoma	7-17	-0/2 -2/2	none	none	na
[82], 1994	Encircling CS	Endocardial and epicardial mapping	33	36-71	IVT	mean 60	-29/32 (91%) -30/32 (94%)	none	1 death 2d. post-op	38 ± 14 vs. 45 ± 12 ($p = 0.02$)
[83], 1997	CS ± aneurysmectomy, ERP, and/or CABG	Endocardial and epicardial mapping	42	32-78	IVT	3-69	-28/38 (74%) -35/38 (92%)	31 required ICD	4 deaths w/in 30 d. - none sudden	na

CS, cryosurgery; EEV, endocardial enciveling ventriculotomy; ERP, endocardial resection procedure; ICM, idiopathic cardiomyopathy; IVT, ischemic ventricular tachycardia; na, data not available
*Surgical success defined as no spontaneous ventricular tachycardia or sudden death, without the need for pharmacological suppression
**Clinical success defined as no spontaneous ventricular tachycardia or sudden death with or without the need for pharmacological suppression.
∞ Statistical comparison demonstrated no additional benefit in patients receiving both CS and ERP vs CS alon

be attributed to cryosurgery per se, or to improved mapping and surgical techniques cannot be distinguished in this grouped analysis. Using cryosurgery alone to treat patients with drug-refractory ventricular tachycardia after inferior wall infarcts, Caceres et al. were able to obtain a surgical cure rate of 79% and a clinical cure rate of 93% [52], which contrasts with a 60% surgical cure rate in that subgroup [51]. Using cryosurgery adjunctively with subendocardial resection in the inferior myocardial infarct subgroup, Hargrove et al. were able to achieve a surgical cure of 93% in 14 patients, compared with a consecutive series of 27 patients in which cryosurgery was not a standard adjunct, where the surgical cure rate was only 54% ($p = 0.01$) (Table 2) [53]. These data suggest that cryosurgery is at least equivalent to and may in fact surpass other surgical modalities for the treatment of drug-refractory VT, a hypothesis that could only be proven in the context of prospective randomized trials.

Typically the populations of patients in whom these techniques have been applied are high risk patients with depressed myocardial function, which is reflected by the high surgical mortality seen in Table 2. The addition of cryosurgery to the treatment of drug refractory ventricular tachycardia has been associated with either a neutral or beneficial effect on cardiac performance (Table 2). Presumably this is a reflection of the ability to preserve more viable myocardium, preclude the need for mitral valve replacement, and protect against tachycardia-induced cardiomyopathy in those patients with frequent tachycardia episodes.

Cryosurgical Mapping in Canine Models of Ventricular Tachycardia

Cryomapping has been used to identify critical portions of reentrant ventricular tachycardia pathways in a canine infarct model, 3 to 5 days following coronary artery ligation [54]. Electrically induced sustained monomorphic ventricualar tachycardia was mapped epicardially in each animal and epicardial sites within the reentrant circuit were exposed to temperatures between –5°C and 5°C for 10-30 s. Application of the cryoprobe to the earliest site of epicardial ventricular activation resulted in a new activation site rather than tachycardia termination. In contradistinction, cooling the distal part of the common reentrant pathway proximal to the earliest site of ventricular activation resulted consistently in tachycardia termination. The epicardial maps confirmed that the zone immediately proximal to the zone of earliest activation was narrow and flanked by arcs of conduction block.

In conjunction with transmural electrical mapping, interesting observations were made regarding the putative effects of cyrothermal energy on myocardial conduction and reentrant circuits. During cooling, progressive conduction delay was identified following an extrastimulus that otherwise reproducibly induced monomorphic ventricular tachycardia at body temperature. This group surmised that cooling temperatures in epicardium overlying necrotic endocardium resulted in transmural conduction delay sufficient to alter the reentrant circuit, either blocking it or redirecting it. Prior to cooling, conduction was noted to spread horizontally through the thin epicardial surface, with synchronous activation in the epicardial-to-endocardial axis. Conduction delay and block following cooling was also observed in the horizontal direction, allowing quantifiable effects of cooling on conduction velocity [54].

Transvenous Cryoablation of Ventricular Tachycardia

The potential application for percutaneous cryocatheters in the treatment of ventricular tachyarrhythmias has been evaluated in sheep and canine ventricular myocardium. Simulating epicardial ventricular tachycardia using multiple epicardial plaque electrodes, Okishige and Friedman (personal communication, May 1998) were able to demonstrate reversible circuit interruption by freezing the right ventricle using an endocardial cryoablation catheter in sheep. Fifty percent of the lesions created in this study were transmural. Dubuc (personal communication, May 1998) has studied right and left ventricular lesions in dogs created by a cryocatheter introduced via the femoral vein and artery. Serial cryoapplications were administered (temperature ranging from –18°C to –60°C) for up to 4 min. At necropsy, lesions with a median volume of 39 mm^3 were identified, comparable to those created using radiofrequency ablation. The potential advantages of cryocatheter ablation in the treatment of ventricular tachycardia are intriguing but as yet untested.

Atrial Fibrillation Ablation

Sustained atrial fibrillation depends on several factors such as atrial geometry, the presence of functional lines of block, dispersion of refractoriness and slowed conduction velocity [55-57]. Surgical compartmentalization of the left and right atria with transmural incisions and cryolesions ("maze procedure") has been demonstrated to eliminate atrial fibrillation while preserving atrial transport. Cox and Sundt reported a surgical cure rate of 93% in a series of 146 patients, with the remaining 7% successfully maintained in sinus rhythm with medical therapy [58]. However, the procedure requires protracted cardiopulmonary bypass time and is associated with a surgical mortality between 1% and 2% which limits its general applicability. Consequently, there is considerable interest in developing a safer transvenous catheter-based maze procedure. The success of such an approach would depend on the ability to create long linear transmural lesions that preserve myocardial integrity and cause minimal thrombogenic substrate.

Table 3 compares current catheter-based systems that can be applied to atrial fibrillation ablation, including catheter cryoablation. To date, only radiofrequency ablation has been used to treat atrial fibrillation in humans. Swartz et al. reported successful treatment of drug-refractory chronic atrial fibrillation in a patient by application of 8 lines of ablation similar to those created in the maze procedure [59]. Subsequently, Haïssaguerre et al. reported a staged procedure in which patients with drug-refractory paroxysmal atrial fibrillation received sequential linear lesions first in the right atrium and if necessary in the left atrium until atrial fibrillation was no longer inducible [60]. Elimination of atrial fibrillation with or without med-

Table 3. Comparison of energy sources currently available for use in ablative therapy for atrial fibrillation. (Reprinted with permission from [85])

	Cryothermy	Radiofrequency	Laser diode	Microwave
Clinical experience	Extensive surgical experience	Extensive catheter-based experience	None	Minimal
Potential for endocardial disruption	Low	High	High	High
Thrombogenicity	Low	High	High	High
Mapping capability	Yes	Limited	No	No
Ability to create transmural lesions	Excellent - contact forgiving	Requires optimal contact	Excellent - contact forgiving	Excellent - contact forgiving
Perforation rate	Low	Low	Potential for endocardial disruption is high	Potential for endocardial disruption is high

ication was ultimately achieved in almost half of the patients treated. Although the average procedure time was 5 h, minimal morbidity was reported. Stable lines of block or conduction delay were demonstrable in only 10% of the patients, indicating the presence of skip lesions in most of the linear burns, which likely reflects the poor efficacy observed in the study. More recently, Haïssaguerre et al. used localized radiofrequency ablation for focally triggered atrial fibrillation, reporting a 62% success rate off medications at 8 months [61]. It remains to be seen whether the patients selected for this study (patients with marked paroxysmal atrial fibrillation and frequent isolated ectopic beats on Holter monitoring) represent a narrow subgroup or whether such an approach may have broader applicability.

As indicated in Table 3, limitations of radiofrequency are in part related to its contact-dependence and the difficulty of establishing continuous linear burns. Additionally, extensive application of radiofrequency may be associated with a considerable amount of thrombus formation at the site of endocardial injury which increases the risk of procedure-related thromboembolism. Using a canine model of chronic atrial fibrillation, Mitchell et al. performed gross analysis of explanted canine hearts after performing radiofrequency ablation [62]. On average, approximately ten applications were required per linear lesion. There were multiple areas of subepicardial coagulation and hemorrhage. One animal that died of ventricular fibrillation during the procedure had evidence of coagulum which had embolized to the mid left anterior descending coronary artery and to a large diagonal branch. Similar to the observations of Haïssaguerre et al., these researchers noted frequent discontinuities within lesions. Additionally, procedure time was prolonged, averaging 8 h per animal.

The creation of lines of conduction block using cryocatheters has also been tested in canine atrial myocardium [63], and in our studies of goat atrial myocardium [64, 65]. In Thibault's study, a 5-cm tip cryocatheter was compared to a radiofrequency catheter that had ten interspersed ring electrodes. With cryoablation, only two 5-min applications of cryothermy at –70°C were required to create complete lines of block. This contrasted with 20 ± 7 radiofrequency applications with a mean duration of 70 s per burn using a target temperature of 70°C. On gross analysis, radiofrequency caused massive endocardial destruction associated with extensive mural thrombus. In contrast, the cryolesions were discete, showed preservation of endocardial contours, and were covered by a thin layer of thrombus. An example of one such lesion from our use of the cryocatheter in goat atria is shown in Fig. 1. The ability of cryocatheters to create

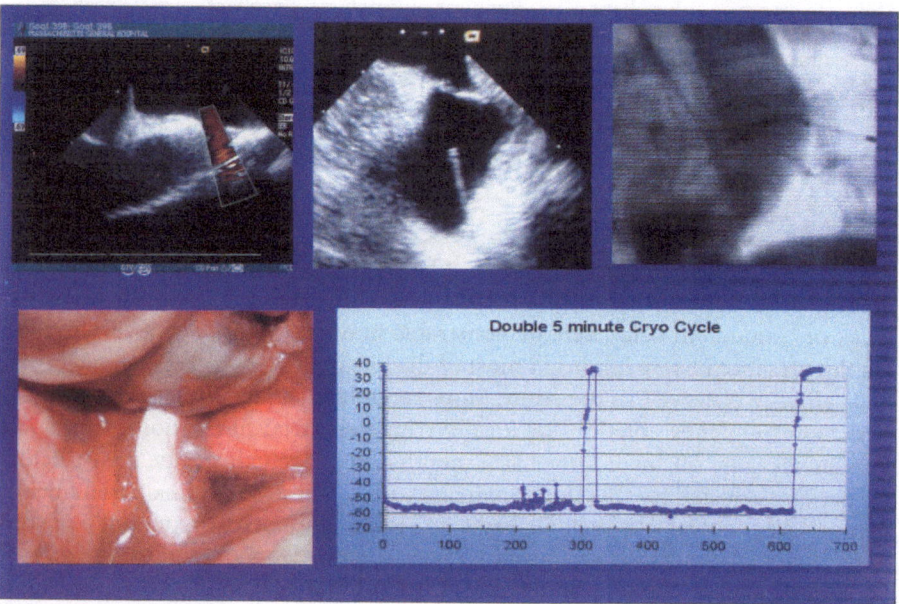

Fig. 1. *Top left:* localization of the left inferior pulmonary vein by phased array intracardiac echo image with color Doppler (Acuson). The intracardiac echo probe is in the right atrium of a 60-kg goat. Imaging across the fossa ovalis identifies the left inferior pulmonary vein with forward flow of blood into the left atrium. *Top center:* phased array intracardiac echo image (Acuson) from the right atrium across the fossa ovalis of a section of a cryoablation catheter (CryoCath) as it traverses the lateral left atrium towards the left inferior pulmonary vein. *Top right:* fluoroscopic image of cryocatheter emerging from the lateral border of the left atrium into the pulmonary vein. The cryocatheter was introduced transvenously and advanced into the left atrium via a transseptal Mullins sheath. The freezing section of the catheter (delimited by the radioopaque markers) advances to reach the proximal portion of the pulmonary vein. *Bottom left:* via a left lateral thoracotomy, ice formation can be seen to form through the pulmonary vein from the intraluminal cryocatheter (the left atrium is at the top of the image while the left lung is at the bottom of the image). *Bottom left:* temperature plot from the cryocatheter's thermocouple during two consecutive 5-min freezing cycles at –60 °C. Temperature is displayed on the *y*-axis and time in seconds on the *x*-axis. The rapidity of the fall in temperature may be important in achieving cell death

long linear lesions efficiently while maintaining the structural integrity of the involved myocardium and its low thrombogenic potential make it ideally suited to a catheter-based maze procedure. For similar reasons, cryothermal ablation may also be better suited for the treatment of focal atrial tachycardias that trigger atrial fibrillation, as recently reported by Haïssaguerre et al. [61]. These localize largely to the pulmonary veins which are thin walled and pose a high risk for perforation and stenosis in response to hyperthermal energy [84]. We are currently testing the effects of cryothermy on canine pulmonary veins using intravenous cryocatheters.

Conclusions

The recent development of steerable electrode-tipped cryocatheters offers a potentially significant alternative to current established ablative therapies, the latter of which depend on hyperthermy which is associated with a significant risk of tissue perforation and thromboembolism. These risks increase in proportion to the extent of tissue destruction required. Cryothermy in contrast causes tissue destruction with preservation of underlying tissue architecture, thereby posing less risk of perforation and thromboembolism. The ability to cryomap yields an additional benefit of testing the safety and efficacy of putative lesion sites prior to creating committed lesions. Finally, current cryocatheters have the capacity to create long functional lines of block in a relatively short amount of time, making it ideally suited to the catheter-based maze procedure.

It remains to be seen whether similar or improved safety and efficacy could be obtained with catheter-based cryothermal ablation relative to the hyperthermal ablative modalities currently in clinical use. Ongoing animal research and clinical trial proposals are being elaborated to address these issues. On the basis of initial observations in this laboratory and in the hands of others, we believe this therapy could have important future applications in the ablation of tachyarrhythmias and may be particularly well suited to the non-pharmacologic treatment of atrial fibrillation.

Note from the Authors: The above has been adapted from a review article published in Progress in Cardiovascular Diseases [85].

References

1. Tsvetkov T, Tsonev L, Meranzov N et al (1985) Functional changes in mitochondrial properties as a result of their membrane cryodestruction. II. Influence of freezing and thawing on Atp complex activity of intact liver mitochondria. Cryobiology 22(2):111-118
2. Petrenko A (1992) A mechanism of latent cryoinjury and reparation of mitochondria. Cryobiology 29(1):144-152

3. Whittaker DK (1984) Mechanisms of tissue destruction following cryosurgery. Ann R Coll Surg Engl 66(5):313-318
4. Gill W, Fraser J, Carter DC (1988) Repeated freeze-thaw cycles in cryosurgery. Nature 219(5152):410-413
5. Mazur M (1965) Causes of injury in frozen and thawed cells. Fed Proc 24:5175-5182
6. Mazur P (1970) Cryobiology: the freezing of biological systems. Science 168(934):939-949
7. McGrath JJ (1993) Low temperature injury processes. In: Roemer RB (ed) Advances in bioheat and mass transfer: microscale analysis of thermal injury processes, instrumentation, modeling, and clinical applications. ASME Odyssey, New Hampshaire, 268:125-132
8. Stewart GJ, Preketes A, Horton M et al (1995) Hepatic cryotherapy: double-freeze cycles achieve greater hepatocellular injury in man. Cryobiology 32(3):215-219
9. Gage AA, Guest K, Montes M et al (1985) Effect of varying freezing and thawing rates in experimental cryosurgery. Cryobiology 22(2):175-182
10. Markovitz LJ, Frame LH, Josephson ME et al (1988) Cardiac cryolesions factors affecting their size and a means of monitoring their formation. Ann of Thorac Surg 46(5):531-535
11. Ghalili K, Roth JA, Kwan SK et al (1992) Comparison of left ventricular cryolesions created by liquid nitrogen and nitrous oxide. J Am Coll Cardiol 20(6):1425-1429
12. Fujino H, Thompson RP, Germroth PG et al (1993) Histologic study of chronic catheter cryoablation of atrioventricular conduction in swine. Am Heart J 125(6):1632-1637
13. Harrison L, Gallagher JJ, Kasell J et al (1977) Cryosurgical ablation of the A-V node-His bundle: a new method for producing A-V block. Circulation 55(3):463-470
14. Gillette PC, Swindle MM, Thompson RP et al (1991) Transvenous cryoablation of the bundle of His. Pacing Clin Electrophysiol 14(4 Pt 1):504-510
15. Ohkawa S, Hackel DB, Mikat EM et al (1982) Anatomic effects of cryoablation of the atrioventricular conduction system. Circulation 65(6):1155-1162
16. Holman WL, Ikeshita M, Douglas JM Jr et al (1983) Ventricular cryosurgery: short-term effects on intramural electrophysiology. Ann Thorac Surg 35(4):386-393
17. Jensen JA, Kosek JC, Hunt TK et al (1987) Cardiac cryolesions as an experimental model of myocardial wound healing. Ann Surg 206(6):798-803
18. Klein GJ, Harrison L, Ideker RF et al (1979) Reaction of the myocardium to cryosurgery: electrophysiology and arrhythmogenic potential. Circulation 59(2):364-372
19. Hunt GB, Chard RB, Johnson DC et al (1989) Comparison of early and late dimensions and arrhythmogenicity of cryolesions in the normothermic canine heart. J Thorac Cardiovasc Surg 97(2):313-318
20. Gallagher JD, Del Rossi AJ, Fernandez J et al (1985) Cryothermal mapping of recurrent ventricular tachycardia in man. Circulation 71(4):732-739
21. Gessman L, Agarwal J, Endo T et al (1983) Localization and mechanism of ventricular tachycardia by ice mapping 1 week after the onset of myocardial infarction in dogs. Circulation 68(3):657-666
22. Wallace A, Mignone R (1966) Physiologic evidence concerning the reentry hypothesis of ectopic beats. Am Heart J 72:60-70
23. Cole JS, Wills RE, Winterscheid LC et al (1970) The Wolff-Parkinson-White syndrome: problems in evaluation and surgical. Circulation 42(1):111-121
24. Slama R, Blondeau P, Aigueperse J et al (1967) Surgical creation of an auriculoventrical block and implantation of a. Arch Mal Coeur Vaisse 60(3):406-422
25. Garcia R, Arciniegas E (1973) Recurrent atrial flutter. Treatment with a surgically induced atrioventricular block and ventricular pacing. Arch Int Med 132(5):754-757

26. Klein GJ, Sealy WC, Pritchett EL et al (1980) Cryosurgical ablation of the atrioventricular node-His bundle: long-term follow-up and properties of the junctional pacemaker. Circulation 61(1):8-15

27. Bredikis J (1985) Cryosurgical ablation of atrioventricular junction without extracorporeal circulation. J Thorac Cardiovasc Surg 90(1):61-67

28. Bredikis JJ, Bredikis AJ (1990) Surgery of tachyarrhythmia: intracardiac closed heart cryoablation. Pacing Clin Electrophysiol 13(12 Pt 2):1980-1984

29. Louagie YA, Guiraudon GM, Klein GJ et al (1991) Closed heart cryoablation of the His bundle using an anterior septal approach. Ann Thorac Surg 51(4):616-619

30. Pritchett ELC, Anderson RW, Benditt DG et al (1979) Reentry within the atrioventricular node. Surgical cure with preservation of atrioventricular conduction. Circulation 60:440-446

31. Holman WL, Ikeshita M, Lease JG et al (1986) Cryosurgical modification of retrograde atrioventricular conduction. Implications for the surgical treatment of atrioventricular nodal reentry tachycardia. J Thorac Cardiovasc Surg 91(6):826-834

32. Holman WL, Hackel DB, Lease JG et al (1988) Cryosurgical ablation of atrioventricular nodal reentry: histologic localization of the proximal common pathway. Circulation 77(6):1356-1362

33. Cox J, Holman W, Cain W (1987) Cryosurgical treatment of atrioventricular node reentrant tachycardia. Circulation 76(6):1329-1336

34. Wood DL, Hammill SC, Porter CB et al (1988) Cryosurgical modification of atrioventricular conduction for treatment of atrioventricular node reentrant tachycardia. Mayo Clin Proc 63(10):988-992

35. Holman WL, Ikeshita M, Lease JG et al (1988) Cardiac cryosurgery: regional myocardial blood flow of ventricular cryolesions. J Surg Res 41(5):524-528

36. Sealy WC, Hattler BG Jr., Blumenschein SD et al (1969) Surgical treatment of Wolff-Parkinson-White syndrome. Ann Thorac Surg 8(1):1-11

37. Iwa T, Mitsui T, Misaki T et al (1986) Radical surgical cure of the WPW syndrome: the Kazawa experience. J Thorac Cardiovasc Surg 91(2):225-233

38. Gallagher JJ, Sealy WC, Anderson RW et al (1977) Cryosurgical ablation of accessory atrioventricular connections: a method for correction of the pre-excitation syndrome. Circulation 55(3):471-479

39. Guiraudon GM, Klein GJ, Gulamhusein S et al (1984) Surgical repair of Wolff-Parkinson-White syndrome: a new closed-heart technique. Ann Thorac Surg 37(1):67-71

40. Guiraudon GM, Klein GJ, Sharma AD et al (1986) Closed-heart technique for Wolff-Parkinson-White syndrome: further experience and potential limitations. Ann Thorac Surg 42(6):651-657

41. Watanabe S, Koyanagi H, Endo M et al (1989) Cryosurgical ablation of accessory atrioventricular pathways without cardiopulmonary bypass: an epicardial approach for Wolff-Parkinson-White syndrome. Ann Thorac Surg 47(2):257-264

42. Bredikis J, Bredikis A (1985) Cryosurgical ablation of left parietal wall accessory atrioventricular connections through the coronary sinus without the use of extracorporeal circulation. J Thorac Cardiovasc Surg 90(2):199-205

43. Lee AW, Crawford FA Jr, Gillette PC et al (1989) Cryoablation of septal pathways in patients with supraventricular tachyarrhythmias. Ann Thorac Surg 47(4):566-568

44. Andress JD, Vander Salm TJ, Huang SK (1991) Bidirectional bundle branch reentry tachycardia associated with Ebstein's anomaly: cured by extensive cryoablation of the right bundle branch. Pacing Clin Electrophysiol 14(11 Pt 1):1639-1647

45. Cox JL, Gallagher JJ, Ungerleider RM (1982) Encircling endocardial ventriculotomy for refractory ischemic ventricular tachycardia. IV. Clinical indications surgical technique mechanism of action and results. J Thorac Cardiovasc Surg 83(6):865-872

46. Guiraudon GM, Guiraudon CM, McLellan DG et al (1989) Mitral valve function after cryoablation of the posterior papillary muscle in the dog. Ann Thorac Surg 47(6):872-876
47. McLellan D, Guiraudon G, Guiraudon C et al (1990) Extensive cryoablation of the left ventricular apex does not impair cardiac function. PACE 134:497 (abstr)
48. Gallagher JJ, Anderson RW, Kasell J et al (1978) Cryoablation of drug-resistant ventricular tachycardia in a patient with a variant of scleroderma. Circulation 57(1):190-197
49. Camm J, Ward DE, Cory-Pearce R et al (1979) The successful cryosurgical treatment of paroxysmal ventricular tachycardia. Chest 75(5):621-624
50. Cox J (1985) The status of surgery for cardiac arrhythmias. Circulation 71:413
51. Miller J, Kienzle M, Harken A et al (1984) Subendocardial resection for ventricular tachycardia: predictors of surgical success. Circulation 70:624-631
52. Caceres J, Werner P, Jazayeri M et al (1988) Efficacy of cryosurgery alone for refractory monomorphic sustained ventricular tachycardia due to inferior wall infarction. J Am Coll Cardiol 11(6):1254-1259
53. Hargrove WCD, Miller JM, Vassallo JA et al (1988) Improved results in the operative management of ventricular tachycardia related to inferior wall infarction. Importance of the annular isthmus. J Thorac Cardiovasc Surg 92(4):726-732
54. El-Sherif N, Mehra R, Gough WB et al (1983) Reentrant ventricular arrhythmias in the late myocardial infarction period. Interruption of reentrant circuits by cryothermal techniques. Circulation 68(3):644-656
55. Moe GK (1962) On the multiple wavelet hypothesis of atrial fibrillation. Arch Int Pharmacodyn Ther 140:183-188
56. Boineau JP, Schuessler RB, Mooney CR et al (1980) Natural and evoked atrial flutter due to circus movement in dogs. Am J Cardiol 45(6):1167-1181
57. Allessie MA, Lammers WJEP, Bonke IM et al (1984) Intra-atrial reentry as a mechanism for atrial flutter induced by acetylcholine and rapid pacing in the dog. Circulation 70(1):123-135
58. Cox JL, Sundt TM 3rd (1997) The surgical management of atrial fibrillation. Annu Rev Med 48(23):511-523
59. Swartz J, Pellersels G, Silvers J et al (1994) A catheter-based curative approach to atrial fibrillation in humans. Circulation 90(4, Part 2):I-335
60. Haïssaguerre M, Jais P, Shah DC et al (1996) Right and left atrial radiofrequency catheter ablation of paroxysmal atrial fibrillation. J Cardiovasc Electrophysiol 7(12):1132-1144
61. Haïssaguerre M, Jaïs P, Shah D et al (1998) Spontaneous initiation of atrial fibrillation by ectopic beats originating in the pulmonary veins. N Engl J Med 339(10):659-666
62. Mitchell MA, McRury ID, Haines DE (1998) Linear atrial ablations in a canine model of chronic atrial fibrillation. Circulation 97:1176-1185
63. Thibault B, Villemaire C, Talajic M et al (1998) Catheter cryoablation is a more effective and potentially safer method to create atrial conduction block: comparison with radiofrequency ablation. PACE 21(4, Part II):944
64. Keane D, Zhou L, Ruskin J (1997) Catheter ablation for atrial fibrillation. Semin Intervent Cardiol 2:251-265
65. Keane D, Zhou L, Haughtaling C et al (1999) Percutaneous cryothermal catheter ablation for the creation of linear atrial lesions. Ir Med J (in press)
66. Camm J, Ward DE, Spurrell RA et al (1980) Cryothermal mapping and cryoablation in the treatment of refractory cardiac arrhythmias. Circulation 62(1):67-74
67. Cox JL, Ferguson TB Jr, Lindsay BD et al (1990) Perinodal cryosurgery for atrioven-

tricular node reentry tachycardia in 23 patients. J Thorac Cardiovasc Surg 99(3):440-449; discussion 449-450

68. Rowland E, Robinson K, Edmondson S et al (1988) Cryoablation of the accessory pathway in Wolff-Parkinson-White syndrome: initial results and long term follow up. Br Heart J 59(4):453-457

69. Plumb V, DC M, JK K et al (1985) Cryosurgery for ventricular tachycardia. J Am Coll Cardiol 5(2):409 (Abstr)

70. Krafchek J, Lawrie GM, Wyndham CR (1986) Cryoablation of arrhythmias from the interventricular septum: initial experience with a new biventricular approach. J Thorac Cardiovasc Surg 91(3):419-427

71. Krafchek J, Lawrie GM, Roberts R et al (1986) Surgical ablation of ventricular tachycardia: improved results with a map-directed regional approach. Circulation 73(6):1239-1247

72. Ott DA, Garson A Jr, Cooley DA et al (1987) Cryoablative techniques in the treatment of cardiac tachyarrhythmias. Ann Thorac Surg 43(2):138-143

73. Vermeulen FE, Hemel NM van, Guiraudon GM et al (1988) Cryosurgery for ventricular bigeminy using a transaortic closed ventricular approach. Eur Heart J 9(9):979-990

74. Page PL, Cardinal R, Shenasa M et al (1989) Surgical treatment of ventricular tachycardia. Regional cryoablation guided by computerized epicardial and endocardial mapping. Circulation 80(3 Pt 1):I124-134

75. Caceres J, Akhtar M, Werner P et al (1989) Cryoablation of refractory sustained ventricular tachycardia due to coronary artery disease. Am J Cardiol 63(5):296-300

76. Lawrie GM, Pacifico A, Kaushik RR (1989) Transannular cryoablation of ventricular tachycardia. Surgical technique and results. J Thorac Cardiovasc Surg 98(6):1030-1035; discussion 1035-1036

77. Rokkas CK, Nitta T, Schuessler RB et al (1994) Human ventricular tachycardia: precise intraoperative localization with potential distribution mapping. Ann Thorac Surg 57(6):1628-1635

78. Graffigna A, Minzioni G, Ressia L et al (1994) Surgical ablation of ventricular tachycardia secondary to congenital ventricular septal aneurysm. Ann Thorac Surg 57(4):921-924

79. Misaki T, Tsubota M, Watanabe G et al (1994) Surgical treatment of ventricular tachycardia after surgical repair of tetralogy of Fallot. Relation between intraoperative mapping and histological findings. Circulation 90(1):264-271

80. Lee R, Mitchell JD, Garan H et al (1994) Operation for recurrent ventricular tachycardia. Predictors of short- and long-term efficacy. J Thorac Cardiovasc Surg 107(3):732-742

81. Gharagozloo F, Porter CJ, Tazelaar HD et al (1994) Multiple myocardial hamartomas causing ventricular tachycardia in young children: combined surgical modification and medical treatment. Mayo Clin Proc 69(3):262-267

82. Guiraudon GM, Thakur RK, Klein GJ et al (1994) Encircling endocardial cryoablation for ventricular tachycardia after myocardial infarction: experience with 33 patients. Am Heart J 128(5):982-989

83. Shumway SJ, Johnson EM, Svendsen CA et al (1997) Surgical management of ventricular tachycardia. Ann Thorac Surg 63(6):1589-1591

84. Robbins IM, Colvin EV, Doyle TP et al (1998) Pulmonary vein stenosis after catheter ablation of atrial fibrillation. Circulation 98(17):1769-1775

85. Lustgarten D, Keane D, Ruskin J (1999) Cryothermal ablation: mechanism of tissue injury and current experience in the treatment of tachyarrhythmias. Progr Cardiovasc Dis (in press)

VENTRICULAR ARRHYTHMIAS

Idiopathic Ventricular Fibrillation: Is the Prognosis Always Bad?

R.N.W. Hauer and C.A. Remme

A minority of cases of ventricular fibrillation (VF) occur in patients in whom no structural heart disease or any other known arrhythmogenic factor can be identified in spite of extensive evaluation. The preferred term for this entity is "idiopathic VF", as suggested by the consensus statement of the steering committees of the Unexplained Cardiac Arrest Registry of Europe (UCARE) and the Idiopathic Ventricular Fibrillation Registry of the United States (IVF-US) [1].

Since survivors of idiopathic VF by definition have a normal left ventricular ejection fraction, many cardiologists thought that the prognosis in these patients should be rather good. However, several reports in the 1990s have shown a high recurrence rate of life-threatening arrhythmic events in this patient category [2-5]. This is important since patients with idiopathic VF are usually young, many of them below the age of 40 years. We have to realize that a long follow-up duration is needed for follow-up evaluation in these patients, since a first recurrence may occur more than 2 years after the index event. Thus, a relatively short follow-up may contribute to the observation that the unfavorable prognosis in survivors of idiopathic VF is still better than in VF patients with structural heart disease.

In our own prospective single-center study, published by Wever et al. [5], 19 consecutive survivors of idiopathic VF were enrolled. The mean age of these patients was 33 years, and 13 patients (68%) were less than 40 years old. During a mean follow-up of 43 months major arrhythmic events occurred in 7 patients (37%). Specific markers predictive of a recurrent event could not be identified, but the numbers were still small.

The data in our previous study were collected between 1985 and 1992 [5]. For the present report we have expanded the data by including additional patients up to January 1999 and extending the follow-up period in all patients referred after surviving idiopathic VF since 1985.

Department of Cardiology, Heart-Lung Institute, University Hospital Utrecht, The Netherlands

Diagnostic Procedures

The diagnosis of idiopathic VF was made after careful cardiological evaluation including patient history, family history, physical examination, two-dimensional and Doppler echocardiography, nuclear scintigraphy, left and right heart catheterization with cineangiography, and right ventricular biopsies at multiple sites. Persistent or transient long QT-syndrome as well as preexcitation were excluded by electrocardiography, Holter recording, electrocardiographic telemetric monitoring, and an electrophysiologic study in all patients.

Patient Population

From 1985 up to 1999, 37 consecutive patients were enrolled: 27 male and 10 female. Mean age was 37 years. The diagnosis of idiopathic VF was made in all patients. None of the patients had identifiable minor cardiac abnormalities such as mild mitral valve prolapse or mild coronary artery disease. A minority of patients showed abnormalities in the electrocardiogram. Most of these were minor and nonspecific: abnormal repolarization or abnormal intraventricular conduction. Prior to the index episode 22 patients had episodes of cardiac arrest, syncope, or presyncope. Four patients (11%) had relatives in whom sudden death had occurred.

Therapy at Discharge

A defibrillator (ICD) was implanted in 25 patients, in 23 as first therapy and in 2 after drug failure. The other 12 patients were treated with drugs because of suppressibility of the arrhythmia evaluated by Holter recording, telemetry, exercise testing, and electrophysiologic study. Drug treatment included either quinidine, flecainide, amiodarone, or a β-blocking agent.

Follow-Up Results

The mean follow-up duration was 68 ± 41 months (range 3-146 months). All patients were followed in the out-patient clinic, once every 3 months for ICD patients, and at least once every 6 months for other patients.

During follow-up the original diagnosis appeared to be erroneous in three patients. One patient with numerous ICD shocks during the first year after the index event appeared to have a positive ergonovine test, indicating coronary artery spasm. After proper drug treatment no more ICD shocks occurred during more than 5 years' follow-up. The second patient developed congestive heart failure due to dilated cardiomyopathy. The third patient developed a right ventricular apical aneurysm. The diagnosis of arrhythmogenic right ventricular dysplasia was made echocardiographically more then 10 years after the index episode. This diagnosis was confirmed at autopsy, 1 year later. In all other patients (92%) no evidence of structural heart disease has been obtained in spite of regular physical examination and echocardiography at least every 2 years.

A major arrhythmic event, defined as documented VF or sustained rapid ventricular tachycardia or sudden death without evidence of non-arrhythmic cause and appropriate ICD shock, occurred in 15 of the total group of 37 patients (41%).

Of the total group two patients died suddenly, one while on quinidine therapy for 3 years without any event and the other while on flecainide after a symptom-free interval of more then 10 years (the patient with arrhythmogenic right ventricular dysplasia). A third patient was succesfully resuscitated from VF, after having been on flecainide without symptoms for about 2 years. None of the patients with an ICD died. Appropriate shocks occurred in 11 of the 25 patients with an ICD (44%). Of the 12 patients without ICD, major arrhythmic events occurred in 5 (42%).

We were not able to identify a risk factor for recurrences. Arrhythmic events prior to the index episode occurred in 10 of 15 patients with recurrences and in 12 of 22 patients without recurrences, which is not significantly different. Two patients were treated with β-blocking agents because of strong evidence that the arrhythmia typically occurred in the setting of exercise and emotion. These patients remained event-free for 10 and 3 years, respectively.

Conclusions

1. Idiopathic VF is associated with a high incidence of life-threatening arrhythmic events during long-term follow-up.
2. Implantable cardioverter defibrillator implantation should be considered as a therapy of first choice, especially in patients without reliable indicators for guiding therapy.
3. In a small minority of patients with the original diagnosis of idiopathic VF, this diagnosis should be corrected because of manifestation of another arrhythmogenic disorder.
4. No risk factor for recurrences could be identified. Further studies are needed to confirm that a very carefully selected group of patients may be treated properly with β-blocking agents.

We have to conclude that at this time it is not possible to answer the question posed in our title. An unselected subgroup of 17 of our 37 patients was studied by body surface mapping by Peeters et al. [6]. Patients with idiopathic VF had either a normal dipolar QRST integral map (29%) or an abnormal dipolar map or even a nondipolar map (71%). Recurrences occurred exclusively in patients with an abnormal QRST integral map. The results of the signal-averaged ECG may also contribute to risk stratification. However, the numbers are too small and the follow-up too short to guide therapy. We will have to wait for the results of the multicenter Unexplained Cardiac Arrest Registry of Europe (UCARE) for additional information.

References

1. Consensus statement of the Joint Steering Committees of the Unexplained Cardiac Arrest Registry of Europe and of the Idiopathic Ventricular Fibrillation Registry of the United States (1997) Survivors of out-of-hospital cardiac arrest with apparently normal heart. Need for definition and standardized clinical evaluation. Circulation 95:265-272
2. Viskin S, Belhassen B (1990) Idiopathic ventricular fibrillation. Am Heart J 120:661-671
3. Siebels J, Schneider MAE, Geiger M, Kuck KH (1991) Unexpected recurrences in survivors of cardiac arrest without organic heart disease. Eur Heart J 12:86 (abstr)
4. Meissner MD, Lehmann MH, Steinman RT, Mosteller RD, Akhtar M, Calkins H, Cannom DS, Epstein AE, Fogoros RN, Liem LB, Marchlinski FE, Myerburg RJ, Veltri EP (1993) Ventricular fibrillation in patients without significant structural heart disease: a multicenter experience with implantable cardioverter-defibrillator therapy. J Am Coll Cardiol 21:1406-1412
5. Wever EFD, Hauer RNW, Oomen A, Peters RHJ, Bakker PFA, Robles de Medina EO (1993) Unfavorable outcome in patients with primary electrical disease who survived an episode of ventricular fibrillation. Circulation 88:1021-1029
6. Peeters HAP, Sippensgroenewegen A, Wever EFD, Potse M, Daniëls MCG, Grimbergen CA, Hauer RNW, Robles de Medina EO (1998) Electrocardiographic identification of abnormal ventricular depolarization and repolarization in patients with idiopathic ventricular fibrillation. J Am Coll Cardiol 6:1406-1413

The Syndrome of Right Bundle Branch Block, ST Segment Elevation in V1 to V3 and Sudden Death. Are Asymptomatic Patients at High Risk for Sudden Death?

J. Brugada[1], P. Brugada[2] and R. Brugada[3]

Introduction

In 1992 a new syndrome consisting of syncopal episodes and/or sudden death in patients with a structurally normal heart and a characteristic electrocardiogram (ECG) with a pattern of right bundle branch block with an ST segment elevation in leads V1 to V3 was described [1]. In 1998 the poor prognosis of patients with this syndrome who were not receiving an implantable defibrillator was reported [2, 3]. In 1998 the genetic nature of the disease and its association with a mutation in the cardiac sodium channel gene was described [4]. Because the diagnosis is easily made by means of the ECG, an increasing number of asymptomatic patients with the ECG pattern are being identified worldwide. This fact has raised the question of whether the presence of an abnormal ECG without symptoms indicates that the patient is affected by the disease and what the prognosis is. In this article we will review our present knowledge concerning asymptomatic patients with the classical ECG pattern of the disease.

In the Brugada syndrome, the diagnosis is based on the history of aborted sudden death with the typical electrocardiographic pattern of ST segment elevation in leads V1-V3, with or without right bundle branch block [1] (Fig. 1). In some cases, however, the diagnosis is different because some individuals present with an abnormal electrocardiogram but are completely asymptomatic or there is a history of sudden death in the family and the electrocardiographic criteria are observed.

Incidence of an Abnormal ECG in the General Population

A prospective study of an adult Japanese population (22,027 subjects) showed an incidence of 0.05% of ECGs compatible with the syndrome (12 subjects) [5]. A

[1]Arrhythmia Unit, Cardiovascular Institute, Hospital Clinic, University of Barcelona, Spain; [2]Cardiovascular Research and Teaching Institute Aalst, Cardiovascular Center, Aalst, Belgium; [3]Department of Cardiology, Baylor College of Medicine, Houston, Texas, USA

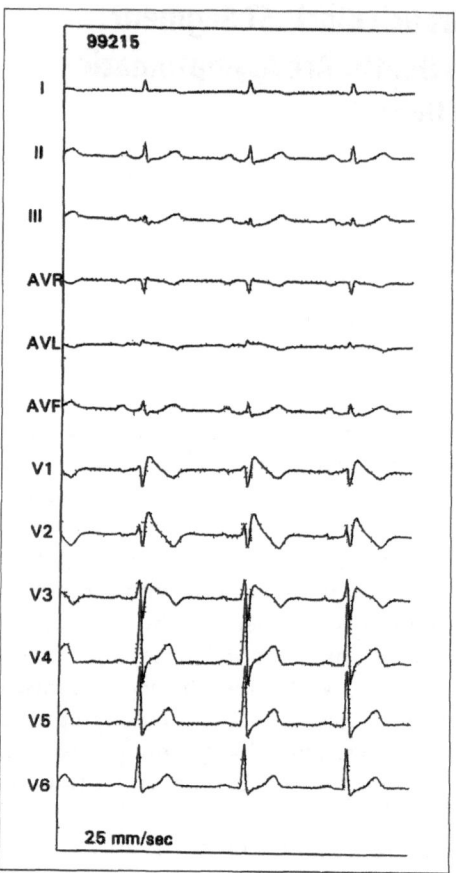

Fig. 1. Typical ECG of the syndrome. Note the pattern resembling a right bundle branch block in lead V1 and the ST segment elevation in leads V1 to V3. Paper speed 25 mm/s

second study of adults in Awa (Japan) showed an incidence of 0.6 % (66 cases out of 10,420) [6]. However, a third study in children from Japan showed an incidence of ECGs compatible with the syndrome of only 0.0006% (1 case in 163,110) [7]. These results suggest that the syndrome manifests primarily during adulthood, which is in concordance with the mean age of sudden death victims (35-40 years).

The presence of concealed and intermittent forms, however, makes the diagnosis difficult in some patients. The ECG can be modulated by changes in autonomic balance and the administration of antiarrhythmic drugs [8]. β-adrenergic stimulation normalises the ECG, while IV ajmaline, flecainide or procainamide accentuate the ST segment elevation and are capable of unmasking concealed and intermittent forms of the disease. These data are very important when we deal with family members of a patient with the syndrome. We know that a normal ECG in the resting state is not sufficient to exclude that a family member is affected with the syndrome. Some family members only manifest the typical ECG pattern after ajmaline or flecainide administration.

Recent data suggest that loss of the action potential dome in the right ventricular epicardium, but not in the endocardium, underlies the ST segment elevation seen in the Brugada syndrome [9, 10]. Also, electrical heterogeneity within the right ventricular epicardium leads to the development of closely coupled extrasystoles via a phase 2 reentrant mechanism, which then precipitate ventricular tachycardia-ventricular fibrillation. Right ventricular epicardium is preferentially affected because of the predominance of transient outward current in this tissue. Antiarrhythmic drugs, such as amiodarone and β-blockers, do not prevent sudden death in symptomatic or asymptomatic individuals.

Clinical Manifestations

The complete syndrome is characterised by episodes of rapid polymorphic VT (Fig. 2) in patients with an ECG pattern of right bundle branch block and ST segment elevation in leads V1 to V3. The manifestations of the syndrome are caused by episodes of polymorphic VT/VF. When the episodes terminate spontaneously, the patient develops syncopal attacks. When the episodes are sustained, full blown cardiac arrest and eventually sudden death occur. Thus, these manifestations can range widely: at one end of the spectrum we have asymptomatic individuals and at the other end of the spectrum those who die suddenly. Many patients who have the disease can appear to be otherwise very healthy and active, vigorously engaging in exertional activity or exercise. Physical examinations are almost always normal.

There exist asymptomatic individuals in whom the atypical ECG is detected during routine examination. This ECG cannot be distinguished from that of symptomatic patients. In other patients, the characteristic ECG is recorded during screening after the sudden death of a family member with the disease. On the other hand, there is the group of symptomatic patients who have been diagnosed as suffering syncopal episodes of unknown cause, or vaso-vagal origin, or have a diagnosis of idiopathic ventricular fibrillation. Some of these patients are diagnosed at follow-up, when the ECG changes spontaneously from normal to the typical pattern of the syndrome. This is also the case for those individuals in whom the disease is unmasked by the administration of an antiarrhythmic drug given for other arrhythmias, for instance atrial fibrillation.

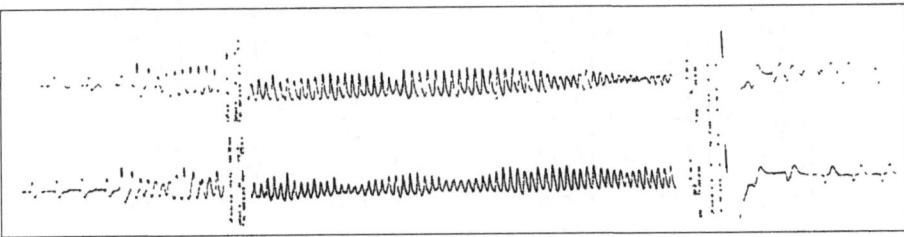

Fig. 2. Two different episodes of polymorphic ventricular arrhythmias documented in one patient with an implantable defibrillator. Note that the arrhythmias occur at different sinus rates and in the absence of short-long sequences or prolongation of the QT interval preceding the episodes

Recent studies indicate that patients displaying the ECG characteristics of the syndrome have a similar incidence of arrhythmia and sudden death to that of patients in whom the ECG manifestation must be unmasked with a sodium-channel blocker. Up to 40% of individuals will develop a new or a first episode of polymorphic VT or sudden death during a 2-3 years follow-up.

Diagnosis

The diagnosis of the syndrome is easily obtained by electrocardiography as long as the patient presents the typical ECG pattern and there is a history of aborted sudden death or syncopes caused by a polymorphic VT. It is difficult to forget such a typical ECG. The ST segment elevation in V1 to V3 with the right bundle branch block pattern is characteristic. The ST changes are different from the ones observed in acute septal ischemia, pericarditis, ventricular aneurysm and in some normal variants, such as early repolarization. There are however ECGs which are not as characteristic, and they are only recognised by a physician who has this syndrome in mind. There are also many patients with a normal ECG in whom the syndrome can only be recognised a posteriori when the typical pattern appears in a follow-up ECG or after the administration of ajmaline, procainamide or flecainide (Fig. 3).

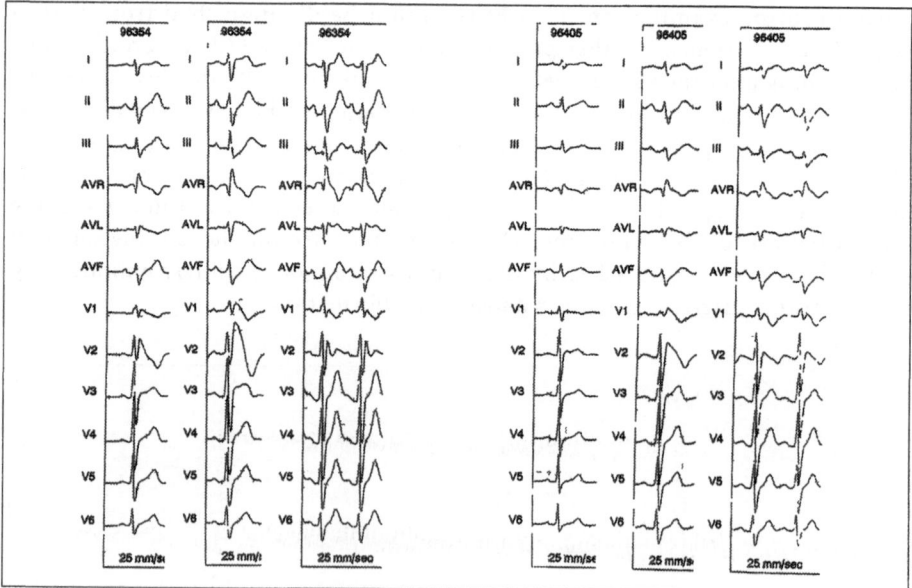

Fig. 3. Effects of the intravenous administration of ajmaline and isoproterenol on the ECG of a patient (left panels) and his brother (right panels). The ST segment elevation in control ECG (left panel) becomes evident after ajmaline administration (middle panel) and normalizes after isoproterenol (right panel)

It is possible that the electrocardiographic patterns are different depending on the genetic abnormality. This is the case in other genetic diseases, such as the long QT syndrome [11]. The mutations that have been discovered in the two families give proof of this fact in Brugada syndrome: their ECGs are similar, but not identical. Even though in both cases the affected gene is the same, the exact mutation is different. It will be necessary to identify more mutations and make a close genotype-phenotype correlation to establish the links. However, we cannot forget the great variability of the ECG in this syndrome, something which will certainly not facilitate analysis.

Additional diagnostic problems are caused by the changes in the ECG induced by the autonomous system and by antiarrhythmic drugs. The study by Miyazaki et al. [8] was the first one to show the variability of the ECG pattern in the syndrome. Despite the fact that we described the syndrome as a persistent ECG pattern, we soon recognised that it is variable over time, depending on the autonomic interaction and the administration of antiarrhythmic drugs. Adrenergic stimulation decreases the ST segment elevation while vagal stimulation worsens it. The administration of class Ia, Ic and III drugs increases the ST segment elevation. Patients with syncope of unknown cause must be challenged with antiarrhythmic drugs in order to exclude the possibility of this syndrome as a cause of ventricular arrhythmias and syncope.

Prognosis and Treatment

This syndrome has a very poor prognosis when left untreated. One-third of patients who suffer syncopal episodes or are resuscitated from near-sudden death develop a new episode of polymorphic VT within 2 years [2, 3]. Unfortunately, the prognosis of asymptomatic individuals with typical ECG is also poor. In spite of not having had any previous symptoms, one-third of these individuals present a first polymorphic VT or ventricular fibrillation within 2 years of follow-up as well. The observations on prognosis of patients with Brugada syndrome from Europe are virtually identical to those for sudden unexplained death syndrome (SUDS) patients in Thailand who show the abnormal ECG pattern. The cumulative proportion of VF or cardiac arrest occurred in approximately 60% of the patients within 1 year and 40% were likely to die suddenly if untreated. Furthermore, patients who have recurrent events but do not die, face the risk of having anoxic encephalopathy, from light to disabling forms.

These data are of extreme importance for the delineation of treatment policies of these patients. Because antiarrhythmic drugs (amiodarone or β-blockers) do not protect against sudden cardiac death [2], the only available treatment is the implantable cardioverter-defibrillator. This device effectively recognises and treats the ventricular arrhythmias. When provided with the implantable defibrillator, total mortality in patients with Brugada syndrome has been demonstrated at 0% with up to 10 years follow-up. These results are not surprising. These patients are young and usually devoid from other diseases. Because their heart is structurally normal, and there is no coronary artery disease, these patients do not die from heart failure or complications of ischemic events. Thus, they are the most ideal candidates for treatment with an implantable cardioverter-defibrillator. All symptomatic patients should receive this device.

On the other hand, major concerns arise in the treatment of asymptomatic individuals. Of the six asymptomatic patients who died suddenly in our previous study [2], four patients were members of affected families, but two were sporadic cases. Data from electrophysiological investigations did not help us to predict prognosis, although this may be caused by a type II error (insufficient number of patients to prove a statistically significant difference). At present, we believe four different groups of patients can be distinguished:

1. Symptomatic individuals with the disease who require an implantable cardioverter-defibrillator. Patients with transient normalisation of the ECG during follow-up have the same prognosis as patients with a permanently abnormal ECG (Brugada J, unpublished observations).
2. Asymptomatic patients with a family history of sudden death, a prolonged HV interval and inducible polymorphic VT or ventricular fibrillation who also require an implantable defibrillator.
3. Asymptomatic individuals without a family history of sudden death but also with inducible sustained polymorphic ventricular arrhythmias, who also require a defibrillator.
4. Asymptomatic individuals without a family history of sudden death and no inducible ventricular arrhythmias who should not be treated but followed-up carefully for development of symptoms suggesting arrhythmias (particularly syncope). One has to realise, however, that these recommendations may change rapidly depending upon the availability of new data.

Conclusions

The syndrome of right bundle branch block, ST segment elevation from V1 to V3 and sudden death is a new entity. This disease is genetically determined and it is different from the long QT syndrome and right ventricular dysplasia. The incidence of sudden death in this syndrome is very high and, at present, sudden death can only be prevented by implanting a cardioverter-defibrillator. The ECG is a marker of sudden death in symptomatic, but also asymptomatic individuals.

References

1. Brugada P, Brugada J (1992) Right bundle branch block, persistent ST segment elevation and sudden cardiac death: a distinct clinical and electrocardiographic syndrome. J Am Coll Cardiol 20:1391-1396
2. Brugada J, Brugada R, Brugada P (1998) Right bundle branch block and ST segment elevation in leads V1-V3: a marker for sudden death in patients with no demonstrable structural heart disease. Circulation 97:457-460

3. Nademanee K, Veerakul G, Nimmannit S et al (1997) Arrhythmogenic marker for the sudden unexplained death syndrome in Thai men. Circulation 96:2595-2600
4. Chen Q, Kirsch GE, Zhang D, Brugada R, Brugada J, Brugada P et al (1998) Genetic basis and molecular mechanisms for idiopathic ventricular fibrillation. Nature 392:293-296
5. Tohyou Y, Nakazawa K Ozawa A et al (1995) A survey in the incidence of right bundle branch block with ST segment elevation among normal population. Jpn J Electrocardiol 15:223-226
6. Namiki T, Ogura T, Kuwabara Y et al (1995) Five-year mortality and clinical characteristics of adult subjects with right bundle branch block and ST elevation. Circulation 93:334
7. Hata Y, Chiba N, Hotta K et al (1997) Incidence and clinical significance of right bundle branch block and ST segment elevation in V1-V3 in 6-to 18-year-old school children in Japan. Circulation 20:2310
8. Miyazaki T, Mitamura H, Miyoshi S, Soejima K, Aizawa Y, Ogawa S (1996) Autonomic and antiarrhythmic modulation of ST segment elevation in patients with Brugada syndrome. J Am Coll Cardiol 27:1061-1070
9. Antzelevitch C (1998) The Brugada syndrome. J Cardiovasc Electrophysiol 9:513-516
10. Gussak I, Antzelevitch C, Bjerregaard P, Towbin JA, Chaitman BR (1999) The Brugada syndrome. Clinical, electrophysiologic and genetic aspects. J Am Coll Cardiol 33:5-15
11. Priori SG, Diehl L, Schwartz PJ (1995) Torsade de pointes. In: Podrid PJ, Kowey PR, (eds) Cardiac arrhythmia. Williams and Wilkins, Baltimore, pp 951-963

Is Atrial Vulnerability Increased In Arrhythmogenic Right Ventricular Cardiomyopathy?

D. Corrado, G. Buja, C. Basso, A. Nava and G. Thiene

Background

Arrhythmogenic right ventricular cardiomyopathy (ARVC) is a heart muscle disease, often familial, that is characterized pathologically by fibro-fatty replacement of the right ventricular (RV) myocardium and clinically by ventricular arrhythmias of RV origin leading to sudden death, mostly in young people and athletes [1-8]. The progressive loss of the RV myocardium has been considered the result of a genetically determined dystrophic process, an inflammatory myocardial injury and death, or a programmed cell death ("apoptosis") [1-6, 9]. The most frequent clinical features of ARVC consist of ventricular arrhythmias with left bundle branch block morphology ranging from isolated premature ventricular beats to sustained ventricular tachycardia or ventricular fibrillation [1-7, 10]. Other common clinical manifestations of the disease include global and/or regional dysfunction and structural alterations of the right ventricle or both ventricles, and ECG depolarization/repolarization changes, mostly localized to right precordial leads [11]; supraventricular arrhythmias (SVA) -mostly atrial fibrillation and flutter- represent a less frequent clinical feature [12-15]. Whatever the etiopathogenetic mechanisms involved, there is definitive clinico-pathological evidence that ARVC is a progressive heart muscle disease [6]. Clinico-pathological investigations and long-term follow-up data from clinical studies indicate that ARVC with time may lead to more diffuse RV changes and left ventricular involvement culminating in heart failure [6, 16, 17]. Therefore, the natural history of ARVC is a function of both the electrical instability of diseased ventricular myocardium, which can precipitate "arrhythmic" cardiac arrest any time during the disease course, and the progressive myocardial loss that results in right or biventricular dysfunction and heart failure. The following clinico-pathological phases can be considered [4]: (1) "concealed disease" characterized by subtle RV structural changes, with or without minor ventricular arrhythmias, during which sudden death may be the first manifestation of the disease, mostly in young people and athletes; (2) "overt electrical disorder" in which severe RV arrhythmias and

Dipartimenti di Cardiologia e Patologia, Università di Padova, Padua, Italy impending cardiac arrest are associated with overt RV functional and structural abnormalites; (3) "right ventricular failure" due to the progression and extension of the RV muscle disease that provokes global RV dysfunction; (4) final stage of "biventricular pump failure" due to significant LV involvement. At this stage, ARVC mimics a biventricular dilated cardiomyopathy leading to congestive heart failure and thromboembolic complications [5, 6].

The present study will address the prevalence of SVA in patients with ARVC and correlate their occurrence with the disease natural history.

Previous Studies on Atrial Electrical Vulnerability In ARVC

The few available studies on the atrial electrical instability in ARVC mostly focused on the spontaneous occurrence of SVA; only one recent investigation addressed the inducibility of SVA by programmed atrial stimulation.

Fitchett et al. [12] reported on 14 patients (9 males and 5 females, aged 9-62 years, mean 28) with "right ventricular dilated cardiomyopathy" (mostly consistent with ARVC), 12 of whom had arrhythmias of either supraventricular or ventricular origin. SVA occurred in 5 patients (36%) and consisted of atrial fibrillation in 3, paroxysmal atrial tachycardia in 2, and atrial flutter in 2. Four of them had angiographic evidence of significant tricuspidal regurgitation into a dilated right atrium, and 3 developed right heart failure (with a cerebrovascular accident in one) that was preceded by SVA by up to 2 years. Among the remaining 9 patients without SVA, only 2 patients showed right atrial dilatation and one had heart failure.

Klein and Horowitz [13] reported on a family with electrocardiographic and echocardiographic evidence of severe RV cardiomyopathy distinctively associated with paroxysmal episodes of SVA, in the absence of ventricular arrhythmias. Paroxysmal episodes of atrial fibrillation and flutter were observed in five out of eight family members; all affected patients showed a dilated right atrium and right ventricle, and one died due to massive stroke.

Among 72 consecutive patients referred for ventricular arrhythmias in the setting of arrhythmogenic right ventricular dysplasia, Tonet et al. [14] documented coexistent SVA in 17 (24%): atrial fibrillation in 10, atrial tachycardia in 7 and atrial flutter in 5. Five of these patients (among 12 with available echocardiogram, 42%), had an enlarged right atrium and 1 also had tricuspid insufficiency. On the other hand, 6 of the 55 patients without SVA had a dilated right atrium (6 of 39 echocardiograms, 15%); 2 of them also had tricuspid insufficiency. It is worth noting that all these 6 patients had been taking antiarrhythmic drugs.

Recently, Brembilla-Perrot et al. [15] reported the prevalence of sustained SVA, both spontaneous and induced at electrophysiologic study, in patients with ARVC. Among 47 patients (33 male and 14 female, aged 21 to 72 years, mean 44 ± 18), 8 (17%) had a history of spontaneous SVA consisting of atrial fibrillation in 5, paroxysmal junctional tachycardia in 2, and atrial flutter in one; all except one (87%) had an enlarged right atrium. Spontaneous ventricular tachycardia were documented in 7 cases: sustained in 5 and nonsustained in 2. SVA preceded the occurrence of ventricular tachycardia by several years. On the other hand, 27 patients (69%) had *inducible* sustained SVA at electrophysiologic study: atrial fibrillation ($n = 14$), atrial flutter or tachycardia ($n = 11$), or AV nodal reentry tachycardia ($n = 2$); 22 of them also had inducible ventricular tachycardia and another one inducible ventricular fibrillation (during isoproterenol infusion in 11). There were no echocardiographic data, including the right atrial size, that correlated with the inducibility of SVA. It is noteworthy that the patients with ARVC and spontaneous SVA were statistically significantly older than patients with electrophysiologically inducible SVA (55 ± 15 vs 42 ± 15 years, $p < 0.05$).

Are SVA a Sign of ARVC Progression?

The mechanism of SVA in ARVC is unknown. SVA may be either an indirect consequence of right and left ventricular dysfunction or the result of a direct atrial involvement. Although fatty infiltration and parchment-like wall have been occasionally observed even in the atrial myocardium, unfortunately there are no studies which systematically addressed the atrial myocardial pathology and correlated morphological and arrhythmological findings. An enlarged right atrium, a right atrial abnormality, or both have been hypothesized to have an important role in the genesis of SVA in ARVC [14, 15].

In order to assess whether SVA are a clinical marker of progression of ARVC to a more diffuse disease leading to heart failure, we reviewed the clinical and pathological findings of the Multicenter Study of the the Council on Cardiomyopathy of the International Society and Federation of Cardiology [6]. The study redefined the anatomo-clinical profile of ARVC with special reference to disease progression and involvement of the left ventricle. The investigation included 42 patients (27 males and 15 females, aged 9 to 65 years, mean 29.6 ± 18), from six collaborative Medical Centers, with clinical and/or pathological diagnosis of ARVC at autopsy or heart transplantation and with the entire heart available for detailed morphological study. Thirty-four patients died suddenly (16 during effort), 2 died and 4 were transplanted because of advanced heart failure; 2 died from other causes. Sudden death was the first sign of disease in 12 patients; the other 30 had palpitations with syncope in 11, heart failure in 8 and stroke in 3. Twenty-seven patients experienced ventricular arrhythmias (ventricular tachycardia in 17), and 5 received a pace-maker. Twelve patients (28%) had SVA consisting of atrial fibrillation ($n = 10$), atrial flutter ($n = 4$), and atrial tachycardia ($n = 3$) (Table 1). According to autopsy findings, 3 subgroups of patients were identified: (1) 10 patients with isolated RV involvement; (2) 15 patients with RV involvement and coexistent fibrofatty left ventricular lesions which were observed only histologically; (3) 17 patients with macroscopic biventricular cardiomyopathy. We compared ARVC patients with (group A, $n = 12$) and without (group B, $n = 30$) SVA with respect to a series of clinical and morphological variables (Table 2). Patients from Group A were significantly ($p < 0.05$) older than patients from group B (48 ± 7 vs 23 ± 3

Table 1. Clinical data of 12 patients with ARVC complicated by SVA

Sex	Age	SVA	Relevant clinical findings	Antiarrhythmic drugs	Pace maker	Clinical oucome
F	58	AF, Afl	Heart failure, SVT, syncope	Digoxine, amiodarone	VVI	Heart transplantation
F	61	AF, AT	Heart failure, SVT	Digoxine, amiodarone	VVIR	Death from congestive heart failure
F	45	AF, Afl	Heart failure, NSVT	Propafenone	–	Sudden death
F	39	AF, Afl	NSVT	Sotalol	–	Sudden death
F	58	AF	Heart failure, stroke	Digoxine, disopiramide	VVIR	Death from congestive heart ailure
M	65	Afl, AF	Heart failure, stroke	Beta-blockers	–	Death from massive cerebral embolism
M	41	AF, AT	Heart failure	Digoxine, amiodarone	–	Heart transplantation
F	38	AF	Heart failure, NSVT, stroke	Digoxine, amiodarone, mexiletine	–	Heart transplantation
M	41	AF	Heart failure, SVT	Sotalol	VVI	Cerebral malignancy
M	42	AF	Heart failure, NSVT	–	–	Heart transplantation
M	51	AF, Afl	Syncope, NSVT	Sotalol	–	Sudden death
M	36	AT	Syncope, SVT	Sotalol	–	Sudden death

ARVC, arrhythmogenic right ventricular cardiomyopathy; SVA, supraventricular arrhythmias; AF, atrial fibrillation; Afl, atrial flutter; AT, atrial tachycardia; SVT, sustained ventricular tachycardia; NSVT, non sustained ventricular tachycardia

years), had significantly longer disease duration (8.9 ± 7 vs 2.1 ± 1 years), significantly more often had inverted T waves until lateral precordial leads (V5 and V6) (67% vs 7%), underwent pacemaker implantation (33% vs 0), and developed stroke (25% vs 0) and heart failure (75% vs 0%). With regard to morphological variables, hearts from group A weighted significantly more than those from group B (495 ± 160 vs 355 ± 60 g), significantly more often had right atrial enlargement (45% vs 3.5%) and macroscopic left ventricular involvement (92% vs 20%). There was no statistically significant difference between the two groups with regard to incidence of syncope and ventricular arrhythmias, presence of RV aneurysms, severity of RV thinning, and occurrence of inflammatory infiltrates.

Therefore, the study suggests that SVA are an important clinical marker for heart failure in longstanding ARVC. SVA appear to reflect the progression of the

Table 2. Clinical characteristics and morphological findings in ARVC patients with (group A) or without (group B) SVA

	ARVC with SVA Group A (n = 12 pts)	ARVC without SVA Group B (n = 30 pts)
Age (years)	48 ± 7	23 ± 3*
Disease duration (years)	8.9 ± 4	2.1 ± 1*
Syncope	3 (25%)	8 (27%)
Inverted T waves:		
- right precordial leads (V1-V4)	12/12 (100%)	15/16 (92%)
- lateral leads (V5,V6)	8 (67%)	2 (7%)*
Ventricular arrhythmias	10 (83%)	20(67%)
Heart failure	9 (75%)	0*
Stroke	3 (25%)	0*
PM implantation	4 (33%)	0*
Heart weight (g)	495 ± 160	355 ± 60*
Significant RV wall thinning ($\leq$ 2 mm)	9 (75%)	18 (60%)
RV aneurysms	6 (50%)	14 (47%)
Left and/or right atrial enlargement	5 (45%)	1 (3.5%)*
Inflammatory infiltrates	10 (83%)	19 (63%)
Gross LV involvement	11(92%)	6(20%)*

RV, right ventricular; LV, left ventricular
*$p < 0.05$

myocardial disease, since it occurred in older patients with a longer clinical history and pathological evidence of more severe cardiomegaly with right atrial enlargement and gross LV involvement.

Whether there is a specific involvement of the atrial myocardium in terms of myocardial loss and inflammation remains to be established.

Conclusions

Spontaneous SVA occur in 24%-36% of patients with ARVC, are age-dependent, and affect patients with longstanding clinical history of ARVC culminating in death or heart transplantation for heart failure. Hearts from patients with ARVC complicated by SVA weigh more, and more often exhibit right or biatrial dilatation as well as left ventricular involvement. All these findings suggest that SVA are a late complication of ARVC course and reflect its progression to a more diffuse disease with right atrial and left ventricular involvement.

Whether programmed atrial stimulation unmasks earlier atrial vulnerability in patients with ARVC remains to be confirmed.

Acknowledgements. This study was supported by the Veneto Region, Venice, and by the National Council for Research, Rome, Italy

References

1. Marcus FI, Fontaine G, Guiraudon G et al (1982) Right ventricular dysplasia. A report of 24 adult cases. Circulation 65:384-398
2. Thiene G, Nava A, Corrado D, Rossi L, Pennelli N (1988) Right ventricular cardiomyopathy and sudden death in young people. N Engl J Med 318:129-133
3. Nava A, Rossi L, Thiene G (eds) (1997) Arrhythmogenic right ventricular cardiomyopathy- dysplasia. Elsevier, Amsterdam
4. Thiene G, Nava A, Angelini A, Daliento L, Scognamiglio R, Corrado D (1988) Anatomoclinical aspects of arrhythmogenic right ventricular cardiomyopathy. In: Baroldi G, Camerini F, Goodwin JF (eds) Advances in cardiomyopathy. Springer Milan, pp 397-408
5. Basso C, Thiene G, Corrado D, Angelini A, Nava A, Valente M (1996) Arrhythmogenic right ventricular cardiomyopathy: dysplasia, dystrophy, or myocarditis? Circulation 94:983-991
6. Corrado D, Basso C, Thiene G et al (1997) Spectrum of clinicopathologic manifestations of arrhythmogenic right ventricular cardiomyopathy/dysplasia: a multicenter study. J Am Coll Cardiol 30:1512-1520
7. Corrado D, Thiene G, Nava A, Rossi L, Pennelli N (1990) Sudden death in young competitive athletes: clinicopathologic correlation in 22 cases. Am J Med 89:588-596
8. Corrado D, Basso C, Schiavon M, Thiene G (1998) Screening for hypertrophic cardiomyopathy in young athletes. New Engl J Med 339:364-369
9. Valente M, Calabrese F, Angelini A, Basso C, Thiene G (1998) In vivo evidence of apoptosis in arrhythmogenic right ventricular cardiomyopathy. Am J Pathol 152:479-484
10. Fontaine G, Frank R, Fontaliran F, Lascault G, Tonet J (1992) Right ventricular tachycardias. In: Parmley WW, Chatteryce K (eds) Cardiology. Lippincott, New York 1:1-17
11. McKenna WJ, Thiene G, Nava A et al (1994) Diagnosis of arrhythmogenic right ventricular dysplasia/cardiomyopathy. Br Heart J 71:215-218
12. Fichett DH, Sugrue DD, Mac Arthur CG, Oakley CM (1984) Right ventricular dilated cardiomyopathy. Br Heart J 51:25-30
13. Klein LW, Horowitz LN (1988) Familial right ventricular dilated cardiomyopathy associated with supraventricular arrhythmias. Am J Cardiol 62:482-483
14. Tonet JL, Castro-Miranda R, Iwa T, Poulain F, Frank R, Fontaine G (1991) Frequency of supraventricular tachyarrhythmias in arrhythmogenic right ventricular dysplasia. Am J Cardiol 67:1153
15. Brembilla-Perrot B, Jacquemin L, Houplon P et al (1998) Increased atrial vulnerability in arrhythmogenic right ventricular cardiomyopathy. Am Heart J 135:748-754
16. Blomström-Lundqvist C, Sabel CG, Olsson SB (1987) A long term follow up of 15 patients with arrhythmogenic right ventricular dysplasia. Br Heart J 58:477-488
17. Pinamonti B, Sinagra G, Salvi A et al (1992) Left ventricular involvement in right ventricular dysplasia. Am Heart J 123:711-724

Is Right Ventricular Outflow Tract Tachycardia a Minor Form of Arrhythmogenic Right Ventricular Cardiomyopathy?

A. Proclemer[1], C. Fresco[1], G. Muner[1], M. De Cristofaro[1] and E. Bertaglia[2]

Introduction

Right ventricular outflow tract (RVOT) arrhythmias show left bundle branch block and inferior axis (LBBB-IA) aspect and include three main clinical forms: (1) repetitive monomorphic (LBBB-IA) nonsustained ventricular tachycardia (VT); (2) paroxysmal stress- and catecholamine-mediated sustained VT; (3) frequent and/or repetitive monomorphic ventricular premature beats [1-7]. Some patients can have both forms of RVOT-VT, and during exercise stress testing they may show initial suppression of nonsustained VT, final induction of sustained VT or relapse of the arrhythmia immediately after the peak exercise. The mechanism of RVOT-VT is due to catecholamine-mediated delayed after-depolarizations [8]. This model of triggered activity depends on the stimulation of cAMP, which causes an increase in intracellular calcium. The mechanism of triggered activity is supported by the difficult induction of RVOT-VT with programmed ventricular stimulation, by the facilitating effect of isoproterenol infusion on VT induction by ventricular pacing and by the cycle-length dependence of VT appearance [3, 8].

RVOT arrhythmias may be either idiopathic [1-9] or take the form of arrhythmogenic right ventricular cardiomyopathy [10, 11]. Table 1 summarizes the principal distinguishing clinical and instrumental characteristics of the two syndromes.

Substrate of Idiopathic RVOT Arrhythmias

Conventional noninvasive and invasive diagnostic studies are usually normal, and only few cases reveal mild or nonspecific abnormalities, whose pathophysiological significance is unclear. These abnormalities are probably benign, because patients with idiopathic RVOT-VT show a favorable long-term prognosis and do

[1]Istituto di Cardiologia e di Radiologia, Azienda Ospedaliera Santa Maria della Misericordia, Udine, Italy; [2]Divisione di Cardiologia, Azienda Ospedaliera Mirano, Venice, Italy

Table 1. Main characteristics distinguishing between idiopathic RVOT arrhythmic syndrome (IDIO RVOT) and arrhythmogenic right ventricular dysplasia/cardiomyopathy (ARVD/C)

	IDIO RVOT-VT	ARVD/C
Possible genetic defect	No	Yes
QRS and ST-T abnormalities of sinus beats	No	Yes
Signal-averaged ECG	Normal	Abnormal
Echo-angiographic aspect of RV	Normal	Abnormal
RV histology	Normal	Abnormal
RV abnormalities by MRI	Localized	Diffuse
VT mechanism	Triggered activity	Reentry
VT induction	Difficult	Easy
Adenosine sensitive	Yes	No
QRS duration of VT beats	120 ms	>120 ms
QRS aspect of VT beats	Monomorphic	Mono-polimorphic
RS ablation methods	Endocardial and pace mapping	Concealed entrainment and endocardial mapping
ICD indication	No	Possible
Prognosis	Favorable	Unfavorable
Arrhythmia disappearence	Possible	Unusual

VT, ventricular tachycardia

not reveal progressive heart disease during the follow-up [1-7]. RV endomyocardial biopsy, even targeted at various sites of the RVOT, do not show particular abnormalities [8].

In contrast, cardiac magnetic resonance imaging (MRI) study of the RV appears as a very useful diagnostic technique in patients with apparently idiopathic LBBB-IA arrhythmias (Tables 2, 3). In the series of Carlson et al. [12] cine and gradient MRI sequences revealed structural and functional abnormalities of the right ventricle in 22 of 24 patients with RVOT-VT (95%), in 17 of 44 persons with other cardiovascular diseases (39%), and in only 2 of 16 normal subjects (12.5%). In patients with RVOT-VT most of these abnormalities were characterized by focal areas of decreased systolic wall thickening confined to the RVOT. In

Table 2. Cardiac MRI results: idiopathic RVOT arrhythmias

Author	Cases	Controls	Arrhythmia	RV abnormalities		P
				Cases	Controls	
Carlson et al. [12]	22	16	S-nSVT	95%	12%	0.0001
Globits et al. [13]	20	10	VT	65%	0%	0.001
Markowitz et al. [16]	14	18	S-nSVT	71%	6%	0.001
Proclemer et al. [18]	19	10	VPB-sSVT	84%	0%	0.008
White et al. [15]	35	15	S-nSVT	76%	0%	0.008

S, sustained; nS, nonsustained; VT, ventricular tachycardia

Table 3. Right ventricular defects in patients with apparently idiopathic RVOT arrhythmias and abnormal cardiac MRI findings

Author	Focal thinning	Wall motion abnormalities	Fatty infiltration	RVOT abnormalities
Carlson et al. [12]	66%	100%	na	95%
Markowitz et al. [16]	60%	40%	40%	21%
Globitz et al. [13]	45%	20%	25%	40%
Proclemer et al. [18]	87%	100%	na	100%
White et al. [15]	84%	97%	25%	100%

the two control groups such abnormalities were not localized in the RVOT and appeared qualitatively different. Globits et al. [13] examined by MRI 20 patients undergoing radiofrequency catheter ablation for symptomatic RVOT-VT. Echocardiogram was normal in all patients. Right ventricular volumes and ejection fraction of patients with RVOT-VT showed no difference from normals, but in 13 (65%) of 20 arrhythmic patients cardiac MRI demonstrated various structural abnormalities of the right ventricular free wall, including focal wall thinning ($n = 9$), dyskinetic wall segments ($n = 4$), and fatty tissue infiltration ($n = 4$). Eight of these patients had additional and similar abnormalities in the RVOT, corresponding with the ablation site in six. In the Gill et al. study [14], including 16 patients with sustained VT, the MRI scan was abnormal in three of seven patients with normal echo and angiogram. The most frequent abnormality was a thin area of the RVOT wall with dyskinesis and failure to thicken during systole.

White et al. [15] evaluated 58 consecutive patients (mean age 43 years), with ventricular arrhythmias of LBBB morphology but without clear evidence of arrhythmogenic right ventricular dysplasia. On 2D echocardiography, results were negative for myocardial abnormalities in 50 patients (94%) and equivocal in 3 (6%). Positive electrophysiologic study was documented in 35 of the 44 tested patients (80%), and monomorphic VT was identified as originating in the right ventricle in 28. MRI revealed myocardial abnormalities of the anterior wall of the right ventricle in 32 cases (60%); fixed thinning was demonstrated in 27 (84%), focally increased signal intensity that suggested fatty replacement of the myocardium in 8 (25%) and focally reduced systolic wall thickening in 31 (97%). Among the 35 patients with a consensus diagnosis of idiopathic RVOT-C VT, defects confined to the right ventricular anterior wall were detected in 25 (71%). Among the 18 cases with VT of indeterminate origin, MRI revealed right ventricular abnormalities in only 7 (39%, $p = 0.022$). Right ventricular abnormalities were not shown in the control subjects or in the patients with unrelated cardiac diseases (100% specificity). Zone IB (lower infundibulum) was the region most often abnormal (94%). Cranial extension of these defects into the subpulmonic region of the outflow tract (zone IA) was evident in only 7 (21%) of the 33 patients with zone IB abnormalities, while caudal extension into the subparietal region of the anterior wall of the right ventricular body (zone IIB) was noted in 24 cases (73%). In particular, zone IIB was the second most common location of MRI defects. Further extension into the lower region of the anterior wall of the right ventricle was found in 8 (33%) of 24 patients with combined abnormalities in zones IB and IIB. Among the total population with idiopathic RVOT arrhythmias, no specific relationships were found between the individual arrhythmia (VPBs, nonsustained VT, or sustained VT) and either the presence of MRI defects in the right ventricle or the extent of MRI abnormalities. Because the nature of the subtle right ventricular defects at MRI did not correlate with either the severity or inducibility of the arrhythmias, the authors [15] hypothesized that the area of myocardial abnormality could exceed that of electrical activity and that the latter could originate between the more damaged lower infundibulum (zone IB) and the less damaged upper infundibulum (zone IA).

Markowitz et al. [16] used cardiac MRI to screen a homogeneous group of 14 patients with apparently idiopathic adenosine-sensitive VT for possible abnormalities in the right ventricular morphology and function. VT was sustained in three, repetitive and monomorphic in seven, and both in four; VT was terminated with adenosine, vagal maneuvers, and verapamil in most patients. The origin of VT was confined to the RVOT in ten, to the apex in one, and the left ventricular septum in three. Radiofrequency ablation was performed in 11 patients. Signal-averaged ECGs did not demonstrate late potentials, and echocardiography revealed normal right ventricle in all cases. In contrast, MRI was abnormal in 10 patients (71% vs 6% of control subjects; $p = 0.0001$). Particularly, focal thinning was detected in six, fatty infiltration in four, and wall motion abnormalities in four. The most common site of such defects was the right ventricular free wall (nine cases), and only three patients showed outflow tract defects. The presence of MRI abnormalities did not correlate with age, clinical presentation, duration of symptoms, or number of radiofrequency applications. Because there was poor correlation between the origin of VT and the site of MRI defects, the authors considered unlikely that MRI abnormalities are causally related to adenosine-sensitive VT.

To test the hypothesis that arrhythmogenic substrate of repetituive monomorphic RVOT tachycardia is related to an early or localized form of arrhythmogenic right ventricular cardiomyopathy, Grimm et al. [17] performed cardiac MRI and signal-averaged ECG on 23 patients with this arrhythmia, normal standard electrocardiogram of conducted sinus beats, and normal 2D echocardiography. MRI was performed using ECG-gated turbo spin-echo images in order to detect localized wall thickness reductions, signal intensity increase suggesting fatty tissue infiltrates, and regional bulgings or aneurysms. MRI appeared normal in 22 patients (96%) and revealed signal intensity increase in the interventricular septum in only one. Time-domain analysis of the SA-ECG was normal in 21 (91%), frequency-domain analysis in 22 (96%). The conclusion is that normal MRI findings and absence of ventricular late potential in the majority of patients with repetitive RVOT-VT do not prove that an early or concealed form of right ventricular cardiomyopathy creates the arrhythmogenic substrate. Considering the MRI results, the wide discrepancy between this study [17] and previous series may be related to the use of ECG-gated turbo spin-echo sequence rather than cine MRI scans, which appear very useful for detection of the right ventricular wall motion defects.

In our recent series, including the study population previously published [18], we assessed the value of MRI scans in 23 patients with frequent (> 100/h), monomorphic RVOT extrasystoles ($n = 22$) and in 9 patients with frequent RVOT ventricular premature beats (VPBs) and nonsustained RVOT-VT. Fifteen of these patients were totally asymptomatic, 17 reported mild palpitations. The ECG aspect of the sinus beats and the echocardiography were normal in all cases. The mean number of RVOT VPBs/h was 566 ± 251, while the length of runs of RVOT nonsustained VT ranged from 4 to 20 beats. Mean age was 37.9 years ± 4.9 years. MRI studies included spin-echo and gradient-echo sequences in the standard planes. Patients with RVOT arrhythmias showed wider dimensions of RVOT than the control group (10 healthy subjects). Mean anteroposterior and transverse diameters were 37.2 ± 2.2 mm versus 29.7 ± 4.8 mm ($p < 0.01$) and 26.1 ± 4.2 mm versus 20.5 ± 2.5 mm. ($p < 0.01$), respectively. Wall motion and morphological abnormalities were present in 26/32 (81%) patients, and were confined to the anterolateral and lateral walls in 22/26 (85%) cases. All normal subjects had normal MRI findings ($p = 0.008$). No clear correlation was found between the site of wall motion abnormalities and the QRS pattern of ectopies on the frontal plane and on precordial leads. Patients with anterolateral and lateral wall abnormalities of the RVOT showed both right and left inferior axis configuration and either early or late transition. The similarities concerning the results obtained in our series and in previous studies [12, 15, 16, 24] suggest that VT and extrasystoles arising in the RVOT may share the same substrate and represent two expressions of a single arrhythmic syndrome. Other reported similarities include the site of origin, identified by both earliest endocardial activity and pace-map, electrophysiological results and response to radiofrequency ablation therapy [3, 19-25].

The involvement of the cardiac sympathetic nervous system in the pathophysiology of idiopathic RVOT-VT was recently investigated in eight patients by positron emission tomography [26]. This study showed that presynaptic reuptake of norepinephrine and postsynaptic beta-adrenoceptor density are globally reduced in the left ventricular myocardium and that myocardial perfusion at rest was normal. As a consequence, the authors hypothesized that the increased catecholamines levels in the synaptic cleft may have an important role in the pathophysiology of the VT. However, the impossibility of performing the measurements in the thin right ventricular wall constitutes the main limitation of this study.

The origin and the functional significance of the RVOT abnormalities are unclear. The first explanation is that the anatomic and functional abnormalities of the RVOT could be due to the electromechanical influence of frequent ectopy and/or VT runs on RVOT geometry. In other words, this RVOT remodelling can be considered a secondary response to recurrent RVOT arrhythmias as previously documented in patients with idiopathic atrial fibrillation and associated atrial enlargement [27]. For this theory, calcium overload at the cellular level may be responsible of RVOT-VT/VPBs induced electrical remodeling and mechanical dysfunction of RVOT. This hypothesis, however, could be tested properly by repetition of cardiac MRI after long-term suppression of RVOT ectopies by drugs or radiofrequency ablation.

A second hypothesis is that RVOT defects may represent a concealed or a variant form of arrhythmogenic RV cardiomyopathy [10, 15, 28, 29]. In our opinion, however, the substantial difference in the main clinical and instrumental characteristics (Table 1) associated with the favorable long-term prognosis of patients with idiopathic RVOT arrhythmic syndrome compared with patients with arrhythmogenic RV cardiomyopathy do not support this hypothesis.

A third explanation may be related to a unique pathologic process that causes the structural abnormalities of the RVOT and results in triggered activity. The above-mentioned involvement of the cardiac sympathetic nervous system, characterized by sympathetic denervation and catecholamines hypersensitivity, could be responsible for this process [16, 26].

Conclusions

RVOT arrhythmic syndrome includes VPBs and sustained or nonsustained VT episodes with LBBB-IA morphology. The common substrate is characterized by subtle morphological and functional abnormalities, localized to the RVOT, that are detectable by cardiac MRI in the vast majority of this patient population (Tables 2, 3). The pathophysiological role of these abnormalities, however, is still unknown. The favorable long-term prognosis of patients with this syndrome and the absence of documented evolution into a clear form of arrhythmogenic right ventricular cardiomyopathy support the hypothesis that the two syndromes are separate entities. In our opinion, no evidence is available supporting the consideration of idiopathic RVOT arrhythmic syndrome, so defined, as a minor form of "classic" arrhythmogenic cardiomyopathy.

References

1. Brooks R, Burgess JH (1988) Idiopathic ventricular tachycardia: a review. Medicine 67:271-294
2. Proclemer A, Facchin D, Miani D, Feruglio GA (1994) Tachicardia e fibrillazione ventricolare idiopatiche. Inquadramento, diagnosi, terapia e prognosi. G Ital Cardiol 24:1027-1041
3. Lerman BB, Stein KM, Markowitz SM (1996) Idiopathic right ventricular outflow tract tachycardia: a clinical approach. PACE 19:2120-2137

4. Rahilly GI, Prystovsky EN, Zipes DP, Naccarelli GV, Jackman WM, Heger JJ (1982) Clinical and electrophysiological findings in patients with repetitive monomorphic ventricular tachycardia and otherwise normal electrocardiogram. Am J Cardiol 50:459-468

5. Buxton AE, Waxman HL, Marchlinski FE, Simson MB, Cassidy D, Josephson ME (1983) Right ventricular tachycardia: clinical and electrophysiological characteristics. Circulation 68:917-927

6. Proclemer A, Ciani R, Feruglio GA (1989) Right ventricular tachycardia with left bundle branch block and inferior axis morphology. Clinical and arrhythmological characteristics in 15 patients. PACE 12:977-989

7. Mont L, Seixas T, Brugada P et al (1992) The electrocardiographic, clinical and electrophysiologic spectrum of idiopathic monomorphic ventricular tachycardia. Am Heart J 124:746-753

8. Lerman BB, Stein K, Engelstein ED et al (1995) Mechanism of repetitive monomorphic ventricular tachycardia. Circulation 92:421-429

9. Proclemer A, Fresco C (1998) L'infundibolo del ventricolo destro, sede trascurata di displasia aritmogena? Cardiologia 43:805-810

10. Martini B, Nava A, Thiene G et al (1988) Accelerated idioventricular rhythm of infundibular origin in patients with a concealed form of arrhythmogenic right ventricular dysplasia. Br Heart J 59:564-571

11. Marcus FI, Fontaine G (1995) Arrhythmogenic right ventricular dysplasia/cardiomyopathy: a review. PACE 18:1928-1314

12. Carlson MD, White RD, Trohman RG, Adler LP, Biblo LA, Merkatz KA, Waldo AL (1994) Right ventricular outflow tract ventricular tachycardia: detection of previously unrecognized anatomic abnormalities using cine magnetic resonance imaging. J Am Coll Cardiol 24:720-727

13. Globits S, Kreiner G, Heinz G, Frank H, Klaar U, Gossinger H (1995) Morphologic abnormalities by magnetic resonance imaging in relation to successful ablation sites in right ventricular outflow tract tachycardia. Circulation 92:I-684 (abstr)

14. Gill JS, Rowland E, de Belder M, Rees S, Ward DE, Underwood R, Camm AJ (1993) Cardiac abnormalities not visualised by echocardiography and angiography are detected by magnetic resonance imaging in patients with idiopathic ventricular tachycardia. Eur Heart J 14[Suppl]:7 (abstr)

15. White RD, Trohman RG, Flamm SD et al (1998) Right ventricular arrhythmia in the absence of arrhythmogenic dysplasia: MR imaging of myocardial abnormalities. Radiology 207:743-751

16. Markowitz SM, Litvak BL, Ramirez EA, Markisz JA, Stein KM, Lerman BB (1997) Adenosine-sensitive ventricular tachycardia. Right venticular abnormalities delineatede by magnetic resonance imaging. Circulation 4:1192-1200

17. Grimm W, Hellwig EL, Hoffmann J, Manz V, Hahn-Rinn R, Klose KJ (1997) Magnetic resonance imaging and signal-averaged electrocardiography in patients with ripetitive monomorphic ventricular tachycardia and otherwise normal electrocardiogram. PACE 20:1826-1833

18. Proclemer A, Basadonna PT, Slavich GA, Miani D, Fresco C, Fioretti PM (1997) Cardiac magnetic resonance imaging findings in patients with right ventricular outflow tract premature contractions. Eur Heart J 18:2002-2010

19. Gursoy S, Brugada J, Souza O, Steurer G, Andries E, Brugada P (1992) Radiofrequency ablation of symptomatic but benign ventricular arrhythmias. PACE 15:738-741

20. Gumbrielle T, Bourke JP, Furniss SS (1994) Is ventricular ectopy a legitimate target for ablation? Br Heart 72:492-494

21. Zhu DW, Maloney JD, Simmons TW et al (1995) Radiofrequency catheter ablation for management of symptomatic ventricular ectopic activity. J Am Coll Cardiol 26:843-849

22. Wilber DJ, Baerman J, Olshansky B, Kall J, Kopp D (1993) Adenosine-sensitive ventricular tachycardia. Clinical characteristics and response to catheter ablation. Circulation 87:126-134

23. Klein LS, Shih HT, Hackett FK, Zipes DP, Miles WM (1992) Radiofrequency catheter ablation of ventricular tachycardia in patients without structural heart disease. Circulation 85:1666-1674

24. Merino JL, Jimenez-Borreguero J, Peinado R, Merino SV, Sobrino JA (1998) Unipolar mapping and magnetic resonance imaging of "idiopathic" right ventricular outflow tract ectopy. J Cardiovasc Electrophysiol 9:84-87

25. Lauck G, Burkhardt D, Manz M (1999) Radiofrequency catheter ablation of symptomatic ventricular ectopic beats originating in the right outflow tract. PACE 22:5-16

26. Schafers M, Lerch H et al (1998) Cardiac sympathetic innervation in patients with idiopathic right ventricular outflow tract tachycardia. J Am Coll Cardiol 32:181-186

27. Goette A, Honeycutt C, Langberg JJ (1996) Electrical remodeling in atrial fibrillation. Time course and mechanisms. Circulation 94:2968-2974

28. Blake LM, Scheinman MM, Higgins CB (1994) MR features of arrhythmic right ventricular dysplasia. Am J Radiol 162:809-812

29. Pennell D, Casolo G (1997) Right ventricular arrhythmia: emergence of magnetic resonance imaging as an investigative tool. Eur Heart J 18:1843-1845

Electrophysiologic Mechanisms of Polymorphic Ventricular Tachycardia/Torsade de Pointes in the Presence of Normal or Long QT

G. Turitto and N. El-Sherif

Torsade de pointes (TdP) is an ear-pleasing term that describes an eye-catching pattern of polymorphic ventricular tachycardia (PVT) with continually changing morphology of the QRS complexes that seem to twist around an imaginary baseline [1]. The quasi-musical term and the intriguing ECG pattern have caught the attention of electrophysiologists for years and have been, to some extent, a driving force behind the recent focused interest in the role of genetics and ion channelopathy in cardiac arrhythmias. More importantly, this is helping to refocus attention on the role of dispersion of ventricular repolarization in the genesis of malignant ventricular tachyarrhythmias [2].

The most common type of PVT is that associated with structural heart disease and normal QT interval [3] (Fig. 1). The arrhythmia can be asymptomatic and discovered on Holter monitor ECG, but prolonged episodes can degenerate into ventricular fibrillation (VF). PVT can also occur in the setting of acute myocardial ischemia, including coronary artery spasm and Prinzmetal angina [4]. However, considerable interest in recent years has focused on the electrophysiologic mechanisms of PVT/VF in normal hearts (better defined as hearts with no or minimal discernible structural disease). There is more than one electrophysiologic mechanism for PVT/VF in normal hearts (sometimes referred to as idiopathic PVT/VF). An understanding of these mechanisms can be crucial for the proper management of individual patients. The most appropriate way to classify PVT is according to whether it is associated with normal or prolonged QT (or QTU) interval (Fig. 1). The electrophysiologic mechanisms of these two types of PVT may be different.

PVT in the presence of long QT is seen in both the congenital and acquired long QT syndrome (LQTS). The syndrome is due to abnormalities (intrinsic and/or acquired) of ionic currents underlying cardiac repolarization [2]. The in vivo electrophysiologic mechanism of PVT in this syndrome has recently been described in detail utilizing a surrogate experimental model of LQT3 [5-8]. On the other hand, the electrophysiologic mechanism of PVT/VF in normal heart in the presence of normal QT is less well understood and several clinical syndromes

Cardiology Division, Department of Medicine, State University of New York; Health Science Center and Veterans Affairs Medical Center, Brooklyn, NY, USA

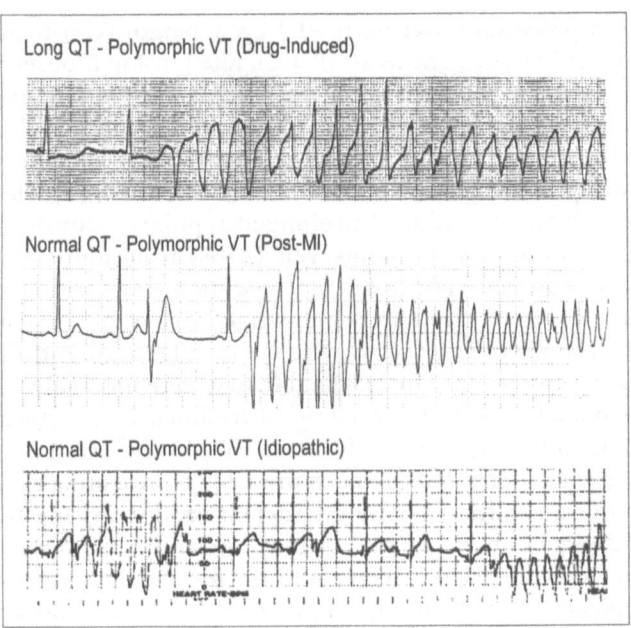

Fig. 1. Electrocardiographic recordings showing the onset of polymorphic ventricular tachycardia (PVT) in: a patient with procainamide-related acquired long QT syndrome (*top tracing*), a patient 3 weeks following inferior wall myocardial infarction (*middle tracing*), and a patient with no detectable structural heart disease and normal QT interval (idiopathic polymorphic VT/VF) (*bottom tracing*). The tachyarrhythmia that started in the second half of the tracing had an averaged rate of 420 beats/min and lasted for 2.5 min before terminating spontaneously. Note the short-coupled ventricular premature beat (VPB) that initiated PVT in the middle and bottom tracings, compared to the long-coupled VPB that initiated the torsade de pointes in the top tracing. (Modified from [3])

have been described. These include cathecholamine-dependent PVT [9], short-coupled variant of TdP [10], PVT/VF in the presence of right bundle branch block pattern (RBBBP) and ST elevation in the precordial leads V1 through V3 (so-called Brugada syndrome) [11], syndrome of nocturnal sudden death in Southeast Asian males [12, 13], and finally idiopathic PVT/VF that does not fit into any of the above syndromes [14]. It is expected that considerable overlap exists among these different syndromes. For instance, many victims of sudden nocturnal death in Southeast Asia have the characteristic ECG pattern of Brugada syndrome [13]. The following is a brief review of the electrophysiologic mechanisms of PVT in normal heart in the presence of normal or prolonged QT.

Electrophysiologic Mechanisms of PVT in the LQTS

In vitro observations have shown differences in ion channel constituents, rate dependence, and pharmacologic sensitivity of midmyocardial M cells, compared to subepicardial and subendocardial cells [15, 16]. The M cells have the steepest action potential duration (APD)-cycle length (CL) relationship, followed by endocardial cells. The least APD-CL relationship is observed in epicardial cells. This APD-CL relationship is exaggerated in situations associated with prolonged cardiac repolarization. This occurs in the congenital LQTS, due to genetic defects resulting in a decrease of repolarizing K^+ currents (LQT1, LQT2, LQT5) or in delayed inactivation of the Na^+ current (LQT3) [2]. This is also seen with pharmacologically induced prolonged repolarization in the acquired LQTS. Using activation-recovery intervals (ARIs) from unipolar extracellular electrograms as a measure of cardiac repolarization and a tridimensional mapping technique, it was possible to demonstrate in vivo the existence of spatial dispersion of repolarization across the ventricular wall and differences in regional recovery in response to CL changes that were markedly exaggerated in the surrogate model of LQT3 [5]. Analysis of tridimensional activation patterns showed that the initial one or two beats of PVT in the LQTS arose as a focal activity from a subendocardial site most probably representing the extracellular manifestation of a conducted early afterdepolarization arising from Purkinje fibers. The subsequent beats of PVT were consistently due to reentrant excitation. The latter was due to infringement of the focal activity on the spatial dispersion of repolarization, resulting in functional conduction block and circulating wavefronts. The polymorphic QRS configuration of VT was due to the varying orientation of the circulating wavefronts. A twisting QRS axis typical of TdP correlated with the bifurcation of a predominantly single rotating wavefront (scroll) into two separate simultaneous wavefronts rotating around the left and right ventricular cavities or with termination of the right ventricular circuit and the reestablishment of a single left ventricular circulating wavefront [6].

Two characteristic ECG markers frequently presage the onset of PVT in the LQTS: one, a tachycardia-dependent QT/T wave alternans, especially in the congenital LQTS, and, two, a short-long (S-L) cardiac sequence usually the result of a ventricular bigeminal rhythm which is seen in both the congenital and acquired LQTS. Recent studies have convincingly shown that both markers are associated with increased spatial dispersion of repolarization [7, 8]. The arrhythmogenicity of QT/T alternans was primarily due to the greater degree of spatial dispersion of repolarization during alternans than during slower rates associated with longer QT but no alternans [7]. The dispersion of repolarization was most marked between midmyocardial and epicardial zones in the left ventricular free wall. In the presence of a critical degree of dispersion of repolarization, propagation of the activation wavefront could be blocked between these zones to initiate reentrant excitation and PVT. Two factors contributed to the modulation of repolarization during QT/T alternans, resulting in a greater magnitude of dispersion of repolarization between midmyocardial and epicardial zones at critical short CLs: (1) differences in restitution kinetics at midmyocardial sites, characterized by larger ΔARI and a slower time constant (τ) compared with epicardial sites, and (2) differences in the diastolic interval that would result in different input to the restitution curve at the same constant CL. An important observation was that marked repolarization alternans could be present in local electrograms without manifest alternation of the QT/T segment in the surface ECG. The latter was seen at critically short CLs associated with reversal of the gradient of repolarization between epicardial and midmyocardial sites, with a consequent reversal of polarity of the intramyocardial QT wave in alternate cycles. This observation provides the rationale for the recent digital signal-processing techniques that attempt to detect subtle degrees of T wave alternans.

A recent study described two different electrophysiologic mechanisms that underlie the relationship between the S-L sequence and the onset of PVT in LQTS [8]: (1) a second subendocardial focal activity (always from a different site) could infringe on the dispersion of repolarization of the first focal activity to initiate reentrant excitation; and (2) a slight lengthening (50-150 ms) of one or more preceding CLs could result in alterations of the spatial pattern of dispersion of repolarization at key sites to promote reentry. The lengthening of the preceding CL produced differentially a greater degree of prolongation of repolarization at midmyocardial and endocardial sites compared with epicardial sites with consequent increase in dispersion of repolarization. The increased dispersion at key adjacent sites could result in the development of de novo zones of functional conduction block and/or slowed conduction to create the necessary prerequisites for successful reentry (Fig. 2).

Electrophysiologic Mechanisms of PVT in Normal Heart in the Presence of Normal QT

Insights into the in vivo electrophysiologic mechanisms of PVT in the so-called Brugada syndrome come primarily from experimental work of Antzelevitch and associates [17, 18]. The Brugada syndrome is characterized by ST segment elevation (unrelated to ischemia, electrolyte abnormalities, or structural heart disease) in the right precordial (V1-V3) ECG leads, often but not always accompanied by a RBBBP [11]. A familial occurrence has long been recognized, and an autosomal dominant mode of inheritance with variable expression has been described. The Brugada syndrome appears unrelated to any gene abnormality thus far described for arrhythmogenic right ventricular dysplasia.

The proposed underlying mechanisms of the syndrome suggest that mutations in the gene encoding the cardiac Na^+ channel, the transient outward channels, and/or Ca^{++} channels are candidates to explain the hereditary transmission of the disease [18, 19]. Mutations have been identified in the cardiac Na^+ channel gene (SCN5A) in three small families and individual patients with a history of VF in the presence of the described ECG abnormalities [19, 20]. Although these initial data have not yet provided a complete explanation for the manifestations of the disease and lack genetic linkage, they form a very encouraging first step for future research [19].

Both theoretical considerations and in vivo experiments support the idea that heterogeneity of repolarization across the wall of the right ventricular outflow tract contributes to the ECG pattern and the genesis of arrhythmias in Brugada syndrome. It is now well established that a transient outward current (I_{to})-medi-

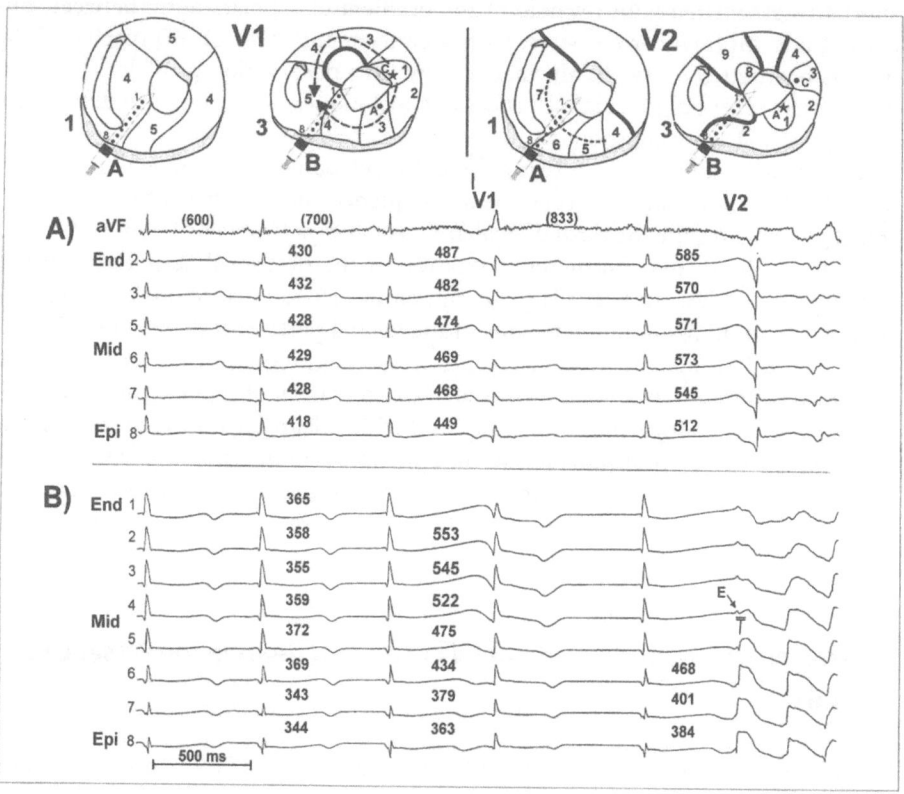

Fig. 2. Recordings from a canine surrogate model of LQT3 induced by infusion of anthopleurin-A showing the onset PVT following a short-long cardiac sequence. Shown are surface ECG lead aVF and unipolar electrograms recorded from two plunge needle electrodes inserted at a basal (**A**) and mid (**B**) cross sections of the ventricles, respectively. Also shown are the activation maps from these two sections (*1* and *3*, respectively). The activation maps are drawn as closed contours at 20-ms intervals and labeled as 1-9 make it easier to follow the activation sequence. The *heavy solid lines* represent arcs of functional conduction block. The *numbers* on the electrograms represent local activation-recovery intervals (ARI) in milliseconds. The *numbers in parentheses* are the cardiac cycle lengths (CLs) in milliseconds. V1 and V2 are two ventricular premature beats that arose from two different subendocardial sites in section 3 (marked by stars). The surface ECG shows that, following a series of relatively regular sinus rhythm at a CL of 600-620 ms, there was a sudden increase of the sinus CL to 700 ms with obvious lengthening of the QT interval of the sinus beat and the occurrence of a single ventricular premature beat (V1). The premature beat was followed after a compensatory pause of 830 ms by a sinus beat, thus creating a short-long sequence. The sinus beat that followed the short-long sequence showed further prolongation of the QT interval and the occurrence of a ventricular premature beat with a different QRS configuration (V2) that initiated VT. The recordings illustrate the alterations in the repolarization pattern and dispersion of repolarization that followed the lengthening of preceding CL and that created the substrate for reentrant excitation. Needle A shows that the increase in the sinus CL preceding V1 resulted in lengthening of ARI at all epicardial (Epi), midmyocardial (Mid), and endocardial (End) sites compared with preceding sinus beats with shorter and relatively constant CLs. The longer compensatory CL after V1 resulted in further lengthening of ARI of the next sinus beat. Critical analysis revealed that the degree of lengthening of ARI at epicardial sites was less than at subepicardial, midmyocardial, and endocardial sites, resulting in greater dispersion between these sites. For needle A, the dispersion of ARI between epicardial site 8

ated phase 1, responsible for the notched appearance of the action potential, is much more prominent in epicardium than in endocardium of the ventricles of many species including man [18]. A prominent action potential notch in epicardium but not endocardium gives rise to a transmural voltage gradient during ventricular activation, which is responsible for the J wave and J point elevation in the ECG [21] (Fig. 3). A prominent I_{to}-mediated notch also predisposes canine right ventricular epicardium to all-or-none repolarization under a variety of conditions, including Na$^+$ channel blockade and ischemia [22].

The loss of the action potential dome (plateau) in epicardium but not endocardium has been shown in arterially perfused wedges of canine right ventricle to lead to the development of a transmural voltage gradient during ventricular repolarization, resulting in ST segment elevation very similar to that observed in patients with the Brugada syndrome. Steep voltage gradients also develop in right ventricular epicardium between sites at which the dome is lost and those at which is maintained, giving rise to phase 2 reentry and the generation of a very early (closely coupled) premature beat, which is then able to precipitate circus movement reentrant VT and VF [22] (Fig. 3). The arrhythmia at times has the appearance of a rapid PVT resembling TdP. All-or-none repolarization of the right ventricular epicardial action potential is caused by an outward shift in the balance of currents active at the end of phase 1 of the action potential (principally I_{to} and I_{Ca}). As a consequence, autonomic neurotransmitters such as acetylcholine facilitate loss of the action potential dome by suppressing I_{Ca} and/or augmenting K$^+$ currents, whereas β-adrenergic agonists restore the dome by augmenting I_{Ca}. Na$^+$ channel blockers also facilitate loss of the canine right ventricular epicardial action potential dome [17, 18]. Accentuation of the ST segment elevation in patients with the Brugada syndrome following vagal maneuvers or treatment with class I antiarrhythmic agents and reduction of ST segment elevation following treatment with β-adrenergic agents are consistent with these findings in isolated tissue preparations [23].

An alternative hypothesis for the genesis of the arrhythmia is based on data from signal-averaged electrocardiogram and body surface mapping. These data

and "adjacent" subepicardial site 7, separated by 1 mm, was 10 ms during the stable sinus rhythm at a CL of 600 ms, and increased to 19 ms after the lengthening of the last sinus cycle before V1 to 700 ms. The dispersion of ARI then increased to 37 ms after the longer CL of 833 ms of the short-long sequence. Needle B shows similar directional increases of local ARI after the lengthening of the preceding CL, but the degree of lengthening was more pronounced. Still, the lengthening of ARI at epicardial sites was less marked than at midmyocardial and endocardial sites. The lengthening of the sinus CL from 600 ms to 700 ms resulted in 19-ms and 38-ms increase of the ARI at the two most epicardial sites 8 and 7, respectively, compared with midmyocardial/endocardial sites (ranging from 65 ms at site 6 to 195 ms at site 2). The most illustrative consequence of differential changes in ARI in response to lengthening of preceding CL is seen in the sinus beat after the short-long sequence in needle B. Conduction block occurred between midmyocardial sites 5 and 4. The ARI could only be estimated at sites 6-8 and showed further lengthening compared with the sinus beat before V1. The ARI could not be accurately estimated at sites 1-5 because of superimposition of the local activation potential (site 5) or electrotonic potentials (sites 1-4) on the repolarization wave. However, it is clear that the dispersion of local ARI between sites 5 and 4 was the substrate for the resulting functional conduction block and the initiation of reentrant excitation. (Reproduced with permission from [8])

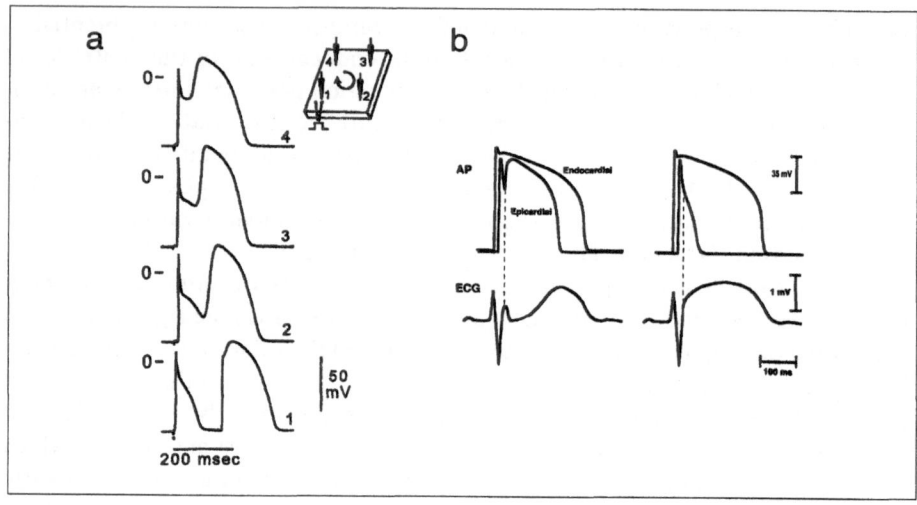

Fig. 3. a Phase 2 reentry. Reentrant activity was induced by exposure of a canine ventricular epicardial preparation to simulated ischemia. Microelectrode recordings were obtained from four sites as shown in the schematic (*upper right*). After 35 min ischemia, the action potential dome develops normally at site 4, but not at sites 1, 2, or 3. The dome then propagates in a clockwise direction, reexciting sites 3, 2, and 1 with progressive delays, thus generating a reentrant extrasystole with a coupling interval of 156 ms at site 1. Basic cycle length = 700 ms. (Adapted with permission from [22]). **b** Difference between epicardial and endocardial action potential morphology. *Top tracings* show epicardial and endocardial action potentials; *bottom* tracing surface ECG. Epicardial action potential is characterized by a pronounced phase 1 which coincides with J wave in surface ECG. Loss of epicardial action potential dome (*top right*) shortens epicardial action potential duration. This causes transmural heterogeneity and ST segment elevation in surface ECG (*bottom right*). (Adapted with permission from [21])

show conduction delay in the area between the anterior wall and the septal region of the right ventricular outflow tract, which is aggravated by accelerated vagal activity [24]. Independent of the presence of a spike-and-dome morphology, significant epicardial conduction delay may give rise to the J wave as well. To explain ST segment elevation, however, substantial shortening of the epicardial action potential is needed. This alternative explanation for the ECG abnormalities may help to explain the preferential occurrence of VF episodes during the night hours [19].

At present the implantable cardioverter defibrillator is the only recommended management strategy in patients with the Brugada syndrome. However, a pharmacologic agent that inhibits I_{to} could be of potential benefit. In this regard, it is interesting to note that quinidine, which is a strong blocker of I_{to} has been reported by Belhassen et al. to be effective in treating patients with idiopathic VF [14, 25]. Reports of the effectiveness of quinidine in idiopathic VF appeared in the literature as early as 1929 [26]. The relationship between those cases of idiopathic VF and the Brugada syndrome remains conjectural.

The mechanism of catecholamine-dependent PVT appears to be different from that of PVT in the Brugada syndrome insofar as in the latter syndrome β-adrenergic agonists can restore the dome of the epicardial action potential and normalize the characteristic ECG pattern. On the other hand, many patients with idiopathic PVT/VF never show the ECG pattern characteristic of the Brugada syndrome. The nature of the underlying electrophysiologic defect in these cases is not well understood at present.

Familial right ventricular cardiomyopathy or arrhythmogenic right ventricular dysplasia can produce a syndrome identical to the Brugada syndrome [27, 28]. Some have even suggested that the Brugada syndrome may be an early manifestation of right ventricular cardiomyopathy. However, it is important to remember that spontaneous and programmed stimulation-induced VT in right ventricular cardiomyopathy is usually monomorphic rather than polymorphic [29].

Conclusions

The electrophysiologic mechanism(s) of PVT/VF in normal heart continue to unravel. This is a prime example of how molecular biology, ion channel, cellular, and organ physiology coupled with clinical observations are the future paradigm for advancement of medical knowledge.

References

1. Dessertenne F (1966) La tachycardie ventriculaire a deux foyers opposes variables. Arch Mal Coeur 59:263-272
2. El-Sherif N, Turitto G (1999) The long QT syndrome. Pacing Clin Electrophysiol 22:91-110
3. Marsani K, Cowley C, Bekheit S, El-Sherif N (1994) Recurrent syncope for over a decade due to idiopathic ventricular fibrillation. Chest 106:1601-1603
4. Wolfe CL, Nibley C, Bandhari A et al (1991) Polymorphous ventricular tachycardia associated with acute myocardial infarction. Circulation 84:1543-1551
5. El-Sherif N, Caref EB, Yin H et al (1996) The electrophysiological mechanism of ventricular tachyarrhythmias in the long QT syndrome: tridimensional mapping of activation and recovery patterns. Circ Res 79:474-492
6. El-Sherif N, Chinushi M, Caref EB et al (1997) Electrophysiological mechanism of the characteristic electrocardiographic morphology of torsade de pointes tachyarrhythmias in the long QT syndrome. Detailed analysis of ventricular tridimensional activation patterns. Circulation 96:4392-4399
7. Chinushi M, Restivo M, Caref EB et al (1998) Electrophysiological basis of the arrhythmogenicity of QT/T alternans in the long QT syndrome: tridimensional analysis of the kinetics of cardiac repolarization. Circ Res 83:614-628
8. El-Sherif N, Caref EB, Chinushi M, Restivo M (1999) Mechanism of arrhythmogenicity of the short-long cardiac sequence that precedes ventricular tachyarrhythmias in the long QT syndrome. J Am Coll Cardiol 33:1415-1423
9. Leenhardt A, Lucet V, Denjoy I et al (1995) Catecholaminergic polymorphic ventricular tachycardia in children. A 7-year follow-up of 21 patients. Circulation 91:1512-1519
10. Leenhardt A, Glaser E, Burguera M et al (1994) Short-coupled variant of torsade de pointes. A new electrocardiographic entity in the spectrum of idiopathic ventricular tachyarrhythmias. Circulation 89:206-215

11. Brugada P, Brugada J (1992) Right bundle branch block, persistent ST segment elevation and sudden cardiac death: a distinct clinical and electrocardiographic syndrome. A multicenter report. J Am Coll Cardiol 20:1391-1396
12. Baron R, Thacker S, Gorelkin L et al (1983) Sudden death among Southeast Asian refugees. An unexplained nocturnal phenomenon. JAMA 250:2947-2951
13. Nademanee K, Veerakut G, Nimmanit S et al (1997) Arrhythmogenic marker for the sudden unexplained death syndrome in Thai men. Circulation 96:2595-2600
14. Belhassen B, Shapira I, Shoshani D et al (1987) Idiopathic ventricular fibrillation: inducibility and beneficial effects of class I antiarrhythmic agents. Circulation 75:809-816
15. Antzelevitch C, Sicouri S, Litovsky SH et al (1991) Heterogeneity within the ventricular wall: electrophysiology and pharmacology of epicardial, endocardial, and M cells. Circ Res 69:1427-1449
16. Sicouri S, Antzelevitch C (1995) Electrophysiologic characteristics of M cells in the canine left ventricular free wall. J Cardiovasc Electrophysiol 6:591-603
17. Antzelevitch C (1998) The Brugada syndrome. J Cardiovasc Electrophysiol 9:513-516
18. Gussak I, Antzelevitch C, Bjerregaard P et al (1999) The Brugada syndrome. Clinical, electrophysiologic, and genetic aspects. J Am Coll Cardiol 33:5-15
19. Alings M, Wilde A (1999) "Brugada" syndrome. Clinical data and suggested pathophysiological mechanisms. Circulation 99:666-673
20. Chen Q, Kirsch GE, Zhang D et al (1998) Genetic basis and molecular mechanisms for idiopathic ventricular fibrillation. Nature 392:293-245
21. Yan G-X, Antzelevitch C (1996) Cellular basis for the electrocardiographic J wave. Circulation 93:372-379
22. Lukas A, Antzelevitch C (1996) Phase 2 reentry as a mechanism of initiation of circus movement reentry in canine epicardium exposed to simulated ischemia. The antiarrhythmic effects of 4-aminopyridine. Cardiovasc Res 32:593-603
23. Miyazaki T, Mitamura H, Miyoshi S et al (1996) Autonomic and antiarrhythmic drug modulation of ST segment elevation in patients with Brugada syndrome. J Am Coll Cardiol 27:1061-1070
24. Kasanuki H, Ohnishi S, Ohiuka M et al (1997) Idiopathic ventricular fibrillation induced with vagal activity in patients without obvious heart disease. Circulation 95:2277-2285
25. Viskin S, Belhassen B (1998) Polymorphic ventricular tachyarrhythmias in the absence of organic heart diseases: classification, differential diagnosis, and implications for therapy. Progr Cardiovasc Dis 41:17-31
26. Dock W (1929) Transitory ventricular fibrillation as a cause of syncope and its prevention by quinidine sulfate. Am Heart J 4:709-714
27. Corrado D, Nava A, Buja G et al (1996) Familial cardiomyopathy underlies syndrome of right bundle branch block, ST segment elevation and sudden death. J Am Coll Cardiol 27:443-448
28. Tada H, Aihara N, Ohe T et al (1998) Arrhythmogenic right ventricular cardiomyopathy underlies syndrome of right bundle branch block, ST-segment elevation, and sudden death. Am J Cardiol 81:519-522
29. Wichter T, Borggrefe M, Haverkamp W et al (1992) Efficacy of antiarrhythmic drugs in patients with arrhythmogenic right ventricular disease. Circulation 86:29-37

Sudden Infant Death Syndrome and Long-QT Syndrome: What is Their Relationship?

H. Wedekind and G. Breithardt

Sudden Infant Death Syndrome

The sudden infant death syndrome (SIDS) is defined as a sudden death in apparently healthy infants which is unexpected from their history and in which a post-mortem examination fails to demonstrate an adequate cause of death. SIDS has a peak rate at between 2 and 3 months of life [1, 2] and is highest among premature babies and male infants.

Despite intensive research and considerable decline in incidence, SIDS is still the leading cause of death among infants between 1 month and 1 year of age [3]. SIDS has an incidence of 1 per 1000 live births, which means one of every 1000 babies dies of SIDS. In 1994, 38% of postneonatal mortality in Germany was caused by the SIDS [4]. Other parts of the world have similar statistics for SIDS. In the United Kingdom, the incidence of SIDS is 2.5 per 1000 live births, and in the United States 1.6 per 1000 live births [3, 5]. Most of the decline in postneonatal mortality in the U.S. from 4.1/1000 live births in 1980 to 2.9 in 1994 is due to interventions for SIDS [6].

A number of theories on causes of SIDS have been proposed in the past but only a few have been proved so far. Respiratory abnormalities, gastrointestinal diseases, metabolic disorders, epidemiological factors (maternal smoking, prone position of the sleeping baby, non-breastfeeding) and child abuse have frequently been discussed as potential mechanisms. Most of them could be easily dismissed as a frequent cause, although lethal enough in rare instances.

Theories of cardiovascular causes include abnormal reflexes (disorder of the "dive reflex") [7] and abnormalities of the cardiac conduction system [8]. In this context, ventricular fibrillation has been proposed as a cause for SIDS for decades, based on the theories of an abnormal postneonatal development of the nerves controlling cardiac rhythm. The sympathetic innervation of the heart is a

Institute for Arteriosclerosis Research and Department of Cardiology/Angiology, Hospital of the University of Münster, Münster, Germany

developmental process and becomes functionally complete by approximately 6 months of life [9, 10]. During this time, different rates of development give rise to an imbalance in innervation which secondarily leads to QT-prolongation as a sign for abnormal repolarization and vulnerability of the myocardium to malignant arrhythmias.

QT Prolongation as a Risk Factor for SIDS

It is reasonable that a disorder which is associated with sudden death in adults and children with absence of abnormal autopsy findings ("normal heart") would be suspected to cause SIDS. Therefore, since 1976 several prospective studies have been initiated with different results (Table 1).

In 1976, Maron et al. from the National Heart Institute announced that they had found a prolonged QT interval in a significant number of parents of SIDS victims (26%) and of siblings of SIDS patients (39%) [11]. In contrast to this study, Kukolich et al. [12] compared the QT interval in first degree relatives of SIDS victims with that in control subjects and found no significant difference, thus ruling out QT-prolongation as a significant factor in SIDS. In 1983, Southall performed Holter ECGs on nearly 7000 full-term and over 2300 pre-term infants during the first 6 weeks of life [13]. Subsequently, 29 died of SIDS. None of these infants showed a prolonged QT interval in comparison with those of the control group.

The second study by Southall et al. in 1986 measured the QT interval of more than 7000 newborn infants using standard ECG recorders. Of the 15 infants who died subsequently of SIDS, 6 infants had a QTc that exceeded the 90th percentile and one of the 15 infants who died of SIDS had a QTc exceeding the 95th percentile in controls matched for age, birth weight and hospital of birth [5]. In 1998, the results of the "Multicenter Italian Study of Neonatal Electrocardiography and SIDS", coordinated by Peter Schwartz [14] of the University of Milan, Italy, were published. In this large prospective study, ECGs from over 34,000 newborns were

Table 1. Studies on QT interval measurements and SIDS

Author	Year of publication	Enrolled infants	SIDS-victims	No. of victims with significant QTc prolongation	Ref.
Schwartz et al.	1982	4205	3	3[1]	[26]
Southall	1983	6914 full-term, 2337 pre-term	29	none	[13]
Weinstein et al.	1985	1000	8	none	[27]
Southall et al.	1986	7254	15	1[2]	[5]
Schwartz et al.	1998	34442	24	12[3]	[14]

[1] Defined as exceeding more than 2 and 3 standard deviations of QTc in the study group
[2] Defined as exceeding the 95th percentile of QTc in its controls
[3] Defined as a QTc exceeding the 97.5th percentile for the study group

recorded on the 3rd and 4th day of their life between 1976 and 1994. There were 34 deaths in the follow up period of 1 year, of which 24 were caused by SIDS. Half of the infants (12 of 24) had QT interval prolongation and none of the survivors or the infants who died of other causes [10] had a prolonged QTc. The authors conclude that there was a strong association between SIDS and prolongation of the QT interval and that infants with QTc prolongation have an increased susceptibility to life-threatening arrhythmias.

The Long-QT Syndrome

The long-QT syndrome is a cardiac disorder characterized by a prolonged QT interval on the surface electrocardiogram, syncope, seizures, and sudden death from ventricular arrhythmias, specifically torsade de pointes. Two inherited forms of LQT exist: the more common form, the autosomal dominant Romano-Ward syndrome, and the autosomal recessive Jervell and Lange-Nielsen syndrome which is associated with sensorineural deafness. Both syndromes are caused by mutations of genes that encode for cardiac ion channels. At present, mutations in at least four potassium channel genes (HERG, KCNQ1, KCNE1 and KCNE2 [15-18]) and one sodium channel gene (SCN5A) [19] have been identified (Table 2). Penetrance and clinical expressivity are highly variable between and even within families depending on the present genotype and the specific mutation.

Table 2. Molecular genetics of inherited long-QT syndrome. Involved genes, encoding ion channels and distribution of mutations

LQTS subtype	Gene	Chromosome	Current	Proportion (%) of all identified mutations
Romano-Ward syndrome				
LQTS 1	KCNQ1	11p15.5	I_{Ks}	40-60
LQTS 2	HERG	7q35-36	I_{Kr}	30-50
LQTS 3	SCN5A	3p21-24	I_{Na}	5-10
LQTS 4	?	?		<1
LQTS 5	KCNE1	21q22.1-q22.2	I_{Ks}	3-5
LQTS 6	KCNE2	21q22.1-q22.2	I_{Kr}	?
Jervell and Lange-Nielsen syndrome				
JLNS 1	KCNQ1	11p15.5	I_{Ks}	80
JLNS 2	KCNE1	21q22.1-q22.2	I_{Ks}	20
Sporadic LQT syndrome				
LQTS 1	KCNQ1	11p15.5	I_{Ks}	?
LQTS 2	HERG	7q35-36	I_{Kr}	?

LQTS, long-QT syndrome; JLNS, Jervell and Lange-Nielsen syndrome

Pathophysiological Mechanism of Lethal Arrhythmias Due to Prolongation of the QT Interval

Mutations in the five different cardiac ion channel genes lead to prolongation of cardiac repolarization, which predisposes to early afterdepolarizations (EADs) by activation of L-type Ca^{2+} channels [20]. If the EADs have sufficient amplitude, they give rise to triggered activity which is the initiating mechanism for the torsade de pointes tachycardia. Beta-adrenergic receptor activation also activates Ca^{2+} channels [21]. The enhancement of EAD amplitude by sympathetic stimulation may be an explanation for the developmental "sympathetic imbalance" theory as a cause for SIDS.

Genetic Implications

Besides the strong clinical evidence of an association between SIDS and the LQTS, there is still controversial discussion on to what extent QT prolongation may cause SIDS. Over many years, the QT prolongation was interpreted as a clinical sign of abnormal repolarization without a clear association to a morphological substrate in the heart. The revolutionary developments in cardiovascular biology over the past 10 years have led to an understanding of the genetic basis of QT prolongation. The long-QT syndrome is considered to be a "channelopathy". We are now able to bring further genetic information to bear on the question of in how many cases of SIDS victims a LQTS mutation is present. But we should keep in mind that QT prolongation may act as a arrhythmogenic substrate, which requires further trigger factors (e.g., epigenetic or environmental) for the development of life-threatening arrhythmias. This may explain the fact that not all infants with prolonged QT interval develop TdP-tachycardia and suffer from SIDS. Although SIDS is not a familial disease like inherited LQTS, absence of mutations in the genetic testing of relatives of the victim does not exclude LQTS as the cause leading to death because spontaneous mutations may occur. Since the risk of death as a first cardiac event ranges between 2% and 15% according to the genotype [22], an infant with LQTS due to a spontaneous mutation may die with the first arrhythmia, and if no electrocardiograms were available, the infant is thought to be a SIDS victim.

Another important issue should be considered when thinking about LQTS and SIDS. Besides genetic heterogeneity, LQTS occurs with variable penetrance and expressivity, referred to as phenotypic heterogeneity [23, 24]. About 10% of patients, mostly males, have a normal QTc interval (< 0.44 s), and 30% have a borderline prolonged QTc (0.45-0.47s) at initial presentation [25]. Thus, a normal QTc does not exclude LQTS. In those families the parents and the siblings may function as gene carriers although they have normal QT intervals and are thought to be unaffected. Genetic testing in those individuals would be an ideal tool to identify families at risk of SIDS because of low penetrance of LQTS. Furthermore, genetic investigation of SIDS victims and electrophysiological studies of identified mutations will help us to determine the proportion of congenital LQTS as an underlying cause for SIDS.

Acknowledgements. This work was supported by a research grant from the Center for Innovative Medical Research (IMF, We-1-2-II/97) of the University of Münster, Münster, Germany.

References

1. Guntheroth WG (1989) Theories of cardiovascular causes in sudden infant death syndrome. J Am Coll Cardiol 14:443-447
2. Froggatt P, Lynas MA, McKenzie G (1971) Epidemiology of sudden unexpected death in infancy ("cot death") in Northern Ireland. Br J Prev Soc Med 25:119-134
3. Dwyer T, Ponsonby AL (1995) SIDS epidemiology and incidence. Pediatr Ann 24:350-352, 354-356
4. Schellscheidt J, Ott A, Jorch G (1997) Epidemiological features of sudden infant death after a German intervention campaign in 1992. Eur J Pediatr 156:655-660
5. Southall DP, Arrowsmith WA, Stebbens V, Alexander JR (1986) QT interval measurements before sudden infant death syndrome. Arch Dis Child 61:327-333
6. Scott CL, Iyasu S, Rowley D, Atrash HK (1998) Postneonatal mortality surveillance - United States, 1980-1994. Mor Mortal Wkly Rep CDC Surveill Summ 47(2):15-30
7. Wolf S (1966) Sudden death and the oxygen conserving reflex. Am Heart J 71:840-841
8. James TN (1968) Sudden death in babies: new observations in the heart. Am J Cardiol 22:457-506
9. Schwartz PJ (1976) Cardiac sympathetic innervation and the sudden infant death syndrome. Am J Med 60:167-172
10. Gootmann PM (1986) Developmental neurobiology of the autonomic nervous system. Humana Press, Clifton, N.J.
11. Maron BJ, Clark CE, Goldstein RE, Epstein SE (1976) Potential role of Q-T interval prolongation in sudden infant death syndrome. Circulation 54:423-430
12. Kukolich MK, Telsey A, Ott J, Motulsky AG (1977) Sudden infant death syndrome: normal Q-T interval in ECGs of relatives. Pediatrics 60:51-54
13. Southall DP (1983) Identification of infants destined to die unexpectedly during infancy: evaluation of predictive importance of prolonged apnoea and disorders of cardiac rhythm or conduction. B M J 286:1092-1096
14. Schwartz PJ, Stramba-Badiale M, Segantini A, Austoni P, Bosi G, Giorgetti R, Grancini F, Marni ED, Perticone F, Rosti D, Salice P (1998) Prolongation of the QT interval and the sudden infant death syndrome. N Engl J Med 338:1709-1714
15. Curran ME, Splawski I, Timothy KW, Vincent GM, Green ED, Keating MT (1995) A molecular basis for cardiac arrhythmias: HERG mutations cause long QT syndrome. Cell 80:795-803
16. Wang Q, Curran ME, Splawski I, Burn TC, Millholland JM, Van Raay TJ, Shen J, Towbin JA, Mon AJ, Atkinson DL, Lander GM, Conners TD, Keating MT (1996) Positional cloning of a novel potassium channel gene: KVLQT1 mutations cause cardiac arrhythmias. Nature Genet 12:17-23
17. Schulze-Bahr E, Wang Q, Wedekind H, Haverkamp W, Chen Q, Sun Y, Rubie C, Hördt M, Towbin JA, Borggrefe M, Assmann G, Qu X, Somberg JC, Breithardt G, Oberti C, Funke H (1997) KCNE1 mutations cause Jervell and Lange-Nielsen syndrome. Nature Genet 17:267-268

18. Abbott GW, Sesti F, Splawski I, Buck ME, Lehmann Mh, Timothy KW, Keating MT, Goldstein SAN (1999) MiRP1 forms IKr potassium channels with HERG and is associated with cardiac arrhythmia. Cell 97:175-187

19. Wang Q, Shen J, Splawski I, Atkinson D, Li Z, Robinson JL, Moss AJ, Towbin JA, Keating MT (1995) SCN5A mutations associated with an inherited cardiac arrhythmia, long QT syndrome. Cell 80:805-811

20. January CT, Riddle JM (1989) Early afterdepolarisations: mechanism of induction and block: a role for L-type Ca^{2+} current. Circ Res 64:977-990

21. Jurevicius J, Fischmeister R (1996) cAMP compartmentation is responsible for a local activation of cardiac Ca^{2+} channels by beta-adrenergic agonists. Proc Natl Acad Sci USA 93:295-299

22. Zareba W, Moss AJ, Schwartz PJ, Vincent GM, Robinson JL, Priori SG, Benhorin J, Locati EH, Towbin JA, Keating MT, Lehmann MH, Hall WJ (1998) Influence of the genotype on the clinical course of the long-QT syndrome. International Long-QT Syndrome Registry Research Group. N Engl J Med 339:960-965

23. Priori SG, Napolitano C, Schwartz PJ (1999) Low penetrance in the long-QT syndrome: clinical impact. Circulation 99:529-533

24. Wedekind H, Schulze-Bahr E, Haverkamp W, Hördt M, Borggrefe M, Assmann G, Breithardt G, Funke H (1997) Reduced penetrance of a missense mutation in chromosome 11-specific long-QT syndrome. Circulation 18[Suppl]:29

25. Vincent GM, Timothy KW, Zhang L (1996) High prevalence of normal QT interval in patients with the inherited long QT syndrome: important implications for diagnosis. Pacing Clin Electrophysiol 19:588

26. Schwartz PJ, Montemerlo M, Facchini M, Salice P, Rosti D, Poggio G, Giorgetti R (1982) The QT interval throughout the first 6 months of life: a prospective study. Circulation 66:496-501

27. Weinstein SL, Steinschneider A (1985) QTc and R-R intervals in victims of the sudden infant death syndrome. Am J Dis Child 139:987-990

Brugada and Long QT Syndrome Are Two Different Diseases: True or False?

S.G. Priori and L. Crotti

Despite the fact that most events of cardiac arrest (CA) occur in individuals with structural heart disease, a significant percentage (estimated around 3%-8% of CA) of young subjects who die suddenly have no demonstrable structural heart disease at autopsy. The term "idiopathic" ventricular fibrillation (IVF) has been adopted to refer to this group of individuals. The world's largest series of individuals resuscitated from CA and labeled as affected by IVF has been collected in a registry called UCARE [1] by a group of European investigators acting under the auspices of the European Society of Cardiology. According to the UCARE's experience [2] based on 153 individuals followed for a mean follow-up of 5 years, the risk of recurrence of CA in IVF is 25%-30%. Accordingly the use of implantable cardiac defibrillator (ICD) appear justified in this population of patients irrespective of the outcome of programmed electrical stimulation. The hypothesis that CA in IVF survivors may be the "early" manifestation of a disease that will progress over time is not supported by the evidence that only a minority (5%) of these individuals develop an overt structural heart disease at follow-up.

We have proposed [2] that patients with IVF may either experience an arrhythmic event caused by a "transient" abnormality that escaped clinical evaluation post-resuscitation (e.g., electrolyte imbalance, myocarditis) or they may have a so-called "primary electrical disease".

Recent data combining clinical and molecular studies have presented evidence that genetic defects of ion channels may predispose individuals with an otherwise normal heart to CA [3]. Two diseases are classified among the "cardiac ion channelopathies": Long QT Syndrome (LQTS) [4] and Brugada Syndrome [5].

Laboratori di Cardiologia Molecolare, Fondazione Salvatore Maugeri, IRCCS, Pavia, Italy

Long QT Syndrome

LQTS is a familiar disease characterized by an abnormally prolonged QT interval (QTc > 440 ms in males, > 460 ms in females) and by stress-mediated life-threatening ventricular arrhythmias.

LQTS usually manifests itself in children and teenagers [4]. Since its original description [6, 7], it has become clear that no clinically relevant structural cardiac abnormality is present in LQTS patients. The trigger for most of the episodes of life-threatening arrhythmias is represented by a sudden increase in sympathetic activity, mostly mediated by the left cardiac sympathetic nerves. Indeed, antiadrenergic therapies provide the greatest degree of protection.

In 1995 and 1996 major developments occurred in the understanding of the genetic basis of LQTS. It rapidly became clear that more than one gene accounts for the disease; genes were in fact identified in chromosomes 3 (LQT3) [8, 9], 7 (LQT2) [8, 10], 11 (LQT1) [11] and 21 (LQT5) [12, 13].

All these genes encode for subunits of cardiac ion channels: SCN5A on chromosome 3 encodes for α-subunit of the cardiac sodium channel, HERG on chromosome 7 encodes for a potassium channel producing the Ikr current and KVLQT1 and KCNE1 encode for two subunits of the channel conducting the slow component of the delayed rectifier (Iks). Within each of these genes, several different mutations have been identified, suggesting that each different mutation has the potential to represent a distinct disease.

Brugada Syndrome

Brugada Syndrome is a recently (1992) described familiar disease [5, 14], characterized by right bundle-branch block and ST-segment elevation in leads V1 through V3, with normal QT interval and no demonstrable structural heart disease. Patients with this disease are at high risk of ventricular fibrillation and sudden death, typically occurring during sleep [5]. The ECG pattern of Brugada Syndrome has been identified in subjects with structural abnormalities of the right ventricle. Martini et al. [15] suggested that this pattern in conjunction with structural heart disease may represent a novel syndrome associated with high risk of sudden death.

Interestingly, the electrocardiographic pattern diagnostic for the disease is intermittently present in affected individuals: a provocative test based on the intravenous administration of sodium channel blockers (mainly ajmaline or flecainide) is used to unmask the ECG features in the concealed forms of the disease [5, 14].

Brugada Syndrome has a mean age of onset of 30-35 years and phenotypic manifestations are more pronounced in males than in females: this is at variance with LQTS which is more frequently manifest in young females [4].

Pharmacological treatment with amiodarone and/or β-blockers does not protect patients against sudden arrhythmic death, and an implantable defibrillator is so far the only alternative for symptomatic patients [5]. The value of programmed electrical stimulation (PES) in the risk stratification process for Brugada Syndrome is still unclear. Accordingly, the decision is still arbitrary of whether it is appropriate to investigate asymptomatic patients by PES and to implant an ICD in all individuals with inducible VF. To define sensitivity and specificity of PES in predicting the outcome of asymptomatic individuals is currently the most important target of research in the field.

When in 1998 Chen et al. [16] identified the first Brugada-related gene, it was with some degree of surprise that it turned out to be SCN5A, the same gene implicated in the "LQT3" variant of Long QT Syndrome. The issue may be raised whether LQT3 and Brugada Syndrome are distinct diseases or whether overlapping exists between some phenotypic manifestations of the two conditions.

SCN5A: Gene for Two Diseases

In 1992 Gellens et al. [17] cloned and characterized the voltage-gated cardiac sodium channel SCN5A, responsible for the initial upstroke of the action potential in the electrocardiogram. This channel protein contains four homologous domains (DI-DIV), each of which has six putative membrane-spanning regions (S1-S6).

SCN5A Mutations in LQTS

Three mutations were initially identified [9, 18] in six families linked to chromosome 3 which involved a 9-base pair deletion (ΔKPQ) and two point mutations (R1644H and N1325S).

All of these three mutations affect a region important for the inactivation of the Na$^+$ current. Subsequently, Bennett et al. [19] characterized the ΔKPQ mutation by expressing in *Xenopus oocytes* the altered cardiac sodium channel. Mutant channels showed a sustained inward current during membrane depolarization which is likely to disrupt the normal balance between inward and outward currents during the plateau phase and hence prolong cardiac action potential (long QT). The explanation of this persistent inward sodium current came from the single-channel recordings showing mutant channel fluctuation between normal and non-inactivating gating modes (multiple reopening) which is not observed in normal channels. Dumaine et al. [20] further characterized the electrophysiological consequences of the ΔKPQ and the two point mutations. Once expressed in *Xenopus oocytes*, all three mutations increased sodium inward current, however ΔKPQ resulted in quantitatively larger changes in the sodium current, suggesting that this mutation may be associated to a more severe phenotype.

Recently novel mutations have been described (T1645M and T1304M) associated with more benign ECG phenotypes [21].

Benhorin et al. [22] reported a novel SCN5A missense mutation (D1790G), located near the C-terminus of the α-subunit, a region not associated with major functional channel properties. An et al. [23] further characterized the electrophysiological consequences of this mutation. They found no significant effect of D1790G on the biophysical properties of monomeric α-subunit. Coassembling α and β1-subunit steady-state inactivation is shifted by -16 mV, but there is no D1790G-induced sustained inward current. So it is not clear how this mutation can be associated to QT prolongation in LQTS.

SCN5A Mutations in Brugada Syndrome

The genetic defect of Brugada Syndrome was described in 1998 when Chen et al. [16] identified the first mutations in the cardiac sodium channel gene SCN5A, R1232W and T1620M, in the extracellular loops of DIII (S1-S2) and DIV (S3-S4), respectively. Once expressed in *Xenopus oocytes*, T1620M showed a shift in the voltage dependence of steady-state inactivation towards more positive potentials, associated with a faster recovery from inactivation, wheras R1232W behaves like normal channels and probably constitutes a rare polymorphism. We (S.G. Priori and R. Kass, personal communication) recently identified in a LQTS patient a mutation on SCN5A that, when expressed in vitro, also presented a shift in the voltage dependence of steady-state inactivation towards more positive potentials associated with a faster recovery from inactivation.

Chen et al. [16] also identified an insertion of two nucleotides in the intracellular loop between S2 and S3 of DI and a single nucleotide deletion in DIII S6. The insertion disrupts a splice-donor site, but the functional consequences of this splicing mutation have not been studied. The deletion introduces a premature in-frame stop codon and mutant m-RNA failed to express I_{Na} in *Xenopus oocytes* [16]. This suggests that affected patients would have a 50% reduction of sodium channels. However, this is a huge decrease, so preferential expression of the normal allele has been advocated [24].

Alshinawi et al. [24] identified other two mutations: A1924T and R1512W, in the highly conserved DIII-IV cytoplasmic linker and in the C-terminal cytoplasmic domain respectively. Once expressed in *Xenopus oocytes* these mutations showed a negative voltage shift of steady-state inactivation, thus reducing sodium current availability, possibly leading to a reduction of the action potential duration (APD).

Yan and Antzelevitch [25] proposed a hypothesis that would link APD shortening due to reduced I_{Na} to the distinctive ECG pattern of the Brugada Syndrome. They speculated that a transmural inhomogeneity in action potential duration could explain the observed ST-segment elevation and might lead to an increase in arrhythmogeneity. In contrast to endocardial cells, action potentials (APs) of epicardial cells display a pronounced phase 1, referred to as "spike-and-dome morphology". The transient outward current, Ito, which is present in epicardial cells and virtually absent in endocardial cells, underlines the difference between the AP configuration [26]. The magnitude and duration of sodium current, I_{Na}, during phase 0 determines the voltage level at which phase 1 begins; this will have an impact on activation/inactivation characteristics of Ito.

Theoretically a reduction in I_{Na}, as observed in some of the mutations identified in Brugada Syndrome patients, such as A1924T and R1512W [24], may cause a loss of AP dome in epicardial cells that shortens epicardial AP duration. This causes transmural heterogeneity and ST-segment elevation as a result of transmural current flow from endocardium to epicardium [25]. It can be hypothesized that, because of the thinness of the right ventricular wall, the relative contribution of epicardial APs to the surface ECG is more prominent in right than left precordial leads. In addition, it has been demonstrated in dogs that Ito-mediated phase 1 is more pronounced in right than left ventricular epicardium [27]. Hence, the impact of changes in epicardial AP morphology will be most pronounced in right precordial leads (V1-V2-V3). The association between in vitro abnormalities and ECG phenotype is still undetermined for point mutations such as T1620M that fail to show a reduction of I_{Na}.

Is there a Clear-Cut Distinction Between LQT3 and Brugada Syndrome?

It is not uncommon in genetic disorders for two distinct clinical diseases to be the manifestation of different mutations of the same gene. Accordingly, when the evidence became available that some Brugada Syndrome patients present mutations in the cardiac sodium channel, the novel information did not elicit much surprise. At that time (March 1998) the current understanding about LQT3 was that mutations leading to QT prolongation were located in a relatively restricted region of the gene (the DIII-DIV intracellular linker) responsible for inactivation of the sodium current. Mutations located in this region would cause a delay in the inactivation leading to APD prolongation . In the past few months, we and others have described a more complex picture. Patients labeled as "LQT3" (i.e. individuals with prolonged QT interval, and carriers of a mutation in the SCN5A gene) have mutations in portions of the gene unrelated to the control of sodium channel inactivation. Furthermore, mutations spaced few base pairs apart may lead to LQT3 or to Brugada syndrome (T1620M leading to Brugada Syndrome, R1623Q leading to LQT3): this evidence contradicts the initial hypothesis that the topology of the mutations accounted for the clinical phenotype. Unpublished data that we have obtained in collaboration with Robert Kass indicate that the patients with the clinical phenotype of long QT interval have sodium channel mutations leading to a faster recovery from inactivation, i.e. the cellular phenotype described by Chen et al. [16] for mutations (T1620M) leading to Brugada Syndrome. This observation raises the possibility that a phenotypic overlapping may exist and that "transitional" defects leading to an intermediate phenotype may occur. It should be noted that the hypothesis formulated by the group of Antzelevitch [25, 26] to link the cellular defect of

Brugada syndrome to the phenotype (ST segment elevation) concerns only those mutations which lead to a loss of function (splice error and truncations) and not the point mutations which cause a faster recovery from inactivation. The evidence that mutations associated to identical functional changes may be present in LQT3 patients adds a degree of complexity and raises the intriguing possibility that "Brugada Syndrome" and "LQT3" may represent the extreme manifestation of a spectrum of sodium channel defects.

Conclusions

Identification of sodium channel mutations has revealed an unforeseen complexity in the clinical genetics of cardiac ion channel diseases. At variance with potassium channels related variants of LQTS, where the loss of function of the mutant proteins accounts for the phenotype, this link is still missing in sodium channel diseases. The understanding of the cellular basis of the abnormal phenotype is not merely an intellectual curiosity but bears important implications for the identification of gene-specific therapies in LQT3 and Brugada Syndrome.

References

1. Priori SG, Borggrefe M, Camm AJ, Hauer NW, Klein H, Kuck KH, Schwartz PJ, Touboul P, Wellens HJJ (1992) Unexplained cardiac arrest. The need for a prospective registry. Eur Heart J 13:1445-1446
2. Priori SG, Paganini V (1997) Idiopathic ventricular fibrillation: epidemiology, pathophysiology, primary prevention, immediate evaluation and management, long-term evaluation and management, experimental and theoretical developments. Cardiac Electrophysiol Review 1:244-247
3. Priori SG, Barhanin J, Hauer RNW, Haverkamp W, Habo JJ, Kleber AG, McKenna WJ, Roden DM, Rudy Y, Schwartz K, Schwartz PJ, Towbin JA, Wilde AM (1999) Genetic and molecular basis of cardiac arrhythmias: impact on clinical management. (part I, II) Circulation 99:518-528
4. Schwartz PJ, Locati EH, Napolitano C, Priori SG (1995) The long QT syndrome. In: Zipes DP, Jalife J (eds) Cardiac electrophysiology. From cell to bedside (2nd edn). W.B. Saunders Philadelphia, pp 788-811
5. Brugada J, Brugada R, Brugada P (1998) Right bundle branch block, ST segment elevation in leads V1-V3: a marker for sudden death in patients without demonstrable structural heart disease. Circulation 97:457-460
6. Romano C, Gemme G, Pongiglione R (1963) Aritmie cardiache rare dell'età pediatrica. La Clin Pediatr 45:656-683
7. Ward OC (1964) A new familial cardiac syndrome in children. J Irish Med Assoc 54:103-106
8. Yiang C, Atkinson D, Towbin JA, Splawski I, Lehmann MH, Li H, Timothy K, Taggart RT, Schwartz PJ, Vincent GM, Moss AJ, Keating MT (1994) Two long QT syndrome loci map to chromosomes 3 and 7 with evidence for further heterogeneity. Nat

Genet 8:141-147

9. Wang Q, Shen J, Splaswki I, Atkinson D, Li Z, Robinson JL, Moss AJ, Towbin JA, Keating MT (1995) SCN5A mutations associated with an inherited cardiac arrhythmia, long QT syndrome. Cell 80:805-811

10. Curran ME, Splawski I, Timothy KW, Vincent GM, Green ED, Keating MT (1995) A molecular basis for cardiac arrhythmia: HERG mutations cause long QT syndrome. Cell 80:795-803

11. Wang Q, Curran ME, Splawski I, Burn TC, Millholland JM, Van Raay TJ, Shen J, Timothy KW, De Jager T, Schwartz PJ, Towbin JA, Moss AJ, Atkinson DL, Landes GM, Connors TD, Keating MT (1996) Positional cloning of a novel potassium channel gene: KvLQT1 mutations cause cardiac arrhythmias. Nat Genet 12:17-23

12. Sanguinetti MC, Curran ME, Zou A, Shen J, Spector PS, Atkinson DL, Keating MT (1996) Coassembly of KvLQT1 and minK (IsK) proteins to form cardiac Iks potassium channel. Nature 384:78-80

13. Barhanin J, Lesage F, Guillemare E, Fink M, Lazdunski M, Romey G (1996) KvLQT1 and IsK (minK) proteins associate to form the Iks cardiac potassium current. Nature 384:78-80

14. Brugada P, Brugada J (1992) Right bundle branch block, persistent ST segment elevation and sudden cardiac death: a distinct clinical and electrocardiographic syndrome. J Am Coll Cardiol 20:1391-1396

15. Martini B, Corrado D, Nava A, Thiene G (1997) Syndrome of right bundle branch block, ST-segment elevation and sudden death. Evidence of an organic substrate. In: Nava A, Rossi L, Thiene G eds: Arrhythmogenic right ventricular cardiomyopathy/dysplasia. Elsevier, Amsterdam, pp 438-453

16. Chen Q, Kirsch GE, Zhang D, Brugada J, Brugada R, Brugada P, Potenza D, Moya A, Borggrefe M, Breithardt G, Ortiz-Lopez R, Wang Z, Antzelevitch C, O'Brien RE, Schulze-Bahr E, Keating M, Towbin JA, Wang Q (1998) Genetic basis and molecular mechanism for idiopathic ventricular fibrillation. Nature 392:293-295

17. Gellens ME, George AL Jr, Chen L, Chahine M, Horn R, Barchi RL, Kallen RG (1992) Primary structure and functional expression of the human cardiac tetrodotoxin-insensitive voltage-dependent sodium channel. Proc Nat Acad Sci 89:554-558

18. Wang Q, Shen J, Li Z, Timoty K, Vincent GM, Priori SG, Schwartz PJ, Keating MT (1995) Cardiac sodium channel mutations in patients with long QT syndrome, an inherited cardiac arrhythmia. Hum Mol Gen 4:1603-1607

19. Bennet PB, Yazawa K, Makita N, George AL (1995) Molecular mechanism for an inherited cardiac arrhythmia. Nature 376:683-685

20. Dumaine R, Wang Q, Keating MT, Hartmann HA, Schwartz PJ, Brown AM, Kirsch GE (1996) Multiple mechanisms of sodium channel-linked long QT syndrome. Circ Res 78:916-924

21. Wattanasirichaigoon D, Vasely MR, Duggal P, Beggs AH (1997) Mutations of SCN5A are infrequent in patients with long QT syndrome. Circulation 97[Suppl]:56 (abstr)

22. Benhorin J, Goldmit M, MacCluer J, Blangero J, Goffen R, Leibovitch A, Rahat A, Wang Q, Medina A, Towbin J, Karem B (1997) Identification of a new SCN5A mutation associated with the long QT syndrome. Hum Genet:153 (on line)

23. An RH, Wang XL, Kerem B, Benhorin J, Medina A, Goldmit M, Kass RS (1998) Novel LQT3 mutation affects Na+ channel activity through interaction between alpha and beta1 subunits. Circ Res 83:141-146

24. Alshinawi C, Mannens M, Wilde A (1998) Mutations in the human cardiac sodium channel gene (SCN5A) in patients with Brugadaís syndrome. Eur Heart J 19 [Suppl]:78 (abstr)

25. Yan GX, Antzelevitch C (1996) Cellular basis for the electrocardiographic J wave. Circulation 93:372-379
26. Litovsky SH, Antzelevitch C (1989) Rate dependance of action potential duration and refractoriness in canine ventricular endocardium differs from that of epicardium: role of transient outward current. J Am Coll Cardiol 14:1053-1066
27. Di Diego JM, Sun ZQ, Antzelevitch C (1996) Ito and action potential notch are smaller in left vs. right canine ventricular epicardium. Am J Physiol 271:H548-H561

Effect of β-Blocker Therapy on the Frequency and Type of Cardiac Events in Patients with the Hereditary Long QT Syndrome

A.J. Moss[1], W. Zareba[1], W.J. Hall[2], J.L. Robinson[3] and M.L. Andrews[3]

The hereditary long QT syndrome (LQTS) is a genetic channelopathy in which affected individuals have prolonged ventricular repolarization, frequent syncopal episodes, and a propensity to sudden arrhythmic cardiac death [1, 2]. β-Blocker therapy is the recommended treatment of choice for this disorder, although other forms of therapy are also used including pacemakers to prevent bradycardia-induced ventricular tachyarrhythmias [3], surgical antiadrenergic therapy with left cervico-thoracic sympathetic ganglionectomy [4], and implantable cardioverter defibrillators [5] in patients refractory to β-blocker therapy.

In the course of our clinical experience, we have noted that β-blockers have not always been effective in preventing cardiac events (syncope, aborted cardiac arrest, or sudden death) in LQTS. In this study, we report on the type and frequency of cardiac events during equal exposure times before and after the initiation of β-blockers in a large population of patients with LQTS. The findings from this study indicate that β-blockers reduce the rate of cardiac events in probands with LQTS, but some patients continue to experience syncope and sudden death while receiving antiadrenergic therapy.

Methods

Study Population

The study population was drawn from the Rochester portion of the International LQTS Registry [1, 2]. Only LQTS patients who had β-blocker therapy prescribed after 1 year but less than 40 years of age, had risk exposure for cardiac events for at least one year before and after initiation of β-blockers, and were less than 41 years of age at follow-up after starting β-blockers were included in this study ($n = 475$).

Departments of [1]Medicine, [2]Biostatistics, and [3]Community and Preventive Medicine, University of Rochester School of Medicine and Dentistry, Rochester, NY, USA

Risk Exposure

Each patient served as his or her own control. For each LQTS patient, the duration of the risk-exposure after initiation of β-blockers was precisely matched to the same duration before starting β-blockers.

β-Blocker Therapy

β-blocker therapy was initiated at the discretion of the patient's attending physician. A variety of β-blockers were prescribed to the LQTS patients, with acebutalol, atenolol, metoprolol, nadolol, propranolol, and timolol making up the vast majority of these medications. During routine yearly follow-up, we recorded the date β-blocker therapy was started. At subsequent yearly contacts we recorded whether or not the patient continued an active prescription for β-blockers. Among patients who died, we retrospectively determined if the patient had an active prescription for β-blockers at the time of death. We do not have complete data on the dosage of the β-blocker or the degree of compliance with the prescribed therapy in all patients.

LQTS-Related Cardiac Events

LQTS-related cardiac events include unexplained syncope, aborted cardiac arrest requiring cardiac resuscitation, and unexpected, sudden death exclusive of a known cause before age 41 years. We refer to the latter as LQTS-related death. The date and character of these events were identified through our routine, yearly follow-up contact with the individual, his or her family, or the personal attending physician.

Data Management and Analysis

Clinical data were recorded on prospectively designed forms and included demographic, historical, family history, electrocardiographic, therapeutic, and cardiac event information. Quality control procedures were in place throughout the study to ensure internal consistency of the recorded data on printed data forms and to minimize missing data when they could be retrieved. The study data were maintained in a relational data-base system (Ingres) on a Sun computer. The reported analyses used the analytic data-base version 9.0 released October 22, 1997.

All statistical analyses were for paired data, comparing occurrence of cardiac events, counts of cardiac events, and rates of cardiac events in patients before and after initiation of β-blocker therapy. As noted above, periods of identical durations before and after therapy were used for each patient. Since β-blocker therapy was frequently initiated following an LQTS-related cardiac event, the last cardiac event in the month prior to initiation of β-blockers was not counted in the paired analyses. We used this approach to minimize therapy-associated bias when comparing pre- and post-β-blocker cardiac events and cardiac event rates. A few patients had unusually large numbers of cardiac events. To prevent these isolated cases from dominating the events analyses, numbers of cardiac events greater than 25 for a given patient before or after β-blockers were counted as 25.

When comparing the numbers of patients with any cardiac events before and after β-blockers, McNemar's X^2 test was used. When comparing counts of cardiac events or rates of cardiac events, Wilcoxon's signed-rank test was used. All p-values are two-sided, and all were confirmed by permutation tests. Analyses involving β-blocker therapy utilized the intention-to-treat principle. That is, we considered a patient to be on β-blocker treatment once this medication was initiated, whether or not the patient complied or was later taken off β-blockers. The time-to-event analyses were estimated by the Kaplan-Meier method.

Results

Population Characteristics

The LQTS study population was subdivided into probands ($n = 308$) and affected family members ($n = 167$) (Table 1). The probands had a higher percentage of females, had a slower heart rate on the first recorded electrocardiogram, and were more likely to have received antiarrhythmic therapy in addition to β-blockers at some time in their clinical course than were affected family members.

Table 1. Characteristics of the LQTS study population

	Probands ($n = 308$)	Affected family members ($n = 167$)
Demographics		
Age at first cardiac event[a] (years)	13 ± 9[b]	13 ± 7
Age β-blockers started (years)	17 ± 10	16 ± 11
Sex (% of females)	71	53
History		
Congenital deafness (%)	6	1
Syncope or aborted cardiac arrest before β-blockers (%)	62	21
ECG findings[c]		
Heart rate (beats/min)	71 ± 19	79 ± 22
QT$_c$ (s)[d]	0.51 ± 0.06	0.50 ± 0.04
Non-β-blocker therapy at any time (%)		
Pacemaker	23	9
Sympathetic ganglionectomy	10	2
Implanted defibrillator	8	1

[a] For patients with at least one cardiac event (syncope or aborted cardiac arrest)
[b] Plus-minus values are mean ± SD
[c] On the first recorded electrocardiogram
[d] QT$_c$, QT interval corrected for heart rate

Cardiac Events and Cardiac Event Rates

The average duration of risk exposure before and after β-blocker therapy was similar in the probands and affected family members (6.7 and 5.5 years, respectively) (Table 2). The number of patients experiencing any cardiac events, as well as the total number of events, the mean number of events per patient, and the mean rate of cardiac events per year were significantly reduced ($p < 0.001$) after β-blocker therapy in probands, but not in affected family members. Aborted car-

Table 2. Cardiac events in probands and affected family members before and after initiation of β-blocker treatment

	Probands ($n = 308$[a])		Affected family members ($n = 167$[a])	
	Before BB	After BB	Before BB	After BB
Risk exposure				
Before and after β-blockers (years)				
Mean ± SD	6.7 ± 4.5		5.5 ± 3.4	
Min., Max	1.0, 19.9		1.0, 15.7	
Person-years	2061		910	
Cardiac events[b]				
Patients with any events (%)	62	39	21	19
p-value (McNemar χ^2 test)	< 0.001		ns	
No. of events	763	329	84	85
Events per patient (mean ± SD)	2.6 ± 4.8	1.1 ± 2.5	0.5 ± 1.6	0.5 ± 2.7
p-value[c]	<0.001		ns	
Aborted cardiac arrest or LQTS-				
related death (n)	19	26	3	7
LQTS-related death (n)	–	7	–	7
Chance of cardiac event within				
5 years after BB[d] (%; SE)	–	37; 3	–	15; 3
Cardiac event rates[+]				
Events/year (mean ± SD)	0.54 ± 1.56	0.20 ± 0.44	0.12 ± 0.73	0.15 ± 0.93
p-value[c]	<0.001		ns	

BB, β-blocker; ns, not significant; SE, standard error
[a]For 11 probands and 3 affected family members, the occurrence but not the count of cardiac events before and after β-blockers was known; these patients were omitted when the number of cardiac events was utilized in the analyses
[b]Cardiac events before β-blockers include syncope or aborted cardiac arrest; after β-blockers cardiac events also include LQTS-related death
The last cardiac event that occurred in the month before initiation of β-blockers was excluded (see text for explanation). If a patient had more than 25 cardiac events in a pre- or post-β-blocker period, the number was counted as 25
[c]Signed-rank, paired t-test, and permutation tests gave similar p values
[d]Estimated by Kaplan-Meier method, using data in the post-β-blocker period only

diac arrest or LQTS-related death occurred in 8.4% (26/308) of probands and 4.1% (7/167) of affected family members after initiation of β-blockers. The likelihood of experiencing at least one cardiac event (syncope, aborted cardiac arrest, or LQTS-related death) within 5 years after initiation of β-blocker therapy was 37% in probands and 15% in affected family members.

LQTS-Related Death

Seven probands and seven affected family members died suddenly and unexpectedly during follow-up after initiation of β-blocker treatment. Females made up 79% of these patients, and QTc values (0.50 ± 0.04) were similar to those in the overall LQTS population. β-Blocker treatment was started mostly in early adolescence, with death on average 6 years later at 19 ± 6 years. A larger percentage of probands than of affected family members had cardiac events before initiation of β-blockers. Of note, 79% (11/14) of those who died had an active prescription for β-blockers from their physician on the day of death. We do not have information on whether the patients were actually taking β-blockers in the 24-h period before death. None of the 14 patients who died had congenital deafness. The overall LQTS-related cardiac death rate after starting β-blockers averaged 0.3% per year for probands and 0.8% per year for affected family members.

Discussion

The current study indicates that β-blocker therapy is associated with a significant reduction in the mean rate of cardiac events in probands. The low cardiac event rate in the affected family members before initiation of β-blockers may explain the absence of β-blocker effect in this lower-risk group. However, this study also points up the limitations of this therapy. Fourteen patients experienced LQTS-related sudden death during follow-up after initiation of β-blocker treatment, with 11 of the 14 patients having an active prescription for β-blockers on the day of death.

Since we have only limited data on the genotype makeup of the study population, we have not included analyses of cardiac events that occurred after β-blocker therapy by specific genotype. It may be that β-blockers are effective in preventing sudden death in the LQT1 genotype as suggested by Vincent et al. in 1996 [6].

This was not a randomized clinical trial, and thus the results are subject to potential bias. We tried to minimize bias by having each patient serve as his/her own control during equal periods of exposure before and after initiation of β-blockers. We attempted to be as conservative as possible and followed an intention-to-treat type of analysis. Because of incomplete data, we have not provided event rates in terms of specific β-blockers or the dose of β-blockers utilized by the study population. Poor compliance or inadequate β-blocker dosage may account for some of the recurrent life-threatening arrhythmic events observed after initiation of β-blocker treatment in this study. On the other hand, β-blockers

Table 3. LQTS-related death after initiation of β-blocker treatment in probands and affected family members[a]

Patient no	Sex	QTc[b] (s)	Age β-blocker started (years)	Age at death (years)	Events before β-blockers		Events after β-blockers		Active prescription for β-blockers at time of death	Other LQTS treatment[c]
					Syncope	ACA	Syncope	ACA		
Probands										
1	M	0.45	8	13	+	-	-	+	Y	PM, LCTSG
2	F	0.45	13	19	+	-	+	-	Y	
3	F	0.46	7	11	+	-	-	-	Y	
4	F	0.46	16	22	+	-	-	-	N	
5	M	0.47	14	25	+	-	+	-	N	
6	F	0.49	14	15	+	-	-	-	Y	
7	F	0.53	10	15	-	-	-	-	Y	PM
Affected family members										
1	F	0.46	18	29	+	-	-	-	Y	
2	F	0.50	8	13	-	-	-	-	Y	
3	F	0.50	18	26	-	-	+	-	N	
4	F	0.52	10	17	+	-	+	-	Y	
5	F	0.52	21	28	+	-	-	-	Y	
6	F	0.57	12	14	+	-	-	+	Y	
7	M	0.58	16	23	-	-	-	-	Y	

QTc, QT interval corrected for heart rate; ACA, aborted cardiac arrest; +, event occurred; -, no event occurred; Y, yes; N, no; PM, pacemaker; LCTSG, left cervicothoracic sympathetic ganglionectomy
[a] None of the 14 patients who died had congenital deafness or had received an implanted cardioverter defibrillator
[b] On the first recorded electrocardiogram
[c] I.e., other than β-blockers

may not be entirely effective in preventing malignant cardiac arrhythmias in all patients with LQTS.

The lack of complete efficacy with β-blocker therapy in LQTS is not surprising. The arrhythmogenic mechanisms associated with LQTS are complex, and hyper-adrenergic phenomena are unlikely to be the sole cause of life-threatening tachyarrhythmias. Furthermore, β-blockers can accentuate sinus bradycardia in LQTS and may contribute to the development of bradycardia-dependent ventricular tachyarrhythmias.

Beta-blocker therapy results in a significant reduction in the frequency of cardiac events in LQTS probands. However, β-blockers have definite limitations since syncope and fatal cardiac events occur in some probands and affected family members while receiving this therapy. Additional studies are indicated to determine which high-risk LQTS patients might benefit from prophylactic ICD therapy.

Acknowledgements. Study supported in part by research grants HL-33843 and HL-51618 from the National Institutes of Health, Bethesda, MD, USA.

References

1. Moss AJ, Schwartz PJ, Crampton RS, Locati E, Carleen E (1985) The long QT syndrome: a prospective international study. Circulation 71:17-21
2. Moss AJ, Schwartz PJ, Crampton RS, Tzivoni D, Locati EH, MacCluer J, Hall WJ, Weitkamp L, Vincent M, Garson A Jr, Robinson JL, Benhorin J, Choi S (1991) The long QT syndrome: prospective longitudinal study of 328 families. Circulation 84:1136-1144
3. Moss AJ, Liu JE, Gottlieb S, Locati E, Schwartz PJ, Robinson JL (1991) Efficacy of permanent pacing in the management of high-risk patients with long QT syndrome. Circulation 84:1524-1529
4. Schwartz PJ, Locati E, Moss AJ, Crampton RS, Trazzi R, Ruberti U (1991) Left cardiac sympathetic denervation in the therapy of the congenital long QT syndrome: a worldwide report. Circulation 84:503-511
5. Priori SG, Zareba WJ, Napolitano C, Locati EH, Robinson JL, Diehl L, Schwartz PJ, Moss AJ (1996) The implantable cardioverter defibrillator (ICD) in the long QT syndrome: data from the international registry. Pacing Clin Electrophysiol 19(2):556
6. Vincent GM, Fox J, Zhang L, Timothy KW (1996) Beta-blockers markedly reduce risk and syncope in KVLQT1 long QT patients. Circulation 94:I-204

Gene Therapy for Long QT Syndrome: Fact or Fiction?

P.J. Schwartz

For many years the therapy for long QT syndrome (LQTS) has been based on simple and sound principles [1, 2]. In essence, therapy had been guided by the time-honored concept that it has to reflect understanding of the mechanisms, underlying or precipitating the main symptoms. In those happy days things were simple, we thought that we were dealing with one disease, and we were assuming that the precipitating events were more or less the same for all patients; the generally accepted common pathway for the initiation of the life-threatening arrhythmias of LQTS was represented by a sudden neural release of norepinephrine secondary to an abrupt activation of the sympathetic nervous system [2].

This concept had logically resulted in the treatment of symptomatic patients with beta-adrenergic blockers and with left cardiac sympathetic denervation [3, 4]. As often happens when logical reasoning is followed, this approach was met with success. As we showed in 1985 [2], the use of antiadrenergic treatment led to a dramatic reduction in mortality among symptomatic patients (from 50% to 4% within 10 years from the first syncope or cardiac arrest) when compared to the outcome in patients left untreated or treated differently.

The identification, between 1995 and 1997, of some of the major genes involved in LQTS opened a new phase and added a new twist, of both excitement and complexity. The realization that all these genes encode cardiac ion channels and, moreover, the understanding of how the specific mutation can alter repolarization [5, 6] appeared to endorse the early enthusiasm for the intriguing possibility of a "gene-specific" therapy [7]. This enthusiasm now needs some reassessing.

A first consequence of the new findings was the realization that we are not dealing with a single disease but that we are actually dealing with different diseases which have a relatively similar phenotype but a markedly different genotype. Put differently, the various genetic defects can all prolong the QT interval but through different alterations in the ionic control of repolarization and probably diverse mechanisms leading to the onset of Torsades-de-Pointes. This resulted in the new terminology currently in use. LQT1 patients are those with mutations on $KvLQT1$, the gene encoding the I_{Ks} current; LQT2 patients have

Dipartimento di Cardiologia, Policlinico S. Matteo, IRCCS e Università di Pavia, Italy

mutations on *HERG*, the gene encoding the I_{Kr} current; LQT3 patients have mutations on *SCN5A*, the gene encoding the cardiac sodium channel gene.

The mutations initially identified on the Na^+ channel gene, *SCN5A*, were found to lead, through a delayed inactivation, to an excess of late inward Na^+ current [8, 9]. Prior to the publication of these data, and actually a few weeks after the identification of *SCN5A* as a LQTS gene, on the basis of the knowledge that the mutations described were in an area important for inactivation, we attempted to shorten the QT interval in a few LQT3 patients by using the Na^+ channel blocker mexiletine [7]. The initial results, extended to LQT1 and LQT2 patients, indicated that mexiletine was producing a differential effect which seemed to be gene-specific: the QT interval of LQT3 patients shortened much more than that of LQT1 and LQT2 (Fig. 1). Our early observations were followed and confirmed by others using lidocaine [10] and more recently using flecainide with apparently striking results, always in LQT3 patients (A.J. Moss, personal communication).

So far, the use of Na^+ channel blockers is regarded by many as the closest thing to "gene-specific" therapy for LQTS. Despite my own initial enthusiasm and the self-complacent use of the word, I am no longer sure that this is the appropriate terminology. Of the mutations subsequently identified on *SCN5A*, not all produce an excess Na^+ inward current [11]. It may be more precise to consider as "mutation-specific" the treatment of some LQT3 patients with Na^+ channel blockers. This concept implies that these compounds may not necessarily be useful for all LQT3 patients. Furthermore, the realization that other mutations on *SCN5A* can produce the Brugada syndrome and that the patients affected by this often lethal disease are exquisitely sensitive to Na^+ channel blockers, which can trigger life-threatening arrhythmias, calls for caution in the

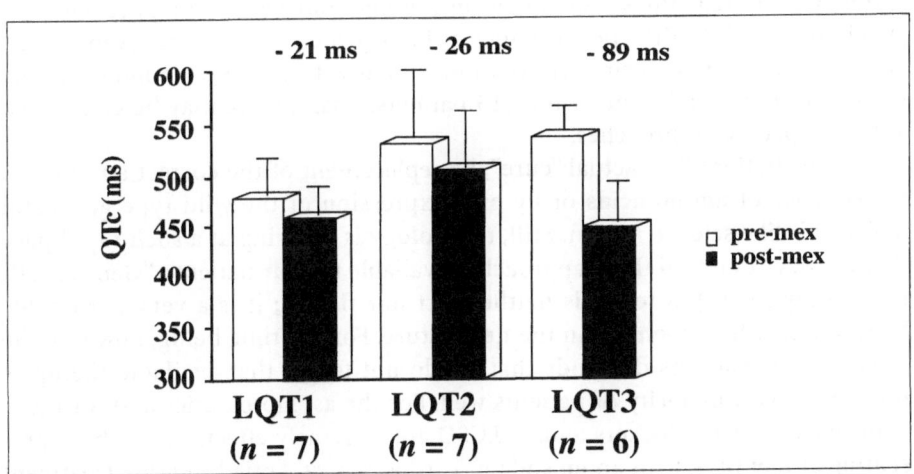

Fig. 1. QTc values in control conditions and during acute oral drug testing with mexiletine in LQT3 (linked to chromosome 3, $n = 6$), in LQT2 (linked to chromosome 7, $n = 7$), and in LQT1 (linked to chromosome 11, $n = 7$) patients. Data are expressed as mean ± SD (Modified from [7])

use of these drugs without a precise knowledge of the electrophysiological consequences of the specific mutations.

Another treatment proposed as "gene-specific" is to increase the extracellular concentration of K^+ in LQT2 patients [12]. The concept is interesting, based on what we know about *HERG* [13], but there is no evidence that the potential beneficial effect would be specific for LQT2 patients, compared to LQT1 and LQT3. Moreover, this approach is hampered by the difficulty in increasing the K^+ level chronically by oral administration [14].

Meanwhile, genotype-phenotype studies have brought significant new information [15, 16]. The data on the relationship between the different genotypes and the triggers for the life-threatening cardiac events are especially relevant here [17]. These data are currently based on more than 700 symptomatic patients of known genotype. In essence, LQT1 patients are at particularly high risk during exercise (69% of the events) and at very low risk (3% of the events) while at rest or during sleep; the remaining events occur under emotional arousal. An almost opposite pattern is present among LQT3 patients who have 51% of their episodes at rest or during sleep without any known arousal and in only 19% of cases during exercise. LQT2 patients do not appear to have a preferential trigger. On this basis, one can logically expect a high success rate with beta-blockers or LCSD among LQT1, and this is exactly what seems to happen. In this group stressful physical exercise should be rigorously avoided. These rather simple and unsophisticated approaches may be taken to represent - in a sense - a true "gene-specific" therapy. By the same token, the knowledge that LQT3 patients can very effectively shorten the QT interval at fast heart rates [16, 18], and that their QT interval is particularly long during long cardiac cycles, raises questions about the use of beta-blockers in this small subgroup and may encourage the simultaneous use of beta-blockers and a pacemaker, to avoid bradycardia, or the performance of LCSD which effectively prevents neural release of norepinephrine without lowering heart rate [19]. We indeed found LCSD very effective in our own LQT3 patients. Again, these may be considered as "gene-specific" approaches.

Fact or fiction? The actual "cure", by replacement of the correct amino acid or sequence of amino acids or by over-expression of the wild type gene, still looks a bit like science fiction. Still, technology is evolving at a such rapid pace that we may soon find these approaches available for our patients. "Gene specific" therapy for LQTS today is neither fact nor fiction; it is a very reasonable hope and it will be looming in the near future. For the time being, however, the safety of our patients demands that we do not forget that available therapies protect the vast majority of patients well. For the asymptomatics and for those with syncope, beta-blockers and/or LCSD are extremely effective; for those presenting at any time with an episode of cardiac arrest, antiadrenergic treatment needs to be complemented by an ICD because it is in this subgroup that beta-blockers are more likely to fail [16].

References

1. Schwartz PJ, Periti M, Malliani A (1975) The long Q-T syndrome. Am Heart J 89:378-390
2. Schwartz PJ (1985) Idiopathic long QT syndrome: progress and questions. Am Heart J 109:399-411
3. Moss AJ, McDonald J (1971) Unilateral cervicothoracic sympathetic ganglionectomy for the treatment of long QT interval syndrome. N Engl J Med 285:903-904
4. Schwartz PJ, Locati EH, Moss AJ, Crampton RS, Trazzi R, Ruberti U (1991) Left cardiac sympathetic denervation in the therapy of congenital long QT syndrome: a worldwide report. Circulation 84:503-511
5. Roden DM, Lazzara R, Rosen MR, Schwartz PJ, Towbin JA, Vincent GM, for the SADS Foundation Task Force on LQTS (1996) Multiple mechanisms in the long-QT syndrome. Current knowledge, gaps, and future directions. Circulation 94:1996-2012
6. Priori SG, Barhanin J, Hauer RNW, Haverkamp W, Jongsma HJ, Kleber AG, McKenna WJ, Roden DM, Rudy Y, Schwartz K, Schwartz PJ, Towbin JA, Wilde AM (1999) Genetic and molecular basis of cardiac arrhythmias: impact on clinical management. Part I and II. Circulation 99:518-528; Part III. Circulation 99:674-681
7. Schwartz PJ, Priori SG, Locati EH, Napolitano C, Cantù F, Towbin AJ, Keating MT, Hammoude H, Brown AM, Chen LK, Colatsky TJ (1995) Long QT syndrome patients with mutations on the SCN5A and HERG genes have differential responses to Na+ channel blockade and to increases in heart rate. Implications for gene-specific therapy. Circulation 92:3381-3386
8. Bennett PB, Yazawa K, Makita N, George AL Jr (1995) Molecular mechanism for an inherited cardiac arrhythmia. Nature 376:683-685
9. Dumaine R, Wang Q, Keating MT, Hartmann HA, Schwartz PJ, Brown AM, Kirsch GE (1996) Multiple mechanisms of Na+ channel-linked long-QT syndrome. Circ Res 78:916-924
10. Rosero SZ, Zareba W, Robinson JL, Moss AJ (1997) Gene-specific therapy for long QT syndrome: QT shortening with lidocaine and tocainide in patients with mutation of the sodium channel gene. ANE 3:274-278
11. An RH, Wang XL, Kerem B, Benhorin J, Medina A, Goldmit M, Kass RS (1998) Novel LQT-3 mutation affects Na+ channel activity through interactions between α- and β1-subunits. Circ Res 83:141-146
12. Compton SJ, Lux RL, Ramsey MR, Strelich KT, Sanguinetti MC, Green LS, Keating MT, Mason JW (1996) Genetically defined therapy of inherited long-QT syndrome. Correction of abnormal repolarization by potassium. Circulation 94:1018-1022
13. Sanguinetti MC, Curran ME, Spector PS, Keating MT (1996) Spectrum of HERG K+-channel dysfunction in an inherited cardiac arrhythmia. Proc Natl Acad Sci USA 93:2208-2212
14. Tan HL, Alings M, Van Olden RW, Wilde AAM (1999) Long-term (subacute) potassium treatment in congenital HERG-related long QT syndrome (LQTS2). J Cardiovasc Electrophysiol 10:229-233
15. Schwartz PJ (1997) The long QT syndrome. In: Camm AJ (ed) Clinical approaches to tachyarrhythmias series. Futura, Armonk, NY
16. Schwartz PJ, Priori SG, Napolitano C. Long QT syndrome. In: Zipes DP, Jalife J (eds) Cardiac electrophysiology. From cell to bedside, 3rd edn. WB Saunders, Philadelphia (in press)

17. Schwartz PJ, Moss AJ, Priori SG, Wang Q, Lehmann MH, Timothy K, Denjoy I, Haverkamp W, Guicheney P, Paganini V, Scheinman MM, Karnes PS (1997) Gene-specific influence on the triggers for cardiac arrest in the long QT syndrome. Circulation 96[Suppl]:212 (abstr)
18. Priori SG, Napolitano C, Locati EH, Cantù F, Stramba-Badiale M, Keating MT, Towbin JA, Colatsky TJ, Chen LK, Schwartz PJ (1996) Long QT syndrome patients genetically linked to defective genes on chromosomes 11, 7 and 3 present differential response to changes in heart rate. J Am Coll Cardiol 27[Suppl A]:171A

An Overview of Secondary Prevention Implantable Cardioverter-Defibrillator Trials: AVID, CIDS and CASH

G.V. Naccarelli, D.L. Wolbrette, H.T. Patel, J. Dell'Orfano and J.C. Luck

Sudden cardiac death, usually due to a ventricular tachyarrhythmia, accounts for 350,000-400,000 deaths annually in the United States. Less than 20% of patients will survive a cardiac arrest and be discharged alive from a hospital [1]. Of the survivors, 50% will be dead within 3 years [1]. Since survivors of a cardiac arrest are at high risk for a recurrent arrhythmic event, aggressive management of this group of patients is mandatory. Unfortunately, patients with previous sustained ventricular tachyarrhythmias only account for < 1% of patients who die suddenly. Given the high subsequent event rate and the low chance of surviving another cardiac arrest, there has been aggressive prescription of antiarrhythmic drugs, in an attempt to prevent arrhythmia recurrence, and of implantable cardioverter-defibrillators (ICDs), to successfully convert a sustained ventricular tachyarrhythmia [2]. Previous trials have suggested that amiodarone and sotalol are the most effective antiarrhythmic agents in patients with sustained ventricular tachycardia (VT)/ventricular fibrillation (VF). Antiarrhythmic approaches in these trials have included empirical and Holter/electrophysiologically guided use of these antiarrhythmic drugs [3]. One study of cardiac arrest survivors demonstrated that class I agents had a deleterious effect on survival [4]. In the same study [4], β-blockers improved survival. The benefits of β-blockers are supported by their known effects in prolonging survival in high-risk patients post-myocardial infarction (MI) or with congestive heart failure (CHF) [5].

Amiodarone has a low incidence of proarrhythmia and has been shown to have neutral-to-improved effects on survival in CHF patients [6, 7] and to decrease arrhythmic mortality in post-MI patients [8-11]. Amiodarone has been reported to be efficacious in over 60% of patients with drug-refractory sustained VT/VF [12, 13]. In the CASCADE trial [14], patients treated with empirical amiodarone had better "cardiac survival" (defined as cardiac mortality, syncope/ICD shock, resuscitated cardiac arrest) than the conventionally treated group guided by serial electrocardiographic or electrophysiological testing ($p = 0.007$). In addition, the amiodarone patients had a higher survival rate free of sustained

Section of Cardiology and Cardiovascular Center, Penn State University College of Medicine, Hershey, Pennsylvania, USA

arrhythmias ($p = 0.001$). There were no significant differences in outcomes between conventionally treated patients whose inducible arrhythmias were or were not suppressed. However, the amiodarone-treated group had a higher incidence of serious side effects including a 10% incidence of pulmonary toxicity over a 3-year period.

The ESVEM trial demonstrated that guided sotalol therapy was superior to other drugs tested in the prevention of VT recurrence [15]. Findings from this study are limited by the lack of a placebo-controlled limb of the study. In addition, active control comparisons against a pure β-blocker or amiodarone were not made. Sotalol's efficacy may be enhanced by its lack of proarrhythmic effects in a post-MI population [16].

ICDs have had a significant impact in the treatment of patients with sustained ventricular tachyarrhythmias. In 1998, over 40,000 ICDs were implanted worldwide. Uncontrolled studies suggested that the ICD reduced the 5-year sudden death rate in high-risk patients to less than 5% [17-20]. Despite this remarkable success rate, critics have claimed that previous ICD data were suspect since they were retrospective and not placebo-controlled. In addition, although the rate of sudden deaths was reduced, there was concern that ICDs converted arrhythmic to non-arrhythmic deaths with little impact on long-term survival [19, 21].

Since sotalol, amiodarone and ICDs have often been used after other antiarrhythmic therapies have failed, little prospective controlled data for these therapies have existed in the past. One small prospective trial [22] demonstrated that early ICD implantation in non-drug responders resulted in a lower number of outcome events including deaths (0.27 Hazard Ratio, $p = 0.02$) than the conventional antiarrhythmic drug arm. In patients with previous sustained VT/VF, data from several studies to determine the best therapy (amiodarone versus other drugs versus ICD) to prolong survival are now available [23-27] and will be discussed in this paper (Table 1).

Antiarrhythmics Versus Implantable Defibrillators (AVID) Study

The AVID trial [23] studied whether "best" class III antiarrhythmic therapy (empirical amiodarone or guided sotalol) or ICD therapy was superior in reducing intention-to-treat all cause mortality in patients with a history of sustained VT/VF. Secondary objectives include quality-of-life assessment and cost-effectiveness of the two study arms. Inclusion criteria included the following arrhythmia patients: survivors of a VF arrest; sustained VT/syncope; sustained VT/ejection fraction < 40%; and, sustained VT/near-syncope.

A total of 1016 patients were randomized (509 antiarrhythmic drug; 507 ICD). Only 2.6% of patients received sotalol long-term and 93% of the ICD group had a nonthoracotomy system implanted. Enrollment was discontinued prematurely (7 April 1997) because of a significant survival advantage in the ICD group. During an 18.2 ± 12.2 months follow-up period, death rates were 22.0% ± 3.7% in the antiarrhythmic drug versus 15.8 ± 3.2% in the ICD group. One, 2 and 3-year sur-

Table 1. Amiodarone/ICD trials in sustained VT/VF

	AVID	CIDS	CASH
n	1016	659	349
Therapy	ICD vs empiric amiodarone or guided sotalol	ICD vs empiric amiodarone	ICD vs empiric amiodarone metoprolol propafenone
Primary endpoint	TM	TM	TM
Drug Event Rate	17.7%	8.3%	9.8%
Principal finding	ICD decreased TM by 39% ($p < .02$) compared to amiodarone or sotalol group	ICD decreased TM by 19.6% ($p = .072$) compared to amiodarone	ICD group decreased TM by 30% ($p = .047$) compared to amio/ metoprolol groups

TM, total mortality

vival rates were 89.3%, 81.6% and 75.4% in the ICD group compared to 82.3%, 74.7% and 64.1% in the drug-treated group ($p < 0.02$), resulting in mortality-relative risk reductions of 39%, 27% and 31% in ICD patients. The majority of the ICD benefit occurred in the first 9 months. Due to the premature termination of the study, survival in the ICD patients was only extended by 2.8 months with benefit most prominent in patients with an ejection fraction of $< 35\%$. Patient characteristics, such as age and ejection fraction, were similar in the two treatment groups. However, the ICD group had a lower incidence of prior atrial fibrillation/flutter, while class III CHF patients had a higher use of concomitant β-blockers. The registry group of patients were clinically similar to the patients randomized into the trial [28, 29]. Recent data [30] from the AVID registry population demonstrated similar high mortality rates in all of the entry subgroups. The average hospital charges for the ICD group was $66,600 vs $34,000 for the drug-treated group. This data suggests that aggressive prescription of an ICD is appropriate for all of these subgroups including: cardiac arrest survivors of ventricular fibrillation, syncopal ventricular tachycardia, symptomatic ventricular tachycardia, stable ventricular tachycardia, ventricular tachycardia/fibrillation with transient/correctable cause and unexplained syncope.

Cardiac Arrest Study Hamburg (CASH)

The CASH trial [24] was initiated to compare the efficacy of empirical antiar-rhythmic therapy versus an ICD in survivors of sudden cardiac death unrelated to myocardial infarction (Table 1). CASH was a prospective, randomized, multi-center open-label trial. The primary endpoint was to assess the effects of therapy on total mortality with secondary endpoints assessing the recurrence of hemody-namically unstable VT, sudden death and the incidence of drug withdrawal. In ICD patients, ICD discharges occurring during syncope were counted as VF recurrences, and those occurring during presyncope and/or documented VT were also counted as VT recurrences. Baseline studies and pre- and post-therapy programmed electrical stimulation were performed although these studies were not used as part of the clinical decision-making process. Patients were random-ized to empirical amiodarone, metoprolol, propafenone or an ICD within 3 months of their cardiac arrest.

In 1992, an interim report of findings from the first 287 patients was pub-lished [24] after the Data and Safety Monitoring Board recommended premature termination of enrollment in the propafenone limb of the study due to a signifi-cantly higher mortality (29.5%) and cardiac arrest/sudden death recurrence (23%) occurring in this group compared to a 11.5% total mortality and 0% sud-den death rate in patients treated with an ICD. At the time of this analysis, sudden cardiac death was lowest in the ICD arm and total mortality was similar in the ICD, amiodarone and metoprolol arms of the study.

The study was continued with enrollment to the amiodarone, metoprolol and the ICD treatment limbs. Preliminary results reported at the 1998 American College of Cardiology meetings [25] noted that the ICD arm decreased total mortality and sudden death by 30% when compared to the combined metoprolol and amio-darone treatment arms of the study ($p = 0.047$). There was no statistical difference in study endpoints between the amiodarone and metoprolol treatment arms.

Canadian Implantable Defibrillator Study (CIDS)

The CIDS trial (Table 1) [26] was a randomized, multicenter trial comparing the efficacy of ICD therapy ($n = 328$) to amiodarone ($n = 331$) in 659 patients with prior cardiac arrest or hemodynamically unstable VT. Enrollment criteria includ-ed: documented ventricular fibrillation, out-of-hospital cardiac arrest requiring defibrillation, documented sustained VT ≥ 150 bpm causing presyncope or angina in a patient with an ejection fraction of ≤ 35% or syncope with documented spon-taneous VT ≥ 10 s or induced sustained VT. The primary endpoint compared the above two therapies in reducing arrhythmic death. Secondary endpoints included quality-of-life assessment and cost-efficacy analyses, all caused mortality, nonfatal recurrence of VF, sustained VT causing syncope or cardiac arrest requiring exter-nal cardioversion or defibrillation. Patients were followed for 3-5 years.

Preliminary results were presented by Dr. Connolly at the 1998 American

College of Cardiology sessions [27]. He reported that all cause mortality was 25% in the ICD versus 30% in the amiodarone group. Thus, the ICD group showed a trend ($p = 0.072$) towards overall improvement in survival of 19.6% compared to amiodarone after 3 years of follow-up. The results are confounded by the high crossover rate of this population, since many of the ICD patients took concomitant β-blockers (four times greater than the amiodarone group), sotalol and amiodarone (30%). In addition, 22% of the amiodarone-treatment group later had an ICD inserted. Thus, survival in the amiodarone arm may have been overestimated.

Clinical Perspective (CASH, AVID, CIDS)

The results of the AVID trial supports the use of ICD therapy as a front-line therapy to prolong survival in patients at high risk of sudden death. Since overall survival was improved, the ICD may prolong life further through some undefined nonarrhythmic mechanism. Despite the smaller size of these trials and other problems in interpreting them, the results of CASH and CIDS support the findings of AVID. The results of all three trials are consistent with previous retrospective studies [2] and small prospective trials such as the Dutch Cost-Effectiveness Study [22].

Although the results of these trials are concordant, some differences in the trials exist. AVID and CIDS were powered to determine the overall survival benefit whereas CASH was not. CIDS had a high treatment crossover rate limiting interpretation of its results. The annual mortality rate was twice as high in the AVID drug-treated group versus CIDS or CASH (Table 1).

Although amiodarone, sotalol and β-blockers appear to have a beneficial effect on survival in the above patient population, the lack of placebo-controlled studies raises the question of whether these drugs have a beneficial, neutral or adverse effect on survival. If these drugs had an adverse effect on survival, some of the ICD benefit could be from the lack of any proarrhythmic effect. Based on these three trials, estimated 2-year mortality rates of survivors of sustained VT/VF episodes are 40%-45% with class I agents, 20%-25% with amiodarone or metoprolol and 12%-20% in ICD patients [31]. Amiodarone discontinuation rates were only about 4% per year, minimizing recurrences through a high antiarrhythmic drug withdrawal rate. The results of all of these studies are confounded by the fact that many of the ICD patients took concomitant β-blockers, sotalol and amiodarone. Future cost-efficacy and quality-of-life analysis will help clinicians in prescribing the most cost-effective therapy.

Myerburg et al. [32] examined the importance of choosing the highest risk yield patient groups for studies and therapies. Although many therapies may be statistically effective, these same therapies may be inefficient and cost-ineffective. Thus in AVID [23, 32], although ICD therapy reduced mortality by 27% (25% in the drug arm vs 18% in the ICD arm), the efficiency of the treatment was only 7%. Preliminary results of cost-efficacy analyses [33] suggest that even in this high risk population, an ICD may be five times less cost-effective than an ICD in the MADIT population [34, 35] who had no history of prior sustained ventricular tachyarrhythmia. The premature termination of AVID underestimates the cost-benefit of the ICD arm of the study.

Based on the above studies, the ACC/AHA recently recommended that ICDs should be prescribed with a class I indication as front-line therapy in patients with hemodynamically destabilizing VT/VF [36]. Since 40%-70% of ICD patients need the use of a concomitant antiarrhythmic agent [37], antiarrhythmic drugs such as β-blockers, sotalol and amiodarone should and will continue to be added when clinically appropriate. Depending on baseline structural heart disease (post-MI, CHF), appropriate nonarrhythmic therapy, such as aspirin, statins, and ACE-inhibitors [5], should be prescribed. Proper revascularization of patients with high risk, occlusive coronary artery disease, should continue to be part of the overall management strategy for preventing sudden cardiac death [38, 39]. Although ICDs have proven to prolong survival in these secondary prevention trials, the use of ICDs in primary prevention [5, 32, 40] will have the largest future potential impact in the fight against sudden death.

References

1. Schaffer WA, Cobb LA (1975) Recurrent ventricular fibrillation as mode of death in survivors of out-of-hospital ventricular fibrillation. N Engl J Med 293:259-262
2. Gilman JK, Jalal S, Naccarelli GV (1994) Predicting and preventing sudden death from cardiac causes. Circulation 90:1083-1092
3. Mason JW, the ESVEM Investigators (1993) A comparison of electrophysiologic testing with Holter monitoring to predict antiarrhythmic drug efficacy for ventricular tachyarrhythmias. N Engl J Med 329:445-451
4. Hallstrom AP, Cobb LA, Yu BH, Weaver WD, Fahrenbruch CE (1991) An antiarrhythmic drug experience in 941 patients resuscitated from an initial cardiac arrest between 1970-1985. Am J Cardiol 68:1025-1031
5. Naccarelli GV, Wolbrette DL, Dell'Orfano JT, Patel HM, Luck JC (1998) A decade of clinical trial developments in postmyocardial infarction, congestive heart failure, and sustained ventricular tachyarrhythmia patients: from CAST to AVID and beyond. J Cardiovasc Electrophysiol 9:864-891
6. Doval HC, Nul DR, Grancelli HO, Perrone SV, Bortman GR, Curiel R, for the Grupo de Estudio de la Sobrevida en la Insuficiencia Cardiaca en Argentina (GESICA) (1994) Randomized trial of low-dose amiodarone in severe congestive heart failure: Grupo de Estudio de la Sobrevida en la Insuficiencia Cardiaca en Argentina (GESICA). Lancet 344:493-498
7. Singh SN, Fletcher RD, Fisher SG, Singh BN, Lewis HD, Deedwania PC, Massie BM, Colling C, Lazzeri D, for the Survival Trial of Antiarrhythmic Therapy in Congestive Heart Failure (1995) Amiodarone in patients with congestive heart failure and asymptomatic ventricular arrhythmia. N Engl J Med 333:77-82
8. Julian DG, Camm AJ, Frangin G, Janse MJ, Munoz A, Schwartz PJ, Simon P, for the European Myocardial Infarct Amiodarone Trial Investigators (1997) Randomized trial of effect of amiodarone on mortality in patients with left-ventricular dysfunction after recent myocardial infarction: EMIAT. Lancet 349:667-674

9. Cairns JA, Connolly SJ, Roberts R, Gent M, for the Canadian Amiodarone Myocardial Infarction Arrhythmia Trial Investigators (1997) Randomized trial of outcome after myocardial infarction in patients with frequent or repetitive ventricular premature depolarisations: CAMIAT. Lancet 349:675-682

10. Sim I, McDonald KM, Lavori PW, Norbutas CM, Hlatky MA (1997) Quantitative overview of randomized trials of amiodarone to prevent sudden cardiac death. Circulation 96:2823-2829

11. Amiodarone Trials Meta-Analysis Investigators (1997) Effect of prophylactic amiodarone on mortality after acute myocardial infarction and in congestive heart failure: meta-analysis of individual data from 6500 patients in randomised trials. Lancet 350:1417-1424

12. Weinberg BA, Miles WM, Klein LS, Bolander JE, Dusman RE, Stanton MS, Heger JJ, Langefield C, Zipes DP (1993) Five-year follow-up of 589 patients treated with amiodarone. Am Heart J 125:109-120

13. Herre J, Sauve M, Malone P, Griffin J, Helmy I, Langberg J, Goldberg H, Scheinman M (1989) Long-term results of amiodarone therapy with recurrent sustained ventricular tachycardia or ventricular fibrillation. J Am Coll Cardiol 13:442-449

14. The CASCADE Investigators (1993) Randomized antiarrhythmic drug therapy in survivors of cardiac arrest (the CASCADE study). Am J Cardiol 72:280-287

15. Mason JW, the ESVEM Investigators (1993) A comparison of seven antiarrhythmic drugs in patients with ventricular tachyarrhythmias. N Engl J Med 329:445-451

16. Julian DG, Prescott RJ, Jackson FS, Szekeley P (1982) Controlled trial of sotalol for one year after myocardial infarction. Lancet 1:1142-1147

17. Winkle R, Mead H, Ruder M, Gaudiani V, Smith N, Buch W, Schmidt P, Shipman T (1989) Long-term outcome with the automatic implantable cardioverter defibrillator. J Am Coll Cardiol 13:1353-1361

18. Lehmann MH, Steinman RT, Schuger CD, Jackson K (1988) The automatic cardioverter defibrillator as antiarrhythmic treatment modality of choice for survivors of cardiac arrest unrelated to acute myocardial infarction. Am J Cardiol 62:803-805

19. Nisam S (1998) Can Implantable defibrillators reduce non-arrhythmic mortality? J Interventional Cardiac Electrophysiol 2:371-375

20. Estes M (1996) Clinical strategies for use of the implantable cardioverter-defibrillator: the impact of current trials. PACE 19:1011-1015

21. Newman D, Sauve J, Herre J, Langberg J, Lee M, Titus C, Scheinman M (1992) Survival after implantation of the cardioverter-defibrillator. Am J Cardiol 69:889-903

22. Wever EFD, Hauer RNW, van Capelle FJL, Tijssen JGP, Crijns HJGM, Algra A, Wiesfeld ACP, Bakker PFA, Robles de Medina EO (1995) Randomized study of implantable defibrillator as first-choice therapy versus conventional strategy in postinfarct sudden death survivors. Circulation 91:2195-2203

23. The Antiarrhythmics versus Implantable Defibrillators (AVID) Investigators (1997) A comparison of antiarrhythmic-drug therapy with implantable defibrillators in patients resuscitated from near-fatal ventricular arrhythmias. N Engl J Med 337:1576-1583

24. Siebels J, Cappato R, Ruppel R, Schneider MAE, Kuck KH, and the CASH Investigators (1993) Preliminary Results of the Cardiac Arrest Study Hamburg (CASH). Am J Cardiol 72:F109-F113

25. Kuck KH, for the CASH Investigators (1998) Cardiac Arrest Study Hamburg (CASH). Presented at the 47th Annual Scientific Sessions of the American College of Cardiology. Late Breaking Clinical Trials I

26. Connolly S, Gent M, Roberts RS, Dorian P, Green MS, Klein GJ, Mitchell LB, Sheldon RS, Roy D (1993) Canadian Implantable Defibrillator Study (CIDS): Study design and organization. Am J Cardiol 72:F103-F108

27. Connolly SJ, for the CIDS Investigators (1998) Canadian Implantable Defibrillator Study. Presented at the 47th Annual Scientific Sessions of the American College of Cardiology. Late Breaking Clinical Trials I

28. Curtis AB, Hallstrom AP, Klein RC, Nath S, Pinski SL, Epstein AE, Wyse DG, Cannom DS, Renfroe E, for the AVID Investigators (1997) Influence of patient characteristics in the selection of patients for defibrillator implantation (the AVID Registry). Am J Cardiol 79:1185-1189

29. Kim SG, Hallstrom A, Love JC, Rosenberg Y, Powell J, Roth J, Brodsky M, Moore R, Wilkoff B, for the AVID Investigators (1997) Comparison of clinical characteristics and frequency of implantable defibrillator use between randomized patients in the Antiarrhythmics versus Implantable Defibrillators (AVID) trial and nonrandomized registry patients. Am J Cardiol 80:454-457

30. Anderson JL, Hallstrom AP, Epstein AE, Pinski SL, Rosenberg Y, Nora MO, Chilson D, Cannom DS, Moore R, and the AVID Investigators (1999) Design and results of the antiarrhythmic vs implantable defibrillators (AVID) registry. Circulation 99:1692-1699

31. Cappato R (1999) Secondary prevention of sudden death: the Dutch study, the Antiarrhythmics versus Implantable Defibrillator Trial, the Cardiac Arrest Study Hamburg, and the Canadian Implantable Defibrillator Study. Am J Cardiol 83:D68-D73

32. Myerburg RJ, Mitrani R, Interian A, Castellanos A (1998) Interpretation of outcomes of antiarrhythmic clinical trials. Design features and population impact. Circulation 97:1514-1521

33. Larsen GC, McAnulty JH, Hallstrom A, Marchant C, Shein M, Akiyama Y, Brodsky M, Baessler C, Pinski S, Jennings CA, Morris M (1997) Hospitalization charges in the Antiarrhythmics versus Implantable Defibrillators (AVID) Trial: the AVID economic analysis study. Circulation 96:I-77 (abstr)

34. Moss AJ, Hall WJ, Cannom DS, Daubert JP, Higgins SL, Klein H, Levine JH, Saksena S, Waldo AL, Wilber D, Brown MW, Heo M, for the Multicenter Automatic Defibrillator Implantation Trial Investigators (1996) Improved survival with an implanted defibrillator in patients with coronary disease at high risk for ventricular arrhythmia. N Engl J Med 335:1933-1940

35. Mushlin AI, Hall WJ, Zwanziger J, Gajary E, Andrews M, Marron R, Zou KH, Moss AJ (1998) Cost-effectiveness of automatic implantable cardiac defibrillators: results from MADIT. Circulation 97:2129-2135

36. Gregoratos G, Cheitlin MD, Conill A, Epstein AE, Fellows C, Ferguson TB, Freedman RA, Hlatky MA, Naccarelli GV, Saksena S, Schlant RC, Silka MJ (1998) ACC/AHA Guidelines for implantation of cardiac pacemakers and antiarrhythmia devices. A report of the American College of Cardiology/American Heart Association Task Force on Practice Guidelines (Committee on Pacemaker Implantation). J Am Coll Cardiol 31:117-1209

37. Naccarelli GV, Dougherty AH, Wolbrette D (1995) Antiarrhythmic drug implantable cardioverter/defibrillator interactions. In: Zipes DP, Jalife J (eds) From cell to bedside. WB Saunders, Philadelphia, pp 1426-1433

38. Holmes DR, Davis KB, Mock MB, Fisher LD, Gersch BJ, Killip T, Pettinger M, Participants in the Coronary Artery Surgery Study (1986) The effect of medical and surgical treatment on subsequent cardiac death in patients with coronary artery disease: a report from the Coronary Artery Surgical Study. Circulation 73:1254-1263

39. Bigger JT, for the CABG Patch Trial Investigators (1997) Prophylactic use of implanted cardiac defibrillators in patients at high risk for ventricular arrhythmias after coronary artery bypass graft surgery. N Engl J Med 337:1569-1575

40. Nisam S, Mower M (1998) ICD trials: an extraordinary means of determining patient risk? PACE 21:1341-1346

What Has Been the Impact on Clinical Practice of Recently Published Postevent ICD Trials?

D.S. Cannom

Introduction

The American electrophysiology community has a 15-year history of active support of the implantable cardioverter defibrillator (ICD) [1-5]. While there have been debates about the nature and extent of the impact of the ICD, few have doubted that the device saves lives. This is in contrast to the European and Far Eastern electrophysiology communities, where the ICD implantation rate is a fraction of what it is in the United States [6]. The recently completed postevent clinical trials have vindicated the early support of the ICD and have led to a dramatic and ongoing increase in ICD utilization in the United States [7-9]. The anticipated completion of a series of pre-event trials will further broaden the appeal of the ICD.

Background

A major theme in the development of American electrophysiology has been the development of techniques which will accurately and reproducibly assess risk in the patient with and without heart disease. Some attempts at assessing risk have fallen out of favor, including the concept of warning arrhythmias popularized briefly by Lown [10], attempts to suppress postinfarction ventricular premature beats with antiarrhythmic drugs (which the CAST trial showed [11] increased risk to treated patients), and the advent of invasive electrophysiologic (EP) testing [12]. By the late 1980s the latter technique, which determines whether ventricular tachycardia (VT) or other arrhythmias can be induced by electrode catheters, was almost uniformly the method of choice for predicting arrhythmic risk. The technique had limitations, including the inability to predict risk in some high-risk patients, especially those with forms of nonischemic cardiomyopathy.

Once invasive testing identified the high-risk patient – usually a person with a reduced (< 40%) ejection fraction and with persistent inducible nonsuppressible

Division of Cardiology, Good Samaritan Hospital, Los Angeles, California, USA

arrhythmias in the EP laboratory – debate often ensued as to what was best therapy. In the 1980s a number of schools of therapy emerged, ranging from those which favored empiric drug therapy (especially amiodarone), to ICD advocates, to groups preferring surgical resection of arrhythmia-generating ventricular aneurysms [13]. Each school presented large retrospective series claiming efficacy and success for carefully selected patient groups.

The most comprehensive of the retrospective series comparing EP-guided drug therapy to the ICD was compiled by Powell et al. in 1993 [5]. In this combined series from the Massachusetts General and the Good Samaritan Hospitals, 331 sudden death survivors received either EP-guided therapy or an ICD. A total of 150 patients received an ICD with a subsequent total mortality of 29%, in contrast to a mortality of 62% in the 181 patients without an ICD. The effect was most striking in patients with left ventricular ejection fraction under 40%. This study also showed that left ventricular function was more important in predicting long-term mortality than the presence of an ICD. Thus, while not a prospective randomized trial, the results of the Powell study were remarkably predictive of the results of the subsequent randomized trials.

Choice of therapy, then, for the high-risk patient in the late 1980s in the United States was highly variable. These variables were determined by interpretation of the literature, experience with particular therapies, investigative interests, the insurance plan of the patient, and the doctor's relationship with the patient. As ICD therapy was expensive, many insurers were reluctant to approve implants; and, as device therapy was new, some patients were reluctant to accept it, especially when it involved a thoracotomy, before 1993.

Clearly a series of prospective clinical trials was necessary to sort out the benefit and cost issues for the ICD. By 1995 the device industry became a one billion dollar industry further magnifying this need.

Results of the Prospective Postevent Clinical Trials

A patient with sustained ventricular tachycardia or out-of-hospital cardiac arrest has an anticipated recurrence rate of 20%-30% [14]. A number of recent postevent trials compared the ICD to various drug therapies (usually amiodarone) and dramatically clarified the role of the ICD in treating high-risk patients. These trials include the AVID trial (Antiarrhythmics Versus Implantable Defibrillator), the CIDS trial (Canadian Implantable Defibrillator Trial), and the CASH trial (Cardiac Arrest Study Hamburg) [7-9]. A detailed summary of these trials is beyond the scope of this paper, but a number of publications summarize them [15, 16]. All three trials showed that the ICD improved survival in the high-risk patients, including those with cardiac arrest, hypotensive VT, or syncopal VT. The statistical power of the AVID trial was more impressive than that of the CIDS or CASH trial, although these issues relate partially to trial design. The trials are summarized in Table 1. A meta-analysis of these trials will be presented at the North American Society of Pacing and Electrophysiology meeting in May, 1999.

Table 1. Postevent trials

Trial	Design	Target population	Therapies randomized	Outcome
AVID [9]	Randomized, total mortality	$N = 1016$ VF, n = 455 VT syncope or VT EF < 40% with Sx, n = 561	ICD vs amiodarone ($N = 488$) or sotalol ($N = 13$)	ICD improved survival by 39% at 1 year for all arrhythmia classes with EF < 35%
CIDS [7]	Randomized, total mortality	$N = 659$ VF VT syncope VT presync > 150 BPM EF ≤ 35%	ICD vs amiodarone	ICD improved survival by 20%
CASH [8]	Randomized, total mortality	$N = 346$ VF	ICD vs amiodarone, metoprolol	ICD improved survival by 37%

VF, ventricular fibrillation; VT, ventricular tachycardia; EF, ejection fraction; Sx, symptoms including syncope or marked light headachers

Trial Dependent Results

The three major postevent trials conclusively show that the ICD improves survival in high-risk patients. The survival benefit for the ICD patient group in the AVID trial was not great. The extent of the benefit in this trial was significantly design-related. The AVID trial was concluded when preset boundaries for survival were exceeded, and perhaps these boundaries underestimated the benefit of the ICD. Early analysis of the AVID trial, and particularly the meta-analyses that are forthcoming, will clarify the true cost of the ICD therapy.

There were a number of surprises in the results of the trials, and probably there will be more as meta-analyses are undertaken. In the AVID trial, the ICD did not benefit patients with an ejection fraction greater than 35%, which means that EP-guided therapy and an ICD are equally effective. This result was anticipated in the Powell retrospective series [5]. In this group the AVID data also diminish the importance of EP testing in selecting high-risk patients. Finally, the ICD showed benefit for the three high-risk groups included in the trial. However, some of the nonrandomized patient populations who were followed in the registry had long-term risk which equalled that of the main trial patients (syncope with subsequent inducible VT, VT/VF due to reversible causes). When this material is widely disseminated and absorbed, it will probably change our approach to such patients and ICD therapy will be used more frequently.

Although the clinical trials have only been completed recently, the American College of Cardiology (ACC) and the American Heart Association (AHA) have already revised their criteria for ICD implantation [17]. Clearly this is a result of the impact of the trials (Table 1). The class I indications (those for which there is general agreement that ICDs are the preferred therapy) closely parallel the AVID criteria, with the exception of indication III (patient with syncope and subsequent inducible VT). This was one of the subgroups of the CIDS trial, although it composed only 10% of the CIDS population. A series of review articles summarizing the trial data have already appeared in the literature informing physicians of new indications [15, 16].

The average EP practice already feels the impact of the trial data. Patients who have sustained VT or have survived VF are referred for an ICD, not for EP testing and best therapy. The ICD manufacturers note a continued rapid growth in ICD implantation rates in the United States. Data from one manufacturer show an increase in ICD implantations just after publication of the MADIT trial and another increase after publication of the AVID results (Fig. 1) [6]. At every major US scientific meeting in the past year there have been detailed analyses of the trials; the overall impression is that the postevent trials have proven that the ICD improves survival in properly selected high-risk patients.

The trials have affected another major constituency in the United States: the medical insurers. Most insurers rely upon the guidelines prepared by the national organizations, e.g., the ACC and AHA. The fact that these organizations have already adopted the trial results means that insurers have little choice but to grant approval for ICD implantation in the properly identified high-risk patient. Already major insurers (e.g., Blue Cross and Blue Shield) have retained EP experts to explain the guidelines and have adopted the guidelines as their standard of care.

Some questions remain unanswered. The AVID trial did not evaluate the role of EP-guided amiodarone in high-risk patients. I doubt that such a trial will ever be done because of recruitment and expense issues.

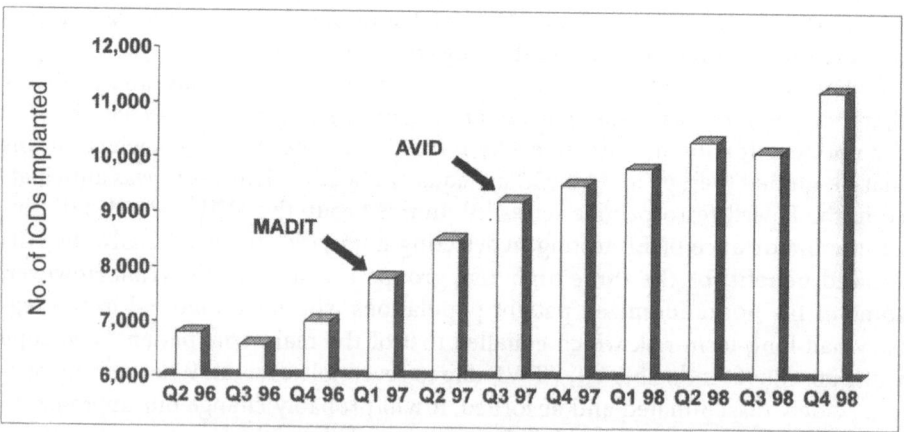

Fig. 1. Growth in the ICD market per quarter over the past 3 years. The figures reflect the entire ICD industry, although they were supplied by Guidant Corporation. The introduction of the MADIT and AVID data resulted in ongoing growth of the ICD implantation rate, but not in any dramatic fashion

Device Dependent Effects

The remarkable evolution of ICD technology has resulted in greater patient acceptance of the ICD. ICDs are now implanted transvenously and are small (40-50 cc) and reliable. In the transvenous era in ICD therapy postoperative complications have virtually disappeared, including infection, atrial and ventricular arrhythmias, and pain, all of which were deterrents to implantation in the open chest era. Even smaller devices are expected and should make implantation easier.

The evolution of dual-chamber ICDs has also improved device acceptance by both physicians and patients. These devices now comprise over 40% of the US market. They both reliably pace (as would any pacemaker) and sense atrial arrhythmias. The precision of the sensing function has eliminated spurious shocks due to atrial tachyarrhythmias; historically this has been one of the most devastating complications of ICD therapy.

Patient Dependent Effects

In the United States awareness of the potential danger of certain symptoms (e.g., syncope) and certain disease states (e.g., long QT, right ventricular dysplasia, and cardiomyopathy) has increased. More and more patients present to cardiologists and electrophysiologists as surviving relatives of families who have lost one or more siblings or relatives to one of these diseases. The press, television shows, and public advocacy groups (e.g., Cardiac Arrhythmias Research and Education Foundation) are responsible for the growing public interest and awareness of these conditions. Counseling such families and recommending therapy is usually very difficult since both the medical facts and the necessary prognostic information are simply not available. The ACC/AHA guidelines list such patients as so-called IIB indications, meaning that ICD implantation in such high-risk patients can be defended but that medical opinion does not favor this. However, many of these patients have such compelling family histories that ICD implantation is recommended and carried out. An effort is being made through the North American Society of Pacing and Electrophysiology (NASPE) to collect a registry of such patients so that the true impact of the ICD (based on firing rates) can be measured and more wide ranging recommendations made for such disease states.

Pre-Event Trials

The next frontier in ICD therapy is the pre-event trials which are currently underway, including Sudden Cardiac Death Heart Failure Trial (SCD-HEFT) and Multicenter Automatic Defibrillator Implantation Trial (MADIT II) (Table 2). These trials are well designed, amply powered and funded to determine accurately whether the next era in ICD therapy will be large-scale prophylaxis. The impor-

Table 2. Pre-event trials

Trial	Design	Target population	Therapies employed	Outcome
MADIT	Randomized, total mortality	$N = 196$ CAD (MI > 3 weeks) LVEF ≤ 35% NSVT EPS inducible PCA-refractory CHF class I-III	ICD vs conventional amiodarone 74%	ICD improved survival by 46%
CABG Patch	Randomized, total mortality	$N = 1000$ CAD with ischemia LVEF < 36% (+) SAEKG CABG candidate	CABG in all ICD vs no therapy	No survival benefit for ICD
MADIT II	Randomized, total mortality	$N = 1200$ CAD EF < 30%	ICD vs conventional therapy	Pending (began summer 1997)
SCD Heft	Randomized, total mortality	$N = 2400$ CAD/CCM EF ≤ 35% CHF class I-III	ICD conventional treatment amiodarone	Pending (began summer 1997)

CABG, coronary artery bypass grafting; CAD, coronary artery disease; CCM, congestive cardiomyopathy; CHF, congestive heart failure; NSVT, nonsustained ventricular tachycardia; PCA, procainamide; SAEKG, signal average electrocardiogram

tance of such trials lies in the large number of sudden deaths that the ICD might prevent. However, the assuredness of a positive result for the ICD in any or all of these trials seems less than in the era of the postevent trials which we have just completed. Nevertheless, not to be optimistic about ICD therapy at the millennium is to deny two decades of extraordinary progress of a technology whose clinical impact and growth has been consistently underestimated.

References

1. Mirowski M, Reid PR, Winkle RA et al (1983) Mortality in patients with implanted automatic defibrillators. Ann Intern Med 98:585-588
2. Winkle RA, Mead RH, Ruder MA et al (1989) Long term outcome with the automatic implantable cardioverter defibrillator. J Am Coll Cardiol 13:1353-1361
3. Kelly PA, Cannom DS, Garan H et al (1988) The automatic implantable cardioverter-defibrillator: efficacy, complications, and survival in patients with malignant ventricular arrhythmias. J Am Coll Cardiol 11:1278-1286

4. Newman D, Suave MJ, Herre J et al (1992) Survival after implantation of a cardioverter defibrillator. Am J Cardiol 69:899-903
5. Powell AC, Fuchs TE, Finkelstein DM et al (1993) Influence of implantable cardioverter defibrillators and long-term prognosis of survivors of out-of-hospital cardiac arrest. Circulation 88:1083-1092
6. Higgins SL (1999) Impact of the Multicenter Automatic Defibrillator Implantation Trial (MADIT) on ICD indication trends. Am J Cardiol II 83:79D-82D
7. Connolly SJ, Gent M, Roberts RS et al, on behalf of the CIDS Co-Investigators (1993) Canadian Implantable Defibrillator study (CIDS): Study design and organization. Am J Cardiol 72:103F-108F
8. Siebels J, Cappato R, Ruppel R, and the CASH Investigators (1993) Preliminary results of the Cardiac Arrest Study Hamburg (CASH). Am J Cardiol 72:109F-113F
9. The Antiarrhythmics Versus Implantable Defibrillators (AVID) Investigators (1997) A comparison of antiarrhythmic drug therapy with implantable defibrillators in patients resuscitated from near-fatal sustained ventricular arrhythmias. N Engl J Med 337:1576-1583
10. Lown B, Wolf M (1971) Approaches to sudden death from coronary heart disease. Circulation 44:130-142
11. The Cardiac Arrhythmia Suppression Trial (CAST) Investigators (1989) Preliminary report: effect of encainide and flecainide on mortality in a randomized trial of arrhythmia suppression after myocardial infarction. N Engl J Med 321:406-412
12. Prystowsky EN (1988) Electrophysiologic-electropharmacologic testing in patients with ventricular arrhythmias. Pacing Clin Electrophysiol 11:225-251
13. Cox JL (1989) Patient selection criteria and results of surgery for refractory ischemic ventricular tachycardia. Circulation 79[suppl]:163-177
14. Mitchell LB (1997) Clinical trials of antiarrhythmic drugs in patients with sustained ventricular tachyarrhythmias. Curr Opin Cardiol 12:33-40
15. Cannom DS, Prystowsky EN (1999) Modern management of ventricular arrhythmias—detection, drugs and devices. JAMA 281:172-179
16. Cannom DS (1998) Implantable cardioverter defibrillator trials: what have we learned? J Card Arrhythm Index (in press)
17. Gregoratos G, Cheitlin MD, Conill A et al (1998) ACC/AHA guidelines for implantation of cardiac pacemakers and antiarrhythmia devices: A report of the American College of Cardiology/American Heart Association Task Force on practice guidelines (Committee on Pacemaker Implantation). J Am Coll Cardiol 31:1175-1209

Is the Implantable Defibrillator Cost-effective?

S. Nisam

Introduction

In the two decades since Mirowski and colleagues introduced the implantable cardioverter defibrillator (ICD) into clinical practice [1], multiple clinical studies have established ICD therapy as the treatment of choice compared to any alternative treatment modality. Specifically, the ICD has been proven to be far superior in terms of overall survival and protection against sudden cardiac death from ventricular tachyarrhythmias in patients resuscitated from ventricular fibrillation or ventricular tachycardia (VF/VT) [2-12] as well as in patients identified as being at high risk despite not yet having suffered spontaneous episodes of VT or VF [13, 14]. However, the relatively high up-front costs – hospitalization and device – have focused much attention on the issue of the cost-effectiveness of ICD therapy [15]. Comparison of the cost-effectiveness of ICD therapy to that of presently well accepted medical therapies, particularly alternatives to ICD therapy, provides results which are enlightening and even surprising. Our article here will cover two main aspects of this question: (1) the conclusions and implications of the published studies on the cost-effectiveness of ICD therapy (ICD C-E); (2) the costs associated with ICD therapy compared to medical management and to other therapies.

ICD Cost-Effectiveness Studies

Table 1 lists the ICD C-E studies, which fall into four classes: (1) mathematical models based on data from the literature; (2) retrospective, nonrandomized studies; (3) studies of costs before and after ICD-implantation; (4) randomized, prospective studies. (For readers interested in the details of these specific studies, the review article by Mushlin et al. [16] provides an excellent overview.) Of greatest scientific credibility are the three randomized studies (MADIT, Dutch, AVID), which we will focus on here.

Guidant European Headquarters, Zaventem, Belgium

Table 1. Overview of ICD cost-effectiveness studies

Mathematical models (data from literature):
  Larsen (1992) [17], Owens (1997) [25], Deering (1998) [18],
  Anderson / Camm (1993) [19]

Retrospective, non randomized studies;
  Kupperman (1990) [20], Kuppersmith (1995) [21], O'Donoghue (1990) [22],
  O'Brien (1992) [23]

Costs before and after ICD implantation:
  Valenti / Kappenberger (1996)[24]

Randomized, prospective studies:
  Dutch study [26]
  MADIT [27]
  AVID [28, 29]

The Dutch study [26], initiated by Hauer and Wever in 1989, was the very first ICD C-E study, and it was carried out expressly for the purpose of obtaining reimbursement for ICD implantation in the Netherlands. Despite the early ICD systems used – with shorter lifetimes and requiring the far costlier thoracotomy implantations – the Dutch study already demonstrated that ICD therapy was cost-effective. In terms of costs per patient life-year saved, it was shown to be a better investment than "conventional therapy" as practiced in the early 1990s (primarily serial antiarrhythmic drug testing, with the ICD as the treatment of "last resort" if patients failed to respond to any of the drugs.) This study provided the initial insight into the impact of "crossovers" when analyzing ICD cost-effectiveness: many of the patients randomized to conventional therapy experienced VT/VF recurrences, and those who survived these recurrences went on to receive ICDs; on an "intention-to-treat" basis, these "crossovers" added substantial costs to the drug-treatment limb (while also prolonging these patients' lives). The most important conclusion from this study was: "the C-E ratio ... was $63 and $94 per patient per day alive in the early ICD and EP-guided groups, respectively ...a net $11, 300 (saved costs) per patient per life-year saved". Patients randomized to ICD therapy were also assessed as having a higher quality of life than those treated by antiarrhythmic drugs, as the latter had more frequent VT/VF recurrences, lower exercise tolerance, more frequent and longer hospitalizations, and more therapy changes. When the quality of life was included in the analysis, the authors emphasized that the cost-effectiveness advantage became even stronger in favor of ICD therapy.

Before reviewing the actual findings of the MADIT C-E Study [27], we draw attention to Table 2, showing how remarkably complete the cost data collection was: 98% (!) of all hospitalization billings; 99.9% (!) of all outpatient diagnostic tests or procedures; 96% of all medications. The primary outcome result of the study was of course directly related to the major outcome criterion of the main

Table 2. MADIT cost-effectiveness study: data completeness. (Reproduced, with permission, from [27])

	Total reported (n)	Conventional therapy[a]	ICD[b]	Total missing (n)
Hospitalizations: patient bills/UB-82/92	697	323 (13)	360 (1)	14
Emergency department visits: UB-82/92	82	30 (3)	46 (3)	6
Physician visits	5203	2275 (0)	2928 (0)	0
Outpatient tests/procedures	6324	3175 (5)	3140 (4)	0
Medications	676	316 (9)	340 (11)	20
Other disease/treatment-related service	214	93 (0)	121 (0)	0

Numbers in parentheses represent numbers of missing data
UB, Uniform billing form; [a]92 Patients in the conventional therapy group, with 2254 person-months of observation; [b]89 Patients in the defibrillator (ICD) group, with 2577 person-months of observation

MADIT study: patients randomized to ICD therapy lived considerably longer. They achieved an overall survival over a 4-year period of 3.66 years, compared to 2.80 years for the drug-randomized cohort. This nearly 1 year extension of life translated to an approximate \$12,500 ICD C-E ratio for currently implanted systems (transvenous, 5-year device longevity). The cost-effectiveness analysis for the AVID study is not yet complete, but the preliminary data [28, 29] seem to show considerably lower efficacy than the MADIT results (Table 3). Part of this difference certainly stems from the far more impressive ICD treatment effect in MADIT compared to AVID, with hazard ratios of 0.46 compared to 0.62, respectively [10, 13]. However, the primary explanation for the apparently large difference in C-E ratio is that the economic numbers published for AVID were based on charges, not costs; whereas, in MADIT, the C-E ratio was calculated from real costs and resource utilization. A second important contributor to this difference is the far shorter follow-up time for patients in the AVID study compared to MADIT: mean 18 months vs 27 months, respectively. As explained by Cannom [29], with a longer follow-up time the AVID C-E ratio could well have been considerably higher. Patient selection in the two studies was certainly another factor, impacting the difference in cost-effectiveness. For example, the AVID hazard ratios showed relatively small benefit for patients with a good ejection fraction (> 0.35). It should be noted, however, that it is particularly in these "healthier" patients, that the protection offered by the ICD against sudden death becomes increasingly more manifest in a longer follow-up period than the mean 18 months in the study.

Table 3. ICD cost-effectiveness studies: AVID and MADIT

Study	ICD	Antiarrhythmic drugs	Comments
AVID [28]	$66 600	$34 000	Implantation hospitalization *charges*
AVID [29]	$85 386	$57 213	3-month follow-up *charges*
MADIT [27]	$44 600	$18 900	Implantation average *costs*
MADIT [27] (transvenous)	$22 800		Cost per life-year saved

ICD Cost-Effectiveness in Comparison to Other Accepted Therapies

Several authors have compared the costs associated with ICD therapy with the costs for other medical interventions. As shown in Table 4 and pointed out by Saksena and others, the ICD is already now as cost-effective, if not more so, than many other currently practiced medical therapies [7, 30].

Another interesting view on this question is given by examining expenditures for antiarrhythmic drugs compared to ICDs. Figure 1 shows a comparison of

Table 4. ICD cost-effectiveness: comparison to other common therapies. (Reproduced, with permission, from [30])

Treatment of hypertension	$23 200
Heart transplantation	$26 900
Estrogen replacement	$32 900
Neonatal intensive care	$5 500-38 800
Renal dialysis	$58 000
Coronary artery bypass	$7 200-44 200
ICD[a]	$7 500

[a]Transvenous/pectoral/increased longevity

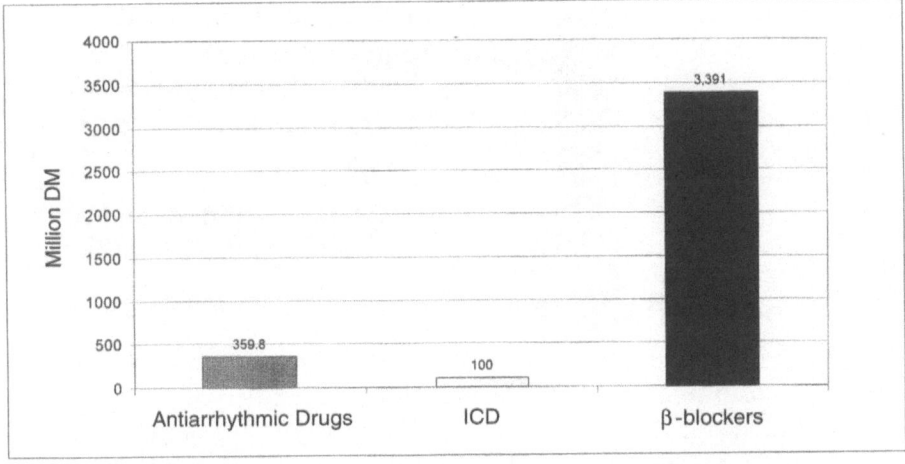

Fig. 1. Expenditure on antiarrhythmic drugs and β-blockers compared to ICDs in Germany in 1997

costs for antiarrhythmic drugs, β-blockers, and ICDs in Germany during 1997 [31]. Compared to ICD expenditure, the ratio approaches 4:1 for antiarrhythmic drugs and over 30:1 for β-blockers. Considering that ICD use is far lower (and antiarrhythmic drug use far higher) in other European countries [32], it is clear that these ratios are even higher in those countries. In light of all that is now known about the relative inefficacy of antiarrhythmic drugs versus the proven efficacy of ICDs, the questions relating to ICD cost-effectiveness should be applied just as critically toward antiarrhythmic drugs.

Valenti et al. reported on costs for patients in the year prior to receiving ICDs compared to costs in the year following implantation [24]. They concluded, on the basis of all the tabulated costs, that an ICD implantation would be "paid off" in about 18 months. The primary factors which contributed to this relatively quick recovery of the "investment" were significant reductions in hospitalization days and number of rehospitalizations following ICD implantation (Fig. 2).

A final cost-effectiveness study we will cite is the important publication by Owens et al. [25]. These researchers used a "Markov model" based on analysis of studies with ICDs and amiodarone in different risk populations and compared three treatment strategies: ICD alone, amiodarone alone, and ICD in combination with amiodarone. They furthermore carried out various sensitivity analyses in order to evaluate each treatment strategy. The effect of crossovers, as mentioned above, also played a major role in this study. It is well known that in both the AVID study and the Canadian Implantable Defibrillator Study (CIDS) approximately 20% of patients assigned to amiodarone were switched to ICDs following VT/VF recurrences [10, 11]. On an "intention-to-treat" basis, these crossovers have the effect of improving the probability of survival of the patients following

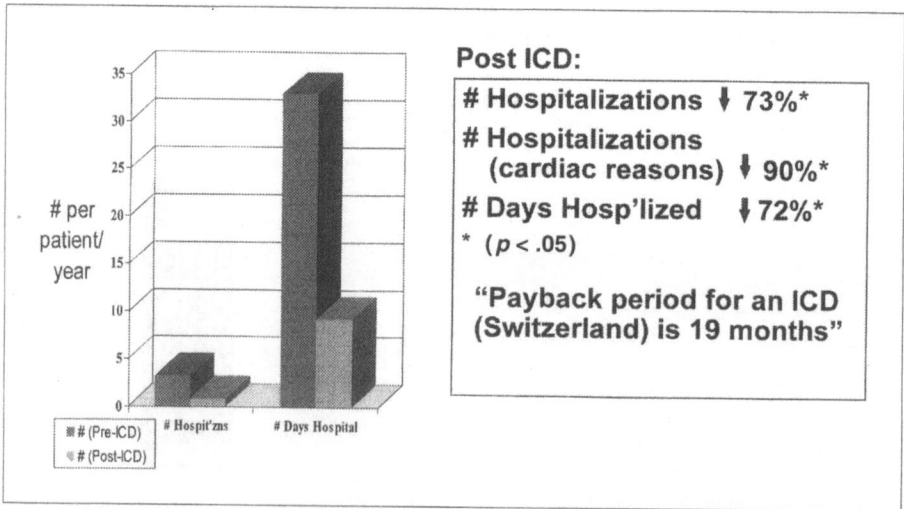

Fig. 2. Impact of ICD therapy on rehospitalization statistics. Numbers of hospitalizations and numbers of days spent in hospital are compared for the year before and the year after ICD implantation

their recurrences. However, in relation to cost-effectiveness, such crossovers considerably increase costs in the antiarrhythmic group. While the Owens study was a theoretical model, applying it to the real data from MADIT shows that that model was quite accurate, yielding an approximate C-E ratio of $20,000 when calculated for devices lasting 5 years. Applying the model to the AVID criteria yields a C-E ratio of approximately $38,000.

Conclusions

The ICD cost-effectiveness studies, whether based on mathematical models or on real data derived from the recently completed randomized, prospective trials, show the cost-effectiveness of ICD therapy to be well within the norms accepted for other medical interventions. Considering that no antiarrhythmic drugs, with the exception of β-blockers, have been shown to prolong life for patients with ventricular tachyarrhythmias – whereas ICDs extend life by 30%-50% – the cost-effectiveness question, until now aimed at ICD therapy, may need to be refocused on antiarrhythmic drugs.

References

1. Mirowski M, Reid P, Mower M et al (1980) Termination of malignant ventricular arrhythmias with an implanted automatic defibrillator in human beings. N Engl J Med 303:322-324
2. Winkle R, Mead H, Ruder M et al (1989) Long-term outcome with the automatic implantable cardiover defibrillator. J Am Coll Cardiol 13:1353-1361
3. Newman D, Sauve MJ, Herre J, Langberg JJ, Lee MA, Titus C, Franklin J, Scheinman MM, Griffin JC (1992) Survival after implantation of the cardioverter defibrillator. Am J Cardiol 69:899-903
4. Böcker D, Block M, Isbruch F, Wietholt D, Hammel D, Borggrefe M, Breithardt G (1993) Do patients with an implantable defibrillator live longer? J Am Coll Cardiol 21:1638-1644
5. Powell AC, Fuchs T, Finkelstein DM, Garan H, Cannom DS, McGovern BA, Kelly E, Vlahakes GJ, Torchiana DF, Ruskin JN (1993) Influence of implantable cardioverter-defibrillators on the long-term prognosis of survivors of out-of-hospital cardiac arrest. Circulation 88:1083-1092
6. Raviele A (1996) Implantable cardioverter defibrillator indications in 1996: have they changed? Am J Cardiol 78(5A):21-25
7. Saksena S, Madan N, Lewis C (1996) Implantable cardioverter-defibrillators are preferable to drugs as primary therapy in sustained ventricular tachyarrhythmias. Prog Cardiovasc Dis 38:445-454
8. Böcker D, Block M, Borggrefe M, Breithardt G (1997) Defibrillators are superior to antiarrhythmic drugs in the treatment of ventricular tachyarrhythmias. Eur Heart J 18:26-30
9. Böcker D, Haverkamp W, Block M, Hammel D, Borggrefe M, Breithardt G (1996) Comparison of D,L-sotalol and implantable defibrillators for treatment of sustained

ventricular tachycardia or fibrillation in patients with coronary artery disease. Circulation 94:151-157

10. The Antiarrhythmics versus Implantable Defibrillators (AVID) Investigators (1997) A comparison of antiarrhythmic-drug therapy with implantable defibrillators in patients resuscitated from near-fatal ventricular arrhythmias. N Engl J Med 337:1576-1583

11. Connolly S, on behalf of the CIDS investigators (1998) The Canadian Implantable Defibrillator Study (CIDS): final results. Oral presentation at the annual session of the American College of Cardiology meeting, Atlanta, 29 March 1998

12. Kuck K-H, on behalf of the CASH investigators (1998) The Cardiac Arrest Study Hamburg (CASH): final results. Oral presentation at the annual session of the American College of Cardiology meeting, Atlanta, 29 March 1998

13. Moss A, Hall WJ, Cannom D et al (1996) Improved survival with an implanted defibrillator in patients with coronary disease at high risk for ventricular arrhythmia. N Engl J Med 335:1933-1940

14. Buxton A (1999) Results from the Multicenter UnSustained Tachycardia Trial (MUSTT). Oral presentation during "Hotline session: new-breaking clinical trials," at the 48th Annual Scientific Sessions of the American College of Cardiology meeting, New Orleans, La, 8 March 1999

15. Levy S (1996) Is the implantable cardioverter-defibrillator cost-effective? Eur Heart J 17:1458-1459

16. Mushlin A, Zwanziger J, Gajary E, Andrews, M, Marron R (1997) Approach to cost-effectiveness assessment in the MADIT Trial. Am J Cardiol 80:33F-41F

17. Larsen G, Manolis A, Sonnenberg F et al (1992) Cost effectiveness of the implantable cardioverter-defibrillator: effect of improved batter life and comparison with amiodarone therapy. J Am Coll Cardiol 19:1323-1334

18. Deering T, Weintraub W (1998) Cost-effectiveness of treatment options for sustained ventricular tachycardia and fibrillation: comparison of the implantable cardioverter-defibrillator without prior electrophysiology testing to other treatment options. PACE 21:767 (abstr)

19. Anderson M, Camm A (1993) Implications for present and future applications of the implantable cardioverter-defibrillator resulting from the use of a simple model of cost efficacy. Br Heart J 69:83-92

20. Kupperman M, Luce B, McGovern B et al (1990) An analysis of the cost effectiveness of the ICD. Circulation 81:91-100

21. Kuppersmith J, Hogan A, Guerrero P et al (1995) Evaluating and improving the cost effectiveness of the implantable cardioverter-defibrillator. Am Heart J 130:507-515

22. O'Donoghue S, Platia E, Brooks-Robinson S, Mispireta L (1990) ICD: is early implantation cost effective? J Am Coll Cardiol 16:1258-1263

23. O'Brien B, Buxton M, Rushby J (1992) Cost effectiveness of the implantable cardioverter defibrillator: a preliminary analysis. Br Heart J 68:241-245

24. Valenti R, Schlapfer J, Fromer M, Fischer A, Kappenberger L (1996) Impact of the implantable cardioverter defibrillator on rehospitalizations. Eur Heart J 17:1565-1571

25. Owens D, Sanders G, Harris R, McDonald K et al (1997) Cost-effectivness of implantable cardioverter defibrillators relative to amiodarone for prevention of sudden Cardiac Death. Ann Intern Med 126:1-12

26. Wever E, Hauer R, Schrijvers G, van Capelle F et al (1996) Cost-effectiveness of implantable defibrillator as first-choice therapy versus electrophysiologically guided, tiered strategy in post-infarction sudden death survivors: a randomized study. Circulation 93:489-496

27. Mushlin A, Hall W, Zwanziger J et al (1998) The cost-effectiveness of automatic implantble cardiac defibrillators: results from MADIT. Circulation 97:2129-2135

28. NIH News Release (1997) NHLBI stops arrhythmia study – ICD reduces deaths. National Institutes of Health, Bethesda, Md, 14 April 1997

29. Cannom D (1998) AVID and Beyond: Lessons learned. J Intervent Cardiol 11:217-226

30. Steinhaus D (1996) Economics: selection of candidates to ICD implant. In: Santini M (ed) Proceedings, progress in clinical pacing 1996. Futura, Armonk, pp 233-240

31. Schwabe U, Paffrath D (eds) (1998) Arzneiverordnungs-Report 1998. Springer, Berlin Heidelberg New York

32. Higgins S (1999) Impact of the multicenter automatic defibrillator trial on implantable cardioverter defibrillator indications trends. Am J Cardiol 83(5B):79-82

What Is the Best Algorithm to Discriminate Between Supraventricular and Ventricular Tachyarrhythmias?

W. Jung, C. Wolpert, S. Spehl and B. Lüderitz

Introduction

Single-chamber ventricular defibrillator implantation has been shown to be an effective and safe treatment for patients with malignant ventricular tachyarrhythmias and to significantly reduce the incidence of sudden cardiac death. However, the high incidence of inappropriate implantable cardioverter defibrillator (ICD) therapy due to supraventricular tachycardias (SVT) is a major challenge and has been reported to affect up to 25% of patients [1, 2]. Enhanced detection criteria such as rate stability, sudden onset, and morphology assessment improve the specificity of ICD therapy, but may place the patient at risk of underdetection of ventricular tachycardia (VT) [3-7]. Recently, it has been shown that algorithms using dual-chamber sensing may significantly improve differentiation between SVT and VT [8-10]. Another beneficial effect of dual-chamber ICD may be the opportunity not only to sense in the atrium, but also to pace in this chamber. Although the beneficial effects of DDD pacing are well known, most of the currently available ICDs provide only fixed ventricular antibradycardia pacing. In a recent retrospective study the need for antibradycardia pacing was analyzed in a consecutive series of 139 ICD patients [11]. The findings of this report indicate that up to 18% of the ICD patients are in need of antibradycardia pacing, with up to 80% of these patients having an indication for DDD pacing. These results are supported by an independent analysis from our center [12].

This report describes the early clinical experience with an ICD capable of dual-chamber detection for arrhythmia diagnosis and dual-chamber pacing function.

Department of Medicine-Cardiology, University of Bonn, Germany

The Device

The Defender (Ela Medical, Montrouge, France) is a tiered-therapy dual-chamber ICD that provides dual-chamber sensing and pacing, antitachycardia pacing modalities, as well as low- and high-energy shock therapies. The Defender model 9001 and its successor model 9201 differ principally in their size and weight as well as in the function of their can. Model 9001, with a weight of 230 g and a volume of 148 ml, has a passive housing and is used for implantation in an abdominal pocket, whereas the case of model 9201, with a weight of 140 g and a volume of 75 ml, serves as a defibrillation electrode and is intended for implantation in the pectoral region. In order to function properly, model 9001 must be connected to at least two defibrillation leads and to one bipolar ventricular sensing and pacing lead. Adding a bipolar atrial lead to the system will allow optimal functioning of the device because delivery of antibradycardia pacing and arrhythmia detection will be performed in dual-chamber configuration. Because the active can of model 9201 serves as a defibrillation electrode, this device must be connected to only one defibrillation lead and to a bipolar ventricular sensing and pacing lead as well as a bipolar atrial sensing and pacing lead. The following leads were proposed in the study: a ventricular lead for sensing, pacing and defibrillation (Biotronik, model SL-ICD 60, Berlin, Germany) and an atrial lead for atrial sensing and pacing (Ela Medical, model Stela BS 45). However, both the choice of lead models and the positioning of the leads was left to the discretion of the managing physician. Both ICD models offer an antibradycardia function that can be programmed in VVI, DDI, or DDD mode.

The Defender stores general quantitative information (statistics) concerning detected or paced events and number of delivered and successful tachycardia therapies since the last counter reset. More detailed information is also available in the Holter function, which allows a complete review of episode mode of onset, evolution, and termination contained in 31 event log summaries of four selected tachyarrhythmia episodes. In general, the device stores the four most recent arrhythmia episodes. However, it will keep, in order of priority, the last episode of VF, the last episode of VT, and the last uncertain or SVT episode. For each episode retained in the Holter memory, the device stores the time and date of the arrhythmia occurrence. It identifies the episode by storing the type of the triggering rhythm. In addition, the device records a pre- and post-AV marker chain of 127 events each and an intracardiac pre-electrogram (ECG) for a maximum duration of 3-4 s preceding the application of the first therapy and a post-ECG for a maximum duration of six cycles after the device has concluded that the applied therapy was successful.

PARAD Classification Algorithm

The Defender uses a sophisticated dual-chamber algorithm for tachyarrhythmia classification [13]. A tiered arrhythmia detection analysis is performed in three consecutive steps: classification of ventricular cycles, majority rhythm identification, and persistence of rhythm. The device first classifies each ventricular cycle according to programmable cycle length criteria as VF or tachycardia (Tachy) or slow rhythm (SR) cycle. Based on this cycle-to-cycle classification, the device applies the majority criterion ($x\%$ of y cycles in a sliding window) to determine the predominant rhythm: VF majority, Tachy majority, SR majority, or No majority. If the rhythm has been identified as Tachy majority, the device uses a new tachycardia sorting algorithm (PARAD) to differentiate between a sinus tachycardia (ST), SVT including AF or flutter or atrial tachycardia, VT, or unsure. This tachycardia sorting depends on the combination of three additional criteria: ventricular rate (RR) stability (stable or unstable), atrioventricular (PR) association (n:1, 1:1, or none), and acceleration at the onset of the tachycardia (atrial origin, ventricular origin, or none). Therapy will be applied only to sustained tachyarrhythmias, if the programmed number of cycles of the persistence counter is met.

The Defender uses the tachycardia sorting template to reclassify rhythms with Tachy majority into three categories: VT (immediate therapy), SVT/ST (exempt from therapy), or unsure (deferred therapy). The Defender provides three predefined tachycardia sorting templates, rate only, standard V, and standard AV, where the latter template takes into account all three criteria (RR stability, PR association, acceleration) by using atrial and ventricular sensing together. In addition to the three standard templates, a "monitoring only" device status can be selected without therapy delivery, and a custom mode is available to the user which allows free programming of any combination of the recognition criteria. Table 1 summarizes the rhythm classification determined by the combination of these three criteria as a function of the three programmable standard tachycardia sorting templates.

The tachycardia recognition criteria are based on parameters programmed to $x\%$ out of y cycles in a sliding window. The Defender constructs a histogram of a programmable number of ventricular intervals and scans its RR interval histogram with a window set to the programmed RR stability window width (nominal setting 63 ms). The stability criterion is fulfilled when the number of RR intervals contained in the window is equivalent to at least $x\%$ of y cycles stored in the histogram. Only cycles faster than the VT detection rate are considered for the calculation of the stability criterion. If the RR stability criterion is met, the device scans its PR interval histogram with a window set to the programmed PR association window width (nominal setting 63 ms). It declares PR association when this number is at least $x\%$ of the number of stable RR intervals. If the number of PR intervals within this window represents at least $x\%$ of the cycles stored in the histogram, the device considers this as 1:1 PR association. Otherwise, if $x\%$ of the number of stored PR intervals is not within the window, it considers this as n:1 association. The device defines an accelerated cycle when its cycle length is shorter than the reference cycle (usually the preceding cycle) decreased by the programmed acceleration prematurity percentage (nominal setting 25%), and when its cycle length is shorter than the programmed Tachy cycle length. Figure 1 depicts the tachycardia classification algorithm.

Table 1. Rhythm classification according to PARAD programming

Combination of criteria			PARAD standard programming		
RP stability	PR association	Acceleration	StdAV	StdV	Rate only
Unstable	-	-	SVT/ST	SVT/ST	VT
Stable	n:1	Ventricular	SVT/ST	VT	VT
Stable	n:1	Atrial	SVT/ST	VT	VT
Stable	n:1	None	SVT/ST	SVT/ST	VT
Stable	1:1	Ventricular	VT	VT	VT
Stable	1:1	Atrial	SVT/ST	VT	VT
Stable	1:1	None	SVT/ST	SVT/ST	VT
Stable	None	Ventricular	VT	VT	VT
Stable	None	Atrial	VT	VT	VT
Stable	None	None	VT	SVT/ST	VT

SVT, supraventricular tachycardia; ST, sinus tachycardia; VT, ventricular tachycardia

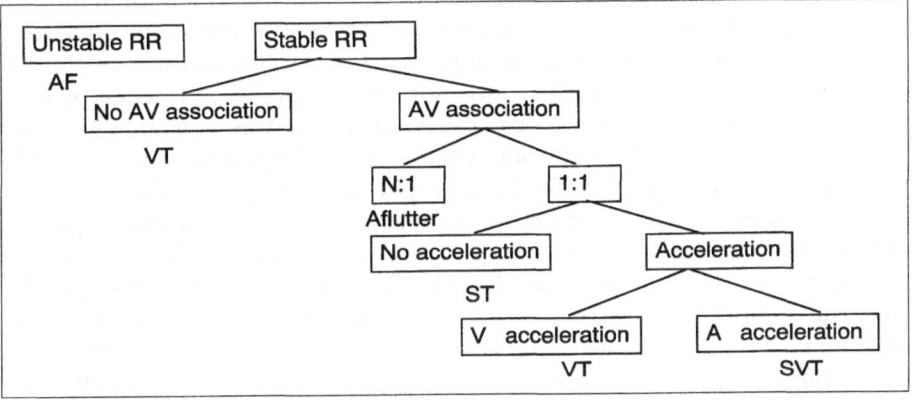

Fig. 1. Tachycardia classification algorithm based on three criteria: ventricular (RR) stability, atrioventricular (AV) association, and acceleration. An unstable ventricular rhythm is always considered to be atrial fibrillation (AF) and therapy is withheld. A stable ventricular rhythm without AV association is declared to be ventricular tachycardia (VT) and is immediately treated. A stable ventricular rhythm with n:1 AV association is interpreted as atrial flutter (Aflutter). A stable ventricular rhythm with 1:1 AV association but without acceleration is considered as sinus tachycardia (ST) and no therapy is delivered. A stable ventricular rhythm with 1:1 AV association and with acceleration of either atrial or ventricular origin is classified as supraventricular tachycardia (SVT) or VT

Results

The diagnostic accuracy of the new tachycardia classification algorithm was evaluated prospectively in 156 episodes of induced sustained tachycardias on the basis of the stability of the RR cycle lengths and AV association [14]. Eighty-nine tachycardias were taken from the Ann Arbor electrogram library; the others were recorded in 50 patients during electrophysiological studies. The atrial and ventricular signals were stored on an external recorder and then injected into an external prototype of a dual-chamber ICD (Defender 9001). The algorithm correctly diagnosed 96% of VT episodes, 100% of ventricular fibrillation (VF) episodes, and 92% of double-tachycardia episodes. The mean detection time for VT was 2.6 ± 0.8 s, and for VF it was 2.1 ± 0.4 s. The positive predictive values for the diagnosis of atrial fibrillation and flutter were 92% and 86%, respectively, and for VT and VF they were 95% and 100%, respectively.

In a recent publication, the sensitivity and specificity of this new tachycardia classification algorithm was evaluated in 18 patients with a mean age of 55 ± 15 years and a mean left ventricular ejection fraction of 35 ± 11% undergoing implantation with the first dual-chamber ICD, the Defender 9001 [15]. One patient with a defibrillation threshold of 34 J was excluded from the primary follow-up analysis because of protocol violation, and a second patient who developed multiple episodes of VF at the end of the implantation procedure died in electromechanical dissociation despite many successful internal and external DC shocks and vigorous resuscitation attempts. Over a mean follow-up period of 7.1 ± 4.5 months, 176 spontaneous tachyarrhythmia episodes were recorded in 11 patients in the device memory. The stored data for each episode were reviewed by independent investigators. A diagnosis was reached by consensus for all but one episode. The physician diagnosis was compared with that by the device. All 122 VT/VF episodes were correctly diagnosed, as were 51 of 53 SVTs. Two episodes of atrial fibrillation with rapid regular ventricular rates were treated as VT, and a third episode, treated as VT, could not be diagnosed with certainty. The time to first therapy delivery was 9.8 ± 3.4 s (range, 2.3-14 s) for VF, and 5.4 ± 1.5 s (range, 2.0-9.5 s) for VT, respectively. All VT/VF episodes were successfully treated with the first ICD shock therapy. The mean tachycardia rate for the spontaneous VT episodes was 153 ± 19 (range, 110-200) beats per minute, for the spontaneous ST episodes was 131 ± 20 (range, 104-180) beats per minute, and for the spontaneous SVT episodes 136 ± 12 (range, 125-153) beats per minute.

During follow-up two atrial lead displacements occurred. In one patient the lead was replaced and in a further patient the device was reprogrammed to ventricular-based pacing and tachycardia detection. One patient developed progressive heart failure and died 8 months after ICD implantation. The patient who was excluded from the primary analysis because of a high defibrillation threshold suffered 19 VT episodes during follow-up, all of which were detected and treated successfully by antitachycardia pacing or with shock therapy. Three months after ICD implant, the patient died in VF despite receiving multiple automatically delivered 34 J shocks. At the end of the follow-up period, 10 DDD ICDs were programmed in DDD mode, 5 in DDI mode, and one in VVI mode. To date 95 patients have received the dual-chamber ICD, the Defender 9001 [16]. Preliminary evaluation of these 95 patients supports the promising early experience with this first dual-chamber ICD with respect to its accuracy in distinguishing SVT from VT.

Conclusions

Dual-chamber ICDs provide efficacy and safety rates equivalent to those of single-chamber ICDs. With the application of the new tachycardia classification algorithm, discrimination of ventricular tachycardia from supraventricular tachycardia is achieved with a specificity of 92% and with a sensitivity of 99.3% for sustained ventricular tachyarrhythmias.

References

1. Hook BG, Marchlinski FE (1991) Value of ventricular electrogram in the diagnosis of arrhythmias precipitating electrical device therapy. J Am Coll Cardiol 19:490-499
2. Grimm W, Flores BF, Marchlinski FE (1992) Electrocardiographically documented unnecessary, spontaneous shocks in 241 patients with implantable cardioverter-defibrillators. Pacing Clin Electrophysiol 15:1667-1673
3. Swerdlow CD, Chen PS, Kass RM, Allard JR, Peter CT (1994) Discrimination of ventricular tachycardia from sinus tachycardia and atrial fibrillation in a tiered-therapy cardioverter-defibrillator. J Am Coll Cardiol 23:1342-1355
4. Swerdlow CD, Ahern T, Chen PS et al (1994) Underdetection of ventricular tachycardia by algorithms to enhance specificity in a tiered-therapy cardioverter-defibrillator. J Am Coll Cardiol 24:416-424
5. Neuzner J, Pitschner HF, Schlepper M (1995) Programmable VT detection enhancements in implantable cardioverter defibrillator therapy. Pacing Clin Electrophysiol 18:539-547
6. Schaumann A, von zur Mühlen F, Gonska BD, Kreuzer H (1996) Enhanced detection criteria in implantable cardioverter-defibrillators to avoid inappropriate therapy. Am J Cardiol 78:42-50
7. Higgins SL, Lee RS, Kramer RL (1995) Stability: an ICD detection criterion for discriminating atrial fibrillation from ventricular tachycardia. J Cardiovasc Electrophysiol 6:1081-1088
8. Schuger CD, Jackson K, Russel TS, Lehmann MH (1988) Atrial sensing to augment ventricular tachycardia detection by the automatic implantable cardioverter defibrillator: a utility study. Pacing Clin Electrophysiol 11:1456-1464
9. Leong PHW, Jabri MA (1992) Arrhythmia classification using two intracardiac leads. IEEE Computer Society Press, Los Alamitos, Calif. pp 189-192 (Proceedings of Computers in Cardiology)
10. Polikaitis A, Arzbaecher R (1995) Sensitivity and specificity of a dual-chamber arrhythmia recognition algorithm for implantable devices. J Electrocardiol 27:78-83
11. Geelen P, Lorga A, Chauvin M, Wellens F, Brugada P (1997) The value of DDD pacing in patients with an implantable cardioverter defibrillator. Pacing Clin Electrophysiol 20:177-181
12. Wolpert C, Jung W, Lilienthal B et al (1997) Ist bei Patienten mit implantierbarem Kardioverter-Defibrillator eine AV-sequentielle Stimulation erforderlich? Systematische Untersuchung an 102 Patienten. Z Kardiol 86:315 (abstr)
13. Korte T, Jung W, Wolpert C, Spehl S, Schumacher B, Esmailzadeh B, Lüderitz B (1998) A new classification algorithm for discrimination of ventricular from supraventricular tachycardia in a dual-chamber implantable cardioverter-defibrillator. J Cardiovasc Electrophysiol 9:70-73

14. Nair M, Saoudi N, Kroiss D, Letac B, for the Participating Centers of the Automatic Recognition of Arrhythmia Study Group (1997) Automatic arrhythmia identification using analysis of the atrioventricular association. Circulation 95:973-967
15. Lavergne T, Daubert JC, Chauvin M et al (1997) Preliminary clinical experience with the first dual-chamber pacemaker defibrillator. Pacing Clin Electrophysiol 20:182-188
16. Jung W, Wolpert C, Spehl S et al (1998) Prospective evaluation of a new arrhythmia classification algorithm for discrimination of ventricular tachycardia from supraventricular tachycardia. Pacing Clin Electrophysiol 21:890 (abstr)

Transthoracic Epicardial Mapping and Ablation of Post-Infarction Ventricular Tachycardia: The Right Solution to the Problem?

E. Sosa, M. Scanavacca and A. D'Avila

Introduction

The majority of sustained ventricular tachycardias after myocardial infarction (post-MI VT) are believed to originate from a reentrant circuit located at the subendocardium [1, 2]. Nevertheless, the functional role of the epicardium in maintaining some reentrant circuits has been well established, and data obtained from intraoperative mapping suggest that epicardial circuits are more common in post-inferior-wall MI [3, 4]. In these circumstances, conventional endocardial pulses of radiofrequency energy may be less effective [5]. Accordingly, subepicardial target sites have been pointed to as one of the reasons for unsuccessful use of catheter ablation to treat patients with VT [6].

Nonsurgical transthoracic epicardial catheter ablation has been recently introduced as an alternative approach to treat patients with recurrent VT related to an epicardial or subepicardial circuit [7-9]. Briefly, this procedure consists of introducing a standard 4-mm-tip ablation catheter into the pericardial space by transthoracic pericardial puncture, similar to the procedure Krikornian and Hancock described for draining pericardial effusions [10].

Given the successful results obtained with this technique in patients with Chagas' disease [7, 8], in whom epicardial circuits predominate, we speculated that transthoracic epicardial catheter ablation could be useful in patients with postinfarction VT related to an epicardial circuit. However, the presence of incidental pericardial adherence associated with transmural myocardial infarction could theoretically impose a limitation for this approach in postinfarction patients.

Transthoracic Mapping and Ablation Technique

We have recently published the preliminary results of this approach [7-9]. However, the way the catheter is inserted into the pericardial space is what has been puzzling other investigators. Actually, this is a main issue, since after the

Heart Institute (InCor), University of São Paulo Medical School, São Paulo, Brazil catheter has been introduced into the pericardial sac, the mapping techniques utilized are the same as for endocardial mapping and ablation. Therefore, it is essential to make clear here the technique used to insert the ablation catheter into the pericardial space.

Transthoracic Puncture

Transthoracic puncture is the most important step in the whole procedure and it can be safely and efficiently undertaken in the electrophysiology laboratory.

Our Approach

After proper aseptic preparation of the subxyphoid area, pericardial puncture is undertaken according to the technique previously described by Krikornian and Hancock [10]. A regular needle used for epidural anesthesia (Tuohy-17G, effective length 79.4 mm, overall lenght 101.6 mm, Abbot I/N# E622; Abbot Ireland Ltd., Sligo, Republic of Ireland) is utilized for this procedure. The needle angle is adjusted according to the region that the operator wishes to access. This region is most frequently the medial third of the right ventricle, where, based on the coronary angiography, no major coronary vessels can be found. In this case, the needle is introduced at a 45° angle and gently advanced under fluoroscopy.

In order to precisely demonstrate the site where the needle tip is, 2 ml contrast medium is injected (loxitalamato of meglumina and sodium; Telebrix Coronar; Gulbert Produções Ltda, Rio de Janeiro, Brazil). When the needle tip has not yet entered the pericardial sac, contrast injection is very helpful in marking the outer limit of the parietal pericardium which will then be utilized to guide needle placement. Delimitation of the parietal pericardium allows clear visualization of the needle and its relations with the heart as the needle is advanced towards the pericardial sac under fluoroscopy. Once the parietal pericardium is defined, it will be as helpful as contrast medium, delimiting the intra-atrial septum during transseptal puncture. In other words, it will be possible to visualize whether the needle is only pushing or has passed through the parietal pericardium as it is advanced.

When the needle tip is inside the pericardial space, contrast medium is injected again and will be seen surrounding the silhouette of the heart. It is crucial to visualize this thin layer of contrast as it confirms that the needle is correctly placed in the pericardial space.

The needle tip can occasionally perforate the right ventricle, which can be easily confirmed by aspirating blood in the syringe. If that happens, the needle is slightly withdrawn and 1-2 ml contrast medium is injected to ensure correct positioning of the needle tip in the pericardium.

In the majority of cases pericardial puncture is achieved without right ventricular perforation. Right ventricular perforation has occurred in 8 of 42 patients, but it has never caused any serious complications to the patient because these perforations are "dry".

The needle tip is very thin and fixed when in contact with the heart, avoiding laceration of the right ventricular wall. Additionally, patients do not receive heparin prior to transthoracic puncture. In only one case a 50-ml hemopericardium occurred, but it was drained with a pigtail catheter.

Finally, after confirming that the needle tip is properly placed in the pericardial space, a soft floppy-tip guide wire is introduced in the pericardial space through the puncture needle. As a rule, the guide wire easily slips into the pericardial space. Perforation of the right ventricle by the guide wire can also happen, but in that case no hemopericardium occurs.

Guide wire position is also monitored through fluoroscopy. An 8-French introducer is then placed in the pericardial space and the guide wire removed. Finally, under fluoroscopy, a quadripolar deflectable catheter with a 4-mm tip is inserted into the pericardial space for mapping and ablation. As soon as the catheter is in the pericardial space, the pericardial fluid is aspirated to check for blood. Normally, only a trivial amount of translucent pericardial fluid is expected.

Once the ablation catheter is introduced in the epicardial space, extensive mapping may be performed without increasing the procedural risk, because there are no papillary muscles or thrombi in the pericardial sac to restrict catheter movement.

Other Approaches to the Pericardial Space

Recently, Verrier et al. have published an interesting paper on transatrial access to the pericardial space, surely an attractive idea [11]. The working hypothesis for this new approach was that pericardial puncture would only be possible in the presence of a sizable pericardial effusion. However, based on our current experience, this supposition should no longer be held as definite fact. It is clear from our data that entering the pericardial space does not require the presence of 200 ml pericardial fluid, as stated by these authors.

So far, 42 patients have undergone the transthoracic approach to the pericardial space. An echocardiogram obtained in all patients 1 week after the procedure showed no effusion, and at long-term follow-up no complications were detected. Three patients complained of mild chest pain, controlled with regular anti-inflammatory drugs. Verrier's approach has been attempted in animals so far, and because only 2 dogs were observed for 24 h, more information is necessary on survival studies before the transatrial access route can be admitted to clinical practice.

Another device has also been recently introduced to allow minimally invasive access to the normal pericardium [12]. It consists of a 21-G needle housed inside a 12-French stainless steel sheath tube 20 cm in length (PerDUCER, Comedicus Inc., Columbia Heights, Minn.). This seems an ingenious device, but it is not clear whether it will be utilized for electrophysiological procedures. It has been reported that placement of the 0.0018-inch J-tipped guide wire in the pericardial space could not be easily confirmed in a series of five patients [13]. Because positioning the guide wire in the pericardial space represents a crucial step in our approach, more has to be learned before the PerDUCER can be utilized for epicardial mapping and radiofrequenty ablation.

Presently, we therefore still recommend the use of a Tuohy-17G epidural needle as the simplest and safest way to reach the pericardial sac in patients without pericardial effusion.

Epicardial Mapping

When the catheter is in the pericardial space (Fig. 1), the operator can easily manipulate it, covering the entire surface of both the right and left ventricles, as well as the atria. The limits of this surface are marked by pericardial reflection. The lateral and posterior left ventricular wall of both ventricles and atria are easier to map than the anterior wall.

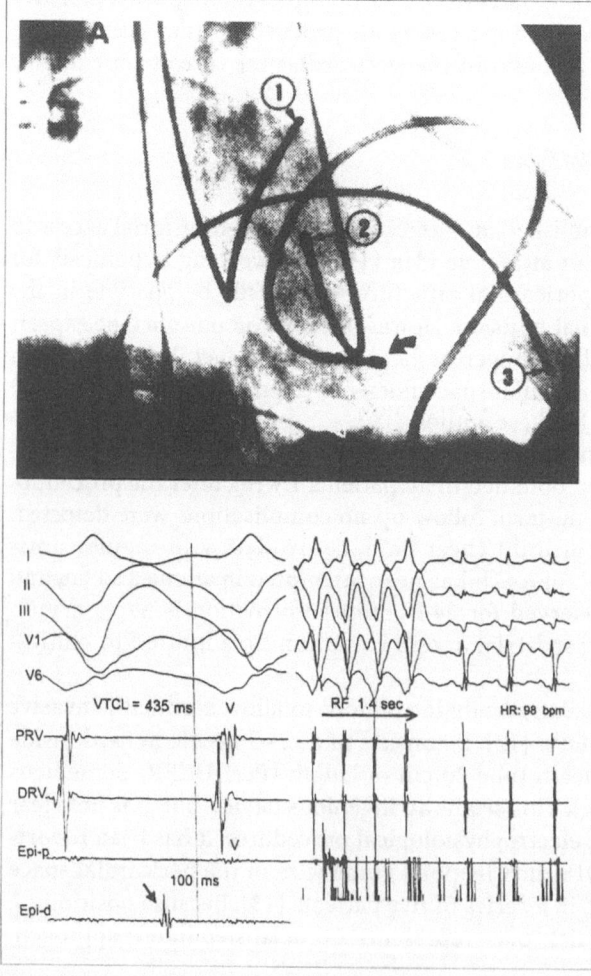

Fig. 1. *Upper panel:* Right anterior oblique view at 60° obtained by fluoroscopy during epicardial mapping procedure. The epicardial catheter (*arrow*) is gently manipulated and placed in different locations of the epicardial space, where epicardial electrograms are obtained. 1, Coronary sinus catheter; 2, endocardial left ventricular catheter; 3, right apical endocardial catheter. *Lower panel:* Activation mapping of ventricular tachycardia obtained during a transthoracic epicardial ablation procedure. A pres-ystolic electrogram fo-und in the distal epicardial vessel (*Epi-d*) precedes the onset of the QRS complex by 100 ms. Application at this site interrupted ventricular tachycardia after 1.4 s, rendering it noninducible. P, Proximal; D, distal; RV, right apical electrogram; VTCL, ventricular tachycardia cycle length; HR, heart rate; V, ventricular electrogram; Epi, epicardial

Another noteworthy peculiarity found in this approach is catheter stability. When the catheter is not being manipulated, it rests stable in a selected site, following ventricular wall motion. Catheter stability is enhanced by the apposition of the two layers of pericardium lying against it. Moreover, the catheter cannot be dislodged to another place as the pericardial space has no room for that. In this sense, the epicardial catheter is easier to manipulate and shows more stability than the endocardial catheter, which tends to be expelled every systole, especially when inside the left ventricular cavity.

Epicardial electrograms are as clear as endocardial electrograms and their interpretation follows the same pattern as that for standard endocardial signs. The possibility of mapping an extensive epicardial surface permits assessment of electrical activity at sites very close together, thus displaying more data about the electrical activity of the heart. This is not usually possible with endocardial mapping, since the presence of papillary muscles and chordae as well as repetitive ventricular systoles prevent free manipulation of the endocardial catheter.

Criteria for the Diagnosis of an Epicardial VT

Due to the high stimulation threshold, entrainment techniques have rarely been used as an indication to select target sites for ablation (Fig. 1). More often, selection has been accomplished by heating the tip of the electrode (thermo mapping) and examining its effect on the VT. This empirical thermo mapping technique consists of radiofrequency pulses of 60 °C for 10 s. If the VT is interrupted within 10 s, application is maintained for 30 s. If the VT is not modified within the first 10 s, the catheter is manipulated until better electrograms are obtained, and new thermo mapping pulses are applied.

The limitations on the use of entrainment and the small lesions produced by empirical use of thermo pulses of 60 °C for 10 s can restrict the ability to distinguish between a bystander site and a common pathway. Therefore, potentially appropriate sites for ablation might fail to be identified. The use of higher temperature pulses for a longer period might identify a larger number of epicardial circuits.

How to Avoid Damaging the Coronary Arteries

In the beginning of our clinical experience, special attention was given to the distance between coronary arteries and the distal electrode of the ablating catheter. Theoretically, the risk of damaging epicardial vessels during the application of radiofrequency energy increases as the catheter approaches the coronary artery. The distance between the vessel and the ablation catheter tip was estimated by either (1) analyzing the distance between the apex of the heart, where large epicardial vessels are unlikely to be present, and the ablating and coronary sinus catheters, (2) observing the distance between the ablating catheter and a coronary artery during left coronary arteriography, or (3) observing the distance between the ablating catheter and epicardial veins of the heart during retrograde injection of contrast medium into the coronary sinus. It was assumed that an important coronary artery is usually close to a major epicardial vein.

Based on the size of the lesion produced by radiofrequency applications in experimental studies, we have empirically established that the smallest acceptable distance between the catheter tip and a major coronary artery should be 12 mm (three times the length of the catheter tip). If the ablation catheter was closer than that to an artery or vein, the radiofrequency pulse was not delivered. Moreover, the ST-T segment was simultaneously monitored in the12-lead electrocardiogram after VT interruption, to detect any possible coronary artery lesion during radiofrequency application.

However, because we have never seen concrete signs of arterial injury produced during epicardial radiofrequency ablation, we have assumed that these pulses are only applied in areas of scar tissue, which means that these applications will be delivered in the vicinity of occluded and previously damaged coronary arteries. Although it is possible to identify and catheterize small coronary arteries responsible for blood supply to the site of origin or pathway of VT in as many as 84% of patients with postinfarction VT, these lesions are unlikely to produce consequences deleterious to the heart [14]. In recent years, occlusion of these vessels by transcoronary chemical ablation has not been found to produce consequences deleterious to ventricular function [15]. Analogously, therefore, applications of radiofrequency pulses close to these vessels should not be expected to give rise to any serious complications. Although further investigation is still needed to clarify this specific point, there is no evidence that this approach should not be implemented at the present time. Actually, preliminary data suggest that it is safe to apply radiofrequency pulses close to the coronary arteries [16], and that selective coagulation necrosis of canine adventitia and media induces extracellular matrix accumulation without neointima formation [17]. However, the long-term effects of radiofrequency pulses delivered in the vicinity of epicardial coronary arteries in human beings remain unclear.

Results

From October 1996 to February 1999, 16 consecutive patients with an old inferior myocardial infarction and recurrent post-MI VT were referred to our group. All patients underwent diagnostic electrophysiologic study and VT was well tolerated, allowing adequate mapping in 14 patients (systolic pressure > 80 mmHg with no signs of low cerebral flow or cardiac output). These patients were selected to undergo radiofrequency ablation. VT was incessant in 1 patient and 2 other patients had previously undergone unsuccessful standard endocardial radiofrequency ablation. Mean age was 56 ± 15 years, 9 patients were male, and mean VT cycle length was 415 ± 48 ms. A total of 23 VTs were induced. Electrophysiologic evidence of an epicardial circuit was present in 7 (30%) of them, and all of them could be successfully ablated by application of an epicardial pulse of radiofrequency (Fig. 1). The procedure was well tolerated in all patients, and none of them experienced creatine kinase MB elevation. Echocardiographic examination on the day of hospital discharge did not reveal pericardial effusion. No complications occurred during hospitalization.

Conclusions

The nonsurgical transthoracic epicardial mapping technique has proved to be a safe and effective approach for identifying and treating epicardial circuits of sustained VT when utilized to guide radiofrequency epicardial catheter ablation. Possible postinfarction pericardial adherences do not preclude its use. Therefore, centers dealing with VT patients on a regular basis should incorporate this procedure into the electrophysiologic routine of mapping and ablation of VT associated with structural heart disease. At the present time, it seems to be the right or at least the best solution for the treatment of post-MI VT related to an epicardial circuit.

References

1. Josephson ME, Marchlinski FE, Buxton AE et al (1984) Electrophysiologic basis for sustained ventricular tachycardia: role of reentry. In: Josephson ME, Wellens HJJ (eds) Tachycardias: mechanism, diagnosis, treatment. Lea and Febiger, Philadelphia, pp 305-323
2. Hadjis TA, Stevenson WG, Harada T, Friedman PL, Sager P, Saxon LA (1997) Preferential locations for critical reentry circuit sites causing ventricular tachycardia after inferior wall myocardial infarction. J Cardiovasc Electrophysiol 8:363-370
3. Svenson RH, Littmann L, Gallagher JJ et al (1990) Termination of ventricular tachycardia with epicardial laser photocoagulation: a clinical comparison with patients undergoing successful endocardial photocoagulation alone. J Am Coll Cardiol 15:163-170
4. Littmann L, Svenson RH, Gallagher JJ et al (1991) Functional role of the epicardium in postinfarction ventricular tachycardia. Circulation 83:1577-1591
5. Blanchard SM, Walcott GP, Wharton JM, Ideker RE (1994) Why is catheter ablation less successful than surgery for treating ventricular tachycardia that results from coronary artery disease? Pacing Clin Electrophysiol 17:2315-2335
6. Kaltenbrunner W, Cardinal R, Dubue M et al (1991) Epicardial and endocardial mapping of ventricular tachycardia in patients with myocardial infarction. Is the origin of the tachycardia always subendocardially localized? Circulation 84:1058-1071
7. Sosa E, Scanavacca M, d'Avila A, Pilleggi F (1996) A new technique to perform epicardial mapping in the electrophysiology laboratory. J Cardiovasc Electrophysiol 7:531-536
8. Sosa E, Scanavacca M, d'Avila A, Piccioni J, Sanchez O, Velarde JL, Silva M, Reolão B (1998) Endocardial and epicardial ablation guided by nonsurgical transthoracic epicardial mapping to treat recurrent ventricular tachycardia. J Cardiovasc Electrophysiol 9:229-239
9. Sosa E, Scanavacca M, d'Avila A, Bellotti G, Pilleggi F (1999) Radiofrequency catheter

ablation of ventricular tachycardia guided by non-surgical epicardial mapping in chronic Chagasic heart disease. Pacing Clin Electrophysiol 22:128-130

10. Krikornian JG, Hancock EW (1978) Pericardiocentesis. Am J Med 65:808-816
11. Verrier R, Waxman S, Lovett E, Moreno R (1998) Transatrial access to the normal pericardial space. Circulation 98:2331-2333
12. Macris M, Igo SR (1999) Minimally invasive access of the normal pericardium: initial clinical experience with a novel device. Clin Cardiol 22:I36-I39
13. Seferovic P, Ristic AD, Maksimovic R et al (1999) Initial clinical experience with PerDUCER device: promising new tool in the diagnosis and treatment of pericardial disease. Clin Cardiol 22:I30-I35
14. Saxon LA, Sherman CT, Stevenson WG, Yeatman LA, Wiener D (1992) Ventricular tachycardia after infarction: sources of coronary blood flow to the infarct zone. Am Heart J 124:84-86
15. Brugada P, de Swart H, Smeets JL, Wellens HJ (1989) Transcoronary chemical ablation of ventricular tachycardia. Circulation 79:475-482
16. Arruda M, Otomo K, Pitha J, Schaer A, Tondo C, Antz M, Bussey J, Nakagawa H, Lazzara R, Jackman W (1997) Epicardial left ventricular recordings and radiofrequency catheter ablation from the coronary veins: a potential adjunct approach for mapping and ablation of ventricular tachycardia. Pacing Clin Electrophysiol 20:1075 (abstr)
17. Hehrlein C, Thompson M, Chuang CH, Splinter R, Tuntelder JR, Littmann L, Svenson RH (1995) Selective coagulation necrosis of canine adventitia and media induces extracellular matrix accumulation without neointima formation. Atherosclerosis 113:109-115

SUDDEN DEATH AFTER MYOCARDIAL INFARCTION

Risk Stratification for Serious Arrhythmic Events in Post-Infarction Patients

N. El-Sherif and G. Turitto

Prologue

In spite of recent improvement in overall cardiovascular mortality, posthospital mortality remains high in survivors of acute myocardial infarction (AMI). Approximately one third of late deaths in survivors of AMI are sudden and unexpected, and the risk of sudden death persists for years after the AMI [1, 2]. Prevention of sudden cardiac death (SCD), which in the majority of cases is due to malignant ventricular tachyarrhythmias (VT, defined as hypotensive ventricular tachycardia/ventricular fibrillation), remains a formidable clinical challenge in survivors of AMI. Management strategy of this major health care problem has centered over the years on two closely related aspects: (1) how to identify those at risk of SCD, and (2) what the best management modalities are – pharmacotherapy or the implantable cardioverter-defibrillator (ICD). Following recent publications of the results of several multicenter studies, pharmacotherapy – mainly antiarrhythmic drugs – has not proven so far to be an effective management modality for those at risk of SCD. This cleared the way for more widespread use of the ICD as the sole or main management modality. Primarily because of the high cost of the ICD, and the invasive nature of this therapeutic modality, the prophylactic use of the device for primary prevention of SCD did not gain momentum until recently. This aspect of management strategy for SCD is still in the clinical research domain, with several primary ICD prevention trials currently underway. However, this trend has highlighted the urgent need for more powerful risk stratification algorithms for SCD in this population.

The most recent results of the MADIT [3] and AVID [4] trials on the one hand and the CABG-PATCH trial [5] on the other underscored the point that the ICD works only when implanted in patients at high risk of arrhythmic death. Besides the invasive electrophysiologic study (EPS), commonly utilized noninvasive risk stratifiers include: left ventricular ejection fraction (LVEF), ventricular arrhyth-

Cardiology Division, Department of Medicine, State University of New York, and Health Science Center and Veterans Affairs Medical Center, Brooklyn, NY, USA

mias on ambulatory Holter recording, signal-averaged electrocardiography (SAECG), heart rate variability (HRV), baroreflex sensitivity (BRS), QT dispersion, and T wave alternans (TWA). In addition, there are a number of other less commonly utilized markers of arrhythmic death. However, with the exception of LVEF, none of the other tests has at present proven to be solely adequate as a powerful risk stratifier. An optimal algorithm that combines more than one index of high risk has not yet been identified or agreed upon.

Left Ventricular Ejection Fraction

LV function is one of the best predictors of cardiac mortality and morbidity in patients with coronary artery disease (CAD), especially after AMI. For example, in the Multicenter Postinfarction Study, patients with an LVEF less than 20% had an approximately 45% 1-year mortality rate, compared to a 4% rate in patients with an LVEF greater than 40% [6]. However, LV systolic dysfunction is not a very sensitive marker of sudden or arrhythmic death [7]. The combination of severely depressed LVEF and NYHA class IV seems to identify patients who will die from pump failure or electromechanical dissociation rather than from malignant VT. On the other hand, of patients with moderate-to-severe LV dysfunction, approximately one third die suddenly, relatively independent of the severity of LV dysfunction [7]. It is important to remember that the extent of LV dysfunction can influence significantly the predictive power of other risk stratifiers, such as the SAECG and EPS.

Ambulatory Holter recording

The finding of complex ventricular arrhythmias on a Holter recording is not specific enough to identify individual patients at high risk of SCD. Spontaneous variation from day to day in the incidence of complex ventricular arrhythmias makes interpretation of the results of therapy guided by Holter recording subject to large errors. A more difficult question that remains unanswered at present is the relationship of asymptomatic complex ventricular arrhythmias to symptomatic VT. It is not clear whether these rhythm disorders are related mechanistically, and therefore whether alterations in spontaneous ectopy by antiarrhythmic therapy will impact on the prognosis.

Signal-Averaged Electrocardiography

The SAECG appears useful in risk stratification of post-MI patients. Late potentials have been shown to predict future arrhythmic events [8, 9]. However, a recent National Institutes of Health study has shown that time-domain (TD)

SAECG indices of late potentials do not provide the best prediction criteria for serious arrhythmic events in the first year after MI, but rather the filtered QRS duration at 40 Hz [10]. The SAECG has some limitations; although it appears to have an excellent negative predictive value, both its sensitivity and positive predictive value are low. Recently, combined time- and frequency-domain analysis of the SAECG was shown to improve its overall predictive accuracy [11, 12]. The rationale for combined time- and frequency-domain analysis of the SAECG is the observation that TD analysis has a high incidence of false positive results in patients with inferior wall MI, while spectral turbulence analysis (STA) has a high incidence of false positive results in anterior MI. In a recent study of 602 post-MI patients, receiver-operated characteristics curves were utilized to optimize cutoff values for each SAECG parameter separately, and also for the combined TD+STA model [12]. The negative predictive accuracy of all three analyses was high (98%). On the other hand, the positive predictive accuracy of TD (19.6%) or STA (18.3%) was quite low, and was significantly improved to 35.8% by combined TD+STA analysis. The best results were obtained in patients with LVEF less than 40%, where the positive predictive accuracy of combined TD+STA analysis was 51.2%. The study concluded that combined TD+STA analysis of the SAECG significantly improves risk stratification power for VT in post-MI patients compared to TD and STA separately.

Heart Rate Variability and Baroreflex Sensitivity

Many studies have revealed an association between the autonomic nervous system and SCD [13]. Both HRV and BRS are measures of the sympathovagal balance. Methods to analyze HRV employ both time- and frequency-domain measurements that quantify periodicities in the data. Prognostic information to risk stratify patients for future VT or other cardiac events leading to premature death may be possible by quantifying HRV [14, 15]. BRS assessed with phenylephrine injection is an alternative noninvasive test to evaluate sympathovagal balance [16]. Two major questions concerning HRV remain to be clarified. First, many methods to measure HRV have been reported, and it is very difficult to conclude which one is most appropriate for establishing normal values and for particular patient subgroups. There is a need to standardize the measurement of HRV and to quantify normal values under various circumstances, including patient age and gender. A recent effort in this regard is the report of the Task Force of the European Society of Cardiology and the North American Society of Pacing and Electrophysiology [17]. Low HRV is associated with increased all-cause mortality in middle-aged and elderly men [18]. HRV did not add independent prognostic value to LV function and ventricular arrhythmias on predischarge Holter recording [19]. On the other hand, in the ATRAMI study, low values of BRS and HRV were significantly associated with an increased mortality risk in a multivariate model in which LVEF and premature ventricular complexes were included [16].

QT Interval and QT Dispersion

Previous studies have shown that prolongation of the QT interval is a risk factor for VT and SCD in patients with previous MI [20], but there has been some controversy as to the predictive accuracy of the prolonged QT interval. QT dispersion may be a more powerful predictor of susceptibility to VT, suggesting that inhomogeneity of repolarization is more closely associated with arrhythmic risk than is prolongation of repolarization itself [21]. Spatial dispersion of recovery times may be a fundamental electrophysiologic substrate for the genesis of reentrant VT. Day et al. first proposed that interlead variability of QT interval in 12-lead electrocardiograms, QT dispersion, reflects dispersion of ventricular recovery time, thus providing a convenient tool for clinical studies [22]. However, the role of QT dispersion for risk stratification of SCD remains controversial, which in large measure may be due to methodologic discrepancies. Some studies suggest that increased QT dispersion is related to susceptibility to VT, independent of the degree of LV dysfunction or clinical characteristics of the patients [21]. Other studies have shown that determination of QT dispersion from the surface ECG, even when performed with the best available methodology, failed to predict subsequent risk in post-MI patients [23]. Some investigators have found an association between measures of dispersion of ventricular repolarization and susceptibility to ventricular fibrillation [24]. However, because of considerable overlap between groups, these measures failed to provide a useful marker for the risk of SCD.

T Wave Alternans

Alternation of the configuration and/or duration of the repolarization wave of the ECG, usually referred to as TWA, is seen under diverse experimental and clinical conditions [25]. Interest in repolarization alternans is attributed to the hypothesis that it may reflect underlying dispersion of repolarization in the ventricle, a well recognized electrophysiologic substrate for reentrant VT. Although overt TWA in the ECG is not common, in recent years digital signal-processing techniques capable of detecting subtle degrees of TWA have suggested that the phenomenon may be more prevalent than previously recognized and could represent an important marker of vulnerability to VT [26]. The electrophysiological basis of arrhythmogenicity of QT/T alternans in long QT syndrome has been recently investigated in an experimental surrogate model of long QT syndrome [27]. The arrhythmogenicity of QT/T alternans was primarily due to the greater degree of spatial dispersion of repolarization during alternans than during slower rates not associated with alternans. The dispersion of repolarization was most marked between midmyocardial and epicardial zones in the LV free wall. In the presence of a critical degree of dispersion of repolarization, propagation of the activation wavefront could be blocked between these zones to initiate reentrant excitation and polymorphic VT. An important observation was that marked repolarization alternans could be present in local electrograms without manifest alternation of the QT/T segment in the surface ECG. The latter was seen at critically short cycle lengths associated with reversal of the gradient of repolarization between epicardial and midmyocardial sites, with a consequent reversal of polarity of the intramyocardial QT wave in alternate cycles. These observations provide a strong impetus for studies that explore the use of microvolt TWA as a strong predictor for SCD.

Recent technical improvements allow the detection of microvolt TWA during sinus rhythm with the heart rate moderately elevated using a bicycle exercise test. Several studies have shown that microvolt TWA detected with heart rate elevation with bicycle exercise is a strong predictor of arrhythmia inducibility at EPS [28, 29]. In a prospective multicenter study of 148 patients, the relationship between TWA and the induction of VT on EPS was assessed. TWA was a moderately sensitive but specific predictor of the results of EPS. However, TWA more accurately predicted future arrhythmic events compared to EPS [29]. TWA compared favorably with EPS and other noninvasive risk markers in predicting recurrence of VT in ICD recipients [30]. The heart rate at the onset of TWA in normal subjects and in patients with VT was also investigated [31]. False positive TWA developed in 7% of age-matched normal subjects at a higher heart rate than in patients with VT. A target heart rate of 110 beats/min was found to be highly sensitive and specific. However, because of their lower symptom-limited heart rate, many patients may not be able to achieve the target heart rate associated with TWA, resulting in an indeterminate test. In these patients, noninvasive or pharmacologic means to increase heart rate may be considered.

Electrophysiologic Study

The role of EPS in risk stratification of post-MI patients with regard to arrhythmic events remains controversial. Inducible VT was reported in 9%-20% of survivors of recent MI by EPS, and after a follow-up period of 1-2 years serious arrhythmic events occurred in 14%-36% of patients with inducible sustained VT [32-34]. In the MADIT study, patients with one or more prior MI, an LVEF of 35% or less, nonsustained VT, and inducible nonsuppressible VT had significantly improved survival with the ICD compared to conventional medical therapy [3]. The MUSTT study investigated a very similar population (the only difference was LVEF ≤ 40%) and found that in patients with inducible VT, EP-guided antiarrhythmic therapy improved survival primarily due to therapy with the ICD rather than "effective" antiarrhythmic drugs (A.L. Buxton, personal communication). In this study, the 5-year incidence of arrhythmic death or cardiac arrest in patients who had no inducible VT was 26%, compared to 32% in patients with inducible VT who were followed on no antiarrhythmic therapy. However, the 5-year total mortality was similar (48%). Both MADIT and MUSTT trials failed to shed light on the one crucial question regarding the future role of EPS in risk stratification, namely, whether noninducibility of VT in post-MI patients is a strong marker of low risk independent of other variables, such as the degree of LV dysfunction or TWA.

In Search of Other Risk Stratifiers for SCD

In addition to the more commonly investigated techniques for risk stratification for SCD, several other risk indices have been reported. For instance, QT dispersion detected by magnetocardiograph [35] or by precordial mapping techniques [36] was reported to be a sensitive marker of susceptibility to malignant VT. However, the prohibitive cost of a magnetocardiography laboratory and the technical demands of precordial mapping techniques are obvious deterrents to their wide application in a clinical setting. Beat-to-beat repolarization lability was found in one study to be a better identifier of SCD than other indicators of abnormal repolarization, including spatial QT dispersion and TWA [37]. Low variability of cycle lengths of nonsustained VT was also suggested as an independent predictor of mortality after AMI [38]. Increased heart rate, assessed from a 24-h Holter recording, or even from a standard ECG tracing, was found to be a strong predictor of mortality after AMI [23, 39]. On the other hand, "nonelectrophysiologic" indices may also be associated with increased risk for SCD, for instance, LV mass and hypertrophy [40].

The practical value of many of the risk stratifiers of SCD remains largely unanswered. Although risk stratification for SCD may be improved by using several variables in combination, one problem that has been alluded to is that dichotomous limits derived from univariate analysis may be different when used in the multivariate setting [41].

Epilogue

At present it remains uncertain how to manage post-MI patients at high risk for arrhythmic death. Although combinatorial algorithms that utilize several noninvasive and invasive tests may provide better risk stratification, there is still no consensus as to what is the best way to characterize the patient's arrhythmic risk and whether anti-ischemic measures, antiarrhythmic pharmacologic therapy, the ICD, or a combination of measures represent the best management strategy. Several randomized controlled studies for primary prevention of SCD are currently underway to answer these questions. Unfortunately these studies still use different risk stratification indices as well as different management strategies. For example, the MADIT-II study [42] randomizes patients with CAD and LVEF below 35% to no antiarrhythmic therapy versus the ICD. The Sudden Cardiac Death in Heart Failure Trial (SCD-HeFT) [43] randomizes patients with congestive heart failure and LVEF below 35% to no antiarrhythmic therapy, amiodarone, or the ICD. On the other hand, the primary objective of the Beta-blocker Strategy plus ICD (BEST+ICD) trial [44] is to establish the value of ICD in patients with recent MI, LVEF of 35% or less, and EPS-inducible sustained VT. The first two studies highlight the current impression in the field that, other than low LVEF, no other "electrophysiologic" marker is powerful enough to be included in the risk stratification strategy for primary prevention of SCD, while the third study continues to explore "conventional" electrophysiologic markers. The validity of either approach remains to be defined.

Acknowledgements. This study was supported in part by Veterans Administration Medical Research Funds.

References

1. Rouleau JL, Talajic M, Sussex B et al (1996) Myocardial infarction patients in the 1980s – their risk factors, stratification and survival in Canada: The Canadian Assessment of Myocardial Infarction (CAMI) Study. J Am Coll Cardiol 27:1119-1127
2. De Vreede-Swagemakers JJM, Gorgels APM, Dubois-Arbouw WI et al (1997) Out-of-hospital cardiac arrest in the 1990s: a population-based study in the Maastricht area on incidence, characteristics and survival. J Am Coll Cardiol 30:1500-1505
3. Moss AJ, Hall WJ, Cannom DS et al (1996) Improved survival with an implanted defibrillator in patients with coronary artery disease at high risk for ventricular arrhythmias. N Engl J Med 35:1933-1940
4. The Antiarrhythmics Versus Implantable Defibrillators (AVID) Investigators (1997) A comparison of antiarrhythmic drug therapy with implantable defibrillators in patients resuscitated from non-fatal ventricular arrhythmias. N Engl J Med 337:1576-1583
5. Bigger JT, for the Coronary Artery Bypass Graft (CABG) Patch Trial Investigators (1997) Prophylactic use of implanted cardiac defibrillators in patients at high risk for ventricular arrhythmias after coronary-artery bypass graft surgery. N Engl J Med 337:1569-1575
6. The Multicenter Post-Infarction Research Group (1983) Risk stratification and survival after myocardial infarction. N Engl J Med 309:331-336
7. Kober L, Torp-Pedersen C, Elming H, Burchardt H, on behalf of the TRACE Study Group (1997) Use of left ventricular ejection fraction or wall-motion score index in predicting arrhythmic death in patients following an acute myocardial infarction. Pacing Clin Electrophysiol 20:2553-2559
8. Kuchar DL, Thornburn CW, Sammel NL (1987) Prediction of serious arrhythmic events after myocardial infarction: signal averaged electrocardiogram, Holter monitoring and radionuclide ventriculography. J Am Coll Cardiol 9:531-538
9. El-Sherif N, Ursell SN, Bekheit S et al (1989) Prognostic value of the signal averaged ECG depends on the time of recording in the postinfarction period. Am Heart J 118:256-264
10. El-Sherif N, Denes P, Katz R et al (1995) Definition of the best criteria of the time-domain signal-averaged electrocardiogram for serious arrhythmic events in the post-infarction period. J Am Coll Cardiol 25:908-914
11. Ahuja RK, Turitto G, Ibrahim B, Caref EB, El-Sherif N (1994) Combined time-domain and spectral turbulence analysis of the signal-averaged electrocardiogram

improve its predictive accuracy in post-infarction patients. J Electrocardiol 27[Suppl]:202-206

12. Vazquez R, Caref EB, Torres F, Reina M, Espina A, El-Sherif N (1999) Improved diagnostic value of the combined time- and frequency-domain analysis of the signal-averaged electrocardiogram after myocardial infarction. J Am Coll Cardiol 33:385-394

13. Baron HV, Lesh MD (1996) Autonomic nervous system and sudden cardiac death. J Am Coll Cardiol 27:1053-1060

14. Kleiger RE, Miller JP, Bigger JT Jr, Moss AJ, and the Multicenter Post-Infarction Research Group (1987) Decreased heart rate variability and its association with increased mortality after acute myocardial infarction. Am J Cardiol 59:256-262

15. Bigger JT, Steinman RC, Rolnitzky LM, Fleiss JL, Albrecht P, Cohen RJ (1996) Power law behavior of RR-interval variability in healthy middle-aged persons, patients with recent acute myocardial infarction, and patients with heart transplants. Circulation 93:2142-2151

16. La Rovere MT, Bigger JT Jr, Marcus FI, Mortara A, Schwartz PJ, for the ATRAMI (Autonomic Tone and Reflexes After Myocardial Infarction) Investigators (1998) Baroreflex sensitivity and heart-rate variability in prediction of total cardiac mortality after myocardial infarction. Lancet 351:478-484

17. Task Force of the European Society of Cardiology and the North American Society of Pacing and Electrophysiology (1996) Heart rate variability. Standards of measurement, physiological interpretation, and clinical use. Circulation 93:1143-1165

18. Dekker JM, Schouten EG, Klootwijk P, Pool J, Swenne CA, Kromhout D (1997) Heart rate variability from short electrocardiographic recordings predict mortality from all causes in middle-aged and elderly men. Am J Epidemiol 145:899-908

19. Lanza GA, Guido V, Galeazzi N et al (1998) Prognostic role of heart rate variability in patients with a recent acute myocardial infarction. Am J Cardiol 82:1323-1328

20. Ahnve S, Gilpin E, Madsen EB, Frolicher V, Henning H, Ross J (1984) Prognostic importance of QT interval at discharge after acute myocardial infarction: a multicenter study of 865 patients. Am Heart J 108:395-400

21. Higham PD, Campbell RFW (1994) QT dispersion. Br Heart J 71:508-510

22. Day CP, McComb JM, Campbell RFW (1990) QT dispersion: an indication of arrhythmia risk in patients with long QT intervals. Br Heart J 63:342-344

23. Zabel M, Klingenheben T, Franz MR, Hohnloser SH (1998) Assessment of QT dispersion for prediction of mortality or arrhythmic events after myocardial infarction. Results of a prospective, long-term follow-up study. Circulation 97:2543-2550

24. Oikarinen L, Toivonen L, Viitasalo M (1998) Electrocardiographic measures of ventricular repolarization: dispersion in patients with coronary artery disease susceptible to ventricular fibrillation. Heart 79:554-559

25. El-Sherif N (1996) T-wave alternans. A marker of vulnerability to ventricular tachyarrhythmias. In: Raviele A (ed) Cardiac arrhythmias 1995. Springer, Milan, pp 12-16

26. Rosenbaum DS, Jackson LE, Smith JM et al (1994) Electrical alternans and vulnerability to ventricular arrhythmias. N Engl J Med 330:235-241

27. Chinushi M, Restivo M, Caref EB, El-Sherif N (1998) Electrophysiological basis of the arrhythmogenicity of QT/T alternans in the long QT syndrome. Tridimensional analysis of the kinetics of cardiac repolarization. Circ Res 83:614-628

28. Estes NAM, Michaud G, Zipes DP et al (1997) Electrical alternans during rest and exercise as a predictor of vulnerability to ventricular arrhythmias. Am J Cardiol 80:1314-1318

29. Gold MR, Bloomfield DM, Anderson KP et al (1998) T wave alternans predicts arrhythmia vulnerability in patients undergoing electrophysiology study. Circulation 98[Suppl I]:647 (abstr)
30. Hohnloser SH, Klingenheben T, Li Y G, Zabel M, Peetermans J, Cohen RJ (1998) T-wave alternans as a predictor of recurrent ventricular tachyarrhythmias in ICD recipients: prospective comparison with conventional risk markers. J Cardiovasc Electrophysiol 9:1258-1268
31. Turitto G, Caref EB, Pedalino R et al (1998) Comparison of heart rate at onset of T-wave alternans in normals and patients with malignant ventricular tachyarrhythmias. Circulation 98[suppl I]:647 (abstr)
32. Roy D, Marchand E, Theroux P, Waters DD, Pelletier GB, Bourassa MG (1985) Programmed ventricular stimulation in survivors of an acute myocardial infarction. Circulation 72:487-494
33. Iesaka Y, Nogami A, Aonuma K et al (1990) Prognostic significance of sustained monomorphic VT induced by programmed ventricular stimulation using up to triple extrastimuli in survivors of acute myocardial infarction. Am J Cardiol 65:1057-1063
34. Bourke JP, Richards ADB, Ross DL, Wallace EM, McGuire MA, Uther JB (1991) Routine programmed electrical stimulation in survivors of acute myocardial infarction for prediction of spontaneous ventricular tachyarrhythmias during follow-up: results, optimal stimulation protocol and cost-effective screening. J Am Coll Cardiol 18:780-788
35. Oikarinen L, Paavola M, Montonen J, Viitasalo M et al (1998) Magnetocardiographic QT interval dispersion in postmyocardial infarction patients with sustained ventricular tachycardia: validation of automated QT measurements. Pacing Clin Electrophysiol 21:1934-1942
36. Hubley-Kozey CL, Mitchell LB, Gardner MJ et al (1995) Spatial features in body-surface potential maps can identify patients with a history of sustained ventricular tachycardia. Circulation 92:1825-1838
37. Atiga Wl, Calkins H, Lawrence JH et al (1998) Beat-to-beat repolarization lability identifies patients at risk for sudden cardiac death. J Cardiovasc Electrophysiol 9:899-908
38. Dabrovski A, Kramarz E, Piotrowicz R (1997) Low variability of cycle lengths in nonsustained ventricular tachycardia as an independent predictor of mortality after myocardial infarction. Am J Cardiol 80:1347-1350
39. Copie X, Hnatkova K, Staunton A, Fei L, Camm AJ, Malik M (1996) Predictive power of increased heart rate versus depressed left ventricular ejection fraction and heart rate variability for risk stratification after myocardial infarction: results of a two-year follow-up study. J Am Coll Cardiol 27:270-276
40. Haider AW, Larson MG, Benjamin EJ, Levy D (1998) Increased left ventricular mass and hypertrophy are associated with increased risk for sudden death. J Am Coll Cardiol 32:1454-1459
41. Redwood SR, Odemuyiwa O, Hnatkova K et al (1997) Selection of dichotomy limits for multifactorial prediction of arrhythmic events and mortality in survivors of acute myocardial infarction. Eur Heart J 18:1278-1287
42. Moss AJ, Cannom DS, Daubert JP et al, for the MADIT-II Investigators (1999) Multicenter Automatic Defibrillator Implantation Trial II (MADIT-II): design and clinical protocol. Ann Noninvasive Electrocardiol 4:83-91
43. Bardy GH, Lee KL, Mark DB and the SCD-HeFT Pilot Investigators (1997) The

Sudden Cardiac Death in Heart Failure Trial: pilot study. Pacing Clin Electrophysiol 20:1148 (abstr)

44. Raviele A, Bongiorni MG, Brignole M et al (1999) Which strategy is "best" after myocardial infarction? The beta-blocker strategy plus implantable cardioverter defibrillator trial: Rationale and study design. Am J Cardiol 83(5B):104D-111D

What Is the Clinical and Prognostic Significance of High-Resting Sinus Rate?

F. Hernández-Bernal[1], L. Mantini[2], R. Latini[1], G. Zuanetti[1] and A.P. Maggioni[1,3]
for the GISSI-Investigators

Introduction

The interest in alterations in the autonomic nervous system as useful markers for risk stratification in patients with acute myocardial infarction (MI) has grown steadily in the last few years [1]. The prognostic significance of non-invasive indexes of autonomic nervous system dysfunction, such as heart rate (HR) variability and baroreflex sensitivity, has been evaluated; however, the application of these techniques in clinical practice has been hindered by methodological and practical limitations so that their use is still mostly limited to a few centers. At the same time, it has become clear that simple and crude indexes of sympathetic-parasympathetic balance as well as left ventricular function, such as HR or blood pressure, may play a major role in the risk stratification during the acute phase and at discharge [2-4].

Furthermore, data from clinical trials showed that drugs with a negative chronotropic effect, such as β-blockers and non-dihydropiridine calcium antagonists, have a beneficial effect on mortality [5, 6], while agents that increase HR, such as short-acting dihydropiridines, have a deleterious effect [7, 8].

These results offer a strong rationale for a systematic reevaluation of the prognostic significance of HR in patients with acute MI, to overcome some of the limitations inherent in previous studies where the lack of use of thrombolytic treatment, small sample size and absence of information on heart rhythm might have affected the reliability of the data.

Role of HR in the GISSI Studies: Methodological Issues

The extensive ECG data-base in the GISSI studies [9-10] with almost 20,000 patients, whose ECG at entry and at discharge was available for analysis, represented a unique opportunity to reassess this issue in a population of patients

[1]Dipartimento di Ricerche Cardiovascolari, Istituto Mario Negri, Milan, Italy; [2]Reparto di Cardiologia, Ospedale di Penne, Italy; [3]Centro Studi ANMCO, Florence, Italy

Table 1. Principal characteristics of the Gruppo Italiano per lo Studio della Sopravvivenza nell'Infarto Miocardico trials

	GISSI-2	GISSI-3
Recruitment period	2/88 - 7/89	6/91 - 7/93
Study treatment	Streptokinase versus alteplase; heparin versus control	Lisinopril versus control; nitrates versus control
Interval from symptom onset to randomization (h)	≤ 6	≤ 24
Exclusion criteria	Contraindication to thrombolysis	Killip class IV; systolic blood pressure < 100
Randomized patients	12,490	19,394
Patients with confirmed myocardial infarction at hospital discharge	10,407	16,958
Number of available ECG at entry	8915	11,267
Number of available ECG at discharge	7831	11,117

mostly treated with fibrinolysis during the acute phase. Characteristics of the GISSI studies are summarized in Table 1.

Heart rythm was evaluated and measured from ECG (electrocardiogram) recordings considering the mean of three consecutive R-R wave intervals from lead D_2. The following variables were collected: heart rhythm (sinus, atrial fibrillation, atrial flutter, other), rate, presence of high-degree atrioventricular blocks. These data were then added to the main data-base of GISSI studies, thus allowing a complete evaluation of the prognostic significance of HR.

Patients with suspected MI who had been initially enrolled in the studies but whose infarct had not been confirmed were excluded. Patients who were not in sinus rhythm or with grade 2-3 atrioventricular blocks were also excluded. Cut-offs for HR were predefined at 60, 80, 100 bpm.

The prognostic significance of HR at entry for in-hospital mortality and at discharge for 6-month mortality was evaluated by univariate analysis in the general population and in predefined subgroups of patients, including the elderly, diabetics, patients with anterior, inferior and non-Q AMI and patients presenting with signs of heart failure (Killip class 2-4 at entry and clinically or instrumentally defined congestive heart failure at discharge).

The logistic regression analysis and Cox proportional hazard model were used to assess the independent prognostic value of HR on subsequent mortality for the in-hospital and post-discharge phases respectively by correcting for those variables that were shown to be associated with total mortality in the univariate analysis.

Heart Rate at Entry

A large sample of patients were suitable for this analysis: 8915 and 11,267 patients from GISSI-2 and GISSI-3 studies respectively (more than 20,000 patients over-all). In GISSI-3, there was a progressive increase in mortality with increasing HR, thus confirming the data obtained in GISSI-2 (Fig. 1); and when the data were analyzed for the pre-defined subgroups at different risk, the increase in mortality with increasing HR was consistently present despite the obvious differences in absolute values of mortality in the different subgroups. Multivariate analysis in both studies showed that HR exerts an independent prognostic significance: patients whose HR was higher than 100 bpm had more than a twofold risk of dying in hospital (Table 2).

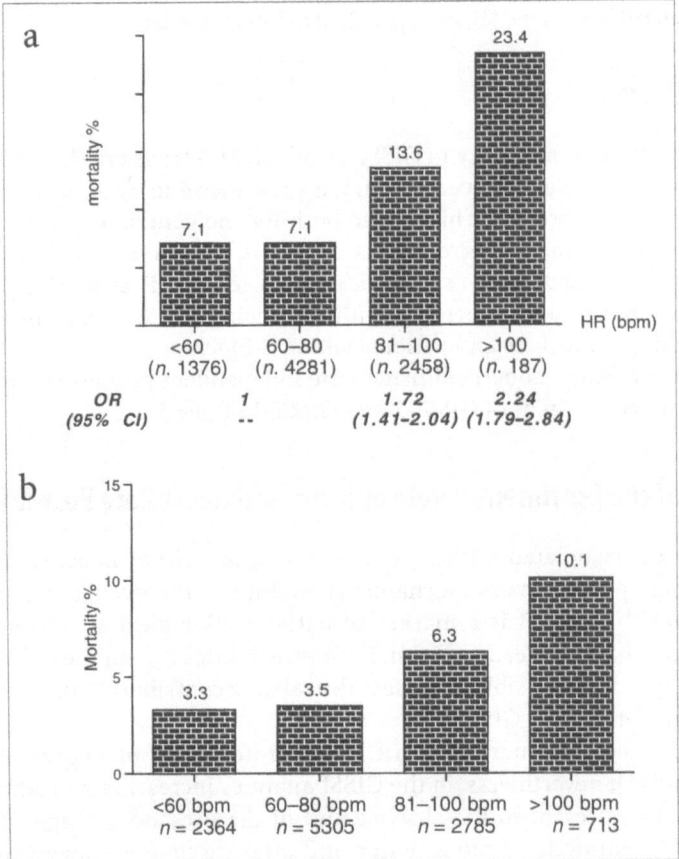

Fig. 1a,b. Heart rate at admission and in-hospital mortality: **a** GISSI-2 study (n. 8915). **b** GISSI-3 study (n. 11,267). CI, confidence interval; HR, heart rate

Table 2. GISSI-2 and GISSI-3 databases: independent predictors of in-hospital mortality

GISSI-2	RR	95% CI
Systolic blood pressure < 100 mmHg	5.42	4.18-7.02
Killip ≥ 2	3.30	2.78-3.91
Age > 70 years	3.02	2.34-3.60
Anterior acute MI	2.64	2.16-3.21
HR > 100 bpm	2.24	1.76-2.85
Female sex	1.75	1.41-2.16
HR 81-100 bpm	1.73	1.42-2.04
Previous acute MI	1.65	1.34-2.02
History of angina	1.45	1.23-1.71
Diabetes	1.28	1.05-1.58
GISSI-3	**RR**	**95% CI**
Systolic blood pressure < 100 mmHg	4.42	3.18-6.02
Age > 70 years	2.80	2.29-3.44
Killip ≥ 2	1.97	1.60-2.45
Anterior acute MI	1.71	1.32-2.22
HR > 80 bpm	1.51	1.21-1.89
Female sex	1.39	1.13-1.72
Hypertension	1.35	1.11-1.65

CI, confidence interval; HR, heart rate; MI, myocardial infarction; RR, relative risk

Heart Rate at Discharge

The relation between HR and mortality in GISSI-2 and GISSI-3 trials are shown in Fig. 2. Consistent with the data observed at entry, a progressive increase of mortality with increasing HR is present. This is true both for the general population and for the different predefined subgroups. As expected, the use of β-blockers (about a third of total population) was associated with lower HR at discharge. However, the increasing 6-month mortality with increasing HR was present in both patients not taking β-blockers and patients taking β-blockers.

Multivariate analysis (Cox model) confirmed the independent prognostic significance of HR on mortality in both GISSI-2 and GISSI-3 (Table 3).

Pathophysiology of the Detrimental Role of Increased Heart Rate Post-MI

Increased HR may be associated with increased mortality either because an accelerated heart beat per se favors mechanisms leading to the occurrence of death, or alternatively because it is a marker of pathophysiological alterations that through other mechanisms lead to death. Both possibilities are supported by previous findings and it is impossible to dissect the relative contribution of these factors from the data obtained in GISSI.

It is usually assumed that increased HR is a manifestation of depressed myocardial function [11]; nevertheless, in the GISSI analyses increasing mortality with increasing HR was present in the absence and in the presence of signs of left-ventricular (LV) dysfunction both at entry and after discharge, suggesting

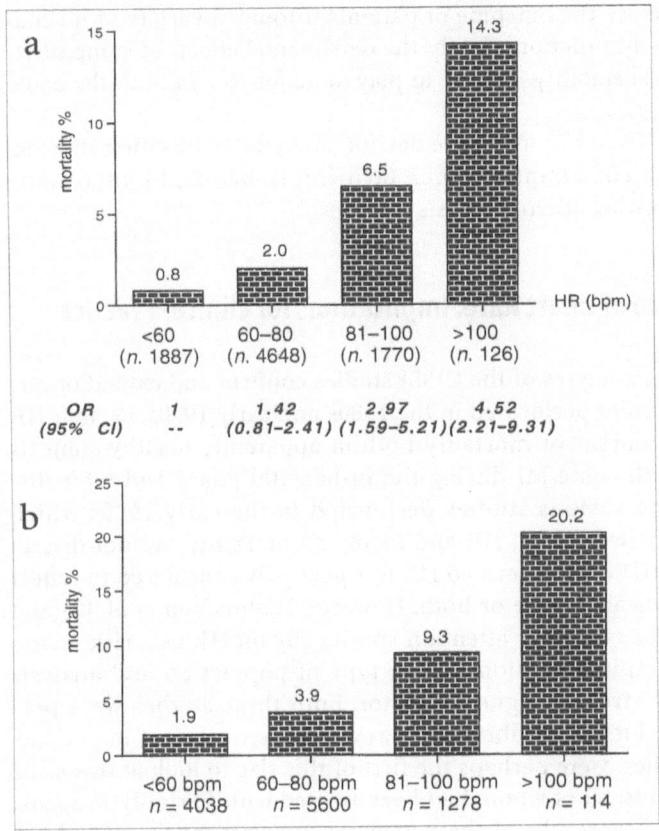

Fig. 2a,b. Heart rate at discharge and 6-month mortality: **a** GISSI-2 study (n. 7831). **b** GISSI-3 study (n. 11,117)

Table 3. GISSI-2 and GISSI-3 databases: independent predictors of 6-month mortality

GISSI-2	RR	95% CI
HR > 100 bpm	4.54	2.21-9.30
Contraindication to stress test	4.10	2.73-6.16
HR 81-100 bpm	2.97	1.68-5.24
Left ventricular dysfunction	1.83	1.33-2.51
Previous acute MI	1.68	1.22-2.34
Killip = 2 at entry	1.65	1.22-2.23
Age (> 70 years)	1.62	1.21-2.18
Complex ventricular arrhythmias	1.55	1.08-2.21
History of hypertension	1.42	1.07-1.70

GISSI-3	RR	95% CI
Contraindication to stress test	2.63	1.92-3.61
Age (> 70 years)	1.98	1.60-2.44
HR > 100 bpm	1.78	1.13-2.80
HR 81-100 bpm	1.75	1.39-2.20
Killip = 2 at entry	1.64	1.32-2.03
Left ventricular dysfunction	1.46	1.10-1.94
Complex ventricular arrhythmias	1.58	1.12-2.23
Diabetes	1.32	1.05-1.64
Hypertension	1.24	1.01-1.52

CI, confidence interval; HR, heart rate; MI, myocardial infarction; RR, relative risk

that high HR may influence the outcome of patients through a variety of mechanisms in addition to LV dysfunction: clearly, the detrimental effects of sympathetic activation on electrical stability appear to play a major role in both the acute and the subacute settings.

On the other hand, HR per se may have detrimental effects, by either increasing myocardial oxygen consumption, thus favoring ischemia, by increasing infarct size or by accelerating atherosclerosis [12].

Prognostic Significance of Heart Rate: Implications for Clinical Practice

The data obtained in the analyses of the GISSI studies confirm and extend observations derived from studies performed in the 1980s and early 1990s, i.e. that HR is a strong prognostic marker of mortality both in apparently healthy subjects [13] and in patients with acute MI during the in-hospital phase and after discharge [2-4, 14-16]. The various studies performed in the early 1980s which showed a relationship between high HR and increased mortality did not dissect the independent role of HR, since elevated HR was generally considered to reflect depressed LV function, heart failure or both. However, Hjalmarson et al. [2] and Disegni et al. [3] have focused their attention specifically on HR as a risk factor. In these two studies, despite variations in the type of population and analysis used, HR emerged as a strong prognostic factor. Both these studies were performed before the introduction of fibrinolysis as a routine treatment in patients with acute MI. Our studies were perhaps the first of this size to look at this issue in a population of patients, all of whom had been treated with fibrinolytic agents during the acute phase. The results of these analyses are very consistent in both studies and show a progressive increase of mortality both in hospital and after discharge with increasing HR. Multivariate analysis showed that there is a specific independent role of HR that is perhaps particularly marked at post-discharge but present also for HR at entry. The results presented by the GUSTO-1 investigators [17], who studied HR among several variables with 30-day mortality as an end-point, are consistent with those obtained in GISSI, with a risk ratio of approximately 1.6 for a HR of 86 vs 62 bpm. However, at variance with our study, in GUSTO-1 a J-shaped relationship was observed, with elevated mortality at very low and at high HR.

Risk stratification of patients with acute MI has evolved in the last few years with the use of several non-invasive and invasive indexes of risk, targeting different aspects of myocardial damage, such as the presence of residual ischemia (exercise and echo stress tests), electrical instability (late potentials, QT dispersion, T-wave alternans), indexes of LV dysfunction (systolic and diastolic volumes, ejection fraction) and sympathetic-parasympathetic imbalance (HR variability, baroreflex sensitivity). Despite the enthusiasm towards the development and implementation of the latter techniques [18, 19], their use is still mostly limited to selected research centers.

The use of simple indexes, such as resting HR for risk stratifying patients, appears as a valuable tool for the clinician, in order to complement information on LV function and residual ischemia. It appears that HR from a resting ECG in patients with sinus rhythm has to be included as a critical variable whenever attempting to quantify the independent prognostic value of more complex analyses.

Finally, although no extrapolation can be made from this observational data to the pharmacological effect of drugs, these data are consistent with observations obtained in clinical trials where drugs able to reduce HR, such as β-blockers [5] or non-dihydropirine calcium antagonists [6], have been usually shown to be effective in reducing morbidity and mortality whereas the opposite has been true for drugs that increase HR, such as short-acting dihydropiridines.

References

1. Task Force of the European Society of Cardiology and the North American Society of Pacing and Electrophysiology (1996) Heart rate variability. Standards of measurement, physiological interpretation, and clinical use. Circulation 93:1043-1065
2. Hjalmarson A, Gilpin EA, Kjekshus J et al (1990) Influence of heart rate on mortality after acute myocardial infarction. Am J Cardiol 65:547-553
3. Disegni E, Goldbourt U, Reicher-Reiss H et al. and the SPRINT Study Group (1995) The predictive value of admission heart rate on mortality in patients with acute myocardial infarction. J Clin Epidemiol 48:1197-1205
4. Copie X, Hnatkova K, Staunton A et al (1996) Predictive power of increased heart rate versus depressed left ventricular ejection fraction and heart rate variability for risk stratification after myocardial infarction. Results of a two-year follow-up study. J Am Coll Cardiol 27:270-276
5. Kjekshus J (1990) Heart rate reduction: a mechanism of benefit? Eur Heart J 8:115-122
6. The Danish Study Group on Verapamil in myocardial infarction (1990) Effect of verapamil on mortality and major events after acute myocardial infarction (the Danish Verapamil Infarction Trial II [DAVIT II]). Am J Cardiol 66:779-785
7. Wilcox RG, Hampton JR, Banks DC et al (1986) Trial of early nifedipine in acute myocardial infarction: the TRENT study. Br Med J 293:1204-1208
8. Goldbourt U, Behar S, Reicher-Reiss H et al (1993) Early administration of nifedipine in suspected acute myocardial infarction: the Secondary Prevention Reinfarction Israel Nifedepine Trial 2 Study. Arch Intern Med 153:345-353
9. Gruppo Italiano per lo Studio della Sopravvivenza nell'Infarto Miocardico (1990) GISSI-2: a factorial randomised trial of alteplase versus streptokinase and heparin versus no heparin among 12490 patients with acute myocardial infarction. Lancet 336:65-71
10. Gruppo Italiano per lo Studio della Sopravvivenza nell'Infarto Miocardico (1994) GISSI-3: effects of lisinopril and transdermal glyceryl trinitrate singly and together on 6-week mortality and ventricular function after acute myocardial infarction. Lancet 343:1115-1122
11. Persky A, Olsson G, Landon C, Faire U de, Theorell T, Hamsten A (1992) Minimum heart rate and coronary atherosclerosis. Independent relations to global severity and rate of progression of angiographic lesions in men with myocardial infarction at a young age. Am Heart J 123:609-616

12. Beere PA, Glagov S, Zarius CK (1984) Retarding effect of lowered heart rate on coronary atherosclerosis. Science 27:180-182
13. Kannel WB, Kannel C, Paffenbarger RS et al (1987) Heart rate and cardiovascular mortality: the Framingham Study. Am Heart J 113:1489-1494
14. Madsen EB, Gilpin E, Henning H et al (1984) Prediction of late mortality after myocardial infarction from variables measured at different time during hospitalization. Am J Cardiol 53:47-54
15. Willems JL, Pardaens J, De Geest H (1984) Early risk stratification using clinical findings in patients with acute myocardial infarction. Eur Heart J 5:130-139
16. Hillis LD, Forman S, Braunwald E, and the Thrombolysis in Myocardial Infarction (TIMI) Phase II Co-Investigators (1990) Risk stratification before thrombolytic therapy in patients with acute myocardial infarction. J Am Coll Cardiol 16:313-315
17. Lee KL, Woodlief LH, Topol EJ et al for the GUSTO-I Investigators (1995) Predictors of 30-day mortality in the era of reperfusion for acute myocardial infarction. Results from an international trial of 41,021 patients. Circulation 91:1659-1668
18. Kleiger RE, Miller JP, Bigger JTJ, Moss AJ (1987) Decreased heart rate variability and its association with increased mortality after acute myocardial infarction. Am J Cardiol 59:256-262
19. Malliani A, Pagani M, Lombardi F et al (1991) Cardiovascular neural regulation explored in the frequency domain. Circulation 84:482-492

What is the Relationship Between Depression, the Autonomic Nervous System and the Risk of Death in Post-Myocardial Infarction Patients?

M.V. Pitzalis[1], O. Todarello[2], A. Fioretti[1], C. Lattarulo[2] and P. Rizzon[1]

Introduction

Several studies have hypothesized a relationship between sudden death and neurophysiological factors. In particular, it has been suggested that there is a complex interrelationship between emotional disturbances (in particular, depression) and cardiovascular mortality in patients who have survived an acute myocardial infarction.

The appearance of psychologic abnormalities in patients who have survived a myocardial infarction is quite frequent [1], depressive symptoms being present in 20-30% [2-4]. Depression in patients with coronary artery disease remains stable over time [5-8] and does not seem to correlate with the severity of cardiac disease [1, 3]. In 1969, Wolf described the possibility of predicting death in 10 patients who had survived myocardial infarction by using psychological tests [9]. Since then, several studies have been drawn up in order to test the prognostic relevance of depression and cognitive impairment in post-myocardial infarction patients [4, 10]. A CAPS substudy suggested that patients at higher risk for mortality and cardiac arrest are not those who appear ambitious, hard driving or engaged in activities (global type A) but rather those who have withdrawn from life's challenges and opportunities [11]. Additionally, patients showing depressive symptoms were characterized by the highest incidence of mortality and/or cardiac arrest [12, 13]. Another multicenter study [14] confirmed the predictive value of depression and showed that depressive symptoms are more prevalent in lower social classes and in patients with lower education, thus underlying the role of socio-economic and psycho-social status in predicting prognosis in post-myocardial infarction patients. Those patients living alone after myocardial infarction have a high incidence of cardiac events during the first 6 months after the acute event [15]. Two recent studies [16, 17] have shown that depressive signs during the acute phase of myocardial infarction are associated with an increase in cardiac mortality. Depression is a prognostic index which is independent from traditional risk factors. The risk is particularly high in those patients who show frequent premature ventricular contractions (>10 PVCs/h).

[1]Istituto di Cardiologia; [2]Istituto di Psichiatria, Università di Bari, Italy

Possible Pathophysiological Implications

The high incidence of arrhythmic events and sudden death in patients with depressive disorders and ventricular arrhythmias suggests the existence of a complex relationship between the central nervous system involved in behavioral control and the cardiovascular system. According to this hypothesis, the interaction between the central nervous system, cardiovascular system and mood might be supported by the dopamine tone of the right hemisphere [18]. In fact, D1 dopamine receptors play an important role in mediating the antidepressant effects of imipramine [19]. Dopamine tone also seems to have a relevant role in sympathetic activation to stressful stimuli [20]. Therefore, it seems possible that mood abnormalities may modify the sympatho-vagal influence on the cardiovascular system, which in turn could facilitate arrhythmic phenomena and sudden death.

In order to evaluate whether a relationship exists between autonomic nervous system activity and psychological alterations, we are performing a study of patients who have survived a myocardial infarction.

Depression and personality characteristics are evaluated using psychological tests and a psychiatric evaluation at defined time points. The psychological tests, which are all self-administered, include Zung's test of anxiety and depression at a clinical level; the State-Trait Anxiety Inventory; the Profile of Mood States (POMS), which evaluates the characteristics of mood from a non-clinical point of view as a component of personality; the Symptom Check List, which evaluates psychiatric symptoms; the Toronto Alexithymia Scale, which evaluates the difficulty patients have in recognizing and expressing their own feelings; and the Minnesota Multiphasic Personality Inventory (MMPI), which explores personality traits. The psychiatric evaluation of depression is made by a psychiatrist using Hamilton's test.

The autonomic nervous system is analyzed by means of time domain parameters obtained from 24-h ECG monitoring. In particular, the standard deviation of the RR interval is evaluated, a parameter that has been shown to have a prognostic role in patients who survived a myocardial infarction, in addition to spectral analysis of short-term oscillations of heart rate and systolic blood pressure. Baroreflex sensitivity, a measure of reflex vagal activity, is also evaluated by using the spectral and phenylephrine techniques.

The interim results of this study, referring to the discharge tests and evaluations of 50 patients, are presented. Clinical evidence of depression was found in 30% of the patients (in line with previously published data), but displayed no significant correlation with the indices of heart rate variability.

The standard deviation of the RR intervals (SDNN) showed a significant correlation with personality abnormalities. In particular, we found significant correlations between the SDNN and the neurotic aspects of the MMPI: depression (Fig. 1), hysteria and hypochondria. All of these were inverse correlations, which means that the greater the heart rate variability, the less serious the psychological abnormalities.

The POMS vigor/activity scale, which concentrates on the patients' own interpretation of their sense of vigor, positively correlates with the SDNN (Fig. 2).

Furthermore, the depressive symptoms evaluated by means of the check list also showed a significant negative correlation with SDNN.

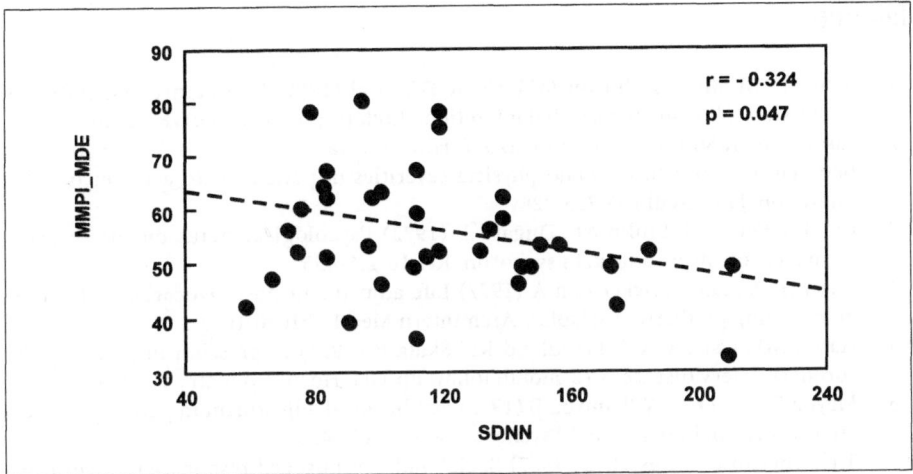

Fig. 1. Relationship between the standard deviation of RR intervals (SDNN) and the values of depression evaluation by means of MMPI. Note that the lower the values of SDNN, the higher the values of depression

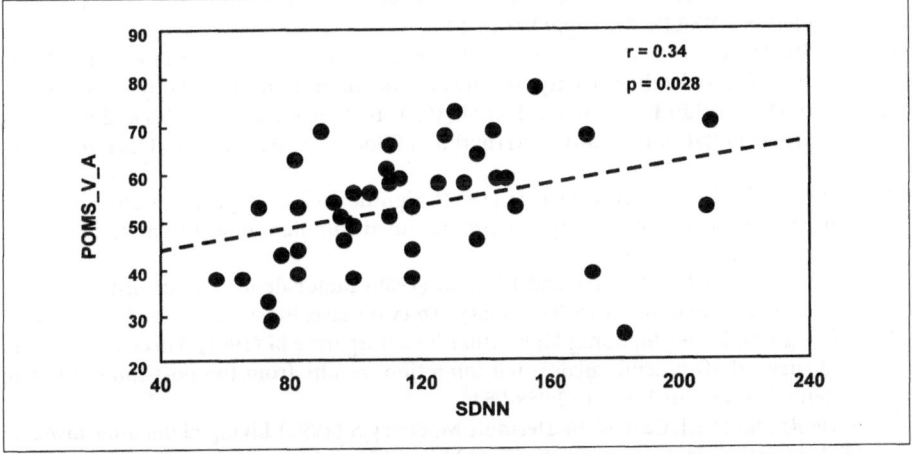

Fig. 2. Relationship between the standard deviation of RR intervals (SDNN) and the values of vigor/activity evaluated by POMS. Note that the higher the values of SDNN, the higher the values of vigor/activity

In conclusion, in patients with acute myocardial infarction, the presence of "neurotic" traits of personality seems to be associated with altered autonomic nervous system activity. Heart rate variability indices are inversely related to the depressive, hysterical and hypochondriac dimensions. These findings may explain the increased risk of sudden death in post-myocardial infarction patients with depression.

References

1. Schleifer SJ, Macari-Hinson MM, Coyle DA et al (1989) The nature and course of depression following myocardial infarction. Arch Intern Med 149:1785-1789
2. Kurosawa H, Shimizu Y, Nishimatzu Y, Hirose S, Takano T (1988) The relationship between mental disorders and physical severities in patients with acute myocardial infarction. Jap Circul J 47:723-728
3. Cay EL, Vetter N, Philip AE, Dugard P (1972) Psycological status during recovery from an acute heart attack. J Psychosom Res 16:425-435
4. Stern JJ, Pascale L, Ackerman A (1977) Life adjustment post myocardial infarction: determining predictive variables. Arch Intern Med 137:1680-1685
5. Hance ML, Carney RM, Freedland KE, Skala R (1996) Depression in patients with coronary artery disease: a 12-month follow up. Gen Hosp Psychiatry 18:61-65
6. Mayou R, Foster A, Williamson B (1978) Psychosocial adjustment in patients one year after myocardial infarction. J Psychosom Res 22:447-453
7. Trelawny-Ross C, Russell O (1987) Social and psychosocial responses to myocardial infarction: multiple determinants of outcome at six months. J Psychosom Res 31:125-130
8. Wells KB, Rogers W, Burnam MA, Camp P (1993) Course of depression in patients with hypertension, myocardial infarction, or insulin-dependent diabetes. Am J Psychiatry 150:632-628
9. Wolf A (1969) Psychosocial forces in myocardial infarction and sudden death. Circulation XXXXIX-XL[Suppl IV]:74-81
10. Garrity TF, Klein RF (1975) Emotional response and clinical severity as early determinants of six-month mortality after myocardial infarction. Heart Lung 4:730-737
11. Ahern DK, Gorkin L, Anderson JL et al (1990) Biobehavioral variables and mortality on cardiac arrest in the Cardiac Arrhythmia Pilot Study (CAPS). Am J Cardiol 66:59-62
12. Kennedy GJ, Hofer MA, Cohen D (1987) Significance of depression and cognitive impairment in patients undergoing programmed stimulation of cardiac arrhythmias. Psychosom Med 49:410-421
13. Carney RM, Rich, MW, Freeland KE et al (1988) Major depressive disorder predicts cardiac events in patients with coronary artery disease. Psychosom Med 50:627-633
14. Ladwig KH, Kieser M, Konig M, Breithardt G, Borggrefe M (1991) Affective disorders and survival after acute myocardial infarction: results from the post-infarction late potential study. Eur Heart J 12:959-964
15. Case RB, Moss AJ, Case N, McDermott M, Ebery S (1992) Living alone after myocardial infarction: impact on prognosis. JAMA 267:515-519
16. Frasure-Smith N, Lesperance F, Talajic M (1995) Depression and 18-month prognosis after myocardial infarction. Circulation 91:999-1005
17. Frasure-Smith N, Lesperance F, Talajic M (1993) Depression following myocardial infarction: impact on 6-month survival. JAMA 270:1819-1825
18. Friedman EH (1995) Depression after MI. (letter) Circulation 92:1668-1669
19. Gambarana C, Ghiglieri O, Tagliamonte A, D'Alessandro N, de Montis GM (1995) Crucial role of D1 dopamine receptors in mediating the antidepressant effect of imipramine. Pharmacol Biochem Behav 50:147-151
20. Friedman EH (1995) Circadian variation of sustained ventricular tachycardia. (letter) Circulation 91:562-563

Does Baroreflex Sensitivity Add Something to Noninvasive Evaluation of Post-Infarction Patients?

M.T. La Rovere

Introduction

In patients recovering from acute myocardial infarction considerable attention has been given for many years to noninvasive measurements of parameters that can identify high risk groups in which further investigation and intervention are needed. The extent of coronary artery disease and of myocardial damage as assessed by exercise stress test and determination of left ventricular ejection fraction together with the presence of electrical instability indentified by the results of 24-h Holter recording have been recognized as the most important pathophysiological determinants of prognosis after myocardial infarction. However, changes in life style and therapeutic interventions have modified the profile of patients with acute myocardial infarction, and the attending improvement in post-discharge survival has affected our ability to identify high risk patients by the use of traditional means.

Although there is a growing awareness that cardiovascular mortality is the final event in a multi-step process and that the autonomic nervous system (particularly its imbalances characterized by an increase in sympathetic and/or a decrease in vagal activity) plays an important role in the chain of events [1], measures of autonomic control have not yet entered the process of risk stratification on a routine basis.

Increased sympathetic activity links several important risk factors for coronary artery disease, and the deleterious effects of the circadian surge in sympathetic activity on platelet aggregability and on vasoconstriction have been recognized as accounting for the increased incidence of myocardial infarction and sudden death [2].

Myocardial infarction can affect the function of the autonomic nervous system, which through its sympathetic and parasympathetic outflows and their

Divisione di Cardiologia, Fondazione "S. Maugeri", IRCCS, Centro Medico Montescano, Pavia, Italy

complex influences can modify cardiac electrophysiology, thus playing a role in the development of life-threatening arrhythmias [3]. An extensive body of experimental evidence has been provided showing both the effects of adrenergic stimulation in reducing the threshold of ventricular fibrillation, particularly in the presence of myocardial ischemia [4], and the role of vagal activation in protection from ventricular fibrillation [5].

The fact that changes in efferent autonomic traffic are largely under baroreceptor control explains why the analysis of baroreceptor function (baroreflex sensitivity, BRS) may represent an indirect marker of the sympatho-vagal interaction to the heart. An increase in arterial blood pressure increases the baroreceptor firing rate, causing vagal excitation and sympathetic inhibition and thus decreasing heart rate, vasoconstriction and contractility with the aim of buffering the blood pressure change. As initially described by Smyth et al. [6], BRS can, therefore, be quantified as the measure of the reflex bradycardia following administration of a pressor agent such as angiotensin or phenylephrine (milliseconds of increase in the RR interval consequent to the increase of 1 mmHg in arterial pressure). Although BRS is generally regarded as a measure of the capacity to increase cardiac vagal efferent activity, the concomitant level of sympathetic activity is critical to reduce the magnitude of the attending bradycardia (i.e. lengthening in RR interval) and possibly it can be viewed as an index of the overall sympatho-vagal interaction to the heart.

The conceptual difficulty concerning the potential link between a measure of the autonomic balance derived from changes in the activity of the sinus node and the actual autonomic activity at the ventricular level has been recently addressed by Mitrani et al. [7]. Ventricular fibrillation was induced in 18 patients with an implantable cardioverter defibrillator both in the control state and after infusion of phenylephrine. It was observed that changes in ventricular fibrillation threshold were obtained almost only in association with increases in sinus cycle length.

Prognostic Value of Baroreflex Sensitivity

The first clinical data suggesting that the analysis of BRS might be of practical value were provided in 1988 [8] as the clinical counterpart of experimental observations [9, 10] showing that a depressed BRS was closely associated with an increased risk for ventricular fibrillation in conscious dogs with a healed myocardial infarction.

BRS was prospectively assessed, by the phenylephrine method, in 78 patients after a first myocardial infarction who were followed for 24 months [8]. BRS averaged 8.2 ± 4.8 ms/mmHg in the 71 patients who survived and 2.4 ± 1.5 ms/mmHg ($p = 0.004$) in the seven patients who died. In this study a cut-off point of 3 ms/mmHg was established by using the value corresponding to one standard deviation below the mean value of BRS in the entire population.

Although all but one of the diseased patients had a left ventricular ejection fraction (LVEF) below 40%, no linear association was found between BRS and several indexes of myocardial damage including the serum creatine kinase peak elevation, LVEF, and mean pulmonary wedge pressure at peak exercise. Despite the limited number of events, it already emerged that within the group of patients with reduced pump function, the risk of death was increased by the coexistence with a depressed BRS. This finding was on the same lines as that found for another autonomic marker (the 24-h normal RR Interval Standard Deviation, SDNN) which was significantly related to cardiac mortality independently of any level of left ventricular function in the large series of the MPIP study [11].

In a subsequent study based on 122 patients [12] a depressed BRS (< 3 ms/mmHg) was significantly associated with life-threatening arrhythmic events. It carried a relative risk of 23.1, which was higher than any other variable tested, including LVEF, ventricular premature contractions (VPCs) > 10/h, late potentials and heart rate variability (HRV).

The value of autonomic markers in adding prognostic information to the well recognized measures of cardiovascular outcome after myocardial infarction has been definitely quantified by the ATRAMI (Autonomic Tone and Reflexes After Myocardial Infarction) study [13]. Patients included in the study had had a recent myocardial infarction, no contraindication to exercise, no unstable angina or ischemia requiring coronary by-pass surgery in the following three months, and no signs or symptoms of congestive heart failure. ATRAMI enrolled 1284 patients who underwent evaluation of LVEF, ventricular arrhythmias and HRV by 24-h Holter recording and BRS by the phenylephrine method. The measure of HRV chosen a priori for the analysis was SDNN.

During the 21 ± 8 months of follow-up the primary endpoint, cardiac death ($n = 44$) or non-fatal cardiac arrest from a documented ventricular fibrillation ($n = 5$) was reached in 49 patients (3.9%). Cardiac mortality rate was higher among patients with low BRS (< 3ms/mmHg) or low SDNN (< 70 ms) than among patients with preserved values (BRS > 6.1 ms/mmHg, SDNN > 105 ms) (9% vs 2% and 10% vs 2%, respectively). The combination of depressed BRS and SDNN further increased risk, being associated with a 2-year mortality of 17% as compared to 2% ($p < 0.0001$) when both were preserved, thus demonstrating that BRS and HRV are not interdependent and that they provide complementary information because they explore different aspects of the neural control of the heart [14]. Both BRS and SDNN were significantly related to cardiac mortality at univariate analyses. At multivariate analysis, when LVEF and VPCs were included, low values of BRS and SDNN remained significantly associated with an increased mortality risk of 2.8 and of 3.2 respectively.

Thus, ATRAMI confirmed that depressed baroreflex sensitivity and/or reduced heart rate variability is a factor influencing risk in addition to better recognized measures of cardiovascular outcome. Indeed, the study points to the critical role of an altered autonomic balance that results in relatively high sympathetic activity and low vagal activity.

The relationship between a depressed BRS and the function of the left ventricle is of particular interest for risk stratification. Figure 1 shows that among patients with reduced LVEF, the 2-year mortality rose from 8% to 18% ($p < 0.01$) in the presence of a depressed BRS. Importantly, mortality did not differ significantly between patients with reduced LVEF and BRS ≥ 3 ms/mmHg and patients with preserved LVEF but BRS < 3 ms/mmHg. This last finding suggests that the preservation of the ability to reflexly augment vagal activity contributes to the survival of patients with low LVEF and strengthens the importance of restoring autonomic balance in patients with depressed ventricular function. The observation that among patients with similarly low ejection fraction values, mortality was greatly influenced by BRS, highlights the importance of factors which modulate a vulnerable substrate.

The practical implication is that in patients with well preserved LVEF the analysis of autonomic markers is of modest value because the difference in mortality between patients with and without signs of autonomic imbalance is not significant, and thus it cannot be recommended. By contrast, when LVEF is depressed the analysis of autonomic markers should be performed because it does discriminate between subgroups at moderate and high risk.

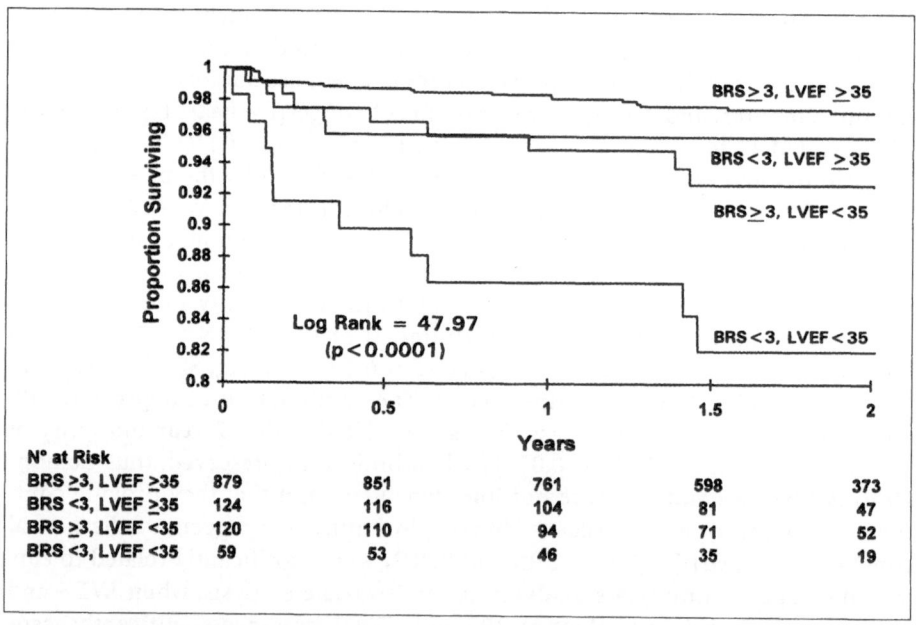

Fig. 1. Kaplan-Meier survival curves for total cardiac mortality according to the association of LVEF and BRS. The total population has been divided into four groups after dichotomization of the variables below and above the lowest 15th percentile (LVEF = 35%, BRS = 3 ms/mmHg). The *p* value refers to differences in events rate between subgroups. In patients with LVEF < 35% cardiac mortality rate at 2 years is affected by the association with BRS < 3 ms/mmHg). (Reproduced with permission from [13])

In light of the expanded indication for the prophylactic use of the implantable cardioverter defibrillator (ICD) currently under evaluation, the combination of autonomic markers with depressed ejection fraction could improve management strategy by reducing the number of unnecessary ICDs.

References

1. Remme WJ (1998) The sympathetic nervous system and ischemic heart disease. Eur Heart J 19[Suppl F]:F62-F71
2. Muller JE, Abela GS, Nesto RW, Tofler GH (1994) Triggers, acute risk factors and vulnerable plaques: the lexicon of a new frontier. J Am Coll Cardiol 23: 809-813
3. Corr PB, Yamada KA, Witkowski FX (1986) Mechanisms controlling cardiac autonomic function and their relation to arrhythmogenesis. In: Fozzard HA, Haber E, Jennings RB et al (eds) The heart and cardiovascular system. Raven Press, New York, pp 1343-1403
4. Lombardi F, Verrier RL, Lown B (1983) Relationship between sympathetic neural activity, coronary dynamics and vulnerability to ventricular fibrillation during myocardial ischemia and reperfusion. Am Heart J 105: 958-965
5. De Ferrari GM, Vanoli E, Schwartz PJ (1995) Cardiac vagal activity, myocardial ischemia and sudden death. In: Zipes DP, Jalife J (eds) Cardiac electrophysiology. From cell to bedside, 2nd edn. Saunders, Philadelphia, PA, pp 422-434
6. Smyth HS, Sleight P, Pickering GW (1969) Reflex regulation of arterial pressure during sleep in man: a quantitative method for assessing baroreflex sensitivity. Circ Res 24:109-121
7. Mitrani RD, Miles WM, Klein LS, Zipes DP (1998) Phenylephrine increases T wave shock energy required to induce ventricular fibrillation. J Cardiovasc Electrophysiol 9:34-40
8. La Rovere MT, Mortara A, Specchia G, Schwartz PJ (1988) Baroreflex sensitivity, clinical correlates and cardiovascular mortality among patients with a first myocardial infarction. A prospective study. Circulation 78:816-824
9. Billman GE, Schwartz PJ, Stone HL (1982) Baroreceptor control of heart rate: a predictor of sudden cardiac death. Circulation 66:874-879
10. Schwartz PJ, Vanoli E, Stramba-Badiale M, De Fearrari GM, Billman GE, Foreman RD (1988) Autonomic mechanisms and sudden death. New insights from analysis of baroreceptor reflexes in conscious dogs with and without a myocardial infarction. Circulation 78:969-979
11. Kleiger RE, Miller JP, Bigger JT Jr, Moss AJ, The Multicenter Postinfarction Research Group (1987) Decreased heart rate variability and its association with increased mortality after acute myocardial infarction. Am J Cardiol 59:256-262
12. Farrell TG, Odemuyiwa O, Bashir Y, Cripps TR, Malik M, Ward DE, Camm AJ (1992) Prognostic value of baroreflex sensitivity testing after acute myocardial infarction. Br Heart J 67:129-137
13. La Rovere MT, Bigger JT Jr, Marcus FI, Mortara A, Schwartz PJ for the ATRAMI (Autonomic Tone and Reflexes After Myocardial Infarction) Investigators (1998) Baroreflex sensitivity and heart rate variability in prediction of total cardiac mortality after myocardial infarction. Lancet 351:487-484

14. Bigger JT Jr, La Rovere MT, Steinman RC, Fleiss JL, Rottman JN, Rolnitzky LM, Schwartz PJ (1989) Comparison of baroreflex sensitivity and heart period variability after myocardial infarction. J Am Coll Cardiol 14:1511-1518
15. La·Rovere MT, Mortara A, Bigger JT Jr, Marcus FI, Malik M, Hohnloser SH, Schwartz PJ (1999) Baroreflex sensitivity contributes to the risk stratification of patients considered for a prophylactic implantable cardioverter defibrillator. Eur Heart J (in press)

Does Electrophysiologic Study Allow Further Risk Stratification in Survivors of Acute Myocardial Infarction?

R.F.E. Pedretti and S. Sarzi Braga

Introduction

Several studies are now available about the possible use of electrophysiologic (EP) study in order to identify, among asymptomatic postinfarction patients, those at risk of malignant ventricular arrhythmias. Most papers clearly showed that a positive EP study represents a strong marker of subsequent life-threatening ventricular arrhythmias, supporting a possible role of programmed ventricular stimulation (PVS) in clinical practice to screen high-risk patients. Nevertheless, despite these promising results, EP testing has not been largely used in the past for risk stratification purposes, probably because EP testing is an invasive procedure and because of the lack of efficacy of antiarrhythmic drugs in preventing arrhythmic death. However, data from recent trials on the implantable cardioverter defibrillator (ICD) has refocused attention on the role of PVS in detecting patients at risk of sudden death after acute myocardial infarction (AMI). In the present paper, some of the most important studies on this topic will be reviewed in order to answer the following questions:
1. Among inducible ventricular arrhythmias, which is predictive of subsequent arrhythmic events?
2. May EP testing prognosticate independently of noninvasive testing in postinfarction patients?
3. May EP testing be used in both early and late postinfarction period to screen for high-risk patients?

Which Induced Ventricular Arrhythmia Is Predictive of Life-threatening Arrhythmic Events After AMI?

The largest experience about prognostic power of EP testing comes from an Australian group which since 1986 has published several papers on this topic.

Divisione di Cardiologia, IRCCS Fondazione Salvatore Maugeri, Clinica del Lavoro e della Riabilitazione, Tradate (VA), Italy

Bourke et al. [1] in 1995 reported data from 502 asymptomatic patients who underwent PVS on average 11 ± 4 days after an uncomplicated AMI; 160 (32%) of these patients did not show any inducible arrhythmia, 44 (9%) showed a monomorphic sustained (longer than 10 s or requiring immediate cardioversion because of hemodynamic collapse) ventricular tachycardia (VT) with a cycle length ≥ 230 ms, 134 (27%) a sustained monomorphic VT with a cycle length <230 ms, and 164 (33%) showed a polymorphic sustained VT or ventricular fibrillation (VF). After a follow-up period of 1 year, incidence of electrical events (i.e. sudden death and nonfatal sustained VT) was 2.2%. In comparison with patients without inducible sustained ventricular arrhythmias, occurrence of electrical events was significantly higher in patients who showed inducible slow sustained monomorphic VT (18% vs 0.6%) but not in those with fast sustained monomorphic VT (0.7%) or sustained polymorphic VT/VF (0.6%).

Similar results were found by Bourke et al. [2] in 1991 in a paper reporting data from EP testing in 1,209 patients with uncomplicated AMI. One year after AMI, patients with sustained monomorphic VT had a 19% incidence of electrical events and a 7% incidence of sudden death, compared to 3% and 1% of patients without inducible arrhythmias. A separate analysis from the same group established that the induction of VF, polymorphic VT or monomorphic VT with a cycle length <230 ms was not associated with a greater incidence of spontaneous ventricular tachyarrhythmias than that observed in patients with no inducible arrhythmias [3]. Therefore, only inducibility of a slow sustained monomorphic ventricular tachycardia is predictive of subsequent electrical events in asymptomatic patients with a recent AMI, while other inducible ventricular arrhythmias should be considered unspecific responses.

Are EP Testing Results Independent of Noninvasive Testing in the Prediction of Arrhythmic Events After Myocardial Infarction?

Several noninvasive markers may be used to predict the risk of malignant ventricular arrhythmias after myocardial infarction:
- Low left ventricular ejection fraction (LVEF), assessed by angiography, radionuclide scanning or two-dimensional echocardiography, which is a measure of left ventricle residual systolic dysfunction and the most important prognostic marker of cardiac mortality in post-AMI patients
- Ventricular late potentials detected on signal-averaged electrocardiogram, which suggest the presence of areas of slow and late depolarization at the border zone level which may be at the basis of re-entry ventricular arrhythmias
- Frequent or repetitive ventricular ectopic beats (VEBs) detected on 24-h Holter monitoring, which represent potential triggers of life-threatening ventricular arrhythmias
- Depressed heart rate variability computed on a 24-h recording or baroreflex sensitivity measured on phenylephrine testing, which measure the residual dysfunction of tonic and reflex cardiac vagal activity after myocardial infarction.

The use of the above-mentioned tests in risk stratification of AMI survivors is supported by several multicenter studies and statements from scientific societies and committees. Nevertheless, the positive predictive accuracy of all markers is very low, in most cases < 15%; thus the combined use of multiple noninvasive tests is requested to increase the positive predictive accuracy of risk stratification algorithms. The combined presence of ≥ 2 risk markers may generally select subgroups of patients with an expected rate of electrical events of approximately 30% at 1-2 years after the index AMI.

Concerning the strength of prognostic power of EP testing, Richards et al. [4] studied survivors of an uncomplicated myocardial infarction who underwent EP testing as well as noninvasive testing based on LVEF measurement, ventricular late potential and VEB detection, respectively. At multivariate analysis, a positive EP testing was the strongest independent predictor of subsequent electrical events; the only other independent risk marker was LVEF. Nevertheless, the positive predictive accuracy of inducible sustained monomorphic VT was not very high, approximately 30%, thus not significantly different from that obtained combining ≥ 2 noninvasive risk markers. These results showed that among the most important risk markers, a positive EP testing was the most powerful predictor of subsequent arrhythmic events after AMI; nevertheless, the relatively low positive predictive accuracy did not support the use of EP study as a screening test in all patients with a recent myocardial infarction.

Based upon these results, in the paper of Bourke et al. [2] data about the possible use of LVEF as a pre-selector of AMI survivors eligible to PVS were reported. In this scenario patients with a preserved LVEF were not considered for EP testing, which was limited only to those patients with left ventricular dysfunction. Results showed that sensitivity, specificity, and positive predictive value of the diagnostic algorithm based upon the combined use of LVEF <40% and PVS were 64%, 96%, and 28%, respectively, thus not significantly different from those obtained by the alternative one (73%, 92%, and 20%, respectively), based upon the execution of EP testing in all AMI survivors. Nevertheless, the number of candidates to PVS in the "two-level" strategy was only 30% of the study population.

Data from Bourke et al. [2] were reported in a paper which summarized the 10-year experience of the Australian group about EP testing; however, some limitations should be underlined: (1) the role of LVEF as a pre-selector for EP testing was assessed in a post-hoc and not in a prospective analysis; (2) LVEF is the most commonly used noninvasive marker, but several other tests may be effectively used in risk stratification of post-AMI patients.

The first prospective study about the prognostic power of a combined use of noninvasive tests and inducible sustained monomorphic VT for the prediction of late arrhythmic events after AMI was published by Pedretti et al. [5] in 1993. At a mean follow-up of 15 ± 7 months, among 303 survivors of an uncomplicated AMI, 54% treated with thrombolysis, 19 (6%) late arrhythmic events occurred. In all patients the following noninvasive risk markers were collected: LVEF < 40% assessed by echocardiography, repetitive VEPs (couplets, unsustained VT) on 48-h Holter monitoring and ventricular late potentials. Of enrolled patients,

67 (22%) were defined as being at high risk after the first level of risk stratification and defined as eligible for PVS. Of 67 eligible patients, 20 (30%) did not perform EP study because the patient or the attending physician did not consent to the procedure. Of the remaining 47, 20 (42%) patients had a positive PVS because a sustained monomorphic VT with heart rate $\leq$ 270 bpm was inducible 25±8 days after AMI. Incidence of late arrhythmic events was significantly higher in patients with positive EP study than in those without (65% vs 4%; p < 0.0001). Moreover, a multivariate analysis was performed in patients selected for EP testing and a positive PVS showed a strong (p < 0.0001) prognostic power independent of noninvasive testing. Incidence of late arrhythmic events was < 1% in patients with $\leq$ 1 noninvasive risk marker after noninvasive testing. This was the first prospective study which clearly showed that a "two-level" strategy may be useful for the prediction of patients at high risk of arrhythmic events after an AMI. Specificity and positive predictive value of the risk stratification algorithm were 88% and 30% after noninvasive testing and increased to 97% and 65% after the execution of EP testing in preselected patients; changes in sensitivity were small, from 87% to 81%. The main conclusion of the paper was that a combined use of noninvasive tests and EP study selected with a good sensitivity a group of postinfarction patients at sufficiently high risk to consider them candidates for implantable cardioverter-defibrillators or therapy guided by EP testing. Another significant conclusion was that PVS had a high negative predictive value, suggesting that no specific treatment appears needed if sustained monomorphic VT is not inducible, despite the presence of different noninvasive risk markers.

Similar results were found by Zoni-Berisso et al. [6] in 1996; three hundred five patients who had survived a recent AMI underwent a risk stratification protocol based upon a "two-level" strategy: after echocardiography, 24-h Holter monitoring, and signal-averaged electrocardiogram, 120 (39%) were found to have $\geq$ 1 of the following risk factors and considered eligible for EP testing: LVEF <40%, repetitive ventricular forms and ventricular late potentials. Of the selected patients, in 17 (14%) EP testing was not performed, in 11 (11%) and 5 (5%) a sustained monomorphic VT with a cycle length $\geq$ 230 ms or a sustained unspecific ventricular tachyarrhythmia was induced, respectively, 11-20 days after AMI. Incidence of arrhythmic events was < 1% in patients with < 1 noninvasive risk marker, 4% in patients with $\geq$ 1 risk marker and negative EP study and 67% in patients with $\geq$ 1 risk marker and positive EP study. From the first to second level, positive predictive accuracy and specificity of the risk stratification algorithm increased from 10% to 67% and from 66% to 99%, respectively, while sensitivity changed from 91% to 55%, respectively.

Pedretti et al. [5] and Zoni-Berisso et al. [6] clearly showed that in patients with a recent uncomplicated AMI not only LVEF but also Holter monitoring and signal-averaged electrocardiogram may effectively be used to limit the execution of EP testing, in 22% and 39% of postinfarction patients if two markers or one marker, respectively, are requested to define arrhythmic risk after noninvasive testing.

Recently, Andresen et al. [7] published a paper which confirmed the two above-mentioned studies. Noninvasive methods as well as PVS were used to identify patients in the late phase after AMI as candidates for prophylactic implantation of a cardioverter defibrillator. A series of 657 patients with AMI underwent Holter monitoring and determination of LVEF. If one of the two methods yielded abnormal findings ($\geq$ 20 VEBs, $\geq$ 10 ventricular pairs or VT, LVEF $\leq$ 40%) PVS was done. Of 657 patients, 304 (46%) had either abnormal Holter monitoring or depressed LVEF. PVS was performed in 146 of 304 patients; it was abnormal in 22 because a sustained monomorphic VT was induced. During a mean follow-up of 37 months, there were 106 (16%) deaths, sudden in 24 (4%), nonsudden cardiac in 45 (7%). The incidence of arrhythmic events (sudden cardiac death, symptomatic VT, cardiac arrest) was 18% in patients with an abnormal PVS and only 4% in those with a normal PVS ($p = 0.03$). Andresen et al. [7] pointed out that two-step risk stratification is helpful in selecting candidates for a defibrillator trial aiming at primary prevention of sudden cardiac death after AMI.

The above-mentioned studies suggest the following question: may a "two-level" risk stratification algorithm be effectively used to screen patients eligible for ICD implantation in survivors of a recent myocardial infarction? The answer is probably yes.

In 1997, Schmitt et al. [8] used a "two-level" risk stratification algorithm similar to that suggested by Pedretti et al. [5] in 1993. In 496 patients with a recent AMI, 74 (15%) were considered eligible for EP testing because of abnormality of the following risk markers: LVEF, signal-averaged electrocardiogram, Holter monitoring and heart rate variability. Of 74 preselected patients, 31 (42%) declined the procedure; of the remaining 43, 13 (30%) had a positive EP testing because a sustained monomorphic VT was induced 10-14 days after AMI; 12 of them received an ICD. After a mean follow-up of 318 days, 7 (58%) of the 12 implanted patients had an appropriate intervention of the ICD, none of the 30 patients with a negative PVS died suddenly, and 3 (10%) of the 31 patients who did not undergo PVS died suddenly. The authors concluded that according to this risk stratification algorithm PVS seems to select patients with a high risk for sudden death which may justify prophylactic ICD implantation after an AMI.

May EP Testing Be Used in Both Early and Late Postinfarction Period to Screen High-Risk Patients?

The above-mentioned studies concern survivors of a recent myocardial infarction. Nevertheless, EP testing may be effectively used to screen high-risk subjects also in subgroups of patients with a late myocardial infarction. In 1990 Wilber et al. [9] evaluated the prognostic power of EP testing in 100 consecutive patients with spontaneous asymptomatic nonsustained VT, chronic postinfarction coronary artery disease and LVEF < 40%. All patients underwent PVS. Fifty-seven patients without inducible sustained ventricular arrhythmias were discharged on no antiarrhythmic therapy, a sustained monomorphic VT was induced in 37 patients and polymorphic VT or VF was induced in 6 patients. Of 43 patients with inducible arrhythmias, 3 were excluded from the analysis because they had spontaneous cardiac arrest during serial drug testing, 20 were discharged on drug therapy resulting in suppression of inducible sustained ventricular arrhythmias, and the remaining 20 patients were discharged on drug therapy resulting in maximal rate slowing of the induced tachycardia. The 1- and 2-year actuarial incidence of cardiac arrest or sudden death was 2% and 6%, respectively, in patients without inducible arrhythmias; 0% and 11%, respectively, in patients in whom inducible arrhythmias were suppressed; and 34% and 50%, respectively, in patients with persistently inducible ventricular arrhythmias. Multivariate Cox analysis identified the persistence of inducible sustained ventricular arrhythmias as the only significant independent predictor of sudden death or recurrent sustained arrhythmias. The authors underlined that therapeutic intervention to prevent sudden death is unnecessary in patients without inducible sustained ventricular arrhythmias, while nonresponders to serial drug testing remain at very high risk for subsequent sudden death.

The results of Wilber et al. [9] represented the background of the MADIT study [10], the first prospective trial which found a significant mortality reduction in still asymptomatic postinfarction patients, all with LVEF < 35%, nonsustained VT, and inducible but nonsuppressible sustained VT when treated with ICD.

Conclusions

Information about the usefulness of EP testing in patients with recent and late myocardial infarction is available in the literature; moreover, PVS may be used to identify a group of asymptomatic patients who will benefit from implantation of an ICD. A positive EP study is apparently the single best predictor of future arrhythmic events in AMI survivors. Since several noninvasive tests are available, PVS should not be advised to the majority of infarct survivors for the mere purpose of risk stratification. PVS should be proposed to patients with one or two noninvasive risk markers; however, before proceeding with invasive EP evaluation, both physician and patient should ask themselves if they are willing to go ahead with ICD implantation in case sustained monomorphic VT is induced. In fact, patients without inducible arrhythmias may be spared long-term treatment in view of their good prognosis. Conversely, patients with inducible sustained monomorphic VT should be implanted with an ICD. This approach is now mandatory for MADIT or MUSST (coronary artery disease, LVEF ≤ 40%, nonsustained VT, and positive PVS) like patients; probably it is the best therapeutic option for inducible patients preselected with different noninvasive markers, as suggested by the data of Schmitt et al. [8]. Conclusive data about this last point will be provided by currently ongoing ICD trials like the BEST-ICD Trial [11].

References

1. Bourke JP, Richards DAB, Ross DL, McGuire MA, Uther JB (1995) Does the induction of ventricular flutter or fibrillation at electrophysiologic testing after myocardial infarction have any prognostic significance? Am J Cardiol 75:431-435

2. Bourke JP, Richards DAB, Ross DL, Wallace EM, McGuire MA, Uther JB (1991) Routine programmed electrical stimulation in survivors of acute myocardial infarction for prediction of spontaneous ventricular tachyarrhythmias during follow-up: results, optimal stimulation protocol and cost-effective screening. J Am Coll Cardiol 18:780-788

3. Denniss AR, Richards DA, Cody DV, Russell PA, Young AA, Cooper MJ, Ross DL, Uther JB (1986) Prognostic significance of ventricular tachycardia and fibrillation induced at programmed stimulation and delayed potentials detected on the signal-averaged electrocardiograms of survivors of acute myocardial infarction. Circulation 74:731-745

4. Richards DAB, Byth K, Ross DL, Uther JB (1991) What is the best predictor of spontaneous ventricular tachycardia and sudden death after myocardial infarction. Circulation 83:756-763

5. Pedretti R, Etro MD, Laporta A, Sarzi Braga S, Carù B (1993) Prediction of late arrhythmic events after acute myocardial infarction from combined use of noninvasive prognostic variables and inducibility of sustained monomorphic ventricular tachycardia. Am J Cardiol 71:1131-1141

6. Zoni-Berisso M, Molini D, Mela GS, Vecchio C (1996) Value of programmed ventricular stimulation in predicting sudden death and sustained ventricular tachycardia in survivors of acute myocardial infarction. Am J Cardiol 77:673-680

7. Andresen D, Steinbeck G, Brüggeman T, Müller D, Haberl R, Steffen B, Hoffman E, Wegscheider K, Dissman R, Ehlers HC (1999) Risk stratification following myocardial infarction in the thrombolytic era: a two-step strategy using noninvasive and invasive methods. J Am Coll Cardiol 33:131-138

8. Schmitt C, Schneider MAE, Zrenner B, Weyerbrock S, Plewan A, Barthel P, Schmidt G (1997) Risk stratification after acute myocardial infarction: the role of programmed ventricular stimulation. Circulation 96:I-716 (abstr)

9. Wilber DJ, Olshansky B, Moran JF, Scanlon PJ (1990) Electrophysiological testing and nonsustained ventricular tachycardia. Use and limitations in patients with coronary artery disease and impaired ventricular function. Circulation 82:350-358

10. Moss AJ, Hall WJ, Cannom DS, Daubert JP, Higgins SL, Klein H, Levine JH, Saksena S, Waldo AL, Wilber D, Brown MW, Heo M (1996) Improved survival with an implanted defibrillator in patients with coronary disease at high risk for ventricular arrhythmia. N Engl J Med 335:1933-1940

11. Raviele A, Bongiorni MG, Brignole M, Cappato R, Capucci A, Gaita F, Mangiameli S, Montenero A, Pedretti R, Salerno J, Sermasi S (1999) Which strategy is "best" after myocardial infarction? The beta-blocker strategy plus implantable cardioverter defibrillator trial: rationale and study design. Am J Cardiol 83:104D-111D

The BEST + ICD Trial: Is ICD Also Effective in the Presence of Optimized β-Blocking Therapy?

R. Cappato, M.G. Bongiorni, M. Brignole, A. Capucci, F. Gaita, S. Mangiameli, A.S. Montenero, R.F.E. Pedretti, A. Raviele, J. Salerno-Uriarte and S. Sermasi

Introduction

Total mortality and sudden death rates during the first year following an acute MI have significantly decreased in the past decade (from 2.8% and 7.1% to 1.9% and 3.0%, respectively) [1, 2] as a result of modern therapy with thrombolytic agents [1-3], aspirin [4], β-blockers [5], angiotensin-converting enzyme (ACE) inhibitors [6], statines [7, 8], and revascularization procedures [9]. Nevertheless, approximately 10% of post-MI survivors remain at high risk of dying in the first months or years following hospital discharge (mortality > 25% at 2 years) [10]. This population accounts for a considerable proportion of deaths every year, approximately 37,500 cases in the USA and 3750 in Italy [11, 12]. Sudden death secondary to sustained ventricular tachycardia (VT) or ventricular fibrillation (VF) accounts for about 50% of all deaths in these high-risk patients [13]. Identification and protection of post-MI patients who are predisposed to develop life-threatening ventricular arrhythmias during follow-up is crucial in order to reduce both sudden death and all-cause mortality.

In order to be beneficial, a measure for preventing sudden death caused by a ventricular tachyarrhythmia should be applied only to the restricted population of patients who are at greater risk of this event [14]. Among predictors of serious arrhythmic events after hospital discharge from MI the following have been identified: a low left ventricular ejection fraction (LVEF), frequent and/or repetitive ventricular premature beats (VPB), ventricular late potentials (LP), reduced heart rate variability (HRV), reduced baroreflex sensitivity, QT prolongation or dispersion, T wave alternans and inducibility of sustained ventricular arrhythmias during electrophysiological study (EPS) [2, 3, 15-33].

Despite the recent progress in risk stratification of post-MI patients, it is still difficult to detect which patient is going to develop VT/VF after an acute MI. Some data suggest that the combination of two or more noninvasive factors, such as low LVEF, frequent and/or repetitive VPB, reduced HRV and ventricular LP, with the inducibility of sustained ventricular arrhythmias at EPS, is able to identify a consistent number of patients with recent MI who are at high arrhythmic risk

Corresponding author: R. Cappato, 2. Med. Abt. AK St. Georg, Hamburg, Germany

in the follow-up [24, 33]. The adequate protection of such patients with preventive measures remains, at the present time, one of the major unresolved problems in cardiology.

The use of class I and, more recently, of class III antiarrhythmic drugs (amiodarone, d-l sotalol and dofetilide) in survivors of MI who are considered to be prone to life-threatening ventricular arrhythmias, has shown no effect, or even a deleterious effect, on total survival [34-41]. Among other currently available antiarrhythmic therapies, only β-blockers and implantable cardioverter defibrillators (ICDs) have proved effective in reducing both sudden death and total mortality after MI. [5, 42]. Despite the clear evidence of their benefit, β-blockers continue to be relatively underused in post-MI patients (31%-45%) [39, 43].

The benefit of ICD therapy used prophylactically was demonstrated in MADIT [42]. In this study, ICDs were compared to non-antiarrhythmic drugs in post-MI patients with LVEF, spontaneous non-sustained VT and inducible non-suppressible sustained ventricular arrhythmias. Therapy with an ICD resulted in a 56% 2-year reduction of all-cause mortality. In another study, the CABG-Patch [44], no benefit was shown if prophylactic ICDs were implanted at the time of surgical revascularization in patients with LVEF and an abnormal signal-averaged electrocardiogram. The different results obtained with these randomized controlled trials underline the need to identify categories of patients at higher risk of sudden death who might benefit most from an ICD. Notably, only a minority of patients enrolled in the MADIT study (8% in the conventional therapy arm and 26% in the ICD arm) received β-blocker therapy [42]. Therefore, at the present time, it is not known whether the prophylactic use of an ICD in inducible patients with recent MI is effective under an optimal treatment with β-blockers. To answer this question, the BEST + ICD trial was planned and enrolment has recently started.

Objectives of the BEST + ICD Trial

The primary objective of the BEST + ICD trial is to establish whether, in patients with recent MI receiving β-blockers, a therapeutical strategy guided by EPS and based on the implantation of an ICD in subgroups with inducible sustained ventricular arrhythmias can improve survival compared to the conventional strategy. The secondary objectives of the study are to investigate: (1) the incidence of sudden death and nonfatal sustained ventricular arrhythmias, and (2) in patients pre-selected by noninvasive testing, the predictive value of EPS regarding major arrhythmic events (sustained VT and/or VF).

Study Design

The BEST + ICD trial is designed as a double-arm observational randomized investigation to evaluate the efficacy of ICD/EPS-guided therapy versus conventional therapy in high-risk patients with recent MI. The trial is aimed to select through noninvasive tests (bi-dimensional echocardiography, 24-h Holter monitoring and signal averaging electrocardiography – SAECG) a group of patients with recent MI in whom the expected all-cause 2-year mortality is greater than 25%. These patients will be considered for treatment with metoprolol if they meet all the other inclusion and exclusion criteria for the study. Patients who tolerate long-term treatment with metropolol will undergo randomization after giving informed consent; a 2:3 ratio will be used for randomization, and patients will be assigned to one of the two following therapeutic alternatives: (1) Conventional Strategy, which is based on the intensive use of metoprolol at optimal doses in conjunction with other therapeutic measures considered effective in post-MI, such as aspirin, ACE-inhibitors and statines; (2) EPS/ICD Strategy, which, in addition to optimal therapy, is based on a further risk stratification by means of an EPS and subsequent implantation of an ICD in patients who have an inducible sustained VT or VF.

Noninvasive Risk Stratification

All survivors of an acute MI, aged $\leq$ 80 years, who are not candidates for a myocardial revascularization procedure, will undergo noninvasive testing 5-21 days after the index MI.

LVEF will be performed by means of two-dimensional echocardiography, ventricular scintigraphy (Tc^{99P1}) or LV angiography. Patients with LVEF $\leq$ 35% will be considered at potential risk [3, 45] and will undergo additional noninvasive evaluation based on: (1) 24-h Holter monitoring to calculate the hourly frequency of VPB and the HRV; (2) SAECG to search for the presence of ventricular LP. A mean hourly frequency of VPB > 10 will be used as a cut-off to identify patients at high risk [16, 18].

The standard deviation of normal R-R intervals (SDNN) will be used to measure the HRV, and a value of < 70 ms will be considered as an indication of reduced HRV [25, 46]. All tests will be performed under no pharmacological wash-out including patients in whom treatment with β-blockers was initiated in the CCU.

Inclusion, Exclusion Criteria

To be eligible for the BEST + ICD trial, patients must meet all the study inclusion and exclusion criteria. Inclusion criteria: (1) recent MI (are 5 to 21 days after the onset), (2) age $\leq$ 80 years, (3) LVEF $\leq$ 35%, (4) presence of one or more of the following additional risk factors: VPB > 10/h and/or SDNN < 70 ms and/or presence of ventricular LP, (5) tolerance to a long-term β-blocker therapy.

Exclusion criteria are: (1) a history of sustained ventricular arrhythmias either associated or not with the acute MI, except for primary VF (occurring within 48 h of the onset of symptoms); (2) nonsustained VT (> 3 consecutive beats) found on standard ECG, 24-h Holter monitoring or ECG stress test; (3) residual myocardial ischemia for which myocardial revascularization (PTCA or CABG procedure) is indicated within a short time period; patients treated with primary PTCA or with rescue PTCA due to inefficacy of thrombolytic therapy during the acute phase of MI can be included in the study; (4) cardiogenic shock, symptomatic hypotension or NYHA functional class IV; (5) contraindications to β-blocking therapy [47-49]; (6) inability of the patients to tolerate a dose of metoprolol of at least 25 mg/day during the run-in phase; (7) presence of any disease associated with a likelihood of survival < 1 year; (8) irreversible brain damage from pre-existing cerebral disease; (9) women of childbearing potential; (10) refusal or inability of the patient to participate in the study; (11) participation in other clinical heart disease trials involving ICD; (12) usual patient residence at long distance from the referring center or other reasons that make the follow-up impossible.

Randomization

An eligible patient who has given written informed consent will be randomized to "conventional strategy" or "EPS/ICD Strategy". The conventional strategy includes treatment with metoprolol in addition to other therapeutic measures considered effective today in post MI patients, such as aspirin, ACE inhibitors, statines, etc. The EPS/ICD strategy is based on a further risk stratification by an EPS and the implantation of an ICD in patients who are inducible into sustained VT or VF; conversely, patients with negative EPS will not receive an ICD and will be treated in the same manner as patients assigned to the conventional strategy.

EPS Protocol

Programmed ventricular stimulation will be performed immediately after the randomization according to the following stimulation protocol: during three drive cycle lengths (600, 460, 375 ms), up to three extrastimuli will be delivered from two different sites in the right ventricle (RV) [30, 31, 42].

ICD Implantation

Because the data analysis will be primarily done on a basis of intention-to-treat, patients assigned to ICD therapy must be implanted as soon as possible, during the same recovery period for acute MI, possibly within a maximum of 3 days after the EPS. It is strongly recommended that patients during this phase be monitored by means of telemetry.

Follow-up

Patients assigned to the two different strategies will be followed every 4 months after enrolment. Administration of any antiarrhythmic drug, including amiodarone, is not allowed. Antiarrhythmic drugs can be used only for treatment of supraventricular arrhythmias, when clinically indicated. Telephone contact with the patient, or his family, will take place monthly to closely monitor the primary end-point (all-cause mortality). At each follow-up visit, a patient history will be taken including a recording of current therapy with particular attention to β-blocker therapy and the prescribed dose; moreover, baseline examination, standard 12-lead ECG and ICD follow-up in patients allocated to ICD therapy will be performed.

Study Endpoints

The primary endpoint of the BEST + ICD trial is all-cause mortality. Secondary endpoints are sudden death, nonsudden death, noncardiac death, resuscitated cardiac arrest, nonfatal sustained VT and appropriate shocks from the ICD in implanted patients. Sudden cardiac death has been defined as occurring within 1 hour from the onset of symptoms, during sleep, or within 24 h of the last contact with the patient when he was seen in a healthy state, and if death occurred in the absence of witnesses.

Analysis of Data

Enrolment Cascade

We have estimated that 14%-25% (average 19%) of patients with recent MI will have a LVEF ≤ 35% [6, 8]. According to Hartikainen et al. [24] and Pedretti et al. [33], it is likely that 80% of these patients, corresponding to around 15% of all patients with recent MI, will present at least one additional noninvasive risk factor, i.e. VPB > 10/h and/or SDNN < 70 ms and/or ventricular LP. Taking into account that 7% of the patients surviving the acute MI phase need myocardial revascularization at short term [3], and that 20% of patients with LVEF ≤ 35% will have nonsustained VT at Holter examination [24], 11% of all patients surviving an acute MI are potentially eligible for this study. According to the large post-MI trials on β-blockers [47-50], 18% of patients will show absolute contraindications to these drugs. Moreover, an additional 5% of this population will not tolerate β-blockers during the run-in phase [51]. Consequently, the percentage of patients potentially eligible for both therapeutic strategies should correspond to 9% of the whole patient population with recent MI. After giving written informed consent, 40% of these patients will be randomized to "Conventional Strategy" and 60% to "EPS/ICD Strategy". Thus, 5.4 % of patients who have survived a recent MI will undergo EPS. Of these, 35% are expected to have a positive EPS [16-18] and will receive an ICD.

Mortality Expectations

It is presumed that patients who survive the acute phase of MI and are at high risk according to the study inclusion criteria will have a 2-year mortality rate > 25% in the absence of extensive use of β-blockers [18, 23-25]. It is expected that β-blockers will reduce all-cause mortality by 21% [5]. Therefore, the 2-year mortality rate during β-blocker therapy in a group of patients like those indicated above is ~ 20%. This is, therefore, the expected all-cause mortality in patients assigned to the "Conventional Strategy" arm. Patients with positive EPS have a 2-year mortality rate of 34% and those with negative EPS of 14 % [30, 31, 42] in the absence of extensive use of β-blockers. Also, in this group of patients β-blockers are presumed to reduce mortality by 21% [5], whereas a further reduction of mortality of at least 35% will occur in patients receiving an ICD [42]. Thus, the expected all-cause mortality in the "EPS/ICD Strategy" arm is 14%.

Statistical Design and Sample Size Calculation

A triangular two-sided sequential design [54] with preset boundaries ($p < 0.05$) will be used for analysis to permit an early termination of the trial, if efficacy, no difference or inefficacy are found. The study will have a 90% ability to detect a 30% reduction (from 20% to 14%) in all-cause mortality at 2-year follow-up, allowing for 3% cross-over [53] from control to EPS-guided therapy and 0.3% per month loss of patients to follow-up. Sample size calculation has been made according to the following data: P1 = 0.20 (probability of all-cause mortality in patients randomized to "Conventional Strategy"); P2 = 0.14 (probability of all-cause mortality in patients randomized to "EPS/ICD Strategy"); r = 2:3; α = 0.05; $1 - \alpha$ = 0.90. This design calls for the enrolment of 1200 patients; assuming a 2:3 randomization ratio, 480 patients will be assigned to the "Conventional Strategy" and 720 to "EPS/ ICD Strategy" arm.

Patient Flow

From the estimation made above, the following "patient flow" may be formulated: 14,000 patients with recent MI will undergo noninvasive testing; 2660 (19%) will have a LVEF ≤ 35%; 1540 (11%) patients will be at high risk after noninvasive testing has been completed and after exclusion of subjects with documented nonsustained VT as well as those who need myocardial revascularization within a short period; 277 (18%) patients will show absolute contraindications to β-blockers. In all, 1263 patients will start metoprolol therapy; of these, 63 (5%) patients will present intolerance to metoprolol during the run-in phase; 1200 patients will be chronically treated with metoprolol and will be randomized after having signed the informed consent; 480 (40%) will be assigned to the "Conventional Strategy" and 720 (60%) to the "EPS/ICD Strategy" and will undergo an EPS; 252 (35%) patients will have a positive EPS and will be implanted with an ICD; 180 (15%) patients will stop metoprolol during the 2-year follow-up period; 6% of patients will need a pacemaker because of a bradyarrhythmia; finally, 2.1%-2.9% will need an ICD because of a nonfatal sustained ventricular arrhythmia.

Time Schedule

A total of 80 centers in Italy and 15 in Germany will participate in the study. It is expected that the 1200 patients will be enrolled into the study over 2 years.

Recruitment started in June 1998. The patients will be stratified by clinical center. Length of follow-up for each patient will depend on the date of entry into the study, since all patients will be followed to a common termination date.

Statistical Analysis

Statistical tests of the difference in the primary endpoint between the two randomized arms will be computed at periodic intervals during the trial by the Data and Safety Monitoring Board as part of the sequential design, and at the conclusion of the study. Data analysis will be done on the basis of both an intention-to-treat (as primary analysis) and an on-treatment principle (as secondary analysis). After having verified the effective balance of the randomized groups, using Student's t-test or nonparametric tests for the qualitative variables, and the chi-squared test or Fisher test for qualitative variables, a survival analysis will be performed using actuarial Kaplan-Meyer curves. If the two groups are unbalanced due to one or more variables, these latter will be introduced as covariates in a multivariate Cox model to verify the possible influence on the outcome of the study. A two-tailed p value < 0.05 will be required for statistical significance.

Registry

Each center will establish a registry to report the data on all patients with acute MI sent to the center during the recruitment period and those who have not been included in the study. Detailed information and specific follow-up data are required for potentially eligible patients who have not been enrolled.

Appendix I: Structure of the Study

Steering Committee: Coordinators: Antonio Raviele, Mestre (Italy); Salvatore Mangiameli, Catania (Italy). *Members:* Maria Grazia Bongiorni, Pisa (Italy); Michele Brignole, Lavagna (Italy); Riccardo Cappato, Amburgo (Germany); Alessandro Capucci, Piacenza (Italy); Fiorenzo Gaita, Asti (Italy); Alessandro Montenero, Roma (Italy); Roberto Pedretti, Tradate (Italy); Jorge Salerno, Castellanza (Italy); Sergio Sermasi, Rimini (Italy).

Data and Safety Monitoring Board: Jackson Hall, Rochester (USA); Helmut Klein, Magdeburg (Germany); Paolo Rizzon, Bari (Italy).

Clinical Advisory Board: Attilio Maseri, Roma (Italy); Massimo Chiariello, Napoli (Italy); Seah Nisam, Brussels (Belgium).

Sponsor: GUIDANT ITALIA, Via Cassanese, 224, Palazzo Raffaello, 20090 Segrate (Italy).

Data Coordination Center: INNOVEX S.r.l. - Centro Direz. Colleoni - Palazzo Taurus - V.le Colleoni, 3 - 20041 Agrate Brianza (Italy).

Appendix II: List of Enrolling Centers

Alboni Paolo, Cento (FE); Arlotti Massimo, Milano; Baldi Nicola, Taranto; Barone Giuseppe, Palermo; Bernabé Daniele, La Spezia; Bertero Giovanni, Genova; Binaghi Giovanni, Varese; Bonatti Vincenzo, Massa; Bongiorni Maria Grazia, Pisa; Bracchetti Daniele, Bologna; Brignole Michele, Lavagna (GE); Bruna Claudio, Cuneo; Buja Gianfranco, Padova; Bulla Vincenzo, Catania; Calculli Giacinto, Matera; Calvi Valeria, Catania; Capucci Alessandro, Piacenza; Cazzin Roberto, Portogruaro (VE); Ceci Vincenzo, Roma; Chiariello Massimo, Napoli; Ciolli Andrea, Roma; Dalmasso Maurizio, Ivrea (TO); De Fabrizio Giuseppe, Avellino; De Simone Antonio, Maddaloni (CE); Del Citerna Federico, Pistoia; Dini Paolo, Roma; Fanelli Raffaele, S.G. Rotondo (FG); Filice Ignazio, Savona; Frabetti Lorenzo, Bologna; Gaita Fiorenzo, Asti; Giani Paolo, Seriate (BG); Gronda Maurizio, Vercelli; Igidbashian Diran, Legnago (VR); Lemme Riccardo, Roma; Leone Giuseppe, Catanzaro; Libero Luigi, Torino; Luise Raffaele, Pescara; Maffei Pietro, Sanremo (IM); Mangiameli Salvatore, Catania; Mantovan Roberto, Treviso; Marchini Anna, Brescia; Marcolongo Marco, Moncalieri (TO); Menozzi Carlo, Reggio Emilia; Musso Giacomo, Imperia; Musto Benito, Napoli; Nicotra Giuseppe/Morgera Tullio, Gorizia/Monfalcone; Occhetta Eraldo, Novara; Pascotto Pietro, Mirano (VE); Pedretti Roberto, Tradate (VA); Pettinati Giacinto, Casarano (LE); Pettini Andrea, Forlì; Petz Eugenio, Trieste; Picarella Bernardo, Palermo; Pistis Gianfranco, Torino; Pizzorno Luigi, Genova Setri P.; Poggio Gianluigi, Tradate (VA); Proclemer Alessandro, Udine; Ravazzi Pier Antonio, Alessandria; Raviele Antonio, Mestre (VE); Renzi Roberto, Ancona; Rognoni Giorgio, Borgosesia (VC); Rolli Angelo, Parma; Salerno Jorge, Castellanza (VA); Sanfelici Daniela, Pietraligure (SV); Sartori Giuseppe, Genova; Scaccia Alberto, Frosinone; Sciré Aldo, Esine (BS); Serio Giovanni, Palermo; Sermasi Sergio, Rimini; Setti Sergio, Rivarolo (GE); Seu Vittorio, Ge Sampierdarena; Sgarbi Ernesto, Pesaro; Terrosu Gianfranco, Sassari; Verlato Roberto, Camposampiero (PD); Vincenti Antonio, Monza (MI); Zaccone Gabriele, Novi Ligure (AL); Zanotto Gabriele, Verona; Zardo Fabio, Pordenone; Zecchi Paolo, Roma; Zennaro Romeo/Pozzetti Daniela, Modena/Mirandola (MO); Zonzin Pietro, Rovigo.

References

1. Califf RM, White HD, Van de Werf F, Sadowski Z, Armstrong PW, Vahanian A, Simoons ML, Simes RJ, Lee KL, Topol EJ (1996) One-year results from the global utilization of streptokinase and TPA for occluded coronary arteries (GUSTO I) trial. Circulation 94:1233-1238
2. Rouleau JL, Talajic M, Sussex B, Potvin L, Warnica W, Davies RF, Gardner M, Stewart D, Plante S, Dupuis R, Lauzon C, Ferguson J, Mikes E, Balnozan V, Savard P (1996) Myocardial infarction patients in the 1990s – their risk factors, stratification and survival in Canada: the Canadian Assessment of Myocardial Infarction (CAMI) study. J Am Coll Cardiol 27:1119-1127
3. Volpi A, De Vita C, Franzosi MG, Geraci E, Maggioni AP, Mauri F, Negri E, Santoro E, Tavazzi L, Tognoni G (1993) Determinants of 6-month mortality in survivors of myocardial infarction after thrombolysis. Results of the GISSI-2 data base. Circulation 88:416-429
4. Antiplatelet Trialists Collaboration (1988) Secondary prevention of vascular disease by prolonged antiplatelet treatment. Br Med J 296:320-331

5. Yusuf S, Peto R, Lewis J, Collins R, Sleight P (1985) Beta blockade during and after myocardial infarction: an overview of the randomized trials. Prog Cardiovasc Dis 27:335-371
6. Latini R, Maggioni AP, Flather M, Sleight P, Tognoni G (1995) ACE inhibitor use in patients with myocardial infarction. Summary of evidence from clinical trials. Circulation 92:3132-3137
7. Scandinavian Simvastatin Survival Study Group (1994) Randomized trial of cholesterol lowering in 4444 patients with coronary heart disease: the Scandinavian Simvastatin Survival Study (4S). Lancet 344:1383-1389
8. Sacks MF, Pfeffer MA, Moye LA, Rouleau JL, Rutherford JD, Cole TG, Brown L, Warnica W, Arnold JMO, Wun CC, Davis BR, Braunwald E (1996) The effect of pravastatin on coronary events after myocardial infarction in patients with average cholesterol levels. N Engl J Med 335:1001-1009
9. Michels KB, Yusuf S (1995) Does PTCA in acute myocardial infarction affect mortality and reinfarction rates? A quantitative overview (meta-analysis) of the randomized clinical trials. Circulation 91:476-485
10. Raviele A, Bonso A, Gasparini G, Themistoclakis S (1998) Prophylactic implantation of implantable cardioverter/defibrillator in post-myocardial infarction patients. In: Vardas PE (ed) Cardiac arrhythmias, pacing and electrophysiology. Kluger Academic Publishers, Dordrecht, pp 305-310
11. ACC/AHA practice guidelines for the management of patients with acute myocardial infarction (1996) J Am Coll Cardiol 28:1328-1428
12. Feruglio GA, Vanuzzo D (1989) La cardiopatia ischemica in Italia: le dimensioni del problema. G Ital Cardiol 19:754-762
13. Uretsky BF, Sheahan RG (1997) Primary prevention of sudden cardiac death in heart failure: will the solution be shocking? J Am Coll Cardiol 30:1589-1597
14. Pratt CM, Waldo AL, Camm AJ (1998) Can antiarrhythmic drugs survive survival trials? Am J Cardiol 81(6A):24D-34D
15. Bigger JT, Fleiss JL, Kleiger R, Miller JP, Rolnitzky LM (1984) The relationships among ventricular arrhythmias, left ventricular dysfunction, and mortality in the 2 years after myocardial infarction. Circulation 69:250-258
16. Mukharji J, Rude RE, Poole WK, Gustafson N, Thomas LJ, Strauss HW, Jaffe AS, Muller JE, Roberts R, Raabe DS, Croft CH, Passamani E, Braunwald E, Willerson JT (1984) Risk factors for sudden death after acute myocardial infarction: two-year follow-up. Am J Cardiol 54:31-36
17. Kostis JB, Byington R, Friedman LM, Goldstein S, Furberg C (1987) Prognostic significance of ventricular ectopic activity in survivors of acute myocardial infarction. J Am Coll Cardiol 10:231-242
18. Maggioni AP, Zuanetti G, Franzosi MG, Rovelli F, Santoro E, Staszewsky L, Tavazzi L, Tognoni G (1993) Prevalence and prognostic significance of ventricular arrhythmias after acute myocardial infarction in the fibrinolytic era. GISSI-2 results. Circulation 87:312-322
19. Denniss AR, Richards DA, Cody DV, Russel PA, Young AA, Cooper MJ, Ross DL, Uther JB (1986) Prognostic significance of ventricular tachycardia and fibrillation induced at programmed stimulation and delayed potentials detected on the signal-averaged electrocardiograms of survivors of acute myocardial infarction. Circulation 74:731-745
20. McClements BM, Adgey AAJ (1993) Value of signal-averaged electrocardiography, radionuclide ventriculography, Holter monitoring and clinical variables for prediction of arrhythmic events in survivors of acute myocardial infarction in the thrombolytic era. J Am Coll Cardiol 21:1419-1427

21. Cain ME, Anderson JL, Arnsdorf MF, Mason JW, Scheinman MM, Waldo AL (1996) ACC expert consensus document. Signal-averaged electrocardiography. J Am Coll Cardiol 27:238-249

22. Kleiger RE, Miller JP, Bigger JT, Moss AJ (1987) Decreased heart rate variability and its association with increased mortality after acute myocardial infarction. Am J Cardiol 59:256-262

23. Farrell TG, Bashir Y, Cripps T, Malik M, Poloniecki J, Bennett ED, Ward DE, Camm AJ (1991) Risk stratification for arrhythmic events in postinfarction patients based on heart rate variability, ambulatory electrocardiographic variables and signal-averaged electrocardiogram. J Am Coll Cardiol 18:687-697

24. Hartikainen JEK, Malik M, Staunton A, Poloniecki J, Camm J (1996) Distinction between arrhythmic and nonarrhythmic death after acute myocardial infarction based on heart rate variability, signal-averaged electrocardiogram, ventricular arrhythmias and left ventricular ejection fraction. J Am Coll Cardiol 28:296-304

25. Zuanetti G, Neilson JMM, Latini R, Santoro E, Maggioni AP, Ewing DJ (1996) Prognostic significance of heart rate variability in post-myocardial infarction patients in the fibrinolytic era. The GISSI-2 results. Circulation 94:432-436

26. La Rovere MT, Bigger JT, Marcus FI, Mortara A, Schwartz PJ (1998) Baroreflex sensitivity and heart-rate variability in prediction of total cardiac mortality after myocardial infarction. Lancet 351:478-484

27. Schwartz PJ, Wolf S (1978) QT interval prolongation as predictor of sudden death in patients with myocardial infarction. Circulation 57:1074-1077

28. Perkiömäki JS, Koistinen MJ, Yli-Mäyry S, Huikuri HV (1995) Dispersion of QT interval in patients with and without susceptibility to ventricular tachyarrhythmias after previous myocardial infarction. J Am Coll Cardiol 26:174-179

29. Rosenbaum DS, Jackson LE, Smith JM (1994) Electrical alternans and vulnerability to ventricular arrhythmias. N Engl J Med 330:235-241

30. Waspe LE, Seinfeld D, Ferrick A, Kim SG, Matos JD, Fisher JD (1985) Prediction of sudden death and spontaneous ventricular tachycardia in survivors of complicated myocardial infarction: value of the response to programmed stimulation using a maximum of three ventricular extrastimuli. J Am Coll Cardiol 5:1292-1301

31. Wilber DJ, Olshansky B, Moran JF, Scanlon PJ (1990) Electrophysiologic testing and nonsustained ventricular tachycardia: use and limitation in patients with coronary artery disease and impaired ventricular function. Circulation 82:350-358

32. Bourke JP, Richards DA, Ross DL, Wallace EM, McGuire MA, Uther JB (1991) Routine programmed electrical stimulation in survivors of acute myocardial infarction for prediction of spontaneous ventricular tachyarrhythmias during follow-up: results, optimal stimulation protocol and cost-effective screening. J Am Coll Cardiol 18:780-788

33. Pedretti R, Etro MD, Laporta A, Sarzi Braga S, Caru B (1993) Prediction of late arrhythmic events after acute myocardial infarction from combined use of noninvasive prognostic variables and inducibility of sustained monomorphic ventricular tachycardia. Am J Cardiol 71:1131-1141

34. Furberg CD (1983) Effect of antiarrhythmic drugs on mortality after myocardial infarction. Am J Cardiol 52:32C-36C

35. The Cardiac Arrhythmia Suppression Trial (CAST) (1989) Investigators. Preliminary report: effect of encainide and flecainide on mortality in a randomized trial of arrhythmia suppression after myocardial infarction. N Engl J Med 321:406-412

36. The Cardiac Arrhythmia Suppression Trial II Investigators (1992) Effect of the antiarrhythmic agent moricizine on survival after myocardial infarction. N Engl J Med 327:227-233

37. Teo KK, Yusuf S, Furberg CD (1993) Role of antiarrhytmic prophylaxis in acute myocardial infarction. Review of clinical results. JAMA 270:1589-1595

38. Waldo AL, Camm AJ, deRuyter H, Friedman PL, MacNeil DJ, Pauls JF, Pitt B, Pratt CM, Schwartz PJ, Veltri EP (1996) Effect of d-l sotalol on mortality in patients with left ventricular dysfunction after recent and remote myocardial infarction. Lancet 348:7-12

39. Julian DG, Camm AJ, Frangin G, Janse MJ, Munoz A, Schwartz PJ, Simon P (1997) Randomized trial of effect of amiodarone on mortality in patients with left-ventricular dysfunction after recent myocardial infarction: EMIAT. Lancet 349:667-674

40. Cairns JA, Connolly SJ, Roberts R, Gent M (1997) Randomized trial of outcome after myocardial infarction in patients with frequent or repetitive ventricular premature depolarisations: CAMIAT. Lancet 349:675-682

41. DIAMOND Study Group (1997) Dofetilide in patients with left ventricular dysfunction and either heart failure or acute myocardial infarction: rationale, design, and patient characteristics of the DIAMOND studies. Clin Cardiol 20:704-710

42. Moss AJ, Hall WJ, Cannom DS, Daubert JP, Higgins SL, Klein H, Levine JH, Saksena S, Waldo AL, Wilber D, Brown MW, Heo M (1996) Improved survival with an implanted defibrillator in patients with coronary disease at high risk for ventricular arrhythmia. N Engl J Med 335:1933-1940

43. GISSI (1996) Six-month effects of early treatment with lisinopril and transdermal glyceril trinitrate singly and together withdrawn six weeks after acute myocardial infarction: the GISSI-3 trial. J Am Coll Cardiol 27:337-344

44. Bigger JT, for the CABG Patch Trial Investigators (1997) Prophylactic use of implanted cardiac defibrillators in patients at high risk for ventricular arrhythmias after coronary-artery bypass graft surgery. N Engl J Med 337:1569-1575

45. Copie X, Hnatkova K, Staunton A, Fei L, Camm AJ, Malik M (1996) Predictive power of increased heart rate versus depressed left ventricular ejection fraction and heart rate variability for risk stratification after myocardial infarction. Results of a two-year follow-up study. J Am Coll Cardiol 27:270-276

46. Task Force of the European Society of Cardiology and the North American Society of Pacing and Electrophysiology (1996) Heart rate variability. Standards of measurement, physiological interpretation and clinical use. Circulation 93:1043-1065

47. The Norwegian Multicenter Study Group (1981) Timolol-induced reduction in mortality and reinfarction in patients surviving acute myocardial infarction. N Engl J Med 304:801-807

48. Beta-blocker Heart Attack Trial Research Group (1982) A randomized trial of propranolol in patients with acute myocardial infarction: mortality results. JAMA 247:1707-1714

49. Viskin S, Kitzis I, Lev E, Zak Z, Zajarias A, Laniado S, Belhassen B (1995) Treatment with beta-adrenergic blocking agents after myocardial infarction: from randomized trials to clinical practice. J Am Coll Cardiol 25:1327-1332

50. Hjalmarson A, Elmfeldt D, Herlitz J, Holmberg S, Malik I, Nyberg G, Ryden L, Swedberg K, Vedin A, Waagstein F, Waldenstrom A, Waldenstrom J, Wedel H, Wilnelmsen L, Wilhelmsson C (1981) Effect on mortality of metoprolol in acute myocardial infarction: a double-blind randomized trial. Lancet 2:823-837

51. Packer M, Bristow M, Cohn JN, Colucci WS, Fowler MB, Gilbert EM, Shusterman NH (1996) The effect of carvedilol on morbidity and mortality in patients with chronic heart failure. N Engl J Med 334:1349-1355

52. The MIAMI Trial Research Group. Metoprolol in acute myocardial infarction (MIAMI) (1985) A randomized placebo-controlled international trial. Eur Heart J 6:199-226

53. Di Pede F, Gasparini G, Raviele A, Piccolo E (1995) Studi elettrofisiologici durante la fase acuta dell'infarto miocardico. Può essere prognostico? In: Caturelli G (ed) Cura intensiva cardiologica. CESI, Rome, pp 495-498

54. Whitehead J (1992) The design and analysis of sequential clinical trials, 2nd edn. Ellis Horwood, Chichester

SEDET Trial: Is Noninvasive Evaluation Sufficient to Identify Patients at High Risk of Arrhythmia?

M. Santini[1], R. Ricci[1] and M. Zoni Berisso[2], on behalf of the Steering Committee of the SEDET Study

Introduction

The superior effectiveness of implantable cardioverter-defibrillator (ICD) therapy as compared to pharmacological therapy in survivors of ventricular fibrillation (VF) and poorly tolerated ventricular tachycardia (VT) was proven by the prematurely terminated Amiodarone Versus Implantable Defibrillator (AVID) study which showed that patients randomized to ICD treatment had a much lower mortality (38% reduction after 1 year, and 25% reduction after 2 and 3 years) than patients randomized to amiodarone treatment [1].

At the same time another study, the Multicenter Automatic Defibrillator Implantation Trial (MADIT) assessed the influence of prophylactic ICD therapy on the outcome of high-risk post-myocardial infarction (MI) patients. This study was also terminated early because of the superiority of ICD therapy over conventional therapy [2]. Patients in MADIT had prior MI (more than 3 weeks previously), left ventricular ejection fraction of 35% or less, and asymptomatic nonsustained VT. A further requirement was that the patients had inducible VT during electrophysiological study (EPS) which was not suppressible by procainamide treatment.

However, invasive EP studies are not routinely performed in daily practice, particularly in asymptomatic patients. Furthermore, the large majority of patients in MADIT had a remote MI, i.e., more than 6 months before enrollment in the study. As yet, it is unknown whether similar reductions in mortality can be achieved with prophylactic ICD implantation if patients are selected on the basis of noninvasive tests and at a much earlier stage, e.g., in the first few weeks after their MI. Therefore, the challenge is to define a patient group with a high risk of life-threatening arrhythmias.

One such group could be the patient population that is ineligible for the standard treatment in the early phase of acute MI, i.e., thrombolysis. Thrombolytic

[1]Dipartimento di Cardiologia, Ospedale San Filippo Neri, Rome, Italy; [2]Dipartimento di Cardiologia, Ospedale Galliera, Genoa, Italy

therapy has been proven to reduce mortality in acute MI patients if administered within the first hours after onset of symptoms. However, many patients arrive late at the hospital, because they are either late in seeking care or late in being diagnosed, or both, and will not benefit from this therapy. Also, patients at increased risk of bleeding or stroke, or other contraindications, and patients with lack of adequate ECG changes, are not eligible for thrombolytic therapy. Thus, many patients – approximately 50% [3-5] – are ineligible to receive the treatment of choice in the acute phase of MI.

Are patients ineligible for thrombolytic therapy at increased risk of arrhythmic events and sudden death? Pedretti et al. [6] showed that late potentials are more prevalent in patients receiving conventional therapy (34%) than in patients receiving thrombolytic therapy (17%). The prevalence of inducibility at EPS is also higher in patients who did not receive thrombolytic therapy compared to patients who did. In another study by Pedretti et al. [7], for example, VT was induced in 20% of patients who had received thrombolytic therapy and in 67% of those who had not. In a study by Sager et al. [8], VT was induced in 8% of thrombolyzed patients at 2 weeks, versus 88% of nonthrombolyzed patients. Thus it appears that the heart of a patient who has not received thrombolytic therapy is less electrically stable than the heart of a patient who has. Indeed, in the 1994 study by Pedretti et al. [7], during a mean follow-up of 23 ± 11 months 13% of the thrombolyzed patients and 43% of the nonthrombolyzed patients had an arrhythmic event.

Several studies report higher in-hospital and long term mortality rates in nonthrombolyzed patients compared to those who were eligible and received thrombolysis [9, 10, GISSI]. However, patients in these trials could be randomized only if they were eligible to receive thrombolysis, and therefore these results cannot be generalized to patients who are ineligible for thrombolytic therapy.

Data on ineligible patients are scarce. However, one study published in 1996 by Behar et al. [11] showed that ineligible patients are worse at baseline and continue to be at greater risk after discharge. The study was a prospective survey carried out during a 2-month period in all 25 coronary care units operating in Israel. All centers participated in the GUSTO study (Global Utilization of Streptokinase and Tissue plasminogen activator for Occluded coronary arteries [12], and patients who were not eligible for thrombolytic therapy (according to the GUSTO criteria) were also followed. Of 1014 patients with acute MI, 383 (38%) were treated with a thrombolytic agent and included in the GUSTO study. Ineligible patients for GUSTO were treated either without any reperfusion therapy ($n = 449$), or with mechanical revascularization ($n = 97$), or with 1.5 million units of streptokinase outside of the GUSTO protocol ($n = 85$). The in-hospital and 1-year post-discharge mortality rates were respectively 6% and 2% in patients included in the GUSTO study, 6% and 5% in those mechanically reperfused, 15% and 10% in those treated with thrombolysis despite ineligibility for the GUSTO trial, and 15% and 13% among patients not treated with any reperfusion therapy. In another study by Wilcox et al. [13] sudden death constituted 49% of all deaths in patients treated with heparin plus placebo, compared to 33% in patients treated with heparin plus alteplase.

From the above data one may conclude that patients who are ineligible to receive thrombolytic therapy during acute MI are at increased risk of arrhythmic events and (sudden) death compared to those who did receive thrombolytic treatment. Yet not all patients who are ineligible for thrombolytic therapy will benefit from prophylactic ICD therapy. As a result, to improve the cost-effectiveness of prophylactic ICD, further risk stratification in this patient group is needed. In the prethrombolytic era, left ventricular dysfunction, extensive coronary artery disease, and the presence of frequent or repetitive ventricular premature complexes on ambulatory monitoring were demonstrated to be independent prognostic factors for subsequent mortality among hospital survivors of acute MI [14, 15]. It seems very likely that employing the same risk stratifiers in patients ineligible for thrombolytic therapy will select a subgroup with an even higher risk of life-threatening arrhythmias and therefore improve the cost-effectiveness of therapy.

The SEDET Study (South European Defibrillator Trial)

The SEDET study has been organized to assess the outcome of prophylactic ICD therapy, as compared to conventional therapy, in patients deemed to be at high risk of developing life-threatening arrhythmias, such as patients who are ineligible for thrombolytic therapy with depressed left ventricular function and asymptomatic ventricular arrhythmias.

The objective of SEDET is to determine whether ICD, as compared to standard treatment, can reduce total mortality of patients with acute MI ineligible for thrombolysis and with depressed left ventricular function at discharge. The primary objective is to demonstrate that ICD is superior to standard treatment in reducing 3-year total mortality. The secondary objective is to compare the effects of ICD versus standard therapy with respect to: sudden death, cardiac and non-cardiac mortality, resource utilization, health-related quality of life, and prevalence of spontaneous sustained VT. Optimization of ICD programming is also aimed at. Two connected subproject studies aim to assess the predictive value for sudden death of heart rate variability and baroreceptor reflex sensitivity in patients with these clinical characteristics.

SEDET is an open, randomized, controlled primary prevention study. Approximately 50 centers from seven Mediterranean countries will be involved in the study. Six hundred fifty patients with acute MI who are ineligible for thrombolysis and have depressed left ventricular function with asymptomatic ventricular arrhythmias will be enrolled in the study. Patients will be randomly assigned to conventional treatment or ICD implantation and followed for at least 2 years. Patients in both groups will receive the best available post-MI pharmacological treatment including β-blockers, aspirin, statins, and ACE-inhibitors, unless contraindicated.

Inclusion criteria are the following: acute MI, age from 18 to 75 years, ineligibility for thrombolytic treatment according to European guidelines for the management of acute MI [16], left ventricular ejection fraction between 15% and 40%, ten or more premature ventricular complexes per hour or at least one episode of nonsustained VT on Holter monitoring. Fullfilment of inclusion criteria must be determined between 6 and 42 days after MI onset. The following are grounds for exclusion: advanced age (> 75 years), thrombolytic therapy not received despite eligibility for it, primary percutaneous transluminal coronary angioplasty (PTCA), spontaneous sustained VT or VF more than 48 h from the acute MI onset, patient undergoing electrophysiological studies, indication for pacing or pacemaker present, indication for PTCA or bypass surgery before randomization present, patient on antiarrhythmic therapy which needs to be continued, prospective survival less than 1 year.

It is estimated that in Europe 40%-50% of acute MI patients are ineligible for thrombolysis. Taking into account that about 30% of them have a depressed left ventricular ejection fraction and, of these, about 30% are expected to have frequent premature ventricular complexes or episodes of nonsustained VT, about 3% of the total acute MI population could meet SEDET enrollment criteria.

References

1. The AVID investigators (1997) A comparison of antiarrhythmic drug therapy with implantable defibrillators in patients resuscitated from near fatal ventricular arrhythmias. N Engl J Med 337:1576-1583
2. Moss AJ, Hall WJ, Cannom DS, Daubert JP, Higgins SL, Klein H, Levine JK, Saksena S, Waldo AL, Wilber D, Brown MW, Heo M, for the Multicenter Automatic Defibrillator Implantation Trial Investigators (1996) Improved survival with an implanted defibrillator in patients with prior myocardial infarction, low ejection fraction and asymptomatic non-sustained ventricular tachycardia. N Engl J Med 335:1933-1940
3. Reikvam A, Ketley D (1997) Thrombolytic eligibility in acute myocardial infarction patients admitted to Norwegian hospitals. Int J Cardiol 61:79-83
4. Juliard JM, Himbert D, Golmard JM, Aubry P, Karillon GJ, Boccara A, Benamer H, Steg PG (1997) Can we provide reperfusion therapy to all unselected patients admitted with acute myocardial infarction? J Am Coll Cardiol 30:157-164
5. European Secondary Prevention Study Group (1996) Translation of clinical trials into practice: a European population-based study of the use of thrombolysis for acute myocardial infarction. Lancet 347:1203-1207
6. Pedretti RF, Laporta A, Etro MD, Gementi A, Bonelli R, Anza C, Colombo E, Maslowsky F, Santoro F, Carù B (1992) Influence of thrombolysis on signal-averaged electrocardiogram and late arrhythmic events after acute myocardial infarction. Am J Cardiol 69:866-872
7. Pedretti RF, Colombo E, Sarzi Braga S, Carù B (1994) Effect of thrombolysis on heart rate variability and life-threatening ventricular arrhythmias in survivors of acute myocardial infarction. J Am Coll Cardiol 23:19-26
8. Sager PT, Perlmutter RA, Rosenfeld LE, McPherson CA, Wackers FJ, Batsford WP (1988) Electrophysiologic effects of thrombolytic therapy in patients with a transmural anterior myocardial infarction complicated by left ventricular aneurysm formation. J Am Coll Cardiol 12:19-24

9. French JK, Williams BF, Hart HH, Wyatt S, Poole JE, Ingram C, Ellis CJ, Williams MG, White HD (1996) Prospective evaluation of eligibility for thrombolytic therapy in acute myocardial infarction. Br Med J 312:1637-1641

10. Ozbek C, Heisel A, Krause M, Berg G, Hammer B, Bay W, Sen S, Schieffer H (1995) Comparison of mortality from acute myocardial infarction in patients receiving anistreplase with those not receiving thrombolysls. Am J Cardiol 76:1103-1107

11. Behar S, Gottlieb S, Hod H, Benari B, Narinski R, Pauzner H, Rechavia E, Faibel HE, Katz A, Roth A, Goldhammer E, Freedberg NA, Rougin N, Kracoff O, Shapira C, Jafari J, Lotan C, Daka F, Weiss T, Kanetti M, Klutstein M, Rudnik L, Barasch E, Mahul N, Blondheim D (1996) The outcome of patients with acute myocardial infarction ineligible for thrombolytic therapy. Israeli Thrombolytic Survey Group. Am J Med 101:184-191

12. GUSTO Investigators (1993) An international randomized trial comparing four thrombolytic strategies for acute myocardial infarction. N Engl J Med 329:673-682

13. Wilcox RG, von der Lippe G, Olsson CG, Jensen G, Skene AM, Hampton JR (1990) Effects of alteplase in acute myocardial infarction: 6-month results from the ASSET study. Anglo-Scandinavian Study of Early Thrombolysis. Lancet 335:1175-1178

14. Moss AJ, Davis HT, De Camilla J, Bayer LW (1979) Ventricular ectopic beats and their relation to sudden and nonsudden cardiac death after myocardial infarction. Circulation 60:998-1003

15. Bigger JT jr, Fleiss JL, Kleiger R, Miller JP, Rolnitzky LM (1984) The relationship among ventricular arrhythmias, left ventricular dysfunction and mortality in the 2 years after myocardial infarction. Circulation 69:250-258

16. Julian DG, Boissel JP, de Bono DP, Fox K, Genomi M, Heikkila J, Lopez-Bescos L, Neuhaus KL, Schroder R, Sleight P, Specchia G, Swedberg K, Turina M, Verheugt FWA, Van de Werf F, Zijlstra F (1996) Task force of the ESC. Management of acute myocardial infarction. Eur Heart J 17:43-63

DINAMIT: Does ICD Implantation Improve Life Expectancy in Survivors of Acute Myocardial Infarction?

S.H. Hohnloser, S. Connolly, K.H. Kuck, P. Dorian and M. Gent for the DINAMIT
Investigators

Mortality After Myocardial Infarction

The last two decades have seen a substantial improvement in the survival of patients with acute myocardial infarction. In-hospital mortality has decreased from around 16% in the late 1970s and early 1980s to 8-10% in the early 1990s, as recently documented in a prospective population-based survey [1]. The main reason for this reduced mortality is the more widespread use of and adherence to contemporary therapeutic modalities such as thrombolysis, administration of aspirin, and β-blockers [1]. The survival of patients discharged alive from hospital after myocardial infarction has also been considerably improved. The 1-year total mortality rate of patients discharged alive from hospital ranges between 3% and 11%.

An important consideration concerns the precise cause of death of survivors of acute myocardial infarction, particularly when risk stratification should result in therapeutic measures to decrease arrhythmogenic death. It is often very difficult to define retrospectively the precise cause of death of a patient enrolled in a controlled trial, particularly where suspected sudden arrhythmogenic death is concerned [2]. This problem becomes even more evident when population-based survey data are considered. The best estimate derived from numerous investigations is that arrhythmogenic death accounts for approximately 40%-50% of total mortality in the first year after myocardial infarction. The risk of dying of an arrhythmia decreases considerably over the next 12-24 months [3]. This time dependence of risk within the higher-risk patient groups limits the opportunity for effective intervention strategies to the early periods after the conditioning cardiovascular events.

J.W. Goethe University, Frankfurt, Germany

Background of Postinfarction ICD Trials: The Value of Risk Stratification

Although ICD therapy has been demonstrated to have the potential for reducing mortality in coronary patients, it will be impossible to offer this treatment to all patients surviving an acute myocardial infarction. The high costs associated with ICD therapy as well as other logistic reasons will continue to exclude this. Accordingly, it is of paramount importance to select for ICD therapy those infarct survivors who are at particularly high risk of dying from an arrhythmic cause. Identifying such patients and carrying out ICD therapy in them would potentially impact on all-cause mortality in the entire postinfarction population.

There are several prerequisites which need to be remembered during the process of risk stratification. In order to impact on clinical strategies, risk stratification methods need to be available in all hospitals. This implies that only noninvasive risk stratification methods can be considered; electrophysiological testing, although apparently effective in selecting high risk patients, cannot be used for widespread risk stratification due to its invasive nature, restriction to specialized centers, and associated costs. Of all noninvasive risk stratifiers, determination of left ventricular function is undoubtedly the single most important one. Reduced left ventricular ejection fraction (LVEF) has repeatedly been demonstrated to identify patients with a significantly increased risk of all-cause mortality [4, 5]. If, however, LVEF is below approximately 15%, the proportion of deaths due to heart failure will be increased quite substantially, and this will reduce the likelihood of demonstration of an ICD-associated survival benefit. Several studies have demonstrated that impairment of autonomic nervous system function is another indicator of increased mortality in patients surviving an acute myocardial infarction [6-8]. A decrease particularly in vagal tone with a subsequent predominance of sympathetic tone has been found to be associated with increased arrhythmic mortality. Accordingly, noninvasive markers of autonomic imbalance such as heart rate variability (HRV) or baroreflex sensitivity should be considered for risk stratification after myocardial infarction. HRV can be easily assessed from Holter recordings obtained at the time of hospital discharge. The value of this method has been clearly demonstrated. An even more easily obtained measure of autonomic nervous system function is 24-h average heart rate. Recently, the clinical usefulness of this risk stratifier has been demonstrated in several independent studies [9, 10]. For instance, in a recent meta-analysis of amiodarone trials, annual mortality was 13.4% in those patients who had a LVEF ≤ 40% and an average 24-h heart rate ≥ 80 bpm. Taken together, these findings indicate that by combining determination of LVEF and a measure of autonomic tone, patients at increased risk of sudden arrhythmic death can be identified.

The DINAMIT Trial

DINAMIT (Defibrillator in Acute Myocardial Infarction Trial) is a propsective trial examining the potential of ICD therapy in the improving prognosis of survivors of acute myocardial infarction. It is a European-Canadian multicenter, open, randomized, parallel group comparison between ICD therapy and no ICD therapy. In accordance with the above described considerations concerning risk stratification, postinfarction survivors will be eligible for participation in DINAMIT if they have had an acute myocardial infarction within the last 40 days, have depressed left ventricular function (LVEF $\leq$ 35%), and show evidence of impaired autonomic nervous system function. The latter will be assessed by determination of HRV (standard deviation of NN interval [SDNN] $\leq$ 70 ms) and/or average 24-h mean RR-interval $\leq$ 750 ms from a Holter recording obtained prior to hospital discharge. Two-year mortality in the control group is assumed to be approximately 30%, with 40% of deaths due to ventricular tachyarrhythmias. It is expected that 80% of sudden deaths could be prevented by the ICD. To demonstrate a reduction in total mortality in the ICD group from 30% to 20.4% (α-error of 0.05, β-error of 0.8), a sample size of 525 patients will be required for the trial. To meet these requirements, approximately 7500 infarct survivors will be necessary for screening. DINAMIT started patient enrollment in late 1998. The trial will help to answer the question whether by means of noninvasive risk stratification survivors of myocardial infarction can be identified who will benefit from prophylactic ICD implantation. If this promise holds true, life expectancy of these patients should improve.

References

1. Le Feuvre CA, Connolly SJ, Cairns JA, Gent M, Roberts RS (1996) Comparison of mortality from acute myocardial infarction between 1979 and 1992 in a geographically defined stable population. Am J Cardiol 78:1345-1349
2. Pratt CM, Greenway PS, Schoenfeld MH, Hibben ML, Reiffel JA (1996) Exploration of the precision of classifying sudden cardiac death. Implications from the interpretation of clinical trials. Circulation 93:519-524
3. Myerburg RJ, Kessler M, Castellanos A (1993) Sudden cardiac death: epidemiology, transient risk, and intervention assessment. Ann Intern Med 119:1187-1197
4. Bigger JT Jr, Fleiss JL, Kleiger R, Miller JP, Rolnitzky LM, and the Multicenter Post-Infarction Research Group (1984) The relationships among ventricular arrhythmias, left ventricular dysfunction, and mortality in the 2 years after myocardial infarction. Circulation 69:250-258
5. Odemuyiwa O, Malik M, Farell T, Bashir Y, Poloniecki J, Camm AJ (1991) Comparison of the predictive characteristics of heart rate variability index and left ventricular ejection fraction for all-cause mortality, arrhythmic events and sudden death after acute myocardial infarction. Am J Cardiol 68:434-439
6. Bigger JT Jr, Fleiss JL, Steinman RC, Rolnitzky LM, Kleiger RK, Rottmann JN (1992) Correlations among time and frequency domain measures of heart period variability two weeks after acute myocardial infarction. Am J Cardiol 69:891-898
7. Zuanetti G, Neilson JMM, Latini R, Santoro E, Maggioni A, Ewing DJ, on behalf of GISSI-2 Investigators (1996) Prognostic significance of heart rate variability in post-myocardial infarction patients in the fibrinolytic era. The GISSI-2 results. Circulation 94:432-436

8. Hohnloser SH, Klingenheben T, Zabel M, Li Y-G (1997) Heart rate variability used as an arrhythmia risk stratifier after myocardial infarction. Pacing Clin Electrophysiol 20(II):2594-2601

9. Copie X, Hnatkova K, Staunton A, Fei L, Camm AJ, Malik M (1996) Predictive power of increased heart rate versus depressed left ventricular ejection fraction and heart rate variability for risk stratification after myocardial infarction. Results of a two-year follow-up study. J Am Coll Cardiol 27:270-276

10. Nul DR, Doval HC, Grancelli HO, Varini SD, Soifer S, Perrone SV, Prieto N, Capin O, on behalf of the GESICA-GEMA Investigators (1997) Heart rate is a marker of amiodarone mortality reduction in severe heart failure. J Am Coll Cardiol 29:1199-1205

What Are the Clinical Implications of MUSTT?

S.L. Higgins

The Multicenter Unsustained Tachycardia Trial (MUSTT) findings have yet to be published. However, as a result of presentation of the preliminary results at two major cardiology meetings, the publication is much anticipated. Since it is unpublished, its true clinical impact has yet to be determined. However, based on the response to similar important trials in arrhythmia management, we can make reasonable projections of the potential clinical relevance of this trial.

Background

Initiated in 1990, the MUSTT trial tested the hypothesis that anti-arrhythmic drug therapy guided by electrophysiological testing would reduce the risk of arrhythmic death in patients with coronary artery disease (CAD) a left ventricular ejection fraction (EF) of 40% or less and asymptomatic ventricular tachycardia (VT), defined as from three beats to 30 s at a rate of over 100 bpm. Over 2200 patients were enrolled from 85 centers, though only 767 patients met the electrophysiology (EP) study inducible critera resulting in randomization. The study results were first presented in March 1999 and will likely not be published until late this year or early 2000. The hypothesis and protocol were first published in 1993 by the principal investigator, Alfred E. Buxton, and other MUSTT investigators [1].

Protocol and Enrollment Results

Patients who met the inclusion criteria discussed above (CAD, EF $\leq$ 0.40, non-sustained VT) were required to undergo evaluation and treatment for myocardial ischemia. A baseline EP study was performed from two right ventricular sites with up to triple stimuli and synchronized burst pacing in a very regimented protocol [1]. Of the 2202 patients enrolled, 1435 were not inducible and 63 of those found inductible refused randomization; all of them were followed prospectively in a registry. A total of 704 patients were randomized between

Regional Cardiac Arrhythmia Center, Scripps Memorial Hospital, La Jolla, California, USA

EP-guided anti-arrhythmic drug therapy and "conservative" therapy. The groups were well matched for demographic criteria such as age, gender and race as well as clinical criteria such as average duration of nonsustained VT (five beats) and ejection fraction (30%). In the EP-guided group, only 45% were discharged on a pharmacological agent which included 9% on Amiodarone, 35% on other class I-III agents and 7% on no drug [failed EP-guided testing and refused implantable defibrillator (ICD)]. The remainder of the EP-guided therapy arm (46%) received an ICD. The conservative therapy patient group was discharged on β-blockers when tolerated (51% vs 38% of EP-guided) and angiotensin-converting enzyme (ACE) inhibitors (about 75% of both groups).

Results

The primary endpoint of the MUST trial was arrhythmic death or cardiac arrest defined by independent data and a safety monitoring board with secondary endpoints being overall mortality and cardiac mortality. The preliminary results for the primary endpoint are shown in Table 1. The results of the overall mortality data are shown in Table 2. Statistical analysis will not be reviewed.

Table 1. Arrhythmic death or cardiac arrest in all randomized patients ($n = 704$) divided into conservative and EP-guided therapy groups with the latter further subdivided to those who received an implantable defibrillation (ICD) within the first 90 days and those who did not. Data are expressed in Kaplan-Meier survival estimates with standard error in parenthesis

	EP-guided therapy ICD within 90 days ($n = 167$)	EP-guided therapy no ICD within 90 days ($n = 184$)	Conservative therapy no anti-arrhythmic ($n = 353$)
2 Years	0.97 (± .01)	0.79 (± .03)	0.82 (± .02)
5 Years	0.91 (± .03)	0.63 (± .04)	0.68 (± .03)

Table 2. Total mortality (all causes) in all randomized patients ($n = 704$) divided into conservative and EP-guided therapy groups with the latter further subdivided to those who received an ICD within the first 90 days and those who did not. Data are expressed in absolute numbers of deaths with percentage of each subgroup in parenthesis

	EP-guided therapy ICD within 90 days ($n = 167$)	EP-guided therapy no ICD within 90 days ($n = 184$)	Conservative therapy no anti-arrhythmic ($n = 353$)
Total mortality	35 (21%)	97 (53%)	158 (45%)

Discussion of Study Results

Although the MUSTT study results are only available in preliminary form, the findings are quite striking. First of all, over half of patients subjected to an EP-guided drug testing failed to have any drug shown to suppress inducible ventricular arrhythmias. The majority of those remaining opted to have an ICD. While it cannot be assumed that these ICD recipients represented a higher risk subgroup, their mortality was dramatically less than the other groups. In the Kaplan-Meier analysis shown in Table 1, 91% of the ICD recipients were free of arrhythmic death or cardiac arrest at 5 years as compared to 63% of those receiving EP-guided drug therapy and 68% of those who did not have any EP-directed therapy. Since arrhythmic death is subject to interpretation, total mortality has often been used as a surrogate "hard" endpoint. However, total mortality was also dramatically different among the three groups: 24% of those with an ICD, 55% with EP-guided drug therapy and no ICD and 48% in those patients receiving no anti-arrhythmic therapy.

Clinical Implications

In an as yet unpublished study, it is difficult to draw conclusions, even with such tantalizing preliminary results. However, one can surmise that patients with coronary disease, asymptomatic non-sustained VT and inducible sustained VT do better when undergoing an EP-guided approach than more traditional therapy. Amazingly, the benefit of this treatment is only realized in the subgroup that received an ICD. MUSTT was not designed to test whether the ICD was superior to anti-arrhythmic drug therapy. In fact, that study has already been completed in a similar subgroup, the Multicenter Automatic Defibrillator Implantation Trial (MADIT) [2, 3]. Consistent with the findings of MUSTT, the MADIT investigators found a 54% reduction in mortality when an ICD is chosen over "conventional" anti-arrhythmic drug therapy in patients with CAD, non-sustained VT and a left ventricular ejection fraction ≤ 0.35.

One unanswered criticism of MADIT was that it applied to only a small portion of patients seen in the typical cardiology practice. Unfortunately, MUSTT can be similarly criticized, though it does extend the population to those with less severe congestive heart failure and the number of patients (704) is substantially greater than the 196 enrolled in MADIT. We and others have discussed the potential extrapolation of good scientific studies such as MADIT and MUSTT to clinical practice [4-9]. At a similar time after scientific presentation, but prior to publication, United States health care officials recommended adoption of the MADIT guidelines into clinical practice [10]. As a result of MADIT as well as technological advances in ICD design and other factors, implantation rates have increased dramatically since publication of the MADIT study in 1996, announced by industry to exceed 52,000 implants in 1998 [11, 12].

Will MUSTT have similar impact on expanding ICD usage? Of course, no one knows. However, based upon past experience, the MUSTT study should further encourage ICD usage. MUSTT suggests a limited value for EP test results, since those who were non-inducible and those who had serial EP testing to determine anti-arrhythmic efficacy both had relatively poor outcomes, substantially worse than those who received ICDs. Physicians faced with the real-world challenge of managing patients who may not fit already published results (so-called evidence-based cardiology) will likely extend the results of MUSTT just as was done for MADIT. Therefore, in certain settings, the role of EP studies may be restricted to that of a diagnostic test, or perhaps therapeutic, only for ablation therapy. Once ventricular tachyarrhythmias are induced, the MUSTT findings suggest that proceeding directly to ICD implantation would be in the patient's best interest. Presumably, this should increase utilization of ICDs, even in those interested in cost-effective approaches to arrhythmia management.

Scientific study results are often slowly accepted in clinical practice. Classic examples include the delayed adoption of β-blockers for post-myocardial infarction or ACE-inhibitor for congestive heart failure [14, 15]. Explanations are numerous and include skepticism, ignorance, a desire to await confirmation, financial pressures and others. All of these issues are likely to play a role in the clinical impact of MUSTT. Skepticism should be less than that seen with MADIT as this represents only one of several recently published studies suggesting an enhanced role for ICD therapy over anti-arrhythmic agents [16-19]. Ignorance is also diminishing as the sheer volume of studies and associated industry marketing efforts have educated even the most reluctant. Similarly, MUSTT is one of the studies often cited as one to "await" before encouraging ICD usage [20]. Apparently, it too appears to corroborate the evidence that ICD implantation should be the management of first choice in selected patients. Thus, many of the forces that discouraged prompt acceptance of new therapy in earlier years may be less valid with publication of MUSTT.

Conclusions

Despite the fact that the primary publication is still pending, there is great interest in the results of MUSTT. Preliminary presentations have suggested that high-risk patients (CAD, EF ≤ 0.40, nonsustained VT) with inducible VT at EP study are best treated with an ICD rather than either conventional therapy or EP-guided anti-arrhythmic drug therapy. The clinical implications of the study are presently unknown but could include a decrease in utilization of EP testing for risk-stratification or serial drug testing. The MUSTT study becomes one more in the ever-increasing list of trials supporting ICD therapy in selected high-risk subgroups. Thus, when further publicized, MUSTT may expand ICD utilization despite traditional reluctance towards acceptance of new therapeutic approaches.

Acknowledgements. The author would like to thank Alfred E. Buxton, MD, Lynnett Voshage-Stahl and the MUSTT investigators for assistance with data utilized in this manuscript and Seah Nisam for editorial assistance.

References

1. Buxton AE, Fisher JD, Josephson ME, Lee KL, Pryor DB, Prystowsky EN, Simson MB, DiCarlo L, Echt DS, Packer D, Greer GS, Talajic M, the MUSTT Investigators (1993) Prevention of sudden death in patients with coronary artery disease: the multicenter unsustained tachycardia trial (MUSTT). Prog Cardiovasc Dis 6:215-226

2. MADIT Executive Committee (1991) Multicenter automatic defibrillator implantation trial (MADIT): design and clinical protocol. PACE 14(II):920-927

3. Moss AJ, Hall WJ, Cannom DS, Daubert JP, Higgins SL, Klein H, Levine JH, Saksena S, Waldo AL, Wilber D, Brown MW, Heo M, for the Multicenter Automatic Defibrillator Implantation Trial (MADIT) Investigators (1996) Improved survival with an implanted defibrillator in patients with coronary disease at high risk for ventricular arrhythmia. N Engl J Med 335:1933-1940

4. Higgins SL (1999) Impact of the Multicenter Automatic Defibrillator Implantation Trial (MADIT) on ICD indication trends: a two-year perspective. Am J Cardiol 83:79D-82D

5. Higgins SL, Klein H, Nisam S (1997) Which device should "MADIT protocol" patients receive? Am J Cardiol 79:31-35

6. Higgins SL, Daubert JL, Akhtar M (1997) Who are the MADIT patients? Am J Cardiol 79(5B):42-46F

7. Higgins SL, Voshage-Stahl L (1997) What have we learned from the US experience on the prophylactic use of ICDs following MADIT? In: Raviele A (ed) Cardiac Arrhythmias. Springer-Verlag, Milan, pp 270-275

8. Higgins S (1997) Will management of atrial arrhythmias be important in MADIT patients? In: Capucci A (ed) Atrial fibrillation, evolving concepts and new therapeutic strategies. Bologna

9. Nisam S (1997) Do MADIT results apply only to "MADIT Patients"? Am J Cardiol 79(6A):27-30

10. National Heart, Lung and Blood Institutes Communications (1997) NHLBI stops arrhythmia study-implantable cardiac defibrillators reduce deaths. NIH press release, April 14

11. Bocker D, Block M, Borggrefe M, Breithardt M (1997) Evidence-based cardiology: defibrillators are superior to anti-arrhythmic drugs in the treatment of ventricular tachyarrhythmias. Eur Heart J 18:26-30

12. Cannom DS (1998) A review of the implantable cardioverter defibrillator trials. Curr Opin Cardiol 13:3-8

13. Mushlin AI, Hall WJ, Zwanziger J, Gajary E, Andrews M, Marron R, Zou KH, Moss AJ (1988) The cost-effectiveness of automatic implantable cardiac defibrillators: results from MADIT: Multicenter Automatic Defibrillator Implantation Trial. Circulation 97:2129-2135

14. Viskins S, Kitzis I, Lev E, Zak Z, Heller K, Villa Y, Zajanas A, Laniado S, Belhassen B (1995) Treatment with beta-adrenergic blocking agents after myocardial infarction: from randomized trials to clinical practice. J Am Coll Cardiol 25:1327-1332

15. Garg R, Yusuf S, Collaborative Group on ACE Inhibitor Trials (1995) Overview of randomized trials of angiotensin-converting enzyme inhibitors on mortality and morbidity in patients with heart failure. JAMA 18:1450-1456

16. The AVID investigators (1997) A comparison of anti-arrhythmic drug therapy with implantable defibrillators in patients resuscitated from near fatal ventricular arrhythmias. N Engl J Med 337:1576-1583

17. Cairns JA, Connolly SJ, Roberts R, Gent M (1997) Randomised trial of outcome after myocardial infarction in patients with frequent or repetitive ventricular premature

depolarisations: CAMIAT. Canadian Amiodarone Myocardial Infarction Arrhythmia Trial Investigators. Lancet 49:675-682

18. Julian DG, Camm AJ, Frangin G, Janse MJ, Munoz A, Schwartz PJ, Simon P (1997) Randomised trial of effect of amiodarone on mortality in patients with left-ventricular dysfunction after recent myocardial infarction: EMIAT. European Myocardial Infarct Amiodarone Trial Investigators. Lancet 49:667-674

19. Maloney JD (1989) Consequences of the Cardiac Arrhythmia Suppression Trial: calamity or clarity? Clev Clin J Med 56:649-653

20. Friedman P, Stevenson W (1996) Unsustained ventricular tachycardia-to treat or not to treat. N Engl J Med 335:1984-1985 (editorial)

ALIVE Trial: How Is This Trial Design Different?

C.M. PRATT

The development of the ALIVE study design is based upon an analysis of previous studies attempting pharmacologic reduction of arrhythmic death after acute myocardial infarction (MI). Historically, antiarrhythmic agents with predominant class I or class III (Vaughan Williams classification) activity have been tested and shown in several post-MI clinical trials to be ineffective, or even harmful, in terms of excessive morbidity and mortality because of proarrhythmic effects or end-organ toxicities [1-6]. Examples of such agents and trials include flecainide and encainide in Cardiac Arrhythmia Suppression Trial (CAST) [1], moricizine in CAST II [2], D-sotalol in the Survival With Oral D-Sotalol (SWORD) trial [3, 4], and amiodarone in the European Myocardial Infarction Amiodarone Trial (EMIAT) [5] and the Canadian Amiodarone Myocardial Infarction Arrhythmia Trial (CAMIAT) [6]. A significant contributing factor to the failures in many of these clinical trials was patient selection. A broad net of patients were enrolled in these studies; even those at low risk for arrhythmic death were included and thus subjected to the potentially adverse effects of these agents. This resulted in antiarrhythmic therapy in a subset of patients in whom no benefit could be gained by exposure to the drug and, in many cases, in whom there was an increased risk of mortality due to drug-related arrhythmogenicity or nonarrhythmic toxicity.

Based upon these trials, the following lessons were considered to be pivotal: (1) Post-MI patients with a left ventricular ejection fraction (LVEF) above 35% or below < 15% are less likely to die of a ventricular tachyarrhythmic death than those whose LVEF is 15%-35%. This statement is most relevant to patients in the first year after MI. (2) Cause-specific mortality changes after acute MI such that, for any level of LVEF, the proportion of patients dying from an arrhythmic death diminishes many years after the MI. Patients are most likely to die an arrhythmic death in the first year after acute MI. (3) The combination of low heart rate variability and LVEF cutoff identifies a high risk group for arrhythmic death after acute MI.

Section of Cardiology, Department of Medicine, Baylor College of Medicine, Houston, Texas, USA

The ALIVE Trial Design

The ALIVE (AzimiLide post-Infarct surVival Evaluation) trial is a double-blind, placebo-controlled, multinational trial that will enroll 5900 patients in approximately 600 centers worldwide. Its objective is to evaluate the potential of azimilide to improve survival in a targeted post-MI population at high risk for sudden cardiac death that is arrhythmic in etiology. The key elements of the trial design are outlined below in Fig. 1 [7]. Complete information on the trial is provided in the ALIVE trial protocol.

Hypothesis

The working hypothesis on which the trial is based is that the novel antiarrhythmic agent azimilide dihydrochloride, by virtue of its unique ability to selectively block both I_{Ks} and I_{Ks} in the human myocardium and its effectiveness in preclinical trials in reducing cardiac tachyarrhythmias, will decrease all-cause mortality in a target population of patients with recent MI who are at risk of sudden cardiac death. Inclusion and exclusion criteria, detailed below, will ensure that enrolled patients will be those at highest risk for death through arrhythmic mechanisms as predicted by markers believed most predictive of such an event.

Objectives

The primary objective of the trial is to evaluate the effects of azimilide dihydrochloride (100 mg) versus placebo on all-cause mortality, based on longitudi-

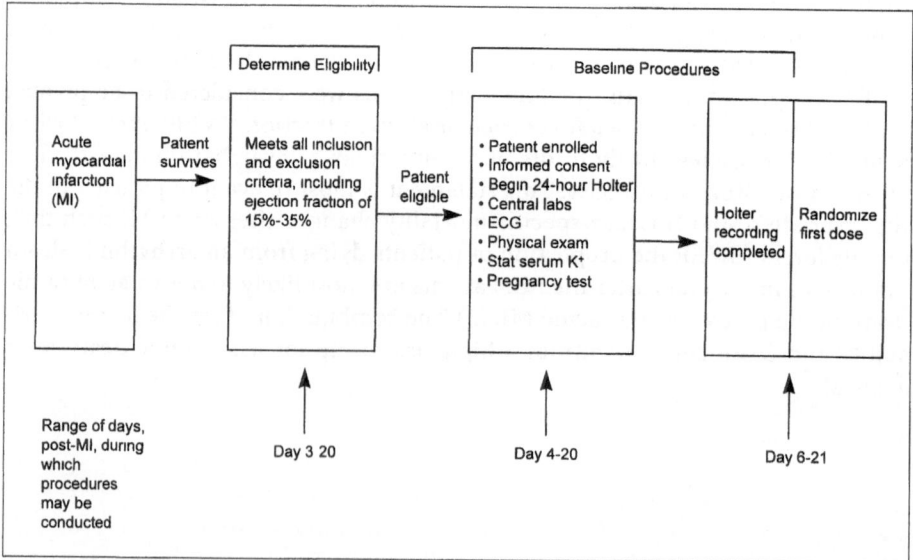

Fig. 1. ALIVE trial study design. (Adapted from [7], with permission of Excerpta Medica Inc)

nal intent-to-treat observations in patients at high risk of sudden cardiac death, namely those with recent (6-21 days) MI, low LVEF (15-35%), and a low heart rate variability (≤ 20 U). Sample size is based on the assumption that the all-cause mortality from sudden cardiac death (heart rate variability ≤ 20 U) is 15% and that azimilide will decrease all-cause mortality by at least 45% in these patients.

Additional objectives of the ALIVE trial are to: (1) evaluate the effects of azimilide on arrhythmic, cardiac, and noncardiac mortality in patients stratified by risk ("at risk" and "at high risk" categories); (2) evaluate the effects of azimilide on all-cause mortality in patients with a single previous MI and in those who have had several previous MIs; (3) determine the effect of concomitant β-blocker and angiotensin-converting enzyme (ACE) inhibitor use on all-cause mortality; (4) identify and compare the cardiovascular-related inpatient utilization patterns and costs of care in post-MI patients randomized to receive 75 mg or 100 mg azimilide or placebo; and (5) determine the relation of each treatment dose or placebo to incidence of patient dropout.

Therapy is discontinued after 1 year of treatment due to concern that cause-specific mortality changes with time after MI, with arrhythmic death gradually diminishing in frequency, thus reducing the theoretical benefit-risk of continuing antiarrhythmic therapy [8].

Summary

The ALIVE trial is an opportunity to utilize many of the lessons from past trials and to test assumptions based on an increased understanding of moderate-risk and high-risk markers of arrhythmia-induced sudden cardiac death. It is expected to test the efficacy and safety of the antiarrhythmic agent azimilide in patients at high risk of sudden cardiac death, a group defined by an LVEF of 15%-35% and heart rate variability ≤ 20 U. The trial proposes to demonstrate improvements in survival in post-MI patients by including only patients at high risk of sudden cardiac death and by excluding those post-MI patients who are unlikely to suffer life-threatening arrhythmia or those who are at risk of non-arrhythmic-generated mortalities (cardiac and noncardiac). Thus, the study seeks to evaluate the potential of azimilide to improve survival in patients at high risk of sudden cardiac death who are most likely to benefit from antiarrhythmic therapy.

References

1. Echt DS, Leibson PR, Mitchell B, Peters RW, Obias-Manno D, Barker AH, Arensberg D, Baker A, Friedman L, Greene HL, Huther ML, Richardson DW, and the CAST Investigators (1991) Mortality and morbidity in patients receiving encainide, flecainide, or placebo. N Engl J Med 324:781-788
2. The Cardiac Arrhythmia Suppression Trial II Investigators (1992) Effect of the antiarrhythmic agent moricizine on survival after myocardial infarction. N Engl J Med 327:227-233

3. Waldo AL, Camm AJ, deRuyter H, Friedman PL, MacNeil DJ, Pitt B, Pratt CM, Rodda BE, Schwartz PJ, for the SWORD Investigators (1995) The SWORD trial. Survival with oral D-sotalol in patients with left ventricular dysfunction after myocardial infarction: rationale, design and methods. Am J Cardiol 75:1023-1027

4. Waldo AL, Camm AJ, deRuyter H, Friedman PL, MacNeil DJ, Pauls JF, Pitt B, Pratt CM, Schwartz PJ, Veltri EP, for the SWORD Investigators (1996) Effect of D-sotalol on mortality in patients with left ventricular dysfunction after myocardial infarction. Lancet 348:7-12

5. Julian DG, Camm AJ, Fragin G, Janse MJ, Munoz A, Schwartz PJ, Simon P, for the European Myocardial Infarct Amiodarone Trial Investigators (1997) Randomized trial of effect of amiodarone on mortality in patients with left-ventricular dysfunction after recent myocardial infarction: EMIAT. Lancet 349:667-674

6. Cairns JA, Connolly SJ, Robert R, Gent M, for the Canadian Amiodarone Myocardial Infarction Arrhythmia Trial Investigators (1997) Randomized trial of outcome after myocardial infarction in patients with frequent or repetitive ventricular premature depolarisations: CAMIAT. Lancet 349:675-682

7. Camm AJ, Karam R, Pratt CM (1998) The azimilide post-infarct survival evaluation (ALIVE) trial. Am J Cardiol 81:35D-39D

8. Pratt CM, Greenway PS, Schoenfeld MH, Hibben ML, Reiffel JA (1996) An exploration of the precision of classifying sudden cardiac death: implications for the interpretation of clinical trials. Circulation 93:519-524

SYNCOPE

What is the Value of Clinical History in Establishing the Cause of Syncope?

P. ALBONI, M. DINELLI, K. BETTIOL AND M. DONATEO

It is commonly accepted that the clinical history is important in the diagnosis of the cause of syncope. For example, pallor, nausea, and diaphoresis are believed to be specific for vasovagal syncope. However, the value of clinical history in the diagnosis of the type of syncope has been little investigated. Wayne et al. [1] analyzed the clinical features of 510 patients with a wide variety of causes of syncope. Particular emphasis was placed on the nature of the prodromal and recovery symptoms, the position prior to syncope and the duration of prodromal and recovery symptoms. Although this study represented the first attempt to critically examine the clinical history in patients with syncope, it was not possible to draw conclusions, because there were several important limitations. In fact, the histories were retrospectively obtained from medical records and precise details were often unavailable. Moreover, many of the diagnoses were established on a presumptive basis due to the absence of clear diagnostic criteria.

A subsequent study prospectively evaluated the role of the clinical history in establishing the cause of syncope [2]. In this study, the clinical histories obtained from 170 patients with syncope presenting to the emergency room were evaluated. A presumed diagnosis was established at the time of emergency treatment. The ability to detect differences in the clinical history in patients with syncope due to a variety of causes was limited in this study because patients were grouped into eight diagnostic classifications, many of which included fewer than ten patients. Despite this limitation, the authors demonstrated that the duration of warning symptoms prior to syncope was greater for neurocardiogenic syncope than for cardiac syncope. Warning symptoms lasting longer than 10 s were seen in about 70% of patients with neurocardiogenic syncope but only in about 30% of patients with cardiac syncope ($p < 0.05$).

Recently, Calkins et al. [3] prospectively investigated the clinical history in the evaluation of patients with syncope, with particular emphasis placed on symptoms and simple demographic variables. However, the historical features of only three causes of syncope were evaluated: neurocardiogenic syncope, syn-

Divisione di Cardiologia, Ospedale Civile, Cento (FE), Italy

cope due to ventricular tachycardia and syncope resulting from atrioventricular block. Eighty patients were studied and each patient was interviewed using a standard questionnaire. For the first time, the relative frequency of each symptom was described and the duration of prodromal symptoms was quantified. The historical features of syncope in the three groups of patients are summarized in Table 1.

Clinical Features of Neurocardiogenic Syncope

Several clinical features of neurocardiogenic syncope, which were previously unrecognized, were observed in this study. Firstly, neurocardiogenic syncope may occur with little or no warning. In fact, among the patients with this type of syn-

Table 1. Comparison of historical features of syncope as reported by Calkins et al. [3]

	NCG (n = 32)	AVB (n = 16)	VT (n = 32)	Overall	p Value NCG vs AVB	NCG vs VT	VT vs AVB
Demographic variables							
Male sex	10 (31%)	13 (81%)	28 (88%)	<0.001	0.002.	<0.001	0.56
Age (years)	44±17	71±7	65±9	<0.01	<0.001	<0.001	0.02
Episodes of syncope	20±29	2.3±1.8	1.9±1.8	<0.001	0.001	<0.001	0.57
Syncope while supine	0 (0%)	0 (0%)	2 (6%)	0.2	1	<0.05	0.54
Syncope only standing	14 (44%)	9 (56%)	16 (50%)	0.7	0.46	<0.05	0.52
Precipitant	12 (38%)	0 (0%)	0 (0%)	<0.001	0.004	<0.001	1
Premonitory signs and symptoms							
Time to onset (s)	89±130	1.4±1.8	34±79	0.01	<0.001	0.04	0.03
Nausea	16 (50%)	0 (0%)	2 (6%)	<0.001	<0.001	<0.001	0.54
Warmth	18 (56%)	1 (6%)	7 (22%)	0.001	0.001	0.005	0.24
Cold	3 (9%)	0 (0%)	0 (0%)	0.1	0.54	0.24	1
Diaphoresis	18 (56%)	0 (0%)	7 (22%)	<0.001	<0.001	0.005	0.04
Lightheadedness	27 (84%)	7 (44%)	20 (63%)	0.01	0.006	0.048	0.21
Palpitations	8 (25%)	0 (0%)	1 (3%)	0.01	0.04	0.03	1
Blurred vision	12 (38%)	0 (0%)	6 (19%)	0.01	0.004	0.1	0.16
Recovery signs and symptoms							
Mild fatigue	9 (28%)	0 (0%)	6 (19%)	0.06	0.02	0.38	0.16
Severe fatigue	21 (66%)	0 (0%)	5 (16%)	<0.001	<0.001	<0.001	0.15
Nausea	7 (22%)	0 (0%)	1 (3%)	0.01	0.08	0.05	1
Confusion	5 (16%)	0 (0%)	4 (13%)	0.26	0.15	1	0.29
Diaphoresis	16 (50%)	1 (6%)	5 (16%)	0.001	0.003	0.003	0.65
Warmth	15 (47%)	0 (0%)	4 (13%)	<0.001	<0.001	0.003	0.29
Palpitations	5 (16%)	0 (0%)	4 (13%)	0.3	0.15	1	0.29
Duration recovery (min)	151±358	1.9±7.5	417±734	0.5	0.025	0.67	0.26
Incontinence	9 (28%)	0 (0%)	4 (13%)	0.03	0.02	0.12	0.29
Major injury	2 (6%)	1 (6%)	6 (19%)	0.2	1	0.26	0.4
Any injury	12 (38%)	7 (44%)	13 (41%)	0.9	0.67	0.8	0.83

AVB, atrioventricular block; NCG, neurocardiogenic; VT, ventricular tachycardia

cope, approximately one-third had less than a 5-s warning. Secondly, lightheadedness was reported by about 80% of patients with neurocardiogenic syncope, whereas the prodromal symptoms of nausea, warmth and diaphoresis were less common and were reported by approximately 50% of the patients. Thirdly, palpitations prior to syncope were not uncommon in patients with neurocardiogenic syncope and were reported by 25% of the patients. Fourthly, mild or severe fatigue were very prominent symptoms following neurocardiogenic syncope, being reported by more than 90% of the patients with this type of syncope. Finally, neurocardiogenic syncope may occur in the absence of an identifiable precipitant. In fact, a clear precipitating factor was identified in only approximately one-half of patients. This contrasts with the generally accepted notion that neurocardiogenic syncope is triggered by a painful, thermal or emotional stimulus.

Clinical Features of Syncope Due to Ventricular Tachycardia

The data reported in Table 1 show some interesting findings. Lightheadedness is frequent prior to loss of consciousness (56% of patients) and diaphoresis and warmth are rather frequent (22%). Strangely, very few patients experienced palpitations (13%). Patients with syncope due to ventricular tachycardia had a marked variability in the duration of the prodromal and recovery symptoms. This most likely reflects a large variation in the cardiac rate of tachyarrhythmia.

Clinical Features of Syncope Due to Atrioventricular Block

Syncope due to atrioventricular block occurred in both standing and supine positions, was associated with short prodromic symptoms (mean duration of warming was less than 2 s) and had a very short duration of recovery symptoms (mean duration of recovery symptoms was 2 min).

Differential Diagnosis

Valuables features of the clinical history in distinguishing syncope due to bradycardia (atrioventricular block) versus tachycardia (ventricular tachycardia) were the duration of the warning and recovery symptoms, the presence of diaphoresis prior to syncope and the presence of mild or severe fatigue following syncope. The two features of the clinical history that could best differentiate these causes of syncope were the duration of warning and recovery symptoms. Patients with syncope due to ventricular tachycardia had a longer duration of warning and recovery symptoms than patients with syncope due to atrioventricular block.

Valuable features of the clinical history in distinguishing syncope due to bradycardia or tachycardia from neurocardiogenic syncope were age, sex, the number of episodes of syncope, the duration of warning and recovery symptoms and the presence of fatigue following syncope. The four features of the clinical history that could best differentiate these causes of syncope were age, sex, the duration of recovery symptoms and the presence of fatigue following syncope. Patients with syncope due to ventricular tachycardia or atrioventricular block were older, more likely to be male, less likely to experience fatigue following syncope and had a shorter duration of recovery symptoms following syncope. The main limitation of the study by Calkins et al. [3] is that the historical features of only three causes of syncope were evaluated and, therefore, it is not possible to define precisely the sensitivity, specificity and predictive value of the historical features. To this purpose we are carrying out a multicentric trial involving 300 consecutive patients referred for evaluation of syncope.

References

1. Wayne HH (1961) Syncope. Physiological considerations and an analysis of the clinical characteristics in 510 patients. Am J Med 30:418-438
2. Martin GJ, Adams SL, Martin HG et al (1984) Prospective evaluation of syncope. Ann Emerg Med 13:499-504
3. Calkins H, Shyr Y, Frumin H, Schork A, Morady F (1995) The value of clinical history in the differentiation of syncope due to ventricular tachycardia, atrioventricular block and neurocardiogenic syncope. Am J Med 98:365-373

Adenosine-Sensitive Syncope: Does it Really Exist?

C. Menozzi[1], M. Brignole[2], G. Gaggioli[2], A. Del Rosso[3], S. Costa[2], A. Bartoletti[2], N. Bottoni[1] and G. Lolli[1]

Adenosine-sensitive syncope has recently been identified as a cause of syncope in some patients affected by unexplained syncope who have an abnormal response to adenosine triphosphate (ATP) test and a negative work-up after complete conventional investigations [1]. Some authors [2-4] have hypothesized that adenosine could be an important modulator in triggering a vasovagal response in susceptible patients. Indeed, the injection of a bolus of adenosine during head-up tilt testing (HUT) has been seen to provoke a vasovagal response in susceptible patients with syncope with a positivity rate comparable to that of isoproterenol [2, 3]. The ATP test has been suggested as a useful tool to identify a subgroup of patients at high risk of severe cardioinhibitory responses of vagal origin [4]. In a recent study [5], we evaluated the possible relationship between adenosine-sensitive syncope and tilt-induced vasovagal syncope. For this purpose, we performed both the ATP and HUT tests in a group of consecutive patients with syncope of uncertain origin, and compared the clinical characteristics of the patients who had a positive response to one or both tests.

ATP Test

ATP (Striadyne, Wyeth, France), 20 mg, was dissolved in 10 cc of saline solution and injected very rapidly (< 3 s) into a suitable antecubital vein with the patient in the supine position. Continuous recordings of electrocardiographic tracing and non-invasive beat-to-beat arterial blood pressure by means of the Finapres method [6, 7] were performed during, and for 2 min after, drug administration. It is well documented in the literature [2, 4, 8-10] that the maximum bradycardic effect following a bolus of ATP usually occurs after 10–20 s (which is the latency time necessary for the drug to reach the heart); this persists for up to 20 s and is followed by sinus tachycardia for up to 2 min; hypotension occurs during and immediately after the bradycardic phase and is sometimes followed by moderate hypertension. Facial flushing, shortness of breath and chest pressure are fre-

[1]Sezione di Aritmologia, Ospedale S. Maria Nuova, Reggio Emilia, Italy; [2]Sezione di Aritmologia, Ospedali Riuniti, Lavagna, Italy; [3]Reparto di Cardiologia, Ospedale S. Pietro Igneo, Fucecchio, Italy

quent side effects, but, owing to the rapid de-activation of the drugs, these are transient and well tolerated by the patient. Positive response to the ATP test was defined as the induction of a complete AV block with a ventricular pause (maximum RR interval) ≥ 6000 ms, which corresponds to the upper 95th percentile of the distribution of values of a control population of subjects without syncope [1].

HUT Test

Patients underwent the standardized protocol of upright tilt testing with nitroglycerin challenge, which is currently used in our department for the diagnosis of unexplained syncope [11-13]. This consisted of 60-degree tilt for 45 min or until syncope occurred. If the test did not induce syncope, 0.4 mg oral spray nitroglycerin was administered while the patient remained in the same tilted position, and the test was continued for a further 20 min. During the test, the beat-to-beat finger arterial pressure was monitored continuously by the Finapres method. Positive response was defined as induction of syncope in the presence of bradycardia, hypotension or both. Cardioinhibitory response was defined as the induction of a pause ≥ 3 s.

Findings

Population

The recruitment process is summarized in Fig. 1. Of a total of 175 patients undergoing ATP and HUT tests, 121 (69%) had a positive response to one or both tests; the final diagnosis remained unestablished in the remaining 54 patients (31%), who had a negative response to both tests. HUT alone was positive in 77 patients, ATP alone was positive in 18 patients and both tests were positive in 26 patients

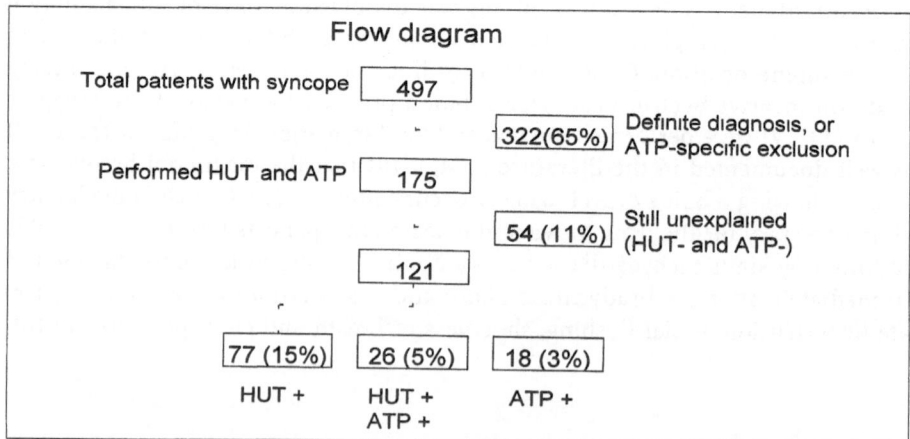

Fig. 1. Diagnostic flow diagram of the patients referred for investigation of syncope. ATP, adenosine triphosphate test; HUT, head-up tilt test

(Fig. 2). Thus, a positive response to the HUT test was about 4 times more frequent than a positive response to the ATP test. An overlap was present in 21% of patients. Owing to the different prevalence of the two forms of syncope, about one-fourth of the patients with tilt-induced syncope also had an adenosine-sensitive syncope, whereas more than half of the patients with adenosine-sensitive syncope also had a tilt-induced syncope.

Clinical Features

The clinical characteristics of these three groups of patients were compared (Table 1). Compared with the patients with isolated positive HUT test, those with

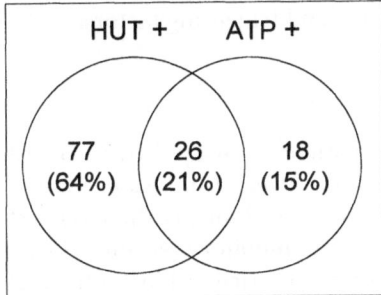

Fig. 2. Distribution of the patients with a positive response to HUT or ATP or both tests

Table 1. Clinical characteristics of the 3 groups of patients with syncope

	HUT+ n = 77	HUT+ ATP+ n = 26	p^a	ATP+ n = 18	p^b
Age (years)	45 ± 20	58 ± 18	0.004	68 ± 10	0.000^c
Women (%)	39 (51%)	19 (73%)	0.03	11 (61%)	ns
Associated diseases:					
- systemic hypertension	4 (5%)	4 (15%)	ns	4 (22%)	0.04
- structural heart diseases	10 (13%)	8 (31%)	0.004	5 (28%)	ns
- ECG abnormalities	7 (9%)	5 (19%)	ns	5 (28%)	0.05
History of syncopal episodes:					
- total number (median)	6 ± 13 (3)	6 ± 7 (4)	ns	3 ± 2 (2)	0.04^c
- duration, mounths (median)	77 ± 107 (36)	120 ± 67 (42)	ns	13 ± 16 (4)	0.003^c
- situational symptoms	14 (18%)	4 (15%)	ns	2 (11%)	ns
- vasovagal symptoms	23 (30%)	5 (19%)	ns	0 (0%)	0.004
- triggering factors	22 (29%)	2 (8%)	0.02	0 (0%)	0.005
- ≥ 1 of the above findings	49 (64%)	8 (31%)	0.004	2 (11%)	0.000
- warnings	55 (71%)	18 (69%)	ns	8 (44%)	0.03
- pre-syncopal episodes	29 (38%)	12 (46%)	ns	4 (22%)	ns
- secondary trauma	32 (42%)	12 (46%)	ns	8 (44%)	ns
- ≥ 1 episode supine/sitting	19 (25%)	9 (35%)	ns	1 (6%)	ns (0.06)^c
- ≥ 1 episode standing	66 (86%)	22 (85%)	ns	17 (94%)	ns

ATP, adenosine triphosphate test; HUT, head up tilt test; ns, not significant
[a] Statistical comparison between HUT+ group and HUT+/ATP+ group
[b] Statistical comparison between HUT+ group and ATP+ group
[c] Statistical comparison between ATP+ group and HUT+/ATP+ group: $p < 0.05$

isolated positive ATP test were older, had a higher prevalence of associated diseases and different clinical characteristics of syncopal episodes. In particular, the patients with isolated positive ATP test had a very much shorter duration and fewer syncopal episodes, a lower prevalence of situational or vasovagal episodes, and a lower prevalence of triggering episodes; the onset of syncopal episodes was more often abrupt, without warning and usually occurred in the standing position. The patients in whom both tests were positive had roughly intermediate characteristics. They differed from those with isolated positive HUT as regards age, sex, associated diseases and lower prevalence of vasovagal, situational and triggering factors. On the other hand, they also differed from those with isolated positive ATP test as regards age, number and duration of syncopal episodes and body position at the time of syncope occurrence; moreover, there was a trend toward a higher prevalence of vasovagal, situational and triggering factors.

The Mechanism of Positive Tests

Atrioventricular block was present in 43 out of 44 patients with a positive ATP test; only one patient had a positive response due to sinus arrest. A mixed or vasodepressor response was the most common response observed during the HUT test, occurring in 74 cases. Among the 29 cases with a cardioinhibitory response during HUT, sinus arrest was more often observed than atrioventricular block (Table 2). Among the patients with positive ATP test, a positive or negative response to HUT test did not influence the type of response to the ATP. Similarly, among the patients with positive HUT response, a positive or negative response to ATP did not influence the response to the HUT. Thus, the cardiac effects of the ATP and HUT tests were quite different and independent of one another, the atrioventricular node being more susceptible to ATP and the sinus node more susceptible to HUT. This is in agreement with the notion that the sites of action are different: membrane purinoceptors for ATP and muscarinic (acetylcholine) receptors for the vagal outflow induced by HUT [8, 9]. Nevertheless, the fact that a positive response to both HUT and ATP was found in 21% of our cases suggests that some common physiopathological mechanism is present (Fig. 2). Indeed, although the receptors are different, the cardiac actions of adenosine are remarkably similar to those of the neurotransmitter acetylcholine. Both acetylcholine and adenosine produce the same effects and share similar receptor-effector coupling systems resulting in the activation of a specific outward potassium current (IK Ach, Ado) from the target effector cells. Moreover, a major role of acetylcholine and adenosine, in addition to their direct effect, is to function in parallel to oppose the cardiac stimulatory action of the sympathetic neurotransmitters norephinephrine and epinephrine on adenilcyclase (cAMP-dependent effect) [8, 9]. Thus, adrenergic, cholinergic and purinergic outflows are integrated at the level of the receptor-effector coupling system, and the final cardiac effect results from the sum of these excitatory and inhibitory effects. A practical consequence might be that a vasovagal syncope could be facilitated by an increased susceptibility to adenosine, and that an adenosine-sensitive syncope could be facilitated by an increased vagal outflow.

Table 2. The characteristics of the positive resposes of ATP and HUT tests in the 3 groups of patients

	HUT+ $n = 77$	HUT+ ATP+ $n = 26$	ATP+ $n = 18$	p
ATP testing				
Atrioventricular block	-	25 (96%)	18 (100%)	ns
Sinus pause	-	1 (6%)	0 (0%)	ns
Maximum RR interval (s)	-	8.2 ± 2.0	7.8 ± 2.6	ns
Systolic blood pressure drop (mmHg)	-	59 ± 22	57 ± 25	ns
HUT testing				
Atrioventricular block	4 (5%)	2 (8%)	-	ns
Sinus pause	18 (23%)	5 (19%)	-	ns
Maximum RR interval, s (median)	8.3 ± 5.5 (6.1)	14 ± 17 (6.8)	-	ns
Mixed or vasodepressor type	55 (71%)	19 (73%)	-	ns

Conclusions

ATP and HUT tests identify different populations of patients affected by syncope. Indeed, different general clinical features, different histories of the syncopal episodes and different sites of action on cardiac effectors were observed. Therefore, adenosine-sensitive syncope and tilt-induced vasovagal syncope are two distinct clinical entities, probably with different etiologies. Nevertheless, an important overlap exists between the two syndromes, which makes it likely that some common physiopathological pathways exist.

The Clinical Features of Adenosine-Sensitive Syncope

Adenosine-sensitive syncope is an uncommon form of syncope, four times less frequent than tilt-induced vasovagal syncope. Indeed, it accounted for 3% of patients referred for investigation of syncope and for 24% of the patients with a negative work-up including HUT. These figures are similar to the 3.4% and 28% rates respectively observed in our previous study [1]. Adenosine-sensitive syncope first manifests itself in old age, though it occasionally occurs in younger patients too [1]. By contrast, tilt-induced vasovagal syncope can occur at any age; typically it begins in the teenage years and there may be a long period of life without recurrences [14]. This explains why, in the present study, we found a great difference in symptom duration and in total number of syncopal episodes between the two groups of patients. There is a female predominance in adenosine-sensitive syncope [1, 4]; the reason is unclear. As the attacks nearly always occur in the standing position, and warning symptoms are frequently absent, loss of consciousness often results in falls that cause injury. The lack of historical findings of vasovagal or situational episodes and the absence of triggering factors characterize this form and clearly differentiate it from vasovagal syncope. However, advanced age, female predominance, sudden onset and frequency of trauma also differentiate adenosine-sensitive syncope from truly unexplained syncope, (ATP- and HUT-negative) [1]. The clinical presentation and the electro-cardiographic manifestation of adenosine-sensitive syncope mimic Stokes-Adams syncope complicating AV block. Indeed, the ATP was able to reproduce the spontaneous episode of paroxysmal AV block in patients who had the fortuitous electrocardiographic recording of a syncopal episode and in whom all the conventional investigations (including electrophysiological study) were unremarkable [1]. In both induced and spontaneous AV blocks, the onset of block was abrupt, and was not preceeded by other rhythm disturbances or sinus bradyarrhythmias. By contrast, when a spontaneous cardioinhibitory neurally mediated syncope was recorded, the pause was caused by either sinus arrest or AV block (as during HUT) and it was usually preceded by other bradyarrhythmias [12].

Other than in patients affected by adenosine-sensitive syncope alone, the ATP test is expected to be frequently positive in patients with vasovagal syncope, and ATP has been shown to be able to trigger a vasovagal reaction in susceptible patients [2, 3]. Indeed, about one-fourth of the patients with tilt-induced syncope also had an adenosine-sensitive syncope, and the ATP test was positive in 15% of the patients with a history of syncope suggestive of a neurally mediated mechanism. The clinical features of the patients who had positive results in both HUT and ATP tests differed both from the patients with tilt-induced syncope alone and from those with adenosine-sensitive syncope alone (Table 1); thus, these patients had clinical features that were atypical both of the vasovagal syndrome and the adenosine-induced syncope. This fact suggests that, in this particular population, more complex, multiple mechanisms are responsible for syncope and that syncopal attacks can be caused alternatively by a vasovagal mechanism or an adenosine-mediated mechanism or both.

References

1. Brignole M, Gaggioli G, Menozzi C, Gianfranchi L, Bartoletti A, Bottoni N, Lolli G, Oddone D, Del Rosso A, Pellinghelli G (1997) Adenosine-induced atrioventricular block in patients with unexplained syncope. The diagnostic value of ATP testing. Circulation 96:3921-3927
2. Shen WK, Hammill S, Munger T, Stanton M, Packer D, Osborn M, Wood D, Bailey K, Low P, Gersh B (1996) Adenosine: potential modulator for vasovagal syncope. J Am Coll Cardiol 28:146-154
3. Mittal S, Stein K, Markowitz S, Lerman B (1997) Can adenosine replace isoproterenol during tilt testing? Circulation 96:1-221 (abstr)
4. Flammang D, Church T, Waynberger M, Chassing A, Antiel M (1997) Can adenosine 5' triphosphate be used to select treatment in severe vasovagal syndrome? Circulation 96:1201-1208
5. Brignole M, Gaggioli G, Menozzi C, Del Rosso A, Costa S, Bartoletti A, Bottoni N, Lolli G (1999) The different clinical features of adenosine-sensitive syncope and tilt-induced vasovagal syncope (in press)
6. Friedman DB, Jensen FB, Matzen S, Secher NH (1990) Non-invasive blood pressure

monitoring during head-up tilt test using the Penaz principle. Acta Anaesthesiol Scand 34:519-522

7. Petersen MEV, Williams TR, Sutton R (1995) A comparison of non-invasive continuous finger blood pressure measurements (Finapres) with intra-arterial pressure during prolonged head-up tilt. Eur Heart J 16:1647-1654

8. Lerman B, Belardinelli L (1991) Cardiac electrophysiology of adenosine. Basic and clinical concepts. Circulation 83:1499-1508

9. Belardinelli L, Linden J, Berne RM (1989) The cardiac effects of adenosine. Prog Cardiovasc Dis 22:73-97

10. Favale S, Di Biase M, Rizzo U, Belardinelli L, Rizzon P (1985) Effect of adenosine and adenosine 5'-triphosphate on atrioventricular conduction in patients. J Am Coll Cardiol 5:1212-1219

11. Brignole M, Menozzi C, Gianfranchi L, Oddone D, Lolli G, Bertulla A (1991) Carotid sinus massage, eye-ball compression test and head-up tilt test in patients with syncope of uncertain origin and in healthy control subjects. Am Heart J 122:1644-1651

12. Brignole M, Menozzi C, Bottoni N, Gianfranchi L, Lolli G, Oddone D, Gaggioli G (1995) Mechanisms of syncope caused by transient bradycardia and the diagnostic value of electrophysiologic testing and cardiovascular reflexivity maneuvers. Am J Cardiol 76:273-278

13. Raviele A, Menozzi C, Brignole M, Gasparini G, Alboni P, Musso G, Lolli G, Oddone D, Dinelli M, Mureddu R (1995) Value of head-up tilt testing potentiated with sublingual nitroglycerin to assess the origin of unexplained syncope. Am J Cardiol 76:267-272

14. Sutton R (1996) Vasovagal syncope: clinical features, epidemiology, and natural history. In: Blanc JJ, Benditt D, Sutton R (eds) Neurally mediated syncope: pathophysiology, investigations, and treatment. Futura, Armonk, NY, pp 71-76

Idiopathic Postural Orthostatic Tachycardia: A Variant of Neurocardiogenic Syncope?

B.P. Grubb

"All beginnings are hard..."
The Talmud

Transient episodes of neurocardiogenically-mediated hypotension and bradycardia have become a well-recognized cause of recurrent syncope and near-syncope [1]. The emergence of tilt table testing as a reliable method for provoking these periods of autonomic decompensation not only provided a useful diagnostic tool but also allowed for a much better understanding of the pathophysiology of these disorders. In the course of investigations, it became apparent that these episodic alterations in autonomic tone could result in varying degrees of systemic hypotension that, while not sufficiently large to cause complete loss of consciousness, were nevertheless great enough to cause symptoms such as near-syncope, lightheadedness, vertigo, and transient ischemic attacks. At the same time, we and other groups identified a large subgroup of patients who have a less severe form of orthostatic intolerance that is characterized by postural tachycardia, exercise intolerance, disabling fatigue, lightheadedness, dizziness, and blurred vision [2]. Detailed investigations of these patients showed that the histories, physical findings, and responses to postural change and head-up tilt were essentially similar. This disorder has become generally known as the postural orthostatic tachycardia syndrome. The present paper will review the clinical characteristics, their responses during head-upright tilt table testing, and the various therapies that can benefit these patients.

Historical Aspects

Starting in the nineteenth century, physicians reported patients suffering from a condition characterized by fatigue and poor exercise tolerance that occurred without an obvious cause (such as prolonged bed rest). Some of the first reports

Division of Cardiology, Department of Medicine, The Medical College of Ohio, Toledo, Ohio, USA

were from the American Civil War by DaCosta, who used the terms "irritable heart syndrome" and "soldier's heart" to describe the condition [3]. At the time of the First World War there were a number of reports of conditions that were labeled as "neurocirculatory asthenia" or "vasoregulatory asthenia", reflecting the idea that these conditions were due to a functional cardiac phenomenon caused by insufficient neural regulation of peripheral blood flow [4]. In 1944 MacLean et al. reported on a group of patients with orthostatic tachycardia that was associated with only a mild drop in blood pressure, who complained of palpitations, lightheadedness, weakness, and exercise intolerance [5]. They hypothesized that a possible mechanism for these problems might be a reduction in venous return to the heart from a disturbance at the capillary venous level.

In the 1960s, Frolich et al. reported two patients who developed a postural tachycardia (with an increase of more than 40 beats/min on standing without hypotension) who experienced extreme postural anxiety, near-syncope, and dizziness [6]. Each patient also displayed an exaggerated heart rate response to isoproterenol and showed symptomatic improvement on receving β-blockers. Much later, in 1982, Rosen and Cryer used the term "postural tachycardia syndrome" to describe a patient who exhibited a greater than 44 beat/min increase in heart rate upon standing (without orthostatic hypotension) associated with complaints of fatigue, exercise intolerance, and palpitations [7]. Shortly thereafter, Fouad et al. described patients with orthostatic intolerance who demonstrated postural tachycardia and only a slight degree of hypotension, referring to the condition as "idiopathic hypovolemia" [8]. Streeten et al. then reported on a similar group of patients who demonstrated orthostatic tachycardia without hypotension [9]. By using gamma camera counting of technetium Tc 99m sodium pertechnetate-labeled erythrocytes over the calf areas of patients while supine and upright they showed evidence of extensive gravity-dependent venous pooling in the lower extremities. Somewhat later, Streeten then published a report of four similar patients who additionally demonstrated a hypersensitivity to noradrenalin infusion [10].

Hoeldtke et al. have described a total of 13 patients with near-syncope, exercise intolerance, fatigue, and cognitive impairment who demonstrated evidence of postural tachycardia [11, 12]. Schondorf and Low, and Low et al. have made a comprehensive analysis of 16 patients who suffered from profound fatigue, an inability to exercise, near-syncope, dizziness, and bowel hypomotility [13, 14]. Many of these patients had been labeled as having psychologic problems such as chronic anxiety or panic attacks. During head-upright tilt table testing these patients had markedly abnormal cardiovascular responses, with heart rates that would frequently climb to as high as 120-170 beats/min, often within the first 2 min of upright tilt. While some of these patients exhibited a mild reduction in blood pressure, most became hypertensive (with up to a 50 mmHg increase in diastolic blood pressure).

These investigators frequently employed the term "postural orthostatic tachycardia syndrome" to describe this condition and postulated that it represented an attenuated form of dysautonomia. Khurana described a group of eight patients who had virtually identical symptoms and tilt responses who also had abnormal sudomotor function [15]. Our group reported on 28 patients who presented with extreme fatigue, lightheadedness, orthostatic tachycardia, exercise intolerance, cognitive impairment, and near-syncope [2]. During head-upright tilt table testing each patient demonstrated an increase in heart rate of at least 30 beats/min (which in each case exceeded 120 beats/min) within the first 10 min of the test. There was a mild fall in systolic blood pressure of 20 mmHg during tilt (although no patient's pressure fell below 85-90 mmHg).

Definitions

Taken together, these observations begin to present a fairly consistent picture of this disorder. While a number of different terms have been coined to describe this phenomenon, we prefer postural orthostatic tachycardia syndrome (or POTS) because it is a fairly descriptive term and easy to remember. These patients manifest an orthostatic intolerance in that they develop symptoms while standing that are relieved by recumbency. POTS patients frequently present with complaints of fatigue, exercise intolerance, lightheadedness, nausea, loss of concentration and memory, tremulousness, and recurrent near-syncope (and sometimes syncope). These patients may frequently be misdiagnosed as having panic attacks or chronic anxiety. Relatively simple activities such as modest exercise, showering (or sometimes even eating), may intensify these symptoms and profoundly limit even the most basic activities of daily life. Because severe autonomic failure is not present, the physical exam is often unrevealing and patients are told that "nothing is wrong".

We define POTS as the development of orthostatic symptoms that are associated with at least a 30 beat/min increase in heart rate or a heart rate of at least 120 beats/min that occurs within the first 10 min of standing or upright tilt. With respect to the age range of patients with POTS (10-60 years), this increase in heart rate exceeds the 99th percentile for control subjects aged 10-83 years [16]. We have tended to focus on heart rate mainly because it is the earliest, most consistent, and easiest-to-measure index of orthostatic intolerance. The disadvantage of focusing on the postural tachycardia is that it does not take into account the nonorthostatic symptoms such as the sudden episodes of autonomic decompensation manifested by marked fluctuations in blood pressure, sinus tachycardia, fatigue, and vasomotor symptoms that many patients experience.

Clinical Features

The majority of POTS patients are within the age range 15-50 years (although we have seen patients as young as 10 and as old as 70 years). The average duration of symptoms prior to presentation seems to be about 1 year. The most common presenting symptoms are palpitations, fatigue, lightheadedness, exercise intolerance, tremulousness, blurring of vision (or tunnel vision), and weakness of the lower extremities. Less frequent complaints include nausea, chest wall pain, hyperventilation, anxiety, cognitive impairment, gastric dysmotility, and headaches. The majority of patient appear to be women, with some studies reporting that the female:male ratio is 5:1 (there may be some degree of referral bias in that women are often more likely to seek medical attention) [17].

In every report of this disorder roughly half of all patients describe having suffered an antecedent febrile illness (presumed to be viral in nature). Based on these observations, several investigators have suggested that in some individuals there may be an immune-mediated pathogenesis [2, 17]. One interesting observation is the cyclic nature of some patients' symptoms. Many women will experience a marked exacerbation of their complaints just prior to their menstrual periods. Some patients will experience periods of intense symptoms that may last for days followed by periods of marked improvement. One of the more interesting complaints will be of episodes of intense symptoms at rest, that are associated with a mild sinus tachycardia (rates ranging from 110 to 130 beats/min) as well as intense fatigue. Some patients report periods of intense fluid loss despite heavy intake. On occasion these patients may develop a hypotension so severe that they require intravenous fluids for stabilization.

Etiology

The etiology of POTS is unclear and most likely represents a heterogenous group of disorders with similar clinical characteristics [15]. The largest group of patients appear to have a mild idiopathic peripheral autonomic neuropathy, in which an inability to increase peripheral vascular resistance during upright posture results in an excessive compensatory postural tachycardia. Venous pooling appears to be present that results in a reduction in ventricular preload, which in turn leads to baroreceptor unloading while upright with a resultant increase in sympathetic outflow [9, 10]. Furlan et al. looked at mean sympathetic nerve activity using microneurography in these patients, as well as heart rate variability indices, and found that they exhibit an overall enhancement of noradrenergic tone at rest and by a postganglionic sympathetic response to standing (with compensatory cardiac sympathetic over-activity) [18]. Interestingly, many of these patients will be noted to develop a bluish discoloration of the lower extremities on prolonged standing [2, 9].

A second group of patients may have a component of β-receptor supersensitivity [17]. Many of these patients complain of extreme tremulousness and anxiety in addition to palpitations and tachycardia while standing. They also demonstrate exaggerated responses to low-dose isoproterenol infusions while supine. It is unclear whether this supersensitivity is primary in nature or due to a secondary denervation supersensitivity.

The term "secondary POTS" is applied in those cases where patients have a known autonomic disorder with preserved cardiac innervation despite peripher-

al autonomic denervation. This can be due to diseases such as diabetes, amyloido-
sis, or Sjögren's syndrome. In occasional patients it may be the presenting sign of
pure autonomic failure or multiple systems atrophy [19].

Evaluation and Management

The first step is a detailed history and physical examination that includes a careful
neurologic examination. Patients should also be evaluated for recognizable causes
of orthostatic intolerance such as anemia, dehydration, or any chronic debilitating
illness. Any drug that the patient may be taking that could cause or aggravate the
problem (such as vasodilators, tricyclic antidepressants, monoamine oxidase
inhibitors, or alcohol) should be identified. Heart rate and blood pressure should
be measured in the supine, sitting, and standing positions. If cardiac causes are
suspected, these should be appropriately evaluated. Sinus tachycardia that is
abrupt in onset and termination unrelated to posture suggests possible sinus
node re-entry and may require electrophysiologic studies.

Tilt table testing is often useful as a standardized measure of response to postural change [1]. Patients are placed on a standard tilt table and, after measurements of baseline blood pressure and heart rate, they are inclined to a 70° head-
up angle. Blood pressure and heart rate measurements are then made every 1-2
min. A heart rate increase greater than 30 beats/min or a rate exceeding 120
beats/min in the first 10 min of passive tilt are considered diagnostic criteria. In
selected patients we will also measure the heart rate response to an intravenous
infusion of 1 µg/min of isoproterenol. Heart rate increases greater than 30
beats/min are considered abnormal. If some POTS patients are kept upright long
enough, they may exhibit a neurocardiogenic-like decompensation with hypotension and syncope.

Therapy begins with first educating the patient as to the nature of the disorder. Any drug that could be causing or aggravating the problem should be
stopped if possible. Next we try to increase salt and fluid intake. Patients are
encouraged to sleep with the head of their beds elevated. Mild aerobic exercise is
strongly encouraged, with an eventual goal of performing 20 min activity three
times a week. Resistance training to build up the lower extremities can be particularly helpful. Elastic support hose are useful in some patients. The hose should
be waist high and provide 30 mmHg ankle counterpressure. Pharmacologic therapy must be tailored to meet the needs of each individual patient, and it should
be remembered that those needs will change over time [1, 20]. Fludrocortisone is
useful in many patients, with the usual dose around 0.2 mg/day. Midodrine is
quite useful due to its peripheral vasoconstrictive action, and is usually given in
5-to 10-mg doses three times a day. Patients with the β-receptor hypersensitivity
form may respond to either β-blocking agents or to clonidine. In patients refractory to other forms of therapy, erythropoietin may be useful. Some groups have
reported that phenobarbital may be useful in selected patients [18]. We have
found the selective serotonin reuptake inhibitors useful in many patients, the

most effective one being venlafaxine [21]. Frequently patients will require a combination of various therapies to be effective. A comprehensive review of potential treatments is beyond the scope of this review and more in-depth discussions of therapy can be found elsewhere [21].

Conclusions

POTS is a potentially recognizable and treatable disorder in which patients present with a marked orthostatic intolerance manifested by postural tachycardia, palpitations, weakness, fatigue, and exercise intolerance. During passive upright tilt these patients demonstrate a heart rate increase of at least 30 beats/min or a peak rate of at least 120 beats/min within the first 10 min, reproducing the patients' symptoms. Some patients may exhibit an exaggerated response to isoproterenol. Therapies directed at correcting autonomic balance can often relieve the severity of the symptoms. Greater efforts will be necessary to better understand this syndrome and provide therapies that will help this group of highly symptomatic patients return to normal life. Continuing research will help provide greater insight into this and other autonomic disturbances associated with chronic orthostatic intolerance [22].

Acknowledgments. The author gratefully acknowledges the continued support of Barbara Straus, MD, without whom little could be accomplished.

References

1. Grubb BP (1998) Neurocardiogenic syncope. In: Grubb BP, Olshansy B (eds) Syncope: mechanisms and management. Futura, Armonk, NY, pp 73-106
2. Grubb BP, Kosinski D, Boehm K, Kip K (1997) The postural orthostatic tachycardia syndrome: a neurocardiogenic variant identified during tilt table testing. Pacing Clin Electrophysiol 20(I):2205-2212
3. DaCosta JM (1871) An irritable heart. Am J Med Sci 27:145-163
4. Holmgren A et al (1957) Low physical work capacity in suspected heart cases due to inadequate adjustment of peripheral blood flow (vasoregulatory asthenia). Acta Med Scand 158:413-415
5. MacLean AR, Allen EV, Magath TB (1944) Orthostatic tachycardia and orthostatic hypotension: defect in the return of venous blood to the heart. Am Heart J 27:145-163
6. Frohlich ED, Dustan HP, Page IH (1966) Hyperdynamic beta adrenergic circulatory state. Arch Intern Med 117:614-619
7. Rosen SG, Cryer PE (1982) Postural tachycardia syndrome. Am J Med 72:847-850
8. Fouad FM, Tadena-Thome L, Braro EL et al (1986) Idiopathic hypovolemia. Ann Intern Med 104:298-303
9. Streeten DHP, Anderson GH Jr, Richardson R et al (1988) Abnormal orthostatic changes in blood pressure and heart rate in subjects with intact sympathetic nervous system function: evidence for excessive venous pooling. J Lab Clin Med 111:326-335

10. Streeten DHP (1990) Pathogenesis of hyperadrenergic orthostatic hypotension: evidence of disordered venous innervation exclusively in the lower limbs. J Clin Invest 86:1582-1588

11. Hoeldtke RD, Dworkin GE, Gaspar SR et al (1989) Sympathotonic orthostatic hypotension: a report of four cases. Neurology 39:34-40

12. Hoeldtke RD, Davis KM (1991) The orthostatic tachycardia syndrome: evaluation of autonomic function and treatment with octreotide and ergot alkaloids. J Clin Endocrinol Metab 73:132-139

13. Schondorf R, Low P (1993) Idiopathic postural orthostatic tachycardia syndrome: an attenuated form of acute pandysautonomia? Neurology 43:132-137

14. Low P, Opfer-Gehrking T, Textor S et al (1995) Postural tachycardia syndrome. Neurology 45:519-525

15. Khurana RK (1995) Orthostatic intolerance and orthostatic tachycardia: a heterogenous disorder. Clin Auton Res 5:12-18

16. Streeten DHP (1987) Orthostatic disorders of the circulation: mechanisms, manifestations, and treatment. Plenum, New York

17. Schondorf R, Low P (1993) Idiopathic postural tachycardia syndromes. In: Low P (ed) Clinical autonomic disorders. Little Brown, Boston, pp 641-652

18. Furlan R, Jacob G, Snell M et al (1998) Chronic orthostatic intolerance: a disorder with discordant cardiac and vascular sympathetic control. Circulation 98:2154-2159

19. Bannister R, Mathias CJ (1992) Clinical features and investigation of the primary autonomic failure syndromes. In: Bannister R, Mathias CJ (eds) Autonomic failure: a textbook of clinical disorders of the autonomic nervous system. Oxford Medical, Oxford, pp 531-547

20. Grubb BP (1998) Dysautonomic syncope. In: Grubb BP, Olshansky B (eds) Syncope: mechanisms and management. Futura Press, Armonk, NY, pp 107-126

21. Grubb BP, Karas BJ (1998) The potential role of serotonin in the pathogenesis of neurocardiogenic syncope and related autonomic disturbances. J Intervent Cardiac Electrophysiol 2:325-332

22. Narkiewicz K, Somers V (1998) Chronic orthostatic intolerance: part of a spectrum of dysfunction in orthostatic cardiovascular homeostasis? Circulation 98:2105-2107

Syncope of Unknown Origin After Electrophysiologic Study and Head-Up Tilt Test: How Useful is an Implantable Loop Recorder?

A. Moya

Syncope is a frequent disorder that can be due to very different etiologies. The etiologic diagnosis of syncope is a complex task. In most of the series in the literature, in 40%-60% [1, 2] of patients the etiology of syncope remains unknown. In most patients, the anamnesis, physical examination and baseline ECG are the most helpful tools in diagnosing the etiology of syncope [1]. In patients in whom the etiology of syncope remains unknown after the initial clinical evaluation, many different additional tests can be performed.

Twenty-four-hour ECG ambulatory monitoring has been used by many authors but its diagnostic yield is low, ranging from 0% to 14% [3]. The most important limitation with conventional ambulatory monitoring is that the majority of the patients do not develop any symptom during the monitoring period, and in addition it is not infrequent to record asymptomatic arrhythmias, either bradyarrhythmias or episodes of non-sustained ventricular tachycardias, that are difficult to interpret.

The electrophysiological study (EPS) has been used to study the conduction properties, mainly of the His-Purkinje system, and the inducibility of ventricular arrhythmias [4]. EPS is mostly useful in patients with organic heart disease or intraventricular conduction defects; its diagnostic contribution in patients with normal ECG and no organic heart disease is low. The head-up tilt test has been used extensively during recent years to recognize vasovagal mechanisms in patients with syncope of unknown origin [5, 6].

Although there are data that suggest that an abnormal finding in EPS or a positive response to the head-up tilt test have a high diagnostic value, it must be considered that EPS and head-up tilt test are provocative tests that can show abnormalities which can be the cause of syncope but they give no definite information about the etiologic correlation between those findings and the syncope. In addition some patients have more than one abnormal finding on these tests, and the diagnostic value of those findings is a matter of clinical judgement.

In 1990 Linzer et al. [7] used a prolonged external ambulatory "loop-recorder" ECG. This device was connected to the patient with external electrodes, similar to those used in conventional ambulatory monitoring. The device could be worn by

Unitat d'Aritmies, Hospital General Vall d'Hebron, Barcelona, Spain

the patient for several weeks, provided that the batteries were replaced every 5-7 days and the electrodes were changed every 2-3 days. When the device was activated by the patient, the system stored the ECG recordings obtained during the previous 5 min and the 1 min after activation. Although this system improved the diagnostic yield of conventional 24- to 48-h Holter monitoring, it had some limitations, mainly related to the fact that the time that the system could be worn was limited to several weeks and to the fact that the duration of the storage capabilities was limited to 5 min. Also the possibility of malfunction of the system was relatively high due to the fact that the system was connected by external electrodes, which were not always connected correctly during the syncopal episode. In this serie, the external loop recorder was used in 57 patients with recurrent syncope of unknown origin. With a follow-up period of 4 weeks, 32 patients (58%) had syncopal events. Of those, in 18 (56%) the recording during the episode was not available, mainly due to problems with the electrode contact or because the patients had the device disconnected or not in use during the syncopal episode. In the remaining 14 patients (24%), the loop recorder showed normal sinus rhythm in seven and some type of arrhythmia in the other seven: ventricular tachycardia in one, supraventricular tachycardia in one, A-V block in two, and bradyarryhthmia that was considered to be neuromediated in three.

During recent years an insertable loop recorder (ILR) system has been developed. This system has some advantages over the external loop recorder: it has an expected life of approximately 14 months; as it is implanted subcutaneously it can be worn continuously and there is not the possibility of contact problems; and the duration of the stored ECG for each episode is longer than with external loop recorder, increasing the possibility of recording arrhythmias during prolonged episodes. The device is small and light (8 cc, 84 x 45 x 16 mm, 40 g), and it can be implanted in subpectoral or submmamary region without additional electrodes. The ECG is recorded between the two tips of the device. The system can be programmed in different modes. In the normal mode the device has a capability of storing 21 min. It can be programmed for only one episode, in which case it stores 20 min pre-event and 1 min after the event, or it can be programmed for three consecutive episodes, storing 6 min pre- event and 1 min afterwards for each episode. It can be programmed in the so-called compressed mode, doubling the time of storing ECG for each episode with less definition in the tracings.

Recently Krahn et al. [8] have published data from 81 patients with syncope of unknown origin in which an ILR was implanted. With a follow-up of 10 ± 4 months, 58 patients (68%) developed syncopal episodes. Of those, in 8 (15%) the recordings of the electrogram during syncopal episode were not available. In the remaining 50 patients (58%) the rhythm during the event was recorded: 29 were in sinus rhythm, in 3 there was supraventricular tachycardia, and in 18 there was some type of "bradyarrhythmia", which was considered to be of neuromediated origin in 7 cases. There were some complications related with the device in four patients, requiring explantation in only one patient.

Another study in progress is the ISSUE [International (Italian and Spanish) Study of Syncope of Unknown Origin] study. The objective of this study is to analyze the diagnostic yield or ILR in different groups of patients with syncope of unknown origin, according to the presence or absence of structural heart disease and abnormalities in ECG. In this study patients were considered to be eligible when they had three or more syncopal episodes in the past 2 years, and when all diagnostic tests, including 24-h Holter monitoring, carotid sinus massage, echocardiogram, EPS, and head-up tilt test, were normal.

To date we have preliminary data from 45 patients with recurrent syncope without apparent structural heart disease and normal ECG (Table 1). These results, with a follow-up of 6.9±4.1 months, show that a syncopal episode was present in 11 patients (24%), a presyncope was present in 3 patients and 1 patient had an episode of angina (Table 1). Three patients (7%) were not able to activate the system during the syncopal event. Of the eight patients with syncope who activated the device during the episode, six showed bradyarrhythmia secondary to sinus arrest (Fig. 1),

Table 1. Electrocardiographic findings recorded in 15 patients from ISSUE who had events at a follow-up of 6.9 ± 4.1 months

Event	N	Finding
Syncope n = 11 (24%)	6	Sinus arrest
	2	Normal sinus rhythm
	3	Not activated
Presyncope n = 3 (7%)	2	Supraventricular tachycardia
	1	Normal sinus rhythm
Angina n = 1 (2%)	1	ST changes → VF

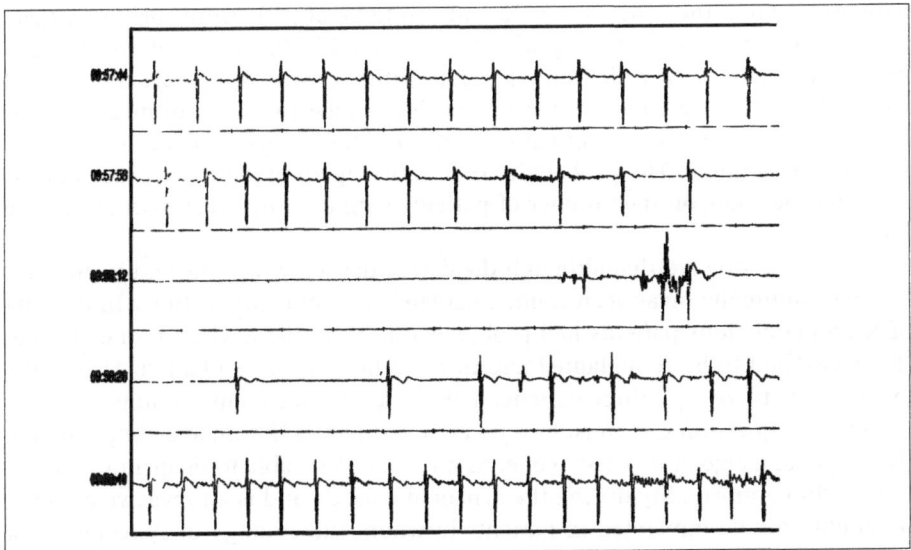

Fig. 1. Tracings obtained from a patient who experienced a syncopal episode. There is a progressive slowing of sinus rhythm, with an asystole of 12 s secondary to sinus arrest. After asystole the patient recovers rhythm with sinus tachycardia. This pattern is highly suggestive of neuromediated syncope

whereas in the remaining two the ECG showed normal sinus rhythm. Two of the three patients who experienced presyncope had paroxysmal supraventricular tachyarrhythmias. In the patient who had angina, there was an elevation of the ST segment. The patient was admitted to hospital, and immediately after admission he experienced an episode of ventricular fibrillation from which he was successfully resuscitated. It can be concluded from this study that the main finding in patients without organic heart disease and with normal ECG with recurrent syncope is sinus arrest. This type of arrhythmia, mainly when it appears in the context of progressive sinus bradycardia after a short period of sinus tachycardia, is highly suggestive of the cardioinhibitory component of a neuromediated response, suggesting that in this group of patients this is the most important etiology of syncope.

When all these results are analyzed some statements can be made. The first is that the probability of failure to activate the system correctly is higher with the external system than with ILR. This is mainly because the stability of the recordings is higher with the ILR than with the external system. When we compare the results obtained with the external recorder and with ILR, we can observe that the diagnostic yield of ILR is higher. This may be due not only to recording problems, but also to the longer life expectancy of the system and the longer recording time for each episode with the ILR.

Another consideration is that the type of findings can differ according to the population studied. In the series of Linzer and Krahn [7, 8], the proportion of patients with structural heart disease was 35% and 62% respectively. In these series the recordings suggested a neuromediated mechanism in 10%-12% of patients, whereas the syncope was considered to be of arrhythmic origin in 12%-22% of patients. In the subgroup of patients of the ISSUE study that are analyzed in this paper, study in which only patients without structural heart disease and with normal ECG were included, the recordings suggestive of neuromediated origin were found in up to 54% of patients, whereas there were no data suggestive of primary arrhythmia. The probability of identifying an arrhythmic cause of syncope thus depends on the number of patients with organic heart disease that are included.

It must be stressed that although the device has a low volume and its implantation is minimally invasive, it is not completely free of complications. In the data of Krahn et al., four patients had problems related to the device: in one of them the device had to be reimplanted and in the others it was explanted. Also in the ISSUE study there were three patients with device-related complications.

Another question that must be answered is when an ILR must be implanted in the diagnostic algorithm of syncope. As an ILR is only able to determine if there is a rhythm abnormality during the syncopal episode and is an invasive method, it should only be implanted in patients in whom the etiology of syncope is not evident after the conventional diagnostic tests for syncope have performed. Once these tests have been carried out, two main criteria should be used to select patients. In patients without organic heart disease and with normal ECG in whom the probability of a severe arrhythmia is low, the IRL should be implanted only in those with recurrent syncope that does not respond to pharmacological treatment, whereas in patients with structural heart disease in whom there is a high probability of severe and even life-threatening arrhythmia, the IRL should be implanted after only one severe syncopal episode, because the identification of the arrhythmia can be crucial in selecting treatment.

Some technological aspects that must be improved are the duration of the stored ECG and the possibility of automatic activation. In all series some patients are not able to activate the device after the episode. In addition some patients may have some asymptomatic arrhythmias that can be relevant for the diagnosis of syncope or that can have some prognostic implications, and in those cases automatic activation of the device, triggered by rhythm abnormalities would be desirable.

References

1. Kapoor WN, Karpf M, Wieand S, Peterson J, Levey GS (1983) A prospective evaluation and follow-up of patients with syncope. N Engl J Med 309:197-204
2. Solverstein MD, Singer DE, Mulley AG, Thibault GE, Barnett GO (1982) Patients with syncope admitted to medical intensive care units. JAMA 248:1185-1189
3. Gibson TC, Heitzman MR (1984) Diagnostic efficacy of 24 hours electrocardiographic monitoring for syncope. Am J Cardiol 53:1013-1017
4. Klein GJ, Gersh BJ, Yee R (1995) Electrophysiological testing. The final court of appeal for diagnosis of syncope? Circulation 92:1332-1335
5. Kenny RA, Ingram A, Bayliss J, Sutton R (1986) Head-up tilt: a useful test for investigating unexplained syncope. Lancet 1:1352-1354
6. Benditt DG, Ferguson DW, Grubb BP, Kapoor WN, Kugler J, Lerman BB et al (1996) ACC expert consensus document. Tilt table for assessing syncope. J Am Coll Cardiol 28:263-275
7. Linzer M, Pritchett ELC, Pontinen M, McCarthy E, Divine GW (1990) Incremental diagnostic yield of loop electrocardiographic recorders in unexplained syncope. Am J Cardiol 66:214-219
8. Krahn AD, Klein GJ, Yee R, Takle-Newhouse T, Norris C (1999) Use of an extended monitoring strategy in patients with problematic syncope. Circulation 99:406-410

Nitrotest Versus Isotest for Vasovagal Syncope: Do They Explore Different Mechanisms?

J. Niño[1] AND C.A. Morillo[2]

Introduction

During the last decade, head-up tilt (HUT) has become the diagnostic method of choice for the evaluation of patients with recurrent vasovagal syncope [1-7]. However, there is still little consensus regarding the ideal HUT protocol. In an attempt to improve the sensitivity and specificity of the test, several approaches have been evaluated, such as varying the degree of inclination and the duration of orthostatic stress as well as the use of provoking agents [8-22]. The sensitivity and specificity of HUT are largely related to the protocol used, and range from 25% to 87%, and from 35% to 100%, respectively [9, 14, 15, 22-24]. The lack of a standard methodology that provides a test with a high sensitivity without sacrificing specificity is largely due to our poor understanding of the mechanisms that mediate neurocardiogenic responses. A wide variety of provoking agents that include sympathomimetics (isoproterenol) and nitrovasodilators (nitroglycerin and isosorbide dinitrate) have been proposed on the basis of the hypothesized mechanisms that trigger the vasovagal response. Orthostatic stress increases venous pooling, leading to a drop in right ventricular filling pressure that causes an increase in catecholamine levels associated with augmented ventricular inotropism. In the susceptible individual, a reduced preload, particularly in the left ventricular cavity, may reflexly activate vagal-C mechanoreceptors, which, associated with impaired baroreflex counter-regulatory mechanisms, precipitate the vasovagal response.

Given the fact that provoking agents have different pharmacodynamic profiles, possibly leading to different clinical responses to HUT, we have recently evaluated the physiologic response to isoproterenol and nitrovasodilators. We hypothesize that the response induced by a specific provoking agent may help identify individual susceptibility to a specific neurocardiogenic response. This

[1]Laboratory of Autonomic Physiology; [2]Department of Cardiology and Cardiovascular Sciences, Fundación Cardiovascular del Oriente Colombiano, Instituto del Corazón, Floridablanca, Santander, Colombia

information may in turn provide a more physiologic target for the selection of therapy in patients with recurrent vasovagal syncope.

Pharmacologic Agents

Isoproterenol is a potent nonselective β-adrenergic agonist with positive chronotropic and inotropic effects, which also reduces vascular peripheral resistance, primarily at the skeletal muscle level [25]. Isoproterenol has an almost immediate effect after initiation of the infusion with prompt restoration of baseline conditions shortly after the infusion is terminated. Isoproterenol was first introduced as a provoking agent during HUT more than a decade ago [4, 5]. Theoretically, increased sympathetic activity may trigger different neurocardiogenic responses during HUT. Isoproterenol administered at high doses (3-5µg/min) increases sensitivity at the expense of reducing specificity [26], however; we have promoted the use of a single-staged low-dose isoproterenol protocol (1-2µg/min) [8].

Nitroglycerine and isosorbide dinitrate are nitrovasodilators that use nitric oxide (NO) as an active intermediate [27]. NO induces venous dilatation and during orthostatic stress increases venous capacitance, leading to reduced preload and reflex activation of sympathetic modulation. In plasma, nitroglycerine has a peak dose around 4 minutes compared with 6 min for isosorbide dinitrate. The autonomic mechanisms related with the induction of neurocardiogenic responses have not been systematically associated to the provoking agent administered. We review here some preliminary information obtained at our laboratory.

Physiologic Aspects

Several investigators have suggested that autonomic disturbances may be involved in the pathophysiology of vasovagal syncope [28-33]. Autonomic function, as assessed by time and frequency domain analysis of heart rate variability in the supine position, showed no differences between syncopal and nonsyncopal subjects [2, 31-33]. Orthostatic stress provokes increases in heart rate variability [2] and impaired vagal tone withdrawal [31-33], most likely reflecting an altered baroreflex gain in syncopal patients. Several investigators have documented a marked reduction in baroreflex sensitivity in patients with recurrent vasovagal syncope [28, 29]. Similarly, impaired vasoconstrictor responses provoked by orthostatic stress [34], as well as during exercise [35], in patients with vasovagal syncope indicate that cardiopulmonary baroreceptors may play an important role in the modulation of the vasodepressor response.

We have recently studied the relationship between sympathovagal balance and the clinical response to HUT using either low-dose isoproterenol or sublingual nitrovasodilators such as isosorbide dinitrate and nitroglycerine [36, 37]. A statistically significant difference in the low-frequency/high-frequency (LF/HF) ratio between nitrovasodilator- and isoproterenol susceptible subjects was found

(Fig. 1). Isoproterenol-susceptible subjects had a higher LF/HF ratio during resting conditions than did nitrovasodilator-susceptible individuals. During the initial orthostatic stress period, this difference was maintained, and a poor activation in LF oscillations of heart rate variability was noted in those patients who
responded to nitrovasodilators, without significant changes in the HF band oscillations (Fig. 1). These data suggest an altered sympathovagal response at rest as
well as during the initial orthostatic stress, with a decreased vagal withdrawal
response. Additionally, we documented an increased baroreflex gain, calculated
by cross-spectral analysis of heart rate and blood pressure variability, in the HF
oscillations, as well as a reduced response in baroreflex latency time in nitrovasodilator-susceptible patients compared with isoproterenol-susceptible subjects
at rest (Fig. 2). These findings suggest that the vasovagal response may be triggered via different mechanisms.

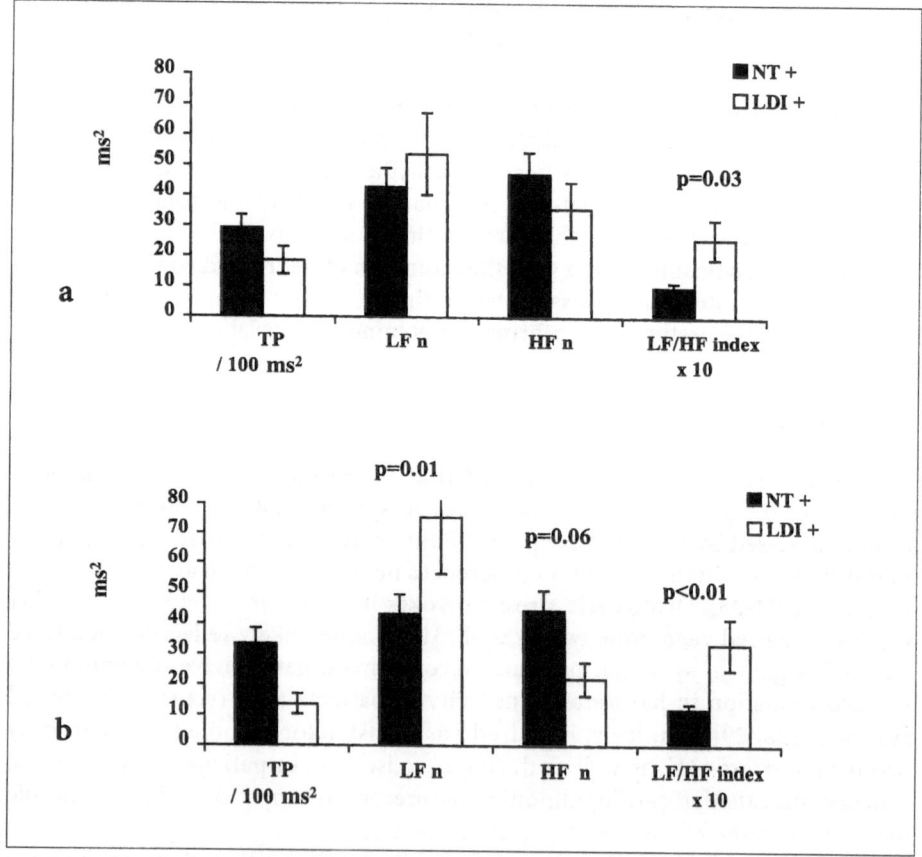

Fig. 1a,b. Heart rate variability at rest (a) and during HUT (b) in the nitrovasodilator (NT)
and isoproterenol (LDI) groups. TP, total power; LF n, normalized power in the low-frequency band; HF n, normalized power in the high frequency band; LF/HF, low-fre-
quency/high-frequency ratio

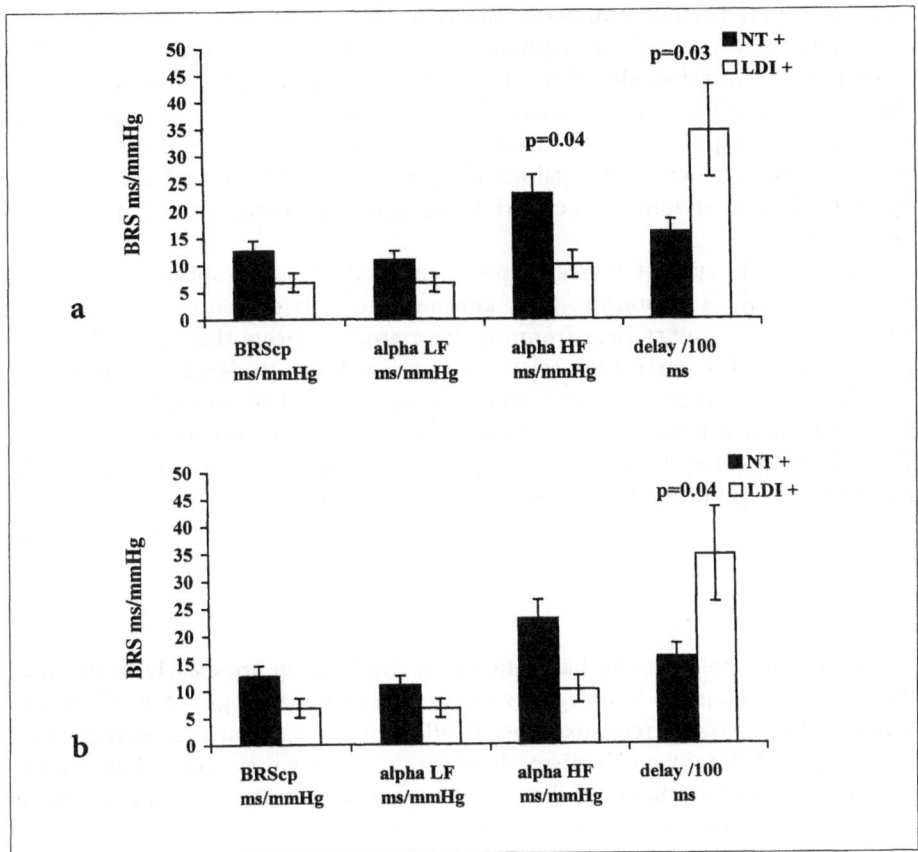

Fig. 2a,b. Baroreflex gain response at rest (a) and during HUT (b) in the nitrovasodilator (NT) and isoproterenol (LDI) groups. BRScp, baroreflex gain with coherence and phase; alpha LF, baroreflex gain in the LF oscillation band; alpha HF, baroreflex gain in the HF oscillation band

Isoproterenol increases sympathetic tone by eliciting its action directly on β-adrenergic receptors. In contrast, nitrovasodilators induce reflex sympathetic activation as a response to capacitance vessel dilatation. It is well known that blocking vagal traffic with atropine prevents bradycardia during the vasovagal response [38, 39]; however, atropine has no effects whatsoever on the vasodilatation response, which is largely dependent on sympathetic baroreflex integrity. Interestingly, there is evidence that NO-mediated vasodilation can be influenced by the baseline level of sympathetic activity, i.e., increased levels of sympathetic tone blunt NO-mediated hyperemia in the human forearm [40]. Syncopal patients who responded to isoproterenol had an increased LF/HF index, suggesting increased sympathetic activity. In contrast, patients responding to nitrovasodilators had a reduced LF/HF index and increased HF, indicative of increased vagal activity. Increased vagal activity in addition to NO release induced by nitrovasodilators may further potentiate the vasodilatory response associated with endothelial NO synthesis precipitated by increased acetylcholine release [41]. Therefore, the pharmacologic agent used to provoke vasovagal syncope during HUT triggers different mechanisms that lead to syncope: namely, isoproterenol mediates the response by increased sympathetic traffic, and nitrovasodilators primarily induce increased vagal activity, which added to NO release triggered by acetylcholine endothelial activation precipitates marked vasodilatation and syncope.

Moreover, the type of clinical response induced by HUT – specifically vasodepressor and mixed responses – may alternatively be triggered by the provoking agent used. Preliminary data from our laboratory indicate that baroreflex coupling during HUT is strongly related to susceptibility to developing mixed or vasodepresor responses. Patients who develop a mixed response have a higher baroreflex gain compared with patients who develop a vasodepressor response. These findings may have further implications for therapy by indicating the potential to target different physiologic responses to HUT.

Summary

Sympathovagal balance and baroreflex gain modulation are clearly involved in the pathophysiology of vasovagal syncope. The pharmacologic agent chosen to provoke the vasovagal response, specifically isoproterenol or nitrovasodilators, may trigger different mechanisms leading to vasovagal syncope. Appropriate knowledge of the mechanisms that lead to syncope with the different provoking agents may have further therapeutic implications.

References

1. Kenny RA, Ingram A, Bayliss J, Sutton R (1986) Head-up tilt: a useful test for investigating unexplained syncope. Lancet 1:1352-1355
2. Abi-Samsara F, Maloney JD, Fouad-Tarazi FM, Castle LW (1988) The usefulness of head-up tilt testing and hemodynamic investigations in the workup of syncope of unknown origin. Pacing Clin Electrophysiol 11:1202-1214
3. Fitzpatrick A, Sutton R (1989) Tilting towards a diagnosis in recurrent unexplained syncope. Lancet 1:658-660
4. Almquist A, Goldenberg IF, Milstein S, Chen MY, Chen X, Hansen R et al (1989) Provocation of bradycardia and hypotension by isoproterenol and upright posture in patients with unexplained syncope. N Engl J Med 320:346-351
5. Waxman MB, Yao L, Cameron DA, Wald RW, Roseman J (1989) Isoproterenol induction of vasodepressor-type reaction in vasodepressor-prone persons. Am J Cardiol 63:58-65
6. Strasberg B, Rechavia E, Sagie A, Kusniec J, Mager A, Sclarovsky S et al (1989) The head-up tilt table test in patients with syncope of unknown origin. Am Heart J 118:923-927

7. Raviele A, Gasparini G, Di Pede F, Delise P, Bonso A, Piccolo E (1990) Usefulness of head-up tilt test in evaluating patients with syncope of unknown origin and a negative electrophysiologic study. Am J Cardiol 65:1332-1337

8. Morillo CA, Klein GJ, Zandri S, Yee R (1995) Diagnostic accuracy of a low dose isoproterenol head-up tilt protocol. Am Heart J 129:901-906

9. Raviele A, Menozzi C, Brignole M, Gasparini G, Alboni P, Musso G et al (1995) Value of head-up tilt testing potentiated with sublingual nitroglycerin to assess the origin of unexplained syncope. Am J Cardiol 76:267-272

10. Cox MM, Perlman BA, Mayor MR, Silberstein TA, Levin E, Pringle L et al (1995) Acute and long-term beta-adrenergic blockade for patients with neurocardiogenic syncope. J Am Coll Cardiol 26:1293-1298

11. Benditt DG, Fergurson DW, Grubb BL, Kapoor WN, Kugler J, Lerman BB et al (1996) Tilt table testing for assessing syncope. J Am Coll Cardiol 28:263-275

12. Khurana RK, Nicholas EM (1996) Head-up tilt test: how far and how long? Clin Auton Res 6:335-341

13. Blanc J, Victor J, Mansourati J, Le Davay M, Dupuis JM, Maheu B (1996) Accuracy and mean duration of different protocols of head-up tilt testing. Am J Cardiol 77:310-313

14. Alehan D, Lenk M, Ozme S, Celiker A, Ozer S (1997) Comparison of sensitivity of tilt protocols with and without isoproterenol in children with unexplained syncope. Pacing Clin Electrophysiol 20:1769-1776

15. Aerts A, Dendale P, Strobel G, Block P (1997) Sublingual nitrates during head-up tilt testing for the diagnosis of vasovagal syncope. Am Heart J 133:504-507

16. Carlioz R, Graux P, Haye J, Letourneau T, Guyomar Y, Hubert E et al (1997) Prospective evaluation of high-dose or low-dose isoproterenol upright tilt protocol for unexplained syncope in young adults. Am Heart J 133:346-352

17. Oribe E, Caro S, Pererera R, Winter SL, Gomes JA, Kaufmann H (1997) Syncope: the diagnostic value of head-up tilt testing. Pacing Clin Electrophysiol 20:874-879

18. Grubb BP, Konsiski D (1997) Tilt table testing: concepts and limitations. Pacing Clin Electrophysiol 20:781-787

19. Benditt DG (1997) Neurally mediated syncopal syndromes: pathophysiological concepts and clinical evaluation. Pacing Clin Electrophysiol 20:572-584

20. Gagglioli G, Bottoni N, Mureddu R, Foglia-Manzillo G, Mascopño G, Bartoli P et al (1997) Effects of chronic vasodilator therapy to enhance susceptibility to vasovagal syncope during upright tilt testing. Am J Cardiol 80:1092-1094

21. Del Rosso A, Bartoli P, Brandinelli-Geri A, Bonechi F, Maioli M, Mazza F et al (1998) Shortened head-up tilt testing potentiated with sublingual nitroglycerin in patients with unexplained syncope. Am Heart J 135:564-570

22. Ammirati F, Colivicchi F, Biffi A, Magris B, Pandozi C, Santini M (1998) Head-up tilt testing potentiated with low-dose sublingual isosorbide dinitrate: a simplified time-saving approach for the evaluation of unexplained syncope. Am Heart J 135:671-676

23. Hou ZY, Yang CY, Ko CC, Lee SS, Chiang HT, Chen CY (1995) Upright postures and isoproterenol infusion for provocation of neurocardiogenic syncope: a comparison of standing and head-up tiltting. Am Heart J 130:1210-1215

24. Raviele A, Gasparini G, Di Pede F, Delise P, Bonso A, Piccolo E (1990) Usefulness of head-up tilt test in evaluating patients with syncope of unknown origin and negative electrophysiologic study. Am J Cardiol 65:1322-1327

25. Hoffman BB, Lefkowitz (1990) Catecolaminas y drogas simpatomimeticas. In: Goodman & Gilman (eds) Las bases farmacológicas de la terapéutica. Editorial Médica Panamericana, Buenos Aires, pp 196-227

26. Kapoor WN (1991) Diagnostic evaluation of syncope. Am J Med 90:91-106

27. Moncada S, Radomski MW, Palmer RM (1988) Endothelium-derived relaxin factor. Identification as nitric oxide and role in the control of vascular tone and platelet function. Biochem Pharmacol 37:2495-2501

28. Morillo CA, Eckberg DL, Ellenbogen KA, Beightol LA, Tahvanainen KUO, Kuusela TA et al (1997) Vagal and sympathetic mechanisms in patients with orthostatic vasovagal syncope. Circulation 96:2509-2513

29. Mosqueda-Garcia R, Furlan R, Fernandez-Violante R, Desai T, Snell M, Jarai Z et al (1997) Sympathetic and baroreceptor reflex function in neurally mediated syncope evoked by tilt. J Clin Invest 99:2736-2744

30. Thomson HL, Wright K, Frenneaux M (1993) Baroreflex sensitivity in patients with vasovagal syncope. Circulation 95:395-400

31. Morillo CA, Klein GJ, Jones DL, Yee R (1994) Time and frequency domain analyses of heart rate variability during orthostatic stress in patients with neurally mediated syncope. Am J Cardiol 74:1258-1262

32. Lepicovska V, Novak P, Nadeau R (1992) Time-frequency mapping in syncope. Clin Auton Res 2:317

33. Lippman N, Stein K, Lerman BB (1995) Failure to decrease parasympathetic tone during upright tilt predicts a positive tilt-table test. Am J Cardiol 75:591-595

34. Sneddon JF, Counihan PJ, Bashir Y, Haywood GA, Ward DE, Camm AJ (1993) Impaired inmediate vasoconstrictor responses in patients with recurrent neurally mediated syncope. Am J Cardiol 71:72-76

35. Thompson HL, Lele S, Atherton JA, Muehle G, Wright KN, McKenna WJ (1995) Abnormal forearm vascular responses during erect dynamic leg exercise in patients with vasodepressor syncope. Circulation 42:2204-2209

36. Villar JC, Niño J, Vega A, Tahvanainen KUO, Morillo CA (1998) Heart rate variability during orthostatic stress identifies the response to sublingual nitroglycerine or isoproterenol head-up-tilt protocols. Pacing Clin Electrophysiol 21:288

37. Niño J, Villar JC, Kuusela T, Tahvanainen KUO, Herrera VM, Guzmán JC, Morillo CA (1998) Baroreflex gain dynamics during oral nitrates or isoproterenol head-up tilt protocols identifies different susceptibility to neurocardiogenic reflexes. Circulation 98:1367

38. Lewis T (1932) A lecture on vasovagal syncope and the carotid sinus mechanism with comments on Gowersís and Nothnagel's syndrome. Br J Med 1:873-876

39. Sra JS, Jazayeri MR, Avitall B, Dhala A, Deshpande S, Black Z et al (1993) Comparison of cardiac pacing with drug therapy in the treatment of neurocardiogenic (vasovagal) syncope with bradycardia or asystole. N Engl J Med 328:1085-1090

40. Engelke KA, Williams MM, Dietz NM, Joyner MJ (1997) Does sympathetic activation blunt nitric oxide-mediated hyperemia in the human forearm. Clin Auton Res 7:85-91

41. Kaufmann H (1995) Neurally mediated syncope: pathogenesis, diagnosis and treatment. Neurology 45:S12-S18

Is the Type of Cardiovascular Response During Tilt Table Testing Useful for the Choice of the Treatment? The New VASIS Classification

M. Brignole[1], C. Menozzi[2], A. Del Rosso[3], S. Costa[1], G. Gaggioli[1], A. Solano[1], N. Bottoni[2], P. Bartoli[3] and R. Sutton[4]

Worldwide experience of more than 10 years of tilt testing has shown that, while it has dramatically reduced the number of patients whose syncope cannot be explained, the population of patients who show a positive response to the test is greatly heterogeneous, raising the possibility that different syndromes can be diagnosed by tilt testing. Many drugs as well as cardiac pacing have been proposed for patients with tilt-induced syncope; however, a consensus on management has not been achieved due to the unsatisfactory results of trials of therapy which have been undertaken. The classification of the Vasovagal Syncope International Study (VASIS) was developed in 1992 in order to facilitate the understanding of the different types of vasovagal reactions that were observed during tilt-induced syncope [1]. This has been recently extended to tilt testing with pharmacological challenge [2, 3]. Like the other current classifications of the positive responses to tilt testing, the VASIS classification is based on the different behaviour of the blood pressure and heart rate observed when the vasovagal reaction and symptoms occur. To date, the cardiovascular patterns preceding the development of the vasovagal reaction have received little study. We believe that the pattern of blood pressure response to tilt may provide more strict diagnostic information and that a more detailed although still arbitrary classification may form the basis of a number of future drug and pacemaker trials and may help us toward a better understanding of the different mechanisms of tilt-induced syncope. We, therefore, propose that the following classification should be used as a complementary classification in addition to the VASIS classification. Moreover, we have tried to correlate this classification with some simple clinical variables.

[1]Sezione di Aritmologia, Ospedali Riuniti, Lavagna, Italy; [2]Sezione di Aritmologia, Ospedale S. Maria Nuova, Reggio Emilia, Italy; [3]Reparto di Cardiologia, Ospedale S. Pietro Igneo, Fucecchio (FI), Italy; [4]Department of Cardiology, Royal Brompton Hospital, London, UK

Method

At the end of 1997, based on a retrospective review of our tilt test traces, we developed a new classification of the positive responses to tilt testing based on the behaviour of blood pressure and heart rate during the pre-syncopal phase of the test. In 1998, we started a prospective validation of this classification in all consecutive patients referred to us for the execution of tilt testing. We planned to stop the study when the data of the first 100 patients suitable for evaluation had been collected.

The study population consisted of patients in whom the cause of syncope had remained uncertain despite a standardized basic evaluation that consisted of careful history, full physical examination, baseline laboratory testing, neurological evaluation, 12-lead electrocardiogram, 24-h ambulatory monitoring, chest X-ray, echocardiography and any other test necessary for a definitive diagnosis of the cause of the syncope. The patients with histories suggestive of vasovagal syncope (considered if a precipitating event such as fear, severe pain, or instrumentation could be identified), or situational syncope (considered if syncope was clearly correlated with coughing, micturition, defecation or swallowing) combined with negative above-mentioned investigations were included. Patients with associated carotid sinus hypersensitivity were also included. Carotid sinus hypersensitivity was defined as the reproduction of syncope in the presence of an abnormal cardioinhibition (asystole > 3 s), vasodepression (fall in systolic blood pressure > 50 mmHg) or both. The carotid sinus massage was performed according to the Method of Symptoms which has been described in previously published reports [4, 5].

Patients underwent the standardized protocol of upright tilt testing with trinitroglycerin (TNG) challenge currently used in our department for the diagnosis of unexplained syncope [3, 4, 6]. This consisted of 60-degree tilt for 45 min or until syncope occurred. If the test did not induce syncope, 0.4 mg oral spray TNG was administered while the patient remained in the same tilt position, and the test was continued for a further 20 min [2]. During the test, the beat-to-beat finger arterial pressure was monitored continuously by the Finapres method [7, 8].

Suggested New Classification of Abnormal Responses

In most patients with an abnormal response during tilt testing, the "syncopal phase" can easily be differentiated from the preceding "pre-syncopal phase" by a clear change in the behaviour of blood pressure and heart rate which correlates with the time of onset of the vasovagal reaction. The time of onset of the syncopal phase varies greatly from patient to patient; it depends also on the passive or TNG phases of occurrence of syncope. The period of time elapsing between the assumption of the upright position and the onset of the syncopal phase constitutes the pre-syncopal phase. We have observed three main patterns:
1. *"Classic (vasovagal) syncope" pattern* (Figs. 1, 2). In this form the behaviour of blood pressure during the pre-syncopal phase is indistinguishable from that

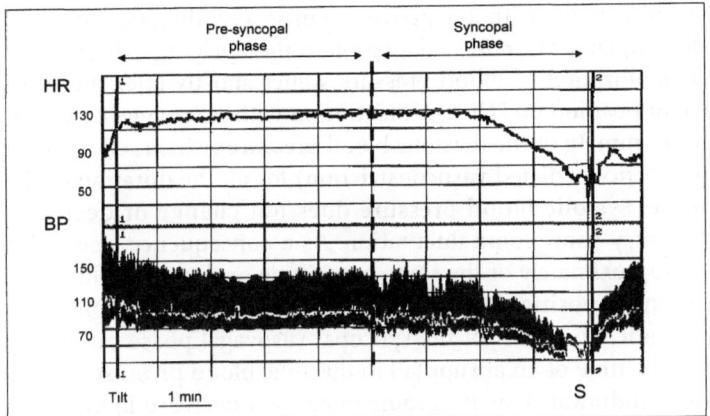

Fig. 1. A case of classic (vasovagal) syncope pattern occurring during the passive phase of tilt testing. *Top trace* shows the heart rate curve; *bottom trace* shows systolic, diastolic and mean blood pressure curves. Blood pressure stabilizes shortly after the assumption of upright position with no changes in diastolic blood pressure for the duration of the preparatory phase (about 4 min); the heart rate immediately rises, than stabilizes. The *vertical dashed line* indicates the time of onset of the vasovagal reaction which is characterized, at first, by fluctuations and mild decrease in diastolic blood pressure without changes in heart rate; later, both blood pressure and heart rate rapidly fall and syncope occurs. The total duration of the vasovagal reaction is about 4 min. HR, heart rate; BP, blood pressure; S, syncope

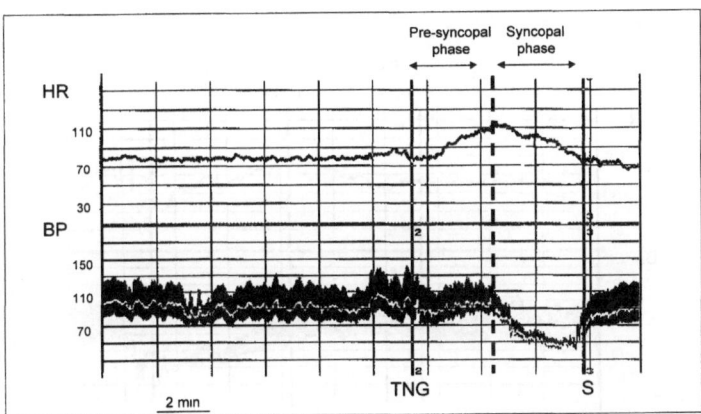

Fig. 2. A case of classic (vasovagal) syncope pattern occurring during trinitroglycerin (*TNG*) challenge. The figure is expanded and the first part of the passive phase of the tilt testing is not shown. The *top trace* shows the heart rate curve; the *bottom trace* shows systolic, diastolic and mean blood pressure curves. Immediately after the administration of 0.4 mg of TNG, there is a mild decrease in blood pressure as a consequence of the haemodynamic effect of the drug. The preparatory phase lasts about 2 min and is characterized by an increase in diastolic blood pressure of 15 mmHg that indicates a full compensatory reflex adaptation with peripheral vasoconstriction. The heart rate rises approximately 35 bpm. The *vertical dashed line* indicates the time of onset of the vasovagal reaction which is characterized by a rapid fall in both blood pressure and heart rate which leads to syncope in about 3 min

observed in patients with a negative response and, therefore, it reflects a rapid and full compensatory reflex adaptation to the upright position. This results in a rapid stabilization of blood pressure values shortly after the assumption of the upright position or TNG administration with no change or a slight increase of about 10 mmHg of the diastolic blood pressure (which reflects the activation of sympathetic-mediated vasoconstriction) for all the duration of the preparatory phase. Systolic blood pressure does not change or decreases slightly, though it may show some fluctuation. As a consequence also pulse pressure remains approximately of the same magnitude or decreases slightly. Compared with the supine position, the heart rate increases during this phase. Patients are asymptomatic. The onset of the syncopal vasovagal phase can easily be determined at the time of an abrupt fall in diastolic blood pressure suggesting sympathetic withdrawal. This is accompanied by a decrease in systolic and pulse pressure. The decrease in heart rate, which is usually present, coincides with or follows shortly after the decrease of blood pressure. Vasovagal symptoms coincide with this phase.

2. *"Dysautonomic (vasovagal) syncope" pattern* (Figs. 3, 4). In this form no steady-state adaption to upright position is present. There is a slow but progressive fall in the diastolic blood pressure which begins immediately after the assumption of the upright position or after the TNG administration and continues till the onset of the vasovagal reaction. The fall in systolic blood pressure is of a even greater magnitude, so that pulse pressure also decreases. Compared with the supine position, the heart rate increases during this phase

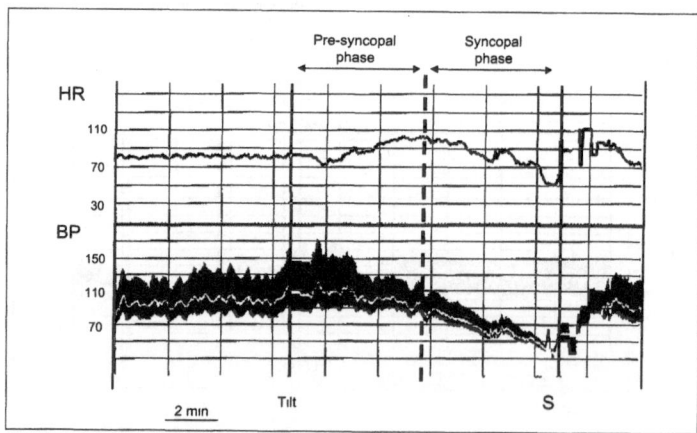

Fig. 3. A case of dysautonomic (vasovagal) syncope pattern occurring during the passive phase of tilt testing. *Top trace* shows the heart rate curve; *bottom trace* shows the systolic, diastolic and mean blood pressure curves. There is an absence of adaptation of blood pressure to the upright position; during the preparatory phase (of about 5 min) blood pressure declines slightly; since systolic pressure decreases more than diastolic, pulse pressure also decreases. The heart rate rises less than in the classic pattern. The *vertical dashed line* indicates the time of onset of the vasovagal reaction which is characterized by a change in the slope of blood pressure decrease as well as a decrease in heart rate

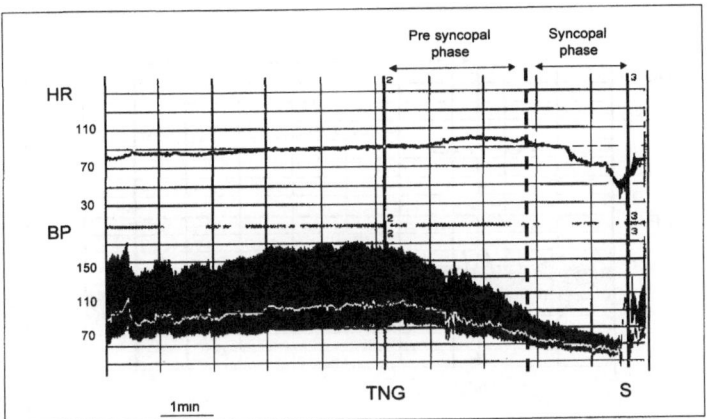

Fig. 4. A case of dysautonomic (vasovagal) syncope pattern occurring during TNG challenge. The figure is expanded and the first part of the passive phase of tilt testing is not shown. The *top trace* shows the heart rate curve; the *bottom trace* shows systolic, diastolic and mean blood pressure curves. There is an absence of adaptation of blood pressure to the upright position; blood pressure declines slightly and progressively throughout the preparatory and the syncopal phase without a change in slope; since systolic pressure decreases more than diastolic, pulse pressure also decreases. During the preparatory phase heart rate rises but less than in the classic pattern. The *vertical dashed line* indicates the time of onset of the vasovagal reaction which, in this case, can be identified only by the decrease in heart rate

by a variable amount. Patients are asymptomatic or develop mild symptoms of hypotension. The vasovagal reaction occurs when a critical value of blood pressure is reached (usually a value of systolic blood pressure of 70-80 mmHg). The onset of the syncopal phase can be appreciated by a change in the slope of decline of blood pressure as well as by a change in heart rate behaviour which usually starts decreasing or, more rarely, stops increasing. Once the vasovagal reaction starts, it is indistinguishable from that observed in the classic syncope pattern.

3. *"Orthostatic intolerance" pattern* (Fig. 5). Also in this form there is a slow but progressive fall in the diastolic blood pressure, which begins immediately after the assumption of the upright position or after the TNG administration, and is indistinguishable from that observed in the dysautonomic syncope pattern. The difference is that there is no clear vasovagal reaction to be discerned and, therefore, the test is characterized only by a long presyncopal phase which lasts until the end of the test. No decrease in heart rate occurs during the test. Systolic pressure decreases to values below 80 mmHg and, therefore, symptoms of hypotension such as dizziness, blurring of the vision, lightheadedness, and sweating occur and persist for several minutes until the end of the test, but complete loss of consciousness does not occur for at least 5 min after the onset of the symptoms, at which time the test is interrupted.

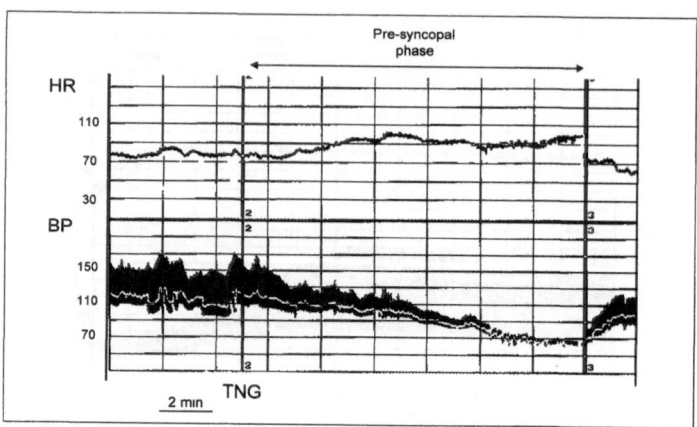

Fig. 5. A case of orthostatic intolerance pattern occurring during TNG challenge. The figure is expanded and the first part of the passive phase of the tilt testing is not shown. The *top trace* shows the heart rate curve; the *bottom trace* shows systolic, diastolic and mean blood pressure curves. There is an absence of adaptation of blood pressure to the upright position; blood pressure declines slightly and progressively throughout the test, as in the dysautonomic pattern, but differs from that by showing no clear vasovagal reaction. The heart rate continuously rises until the end of the test. Thus, the test is characterized only by a prolonged preparatory phase (13 min) which lasts more than in the other two patterns. Systolic blood pressure declines below 80 mmHg for more than 5 min and the patient has symptoms of hypotension but not syncope, then the test is interrupted

Suggested New Classification of the "Syncopal" Phase

The syncopal phase was classified according to a modification of the original VASIS classification [1, 3]:

1. *Type 1-mixed*: Heart rate falls at the time of syncope but the ventricular rate does not fall below 40 bpm or falls below 40 bpm for less than 10 s with or without asystole of less than 3 s. Blood pressure falls before the heart rate falls.
2. *Type 2A-cardioinhibition without asystole*: Heart rate falls to a ventricular rate less than 40 bpm for more than 10 s but asystole of more than 3 s does not occur. Blood pressure falls before the heart rate falls.
3. *Type 2B-cardioinhibition with asystole*: Asystole occurs for more than 3 s. The fall in blood pressure coincides with the heart rate fall or occurs beforehand.
4. *Type 3-vasodepressor*: Heart rate does not fall more than 10% from its peak at the time of syncope.
5. *Exception 1-chronotropic incompetence*: These patients show no heart rate rise during the tilt testing (i.e. less 10% from the pre-tilt rate).
6. *Exception 2-excessive heart rate rise*: These patients show an excessive heart rate rise both at the onset of upright position and throughout its duration before syncope (i.e. greater than 130 bpm).

In the original VASIS classification [1], type 2A was defined as "heart rate falls to ventricular rate less than 40 bpm for more than 10 s or asystole occurs for more than 3 s; blood presure falls before the heart rate falls", and type 2B was defined as "heart rate falls to a ventricular rate less than 40 bpm for more than 10 s or asystole occurs for more than 3 s; blood pressure fall coincides with heart rate fall". The modification was made according to clinical practice, which suggests that asystolic responses may benefit from pacemaker therapy.

Findings

Among 189 patients who underwent tilt testing during the study period, abnormal responses were observed in 115 (Fig. 6). We were able to attribute to one of the 3 classes of the new classification 101 of these patients (88%): classic (vasovagal) syncope in 36, dysautonomic (vasovagal) syncope in 47 and orthostatic intolerance in 18. Fourteen patients (12%) proved impossible to evaluate because of atypical patterns or very short duration of the pre-syncopal phase.

Some details regarding the results of tilt testing are shown in Table 1. Passive tilt testing was more often positive in patients with the classic pattern than in those of the other 2 groups, though the difference was not significant. In the patients with the classic and dysautonomic patterns the mean length of the pre-syncopal phase was 19 ± 15 min for the 17 patients with a positive response during the passive phase and 3.1 ± 1.3 min for the 64 patients with a positive response during the TNG phase. No difference was observed between classic and dysautonomic groups (Table 1). Conversely, the duration of the pre-syncopal phase (during TNG challenge) was longer for the 17 patients with orthostatic intolerance pattern (8.5 ± 4.3 min; $p = 0.000$). The mean duration of the vasovagal syncope phase was slightly

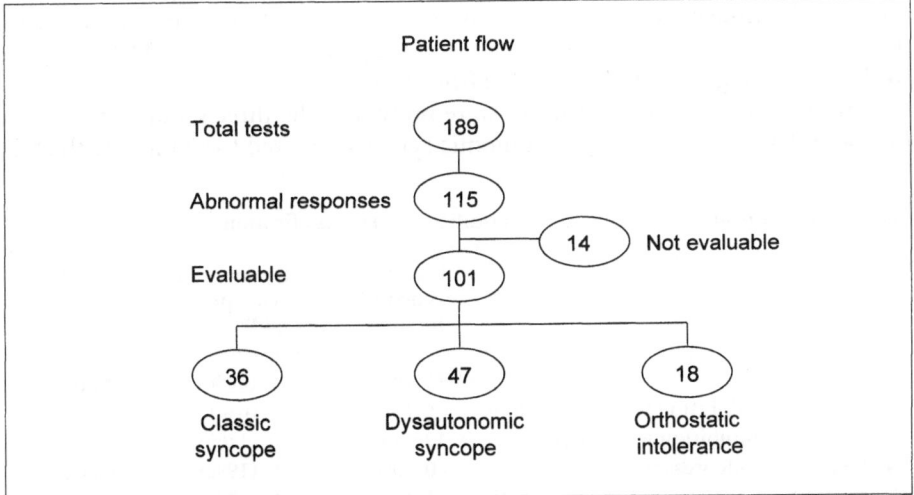

Fig. 6. Patient flow. See text for explanation

Table 1. Tilt test results: details observed in the 3 groups of patients

	Classic syncope $n=36$	Dysautonomic syncope $n=47$	Orthostatic intolerance $n=18$	p value
Phase of the positive response				
Passive phase	12 (33%)	7 (15%)	1 (6%)	ns
TNG phase	24 (67%)	40 (85%)	17 (94%)	(1 vs 3: p=0.07)
Pre-syncopal phase duration (min)				
Passive phase (when positive)	17±16	22±10	-	ns
TNG phase	3.5±1.4	2.9±1.2	8.5±4.3	0.000 (1&2 vs 3)
Syncopal phase duration (min)				
Passive phase (when positive)	2.5±1.4	3.0±1.7	-	ns
TNG phase	2.0±0.8	1.6±0.9	-	ns
Heart rate behaviour				
Maximum heart rate rise (bpm)	105±18	96±20*	93±20**	0.04 (1 vs 2&3)
Difference from baseline (bpm)	37±16	31±15*	30±15**	ns
Max heart rate <90 bpm	7 (19%)	14 (32%)*	8 (47%)**	0.04 (1 vs 3)

TNG, trinitroglycerin
* Evaluated in 44 patients (excluded 3 patients in atrial fibrillation)
** Evaluated in 17 patients (excluded 1 patient in atrial fibrillation)

longer when it occurred during passive than during TNG (2.7 ± 1.5 min and 1.8 ± 0.9 respectively, p = 0.02). No difference was observed between the classic and dysautonomic groups (Table 1). During the pre-syncopal phase, heart rate increased more in the classic group than in the other two groups.

The classification of the syncopal phase is shown in the Table 2. Cardio-inhibitory forms were more frequently observed in the classic group, whereas mixed and vasodepressor forms were more common in those with the dysauto-nomic pattern. The median duration of asystolic pauses was 8.5 s and 8.0 s respectively in the two groups; pauses ranged from 3 s to 41 s.

Several different clinical features were present in the three groups of patients (Table 3). The patients with dysautonomic syncope differed from those with clas-

Table 2. Tilt test results according to the modified VASIS classification

	Classic syncope $n=36$	Dysautonomic syncope $n=47$	p value
Type 1 mixed	15 (42%)	28 (60%)	ns (0.08)
Type 2A cardioinhibition without asystole	6 (17%)	3 (6%)	ns
Type 2B cardioinhibition with asystole	12 (33%)	5 (11%)	0.01
Type 3 pure vasodepressor	0 (0%)	9 (19%)	0.004
Chronotropic incompetence (exception 1)	1 (2%)	2 (4%)	ns
Excessive heart rate rise (exception 2)	2 (6%)	0 (0%)	ns

Table 3. Clinical characteristics of the 3 groups of patients

	Classic syncope n=36	Dysautonomic syncope n=47	p value (vs classic)	Orthostatic intolerance n=18	p value (vs classic)
Age (years)	50±20	65±17	0.000	72±15	0.000
Males	18 (50%)	23 (49%)	ns	10 (50%)	ns
Comorbidities:					
- systemic hypertension	10 (28%)	21 (45%)	ns (0.09)	11 (61%)	0.02
- structural heart diseases	5 (14%)	17 (36%)	0.02	7 (39%)	0.04
- ecg abnormalities	7 (19%)	15 (32%)	ns	9 (50%)	0.02
- diabetes	1 (3%)	2 (4%)	ns	1 (6%)	ns
History of syncopal episodes:					
- total number (median)	4.9±6.4 (3)	3.1±4.5 (2)	ns	2.6±3.4 (1)	ns
- duration, years (median)	13±14 (9)	7±15 (1)	0.003	1±1.5 (0.5)	0.000
- situational symptoms	13 (36%)	12 (26%)	ns	2 (11%)	0.05
- vasovagal symptoms	13 (36%)	9 (19%)	ns (0.06)	0 (0%)*	0.002
- situational or vasovagal	18 (50%)	18 (38%)	ns	2 (11%)*	0.05
- pre-syncopal episodes	20 (56%)	21 (45%)	ns	5 (28%)	0.01
- secondary trauma	11 (31%)	22 (47%)	ns	10 (56%)	ns (0.07)
- vasoactive therapy	9 (25%)	18 (38%)	ns	11 (61%)	0.02
Carotid sinus hypersensitivity	4 (11%)	20 (43%)	0.001	3 (17%)*	ns
- cardioinhibitory form	2	13		1	
- vasodepressor form	2	6		2	

* $p \le 0.05$ vs dysautonomic group

sic syncope in terms of age, prevalence of structural heart disease and duration of syncopal episodes, but had similar prevalence of history of vasovagal or situational events. The patients with orthostatic intolerance were those who differed from those with classic syncope. Carotid sinus hypersensitivity was more frequent in the dysautonomic group than in the other two groups.

Interpretation

This classification is based on some previous observations. For example, the terms "classic" and "dysautonomic" have already been used by Grubb and Samoil [9] to describe anecdotally various phenomena occurring during tilt testing which are similar to those described by us. Patterns that seem similar to our orthostatic intolerance pattern, though not completely overlapping, have been previously described as "exaggerated response" [4, 6] and "progressive orthostatic hypotension" [10, 11]. However, this study is the first that evaluates systematically and prospectively a population of consecutive patients, classifies it according to predefined categories and correlates the classes of patients thus obtained with clinical variables.

The patients with the classic pattern show a full compensatory reflex adaptation to upright position which suggests normal baroreflex function. The onset of the vasovagal reaction cannot be predicted by changes in blood pressure or heart rate and the time of onset is very variable. Once the vasovagal reaction starts, it leads to syncope within a few minutes. The patients with the classic form are largely those who are young and healthy. They have a long history of syncope with long periods of time free of recurrences. Indeed, in our population, these patients had a median of three syncopal episodes during a median 9-year period. In many cases the first syncopal episodes had occurred in the teenage years. Secondary trauma is infrequent and, if it occurs, it is mild. We know from studies of recording of neural activity [12], performed in patients presumably affected by classic vasovagal syncope, that the vasovagal reaction is not preceded by changes of low-frequency sympathetic or vagal rhythms [13] or spontaneous vagal baroreflex gain [14] and that is is ushered in by an abrupt cessation of sympathetic nerve traffic to the skeletal muscle vascular bed. The mechanism responsible for switching from haemodynamic compensation to vasovagal physiology remains largely to be determined [12]. Classic syncope is felt to represent a "hypersensitive" autonomic system which over-responds to various stimuli [9]. For all these reasons we are reluctant to consider this phenomenon as a disease.

The patients with the dysautonomic pattern are unable to achieve a steady-state reflex adaptation to the upright position, suggesting an impaired baroreflex response or an impaired function of the target organs, the heart and the peripheral vasculature. Accordingly, the value of the maximum heart rate reached by this group is lower than that of the classic group. Typically, the vasovagal reaction begins when systolic blood pressure decreases to a critical value of about 70-80 mmHg. Therefore, it seems that prolonged orthostatic hypotension may play a role as a trigger for the vasovagal reaction. This issue has been recently addressed by Gaggioli et al. [15] who demonstrated that treatment with vasodilator drugs, effectively reducing systemic pressure both at rest and upright, was able to increase the positivity rate of tilt testing in predisposed patients. The patients with the dysautonomic pattern are dominantly old, but it may also occur in some younger subjects; many have associated diseases. They have a short history of syncope (median duration of 1 year) with a median of two episodes per patient; therefore, syncopal episodes begin late in life, suggesting they are due to the occurrence of some underlying neural dysfunction. Carotid sinus hypersensitivity is frequently present in these patients, but not in those of the other two groups, suggesting that an impairment at some level of the carotid sinus baroreflex arc is also associated and, therefore, a more complex autonomic dysfunction is present. The cause of this association is not advanced age per se, since carotid sinus hypersensitivity was not associated with the orthostatic intolerance group. On the contrary classic vasovagal syncope and carotid sinus syndrome are two distinct syndromes. For all these reasons, we suppose that dysautonomic syncope is due to a disease of the autonomic function, which begins frequently late in the patient's life and is characterized by a compromised ability to adapt promptly to some external influences ("hyposensitive" autonomic function).

The patients with orthostatic intolerance pattern are a group of patients with syncope in whom tilt testing is unable to elicit a typical vasovagal reaction. The results of the test suggest that the cause of the syncope is an atypical form of orthostatic hypotension. Among the three groups, this form is the most similar to the syndromes of autonomic dysfunction, such as pure autonomic failure, postural orthostatic tachycardia syndrome and chronic fatigue syndrome [16-18]. However, it differs from these with its blunted tachycardia reflex to upright posture and different clinical manifestations. In these patients both the clinical characteristics and the behaviour during the preparatory phase were similar to that in patients with dysautonomic syncope except for the lack of history suggestive of vasovagal or situational episodes and the lack of tilt-induced vasovagal reaction. Thus, it seems that patients with orthostatic intolerance may suffer from some form of autonomic failure and not from vasovagal syncope. Patterns similar to that of orthostatic intolerance are those previously defined as exaggerated responses. These were described during pharmacological tilt testing both with isoproterenol [4] and TNG [6], whereas they have rarely been found during passive tilt testing [4]. Since exaggerated responses were observed also in many control subjects without syncope, their diagnostic value has remained uncertain. The present study is helpful in clarifying the meaning of impaired baroreflex function, which can be observed both in patients with and without syncope. Thus, the term orthostatic intolerance seems preferable to that of exaggerated response.

The "New VASIS Classification" and the Choice of the Treatment

The resulting new VASIS classification may have practical implications. The classic group showed a prevalence of cardioinhibitory forms, whereas the dysautonomic group showed a prevalence of mixed and vasodepressor forms. It seems unlikely that the patients of the three groups may benefit from the same treatment. Future therapy trials should enrol patients taking into account their tilt test patterns. We can anticipate that the dysautonomic patients might benefit from the same therapy usually used for the syndromes of autonomic dysfunction with orthostatic intolerance, namely increasing blood volume (fludrocortisone), reducing blood volume in the lower limb of the body (compression stockings, sleeping with the head of the bed upright) or using new alpha-stimulating agents, midodrine and etilefrine. Recent controlled studies have shown that midodrine is superior to placebo in the syndrome of orthostatic hypotension [19] and in severely symptomatic elderly patients affected by "hypotensive" syncope [20]. If preventive therapy fails, pacemakers may be useful in the cardioinhibitory forms, especially in those with asystole, and when carotid sinus hypersensitivity may be associated. In the latter case, cardiac pacing is definitively of proven efficacy [21, 22]. Most of the patients with classic syncope probably do not need any treatment owing to the benign course of the disease with long periods of absence of recurrences. However, we can expect that the results of pharmacological treatments will be disappointing and similar to those in some placebo-controlled prospective trials that have been unable to show a benefit of the active drug over placebo [23-26]. Cardiac pacing is probably effective in the asystolic forms, as was demonstrated in the recent vasovagal pacemaker study [27] and the pacemaker arm of the VASIS study [28]; however, the role of pacing must be restricted to very severe recurrent forms owing to the benign course of the disease. Tilt training is a new therapeutic strategy which seems to be especially suited to patients with classic vasovagal syncope [29].

Conclusions

Any descriptive classification of pathophysiology at an early stage in its understanding must be expected to receive criticism and undergo modification. It should be remembered that, when we observe nature, we see what we want to see according to our understanding at that time. In order to make some sense of the apparent chaos of nature, we try to classify it into a coherent system that conforms to our expectations. Thus, any system of classification is in some way arbitrary and open to debate [30]. Actually it seems that, more than a clear differentiation, there is a wide spectrum of disorders of orthostatic cardiovascular homeostasis including, on one side, the vasovagal syncope and, on the other side, the syndromes of autonomic dysfunction such as in the postural orthostatic tachycardia syndrome, chronic fatigue syndrome, pure autonomic failure, etc. In this respect the patients with the dysautonomic pattern and those with orthostatic intolerance pattern during tilt testing may represent a link. Future studies should evaluate whether there are different neural and endocrine mechanisms responsible for the different syndromes of tilt-induced orthostatic intolerance.

References

1. Sutton R, Petersen M, Brignole M, Raviele A, Menozzi C, Giani P (1992) Proposed classification for tilt induced vasovagal syncope. Eur J Cardiac Pacing Electrophysiol 2:180-183
2. Del Rosso A, Bartoli P, Bartoletti A, Brandinelli-Geri A, Bonechi F, Maioli M, Mazza F, Michelucci A, Russo L, Salvetti E, Sansoni M, Zipoli A, Fierro A, Ieri A (1998) Shortened head-up tilt testing potentiated with sublingual nitroglycerin in patients with unexplained syncope. Am Heart J 135:564-570
3. Kurbaan AS, Fran'zen AC, Williams T, Wasan BS, Kaddoura S, Sutton R (1998) Vasovagal collapse patterns after the use of glyceryl trinitrate during tilt testing. PACE 21:794 (abstr)
4. Brignole M, Menozzi C, Gianfranchi L, Oddone D, Lolli G, Bertulla A (1991) Carotid sinus massage, eye-ball compression test and head-up tilt test in patients with syncope of uncertain origin and in healthy control subjects. Am Heart J 122:1644-1651
5. Brignole M, Menozzi C, Bottoni N, Gianfranchi L, Lolli G, Oddone D, Gaggioli G (1995) Mechanisms of syncope caused by transient bradycardia and the diagnostic value of electrophysiologic testing and cardiovascular reflexivity maneuvers. Am J Cardiol 76:273-278
6. Raviele A, Menozzi C, Brignole M, Gasparini G, Alboni P, Musso G, Lolli G, Oddone D, Dinelli M, Mureddu R (1995) Value of head-up tilt testing potentiated with sublingual nitroglycerin to assess the origin of unexplained syncope. Am J Cardiol 76:267-272

7. Friedman DB, Jensen FB, Matzen S, Secher NH (1990) Non-invasive blood pressure monitoring during head-up tilt test using the Penaz principle. Acta Anestesiol Scand 34:519-522

8. Petersen MEV, Williams TR, Sutton R (1995) A comparison of non-invasive continuous finger blood pressure measurements (Finapres) with intra-arterial pressure during prolonged head-up tilt. Eur Heart J 16:1647-1654

9. Grubb B, Samoil D (1996) Neurocardiogenic syncope. In: Kenny RA (ed) Syncope in the older patient. Chapman & Hall, pp 91-106

10. Schutzman J, Jaeger F, Maloney J, Fouad-Tarazi F (1994) Head-up tilt and hemodynamic changes during orthostatic hypotension in patients with supine hypertension. J Am Coll Cardiol 24:454-461

11. Betkoski A, Patei C, Halperin A, Jaeger F, Goren H, Fouad-Tarazi F (1995) Reporting on the results of tilt patterns of response offer more information than changes at end-point. Circulation 92:I-203 (abstr)

12. Morillo C, Eckberg D, Ellenbogen K, Beightol L, Hoang J, Tahvanainen K, Kuusela T, Diedrich A (1997) Vagal and sympathetic mechanisms in patients with orthostatic vasovagal syncope. Circulation 96:2509-2513

13. Novak V, Novak P, Kus T, Nadeau R (1995) Slow cardiovascular rhythms in tilt and syncope. J Clin Neurophysiol 12:64-71

14. Glick G, Yu PN (1963) Hemodynamic changes during spontaneous vasovagal reactions. Am J Med 34:42-51

15. Gaggioli G, Bottoni N, Mureddu R, Foglia-Manzillo G, Mascioli G, Bartoli P, Musso G, Menozzi C, MD, Brignole M (1997) Effects of chronic vasodilator therapy to enhance susceptibility to vasovagal syncope during upright tilt testing. Am J Cardiol 80:1092-1094

16. Narkiewicz K, Somers V (1998) Chronic orthostatic intolerance. Part of a spectrum of dysfunction in orthostatic cardiovascular homeostasis? Circulation 98:2105-2107

17. Furlan R, Jacob G, Snell M, Robertson D, Porta A, Harris P, Mosqueda-Garcia R (1998) Chronic orthostatic intolerance. A disorder with discordant cardiac and vascular sypathetic control. Circulation 98:2154-2159

18. Bou-Holaigh I, Rowe P, Kan J, Calkins H (1995) The relationship between neurally mediated hypotension and chronic fatigue syndrome. JAMA 274:961-967

19. Low P, Gilden J, Freeman R, Sheng KN, McElligott MA (1977) Efficacy of midodrine vs placebo in neurocardiogenic orthostatic hypotension. JAMA 277:1046-1051

20. Ward CR, Gray JC, Gilroy JJ, Kenny RA (1998) Midodrine: a role in the management of neurocardiogenic syncope. Heart 79:45-49

21. Brignole M, Menozzi C, Lolli G, Bottoni N, Gaggioli G (1992) Long-term outcome of paced and non-paced patients with severe carotid sinus syndrome. Am J Cardiol 69:1039-1043

22. Gaggioli G, Brignole M, Menozzi C, Devoto G, Gianfranchi L, Gostoli E, Bottoni N, Lolli G (1995) A positive response to head-up tilt test predicts syncopal recurrence in carotid sinus syndrome patients treated with permanent pacemakers. Am J Cardiol 76:720-722

23. Brignole M, Menozzi C, Gianfranchi L, Lolli G, Bottoni N, Oddone D (1992) A controlled trial of acute and long-term medical therapy in tilt-induced neurally-mediated syncope. Am J Cardiol 70:339-342

24. Morillo C, Leitch J, Yee R, Klein G (1993) A placebo-controlled trial of intravenous and oral disopyramide for prevention of neurally-mediated syncope induced by head-up tilt. J Am Coll Cardiol 22:1843-1848

25. Di Gerolamo E, Di Iorio C, Sabatini P, Leonzio I, Barsotti A (1998) Effects of different treatments versus no treatment on neurocardiogenic syncope. Cardiologia 43:833-837
26. Raviele A, Brignole M, Sutton R, Alboni P, Giani P, Menozzi C, Moya A (1999) Effect of etilefrine in preventing syncopal recurrence in patients with tilt-induced vasovagal syncope. A double-blind, randomized, placebo-controlled trial. Circulation (in press)
27. Connolly S, Sheldon R, Roberts R, Gent M (1999) The North American Pacemaker Study (VPS). A randomized trial of permanent cardiac pacing for the prevention of vasovagal syncope. J Am Coll Cardiol 33:16-20
28. Sutton R, Brignole M, Menozzi C, Raviele A, Alboni P, Giani P, Moya A (1999) Dual-chamber pacing is efficacious in treatment of neurally mediated tilt-positive cardioinhibitory syncope. Pacemaker versus no therapy: a multicentre randomized study (in press)
29. Ector H, Reybrouck T, Heidbuchel H, Van de Werf F (1998) Tilt training: a new treatment for neurocardiogenic syncope. Arch Mal Coeur Vaisseaux 91:32 (abstr)
30. Mathias CJ (1995) The classification and nomenclature of autonomic disorders: ending chaos, restoring conflict, and hopefully achieving clarity. Clin Auton Res 5:307-310

Midodrine for Treatment of Vasovagal Syncope

D.G. Benditt, L. Wilbert, G. Fahy, S. Sakaguchi, K.G. Lurie and N. Samniah

Introduction

Most vasovagal fainters who seek medical attention require no more than the reassurance that their physician understands the basis of their symptoms, and education regarding both the nature of the problem and techniques which may avert recurrences. However, when spells are frequent, or are associated with physical injury, or threaten to compromise occupational status, prophylactic treatment measures become a consideration. Unfortunately, the optimum treatment approach remains uncertain.

For the most part, clinical studies of conventional pharmacologic treatment options for vasovagal syncope have yet to provide convincing evidence of treatment benefit [1-10]. Cardiac pacing, on the other hand, although apparently efficacious in selected very symptomatic patients [11-13], is probably not an acceptable option for most vasovagal fainters (especially the young). Consequently, the investigation of alternative treatments remains important. Midodrine, an orally absorbable α_1-agonist, appears to be one of the most promising of the alternatives.

Vasoconstrictor Therapy for Vasovagal Syncope

Among the various classes of drugs which have been considered for prevention of vasovagal spells (e.g., β-adrenergic blockers, mineralocorticoids, serotonin reuptake inhibitors), vasoconstrictors (i.e., drugs that promote vasoconstriction and venoconstriction, and/or counteract rapid vasodilation) are natural contenders. By both mitigating systemic hypotension and maintaining cardiac venous return, these drugs may be expected to eliminate the reflex bradycardia and vasodilatation thought to be at least partly triggered by afferent neural signals from central vascular mechanoreceptors. However, drug-induced hypertension, tachyphylaxis, and inconsistent effectiveness have been major drawbacks.

Cardiac Arrhythmia Center, University of Minnesota Medical School, Minneapolis, Minnesota, USA

Ephedrine, dihydroergotamine, and etilefrine are the vasoconstrictors which, until relatively recently, have been of principal interest for prevention of vasovagal syncope [9, 14, 15]. However, only etilefrine has been subject to rigorous evaluation. In initial non-randomized reports, the effectiveness of etilefrine (a relatively weak α- and β-adrenergic agonist) varied, but overall it appeared to exhibit short-term and long-term effectiveness ranging from 43% to 100%. In contrasting reports, Moya et al. [10] found etilefrine (30 mg/day) to be no better than placebo in preventing tilt-induced syncope, while Raviele et al. [16] did observe apparent benefit in terms of preventing spontaneous events. In the latter study, Raviele et al. [16] compared outcomes in 78 patients; 32 patients were treated with etilefrine (15-125 mg/day) after demonstrating effectiveness during tilt testing, while 46 patients served as untreated controls (it being unclear from the report whether the controls also had had a beneficial response to etilefrine during tilt testing). During a mean follow-up of slightly less than 2 years, syncope recurred in 9% of etilefrine-treated patients, and in 35% of controls ($p = 0.01$). The drug was relatively well tolerated, although 5 of 32 treated patients developed mild hypertension.

In order to better test the effectiveness of etilefrine in vasovagal syncope, a multicenter placebo-controlled trial was initiated in Europe (VASIS trial [19]). However, the etilefrine arm of this study was ultimately terminated after observing no apparent treatment benefit [9]. Occurrence of syncope (etilefrine, 25.9%; control, 23.6%) and time to first syncope recurrence did not differ significantly between active drug and placebo.

Midodrine

Pharmacology

Midodrine [1(2', 5'-dimethoxyphenyl)-2-glycinamidoethanol-HCL] is essentially an inactive prodrug which produces its vasoconstrictor effects via an active metabolite [18, 19]. The outcome is arteriolar constriction and diminished venous pooling due to α-adrenergic receptor agonist activity. Selectivity of midodrine for α_1 and α_2 receptor sites is uncertain, with some claims for α_1 site selectivity being noted in the literature. The drug does not appear to be exerting β-adrenergic agonist activity.

Midodrine is well absorbed from the gastrointestinal tract and achieves a peak plasma concentration within 40 min. After absorption, midodrine undergoes extensive hepatic metabolism, primarily by hydrolysis of the glycine ester to produce the active metabolite desglymidodrine. Only 2%-4% of midodrine is excreted unchanged. Desglymidodrine reaches peak levels in about 1 hour, and is principally responsible for the therapeutic action of the drug by inducing arteriolar and venous capacitance constriction. Peak plasma levels may vary widely, with large differences having been reported between volunteer subjects and patients. Absolute bioavailability of midodrine (in terms of the desglymidodrine) is greater than 90%. Elimination is via the urine, with 75% of a single oral dose being excreted within 24 hours.

The elimination half-life of midodrine in the plasma is only 30 min, whereas desglymidodrine has a half-life in the range of 3 hours. As a result, the overall duration of action of the drug is in the 4-6-h range; thus, the dosing requirement is 3-4 times daily. The initial starting dose is 2.5 mg three times daily, with the maximum dose being in the range of 40 mg daily.

Midodrine is generally very well tolerated. Neither midodrine nor its desglymidodrine metabolite crosses the blood-brain barrier. Consequently, the drug has minimal central nervous system effect. In terms of principal adverse effects, scalp tingling (pilomotor reactions) is perhaps the most common (reported to account for 55% of adverse effects) and annoying side effect [18]. Supine hypertension seems to be uncommon in our experience, although it has apparently been recorded in up to 25% of treated patients in one study. As a rule, side effects are easily managed by dose adjustment.

Clinical Experience

The effects of midodrine have been studied in greatest detail in patients with neurogenic orthostatic hypotension. Gilden [20] reported observations of a dose-ranging placebo-controlled crossover trial in 97 individuals. An almost 30% average increase in standing systolic blood pressure was observed, with the 10-mg administered three times daily dosing seeming to be the most effective. Low et al. [21] used a placebo-controlled crossover design to examine the effect of a 10-mg dose administered three times daily in 171 patients with orthostatic hypotension. Nine patients (three receiving midodrine, six receiving placebo) were excluded for reasons of compliance. Among the others, midodrine was markedly beneficial in terms of improving standing systolic blood pressure and global symptom relief. A compilation of data from 56 published and unpublished clinical studies comprising 3996 patients indicated that midodrine was beneficial in diminishing the effects of orthostatic hypotension in 70%-100% of patients [19].

The use of midodrine in neurally mediated faints such as vasovagal syncope has been addressed in only a few relatively small clinical reports, although the findings of a large multicenter trial should be available soon. Ward and Kenny [22] undertook a double-blind crossover trial of midodrine in one patient with apparently intractable vasodepressor syncope. In that report, symptoms were recorded during comparable periods of no treatment, placebo treatment, and midodrine 5 mg three times daily. In brief, the numbers of days in which dizziness was reported were 13, 13, and 7 respectively. Syncope occurred on 8, 8, and 0 days respectively. Finally, the number of symptom-free days were 14, 13, and 21 respectively. Clearly, this individual demonstrated a very beneficial midodrine effect.

More recently, several reports have attested to the utility of midodrine in small groups of patients with neurally mediated syncope. Sra et al. [23] provided findings in 11 patients (average age 34 years) with recurrent vasovagal syncope whose symptoms had not been adequately controlled on conventional medications. One patient did not tolerate the drug due to headache and the development of hypertension despite a relatively low midodrine dose (7.5 mg/day). Among the remainder, five were symptom-free during the average 17 week follow-up, while four others reported symptom improvement compared to the 3-month baseline period just before entering the trial. Similarly, in a randomized placebo-controlled study (1 month duration) incorporating 16 patients (mean age 56 years) with frequent hypotensive events (fewer than 20 symptom-free days per month), Ward et al. [24] noted a markedly beneficial effect from midodrine treatment. Patients receiving midodrine averaged 7.3 more symptom-free days than those receiving placebo ($p < 0.0001$). Midodrine therapy was also associated with a measurable improvement in quality of life as assessed by standard testing. Finally, in an experience reported from our laboratory comprising 20 patients with recurrent syncope over an average of more than 5 years despite multiple treatment regimens (average of 2.3 drugs), 13 remained completely asymptomatic over 14 months follow-up on midodrine therapy (average daily dose, 22 mg) [25].

Conclusions

Midodrine is a readily absorbed and generally well tolerated drug, which has been demonstrated to be highly effective in the treatment of orthostatic hypotension. More recently, interest has turned toward assessing its efficacy in neurally mediated syncope, and especially in those forms of vasovagal faint in which a prominent vasodepressor effect is present. To date, findings in small studies have been very encouraging. Consequently, it is now reasonable to consider midodrine therapy (in doses usually ranging from 5 mg to 15 mg, three times daily) early in the course of treatment of patients with recurrent troublesome vasovagal faints.

Acknowledgements. The authors acknowledge the valuable assistance of Wendy Markuson in the preparation of the manuscript.

References

1. Almquist A, Goldenberg IF, Milstein S, Chen M-Y, Chen X-C, Hansen R, Gornick CC, Benditt DG (1989) Provocation of bradycardia and hypotension by isoproterenol and upright posture in patients with unexplained syncope. N Engl J Med 320:346-351
2. Fitzpatrick AP, Ahmed R, Williams S, Sutton R (1991) A randomised trial of medical therapy in "malignant vasovagal syndrome" or "neurally-mediated bradycardia hypotension syndrome". Eur J Cardiac Pacing Electrophysiol 2:99-102
3. Brignole M, Menozzi C, Gianfranchi L, Lolli G, Bottoni N, Oddone D (1992) A controlled trial of acute and long-term medical therapy in tilt-induced neurally-mediated syncope. Am J Cardiol 70:339-342
4. Mahananda N, Bhuripanyo K, Kangkagate C, Wansanit K, Kulchot B, Nademanee K, Chaithiraphan S (1995) Randomized double-blind placebo-controlled trial of oral

atenolol in patients with unexplained syncope and positive upright tilt table results. Am Heart J 130:1250-1253

5. Milstein S, Buetikofer J, Dunnigan A, Benditt DG, Gornick C, Reyes WJ (1990) Usefulness of disopyramide for prevention of upright tilt-induced hypotension-bradycardia. Am J Cardiol 65:1339-1344

6. Morillo C, Leitch JW, Yee R, Klein GJ (1993) A placebo-controlled trial of intravenous and oral disopyramide for prevention of neurally mediated syncope induced by head-up tilt. J Am Coll Cardiol 22:1843-1848

7. Kosinski DJ, Grubb BP, Temesy-Armos PN (1994) The use of serotonin re-uptake inhibitors in the treatment of neurally mediated cardiovascular disorders. J Serotonin Res 1:85-90

8. Grubb BP, Wolfe D, Samoil D, Temesy-Armos P, Hahn H, Elliott L (1993) Usefulness of fluoxetine hydrochloride for prevention of resistant upright tilt induced syncope. Pacing Clin Electrophysiol 16:458-464

9. Sutton R, Brignole M, Raviele A, for the Vasis Group Investigators (1998) Randomised controlled trial of etilefrine therapy for vasovagal syncope. Arch Mal Coeur 91(special III):242 (abstr)

10. Moya A, Permanyer-Miralda G, Sagrista-Sauleda J, Carne X, Rius T, Mont L, Soler-Soler J (1995) Limitations of head-up tilt test for evaluating the efficacy of therapeutic interventions in patients with vasovagal syncope: results of a controlled study of etilefrine versus placebo. J Am Coll Cardiol 25:65-69

11. Petersen MEV, Chamberlain-Webber R, Fizpatrick AP, Ingram A, Williams T, Sutton R (1994) Permanent pacing for cardio-inhibitory malignant vasovagal syndrome. Br Heart J 71:274-281

12. Connolly SJ, Sheldon R, Roberts RS, Gent M (1999) The North American vasovagal pacemaker study (VPS): a randomized trial of permanent cardiac pacing for the prevention of vasovagal syncope. J Am Coll Cardiol 33:16-20

13 Benditt DG (1999) Cardiac pacing for prevention of vasovagal syncope. J Am Coll Cardiol 33:21-23 (editorial)

14. Almquist A, Gornick CC, Benson DW Jr et al (1985) Carotid sinus hypersensitivity: evaluation of the vasodepressor component. Circulation 67:927-936

15. Grubb BP, Kosinski D (1996) Current trends in etiology, diagnosis, and management of neurocardiogenic syncope. Curr Opin Cardiol 11:32-41

16. Raviele A, Themistoclakis S, Gasparini G (1996) Drug treatment of vasovagal syncope. In: Blanc JJ, Benditt DG, Sutton R (eds) Neurally-mediated syncope: pathophysiology, investigations, and treatment. Futura, Armonk, NY, pp 113-117

17. Vasovagal Syncope International Study (VASIS) Group (1993) Double-blind randomised study of etilefrine versus placebo in patients with tilt-induced recurrent vasovagal syncope. Eur J Cardiac Pacing Electrophysiol 3:64

18. McTavish D, Goa KL (1989) Midodrine. A review of its pharmacological properties and therapeutic use in orthostatic hypotension and secondary hypotensive disorders. Drugs 38:757-777

19. Anonymous (1996) Midodrine hydrochloride: clinical investigator's brochure. Roberts Pharmaceutical Corp

20. Gilden JL (1993) Midodrine in neurogenic orthostatic hypotension. Int Angiol 12:125-131

21. Low PA, Gilden JL, Freeman R, Sheng K-N, McElligott MA (1997) Efficacy of midodrine vs placebo in neurogenic orthostatic hypotension. JAMA 13:1046-1051

22. Ward C, Kenny RA (1995) Observations on midodrine in a case of vasodepressor neurogenic syncope. Clin Autonom Res 5:257-260

23. Sra J, Maglio C, Biehl M, Dhala A, Blanck Z, Deshpande S, Jazayeri MR, Akhtar M

(1997) Efficacy of midodrine hydrochloride in neurocardiogenic syncope refractory to standard therapy. J Cardiovasc Electrophysiol 8:42-46

24. Ward CR, Gray JC, Gilroy JJ, Kenny RA (1998) Midodrine: a role in the management of neurocardiogenic syncope. Heart 79:45-49

25. Benditt DG, Samniah N, Sakaguchi S, Fahy G, Wilbert L (1998) Midodrine is effective in patients with refractory neurally-mediated syncope. Circulation 98[Suppl I]:706 (abstr)

Vasovagal Syncope: To Pace or not to Pace?

R.S. Sheldon

Most patients with vasovagal syncope faint infrequently and require only reassurance and advice about dietary and lifestyle modifications. However, there is a minority of patients who are considerably more distressed. Patients with recurrent vasovagal syncope may seriously injure themselves, may not be able to drive a car or to perform their jobs, and have a significant drop in objectively measured quality of life [1].

Selecting Patients for Treatment

Many patients appear to improve following assessment, even without specific measures. The patients most appropriate for treatment are those at particularly high risk of frequent syncope following assessment. Several studies taken together showed that patients have a 25% chance of fainting at least once during the 18 months after initial assessment [2].

How can we predict which patients will continue to faint? The time to the first recurrence of syncope following a positive tilt test can be predicted from simple variables such as the number and frequency of preceding syncopal spells [3]. In addition, the time to the first syncopal spell following the tilt test accurately predicts the eventual frequency of syncope in that particular patient [4]. This allows the clinician to pursue a conservative course by simply waiting until syncope recurs, if it does. However, patients who have fainted at least 6 times or who suffer recurrence within 1 year will continue to faint frequently.

Therapies are best understood in light of the current pathophysiologic model of vasovagal syncope. This model has many limitations and we present it only to put in perspective the various drugs. The initial event is orthostatic stress, which reduces left ventricular volumes and elevates sympathetic tone. This in turn causes either increased contractility or increased gain of the ventricular baroreceptors. This causes paradoxically increased firing of the baroreceptors, which in turn triggers a bradycardic and hypotensive response. Bradycardia is caused by

Cardiovascular Research Group, University of Calgary, Calgary, Alberta, Canada

increased vagal tone and hypotension is caused by withdrawal of α-adrenergic tone. The most promising treatments are salt loading, α-adrenergic agonists, β-receptor antagonists, and permanent pacing.

The Evidence for Drug Treatment

Salt and fluid loading. Salt loading increases plasma volume, and therefore might improve orthostatic tolerance and prevent syncope. Simple salt loading increases orthostatic tolerance [5, 6], and salt loading with or without the use of the mineralocorticoid fludrocortisone reduces the probability of a positive tilt test and of syncope in follow-up in young patients [7-9]. Although there are no hard clinical data to support this, many clinicians have adopted it as the first line of treatment. It carries low morbidity and a reasonable chance of success, and seems a practical and useful option.

α-*Adrenergic agonists.* The potential usefulness of α-adrenergic agonists was suggested by the fact that withdrawal of sympathetic tone was responsible for the vasodepression associated with vasovagal syncope. Pseudoephedrine, etilefrine, and midodrine all seemed effective in open label studies. These initially promising results have been tested by two prospective randomized trials. The European VASIS group randomized 126 patients with frequent vasovagal syncope to either placebo or high-dose etilefrine [10]. The patients who received etilefrine did no better than those who received placebo. In contrast, Natale et al. randomized 61 patients with frequent vasovagal syncope to either fluid therapy or escalating doses of midodrine [11]. The patients who received midodrine reported a marked and highly significant reduction in the number of presyncopal and syncopal spells compared to the patients who received only fluid therapy. Therefore the role of α-agonists in preventing vasovagal syncope remains unclear. However many clinicians believe that this is a reasonable empiric option if salt and fluid loading is not successful or not tolerated.

β-*Blockers.* Three recent controlled studies have provided conflicting information about the usefulness of empiric β-blockade in preventing syncope recurrence. One nonrandomized study of 118 patients who were followed for about 2 years showed that 10%-23% of persistently treated patients and 42%-58% of partially or completely untreated patients had at least one recurrence of syncope [12]. A second nonrandomized study of 153 syncope patients with positive tilt tests followed for up to 3 years showed that syncope recurred in the same proportion of treated and untreated patients, and the actuarial probability of remaining free of syncope was similar in both groups [13]. Finally, a small placebo-controlled randomized trial that lasted only 1 month reported that patients treated with atenolol had 83% fewer presyncopal and syncopal spells than did patients treated with placebo [14]. There remains uncertainty about the efficacy of chronic β-blockade in the prevention of syncope.

Taken together, these data begin to give us an insight into the usefulness of drug therapy. Most clinicians begin treatment with fluid and salt loading.

Although there are relatively sparse data to substantiate this approach, it is inexpensive, rational, practical, and probably carries little risk of morbidity. If this is unhelpful, both α-agonists and β-blockers are promising treatments. The data are strong enough to support their use although neither is proven to be useful.

The Evidence for Pacemaker Treatment

What can be done to help patients who either do not respond to medical therapy, or do not tolerate it? The American College of Cardiology/American Heart Association Task Force [15] and the British Pacing and Electrophysiology Group [16] recommend pacing for neurally mediated syncope, as either equivocal or firm recommendations. The clinical data to support these recommendations are as follows. Temporary transvenous pacing is partially effective in reducing the proportion of patients who faint during tilt table testing. The results of four reports taken together [17] showed that temporary dual chamber pacing prevented the development of syncope on tilt table testing in 24/41 subjects (57%), although most conscious subjects became lightheaded. These acute pacing studies suggested that permanent pacing might be helpful.

Several groups have reported studies of the usefulness of chronic pacing in the prevention of neurally mediated syncope. Petersen et al. [18] reported a pioneering study of dual chamber pacing in 37 syncope patients. They were a moderately symptomatic population, having had a median of 6 syncopal spells at a median frequency of 2 syncopal spells per year, and had a positive tilt test ending in a heart rate less than 60 beats/min. Of the 37 patients, 31 received pacemakers with rate hysteresis. Over a mean follow-up of 50 months 62% of the patients remained free of syncope, and 89% reported symptomatic improvement. The number of syncopal spells in the total population fell from an expected number of 136 to only 11. These results were very encouraging for the development of pacemaker therapy for syncope patients.

Several years later Benditt et al. [19] reported equally encouraging results in a study of 36 patients with predominantly vasovagal syncope. They were very symptomatic, having had a median of 10 syncopal spells over a median of 24 months, or about 5 spells yearly. All patients received a novel pacemaker with automatic rate drop responsiveness. This pacemaker can be programmed to sense small drops in heart rate and respond with temporary high rate pacing at rates of 100-120 beats/min. They were followed for a mean of 6 months. During this time, syncope recurred in only 6 patients, compared to an expected rate of recurrences in about 30 patients. Therefore in this relatively short-term study, pacing may have benefited about 80% of patients.

Finally, we studied 12 extremely symptomatic patients who had had a median syncope frequency of 3 spells/month [20]. All had had recurrent syncope after tilt testing and while on medical therapy. All received a pacemaker with a unique rate-smoothing feature that prevented abrupt drops in heart rate, but did not have a high rate response. Following implantation of the pacemaker, the actuarial syncope-free survival increased 20-fold, the syncope frequency dropped by 93%, and quality of life improved highly significantly. The patients had been selected on the basis of highly frequent syncope, and all had syncope early after tilt testing.

These studies provided hope that pacemaker therapy would be helpful to patients with frequent and highly symptomatic vasovagal syncope. Interestingly, the 3 programming modes – rate hysteresis, rate-drop responsiveness, and rate smoothing – appeared to be comparably effective. In the total population of 79 patients the pacemakers provided partial or complete symptomatic relief to at least 80% of patients.

These reports led to the Vasovagal Pacemaker Study (VPS), which was a randomized clinical trial of permanent pacemaker in patients with frequently recurrent vasovagal syncope [21]. There were 54 patients enrolled in this trial. All had fainted at least 6 times, and all had a positive tilt test with development of a relative bradycardia. They had had a median of 14-35 syncopal spells before pacemaker insertion. Half received a dual-chamber pacemaker with rate-drop responsiveness and half received conventional medical therapy. Of the 27 patients in each arm, 19 control patients fainted and 6 paced patients fainted. There was a relative reduction in the risk of syncope of 85% in the paced patients ($p = 0.00002$). In contrast, pacing did not reduce the number of presyncopal spells. This was the first randomized controlled trial of pacemaker therapy in vasovagal syncope, and showed that permanent pacing markedly reduces the recurrence of syncope in severely symptomatic patients.

Although it now seems clear that insertion of a permanent pacemaker provides considerable symptomatic relief to most patients with frequent vasovagal syncope, several important issues remain. The VPS I population was a highly selected, highly symptomatic patient group. They had fainted often, had a relative bradycardia on tilt testing, and were willing to participate in a protocol with a 50% chance of receiving a pacemaker. Whether these results can be extrapolated to other patients with vasovagal syncope is not known. Strictly speaking, the studies have only shown that implanting a pacemaker reduces the frequency of vasovagal syncope. We do not know how much of the benefit is due to a placebo effect, or to what extent specific programming features are required to obtain a benefit from pacemaker therapy. Clinical experience suggests that anxiety may play a role in inducing some episodes of vasovagal syncope, and anxiety reduction may have been beneficial. However, if this were the case one might have expected to see a reduction in presyncope, which did not occur.

Pacemaker and Medical Therapies

For most patients, education and reassurance are enough. Many patients appear to restrict their dietary salt intake, and having them increase their salt intake with the possible adjunctive use of fludrocortisone is prudent. If these simple measures are ineffective then the most reasonable next therapy is either a β-blocker or an α-agonist. These are simple, noninvasive, inexpensive treatments that can be readily discontinued if necessary. Despite these measures, however, some patients will continue to faint. For these highly symptomatic and drug-resistant patients, permanent pacing is now a reasonable option.

There may be special circumstances to consider when selecting patients for pacing. Physicians may have a lower decision threshold for inserting a pacemaker in patients for whom a faint might pose particularly severe risks, such as commercial drivers, pilots, scaffold workers, roofers, and so on. In contrast, there is no evidence that the degree of bradycardia developed on a tilt test either identifies patients at increased risk of recurrent syncope or death, or patients more likely to respond to pacing [22]. Finally, pacemaker therapy could be considered for patients who do not tolerate medical therapies.

References

1. Rose S, Koshman M, McDonald S, Sheldon R (1996) Health-related quality of life in patients with neuromediated syncope. Can J Cardiol 12:131E (abstr)
2. Sheldon RS (1995) What do we know today about the outcome of vasovagal syncope? In: Raviele A (ed) Cardiac Arrhythmias 1995. Springer, New York Berlin Heidelberg, pp 122-126
3. Sheldon R, Rose S, Flanagan P, Koshman ML, Killam S (1996) Risk factors for syncope recurrence after a positive tilt table test in patients with syncope. Circulation 93:973-981
4. Malik P, Koshman ML, Sheldon RS (1997) Timing of first syncope recurrence predicts syncope frequency following a positive tilt table test. J Am Coll Cardiol 29:1284-1289
5. El-Sayed H, Hainsworth R (1996) Salt supplement increases plasma volume and orthostatic tolerance in patients with unexplained syncope. Heart 75:134-140
6. Mangru NN, Young ML, Mas MS, Chandar JS, Pearse, LA, Wolff GS (1996) Usefulness of tilt table test with normal saline infusion in management of neurocardiogenic syncope in children. Am Heart J 131:953-955
7. Scott WA, Giacomo P, Bromberg BI, Schaffer MS, Deal BJ, Fish FA, Dick M (1995) Randomised comparison of atenolol and fludrocortisone acetate in the treatment of pediatric neurally mediated syncope. Am J Cardiol 76:400-402
8. Grubb BP, Temesy-Armos P, Moore J, Wolfe D, Hahn H, Elliot L (1992) The use of head-upright tilt table testing in the evaluation and management of syncope in children and adolescents. Pacing Clin Electrophysiol 15:742-748
9. Balaji S, Oslizlok PC, Allen MC, McKay CA, Gillette PC (1994) Neurocardiogenic syncope in children with a normal heart. J Am Coll Cardiol 23:779-785
10. Giada F, Raviele A, Brignole M, Sutton R, Alboni P, Giani P, Menozzi C, Moya A (1999) Effect of etilefrine in preventing syncopal spells in patients with recurrent vasovagal syncope: a double-blind, randomized trial. J Am Coll Cardiol 33:269A
11. Natale A, Beheiry S, Tomassoni GF, Leonelli FM, Pisano E, Fanelli R, Zimmerman L, Kim VH (1999) Randomized placebo control assessment of midodrine in the treatment of neurocardiogenic syncope. J Am Coll Cardiol 33:269A
12. Cox MM, Perlman BA, Mayor MR, Silberstein TA, Levin E, Pringle L, Castellanos A, Myerburg R (1995) Acute and long-term beta-adrenergic blockade for patients with neurocardiogenic syncope. J Am Coll Cardiol 26:1293-1298

13. Sheldon RS, Rose S, Flanagan P, Koshman ML, Killam S (1997) Effect of beta blockers on the clinical outcome of patients after a positive isoproterenol-tilt table test. Am J Cardiol 78:536-539

14. Mahanonda N, Bhuripanyo K, Kangkagate C, Wansanit K, Kulchot B, Nademanee K, Chaithiraphan S (1995) Randomized double-blind, placebo-controlled trial of oral atenolol in patients with unexplained syncope and positive upright tilt table test results. Am Heart J 130:1250-1253

15. Derives LS, Fisch C, Griffin JC, Gillette PC, Mason JW, Parsonnet V (1991) Guidelines for implantation of cardiac pacemakers and antiarrhythmia devices. A report of the American College of Cardiology/American Heart Association Task Force on Assessment of Diagnostic and Therapeutic Procedures (Committee on Pacemaker Implantation). J Am Coll Cardiol 18:1-13

16. Clarke M, Sutton R, Ward D, Camm AJ, Rickards A, Ingram A, Perrins EJ, Charles R, Jones S, Cobbe S (1991) Recommendations for pacemaker prescriptions for symptomatic bradycardia. British Pacing and Electrophysiology Group Working Party report. Br Heart J 66:185-191

17. Benditt DG, Petersen M, Lurie KG, Grubb BP, Sutton R (1995) Cardiac pacing for the prevention of recurrent vasovagal syncope. Ann Intern Med 122:204-209

18. Petersen MEV, Chamberlain-Webber R, Fitzpatrick AP, Ingram A, Williams T, Sutton R (1994) Permanent pacing for cardioinhibitory malignant vasovagal syndrome. Br Heart J 71:274-281

19. Benditt DG, Sutton R, Gammage M, Fetter J, Markowitz T and the Rate-drop Response Investigators (1997) Clinical experience with Thera DR rate drop response pacing algorithm in carotid sinus syndrome and vasovagal syncope. Pacing Clin Electrophysiol 20:832-839

20. Sheldon RS, Koshman ML, Wilson W, Kieser T, Rose S (1997) Effect of dual-chamber pacing with automatic rate-drop sensing on recurrent neurally mediated syncope. Am J Cardiol 81:158-162

21. Connolly SJ, Sheldon RS, Roberts RS, Gent M (1999) The North American Vasovagal Pacemaker Study. A randomized trial of permanent cardiac pacemaker for the prevention of vasovagal syncope. J Am Coll Cardiol 33:16-20

22. Menozzi C, Brignole M, Lolli G, Bottoni N, Oddone D, Gianfranchi L, Gaggioli G (1993) Follow-up of asystolic episodes in patients with cardioinhibitory, neurally mediated syncope and VVI pacemaker. Am J Cardiol 72:1152-1155

Patient-Activated Implantable Drug Delivery System for Treatment of Vasovagal Syncope: A Simple Solution?

A. RAVIELE, F. GIADA, G. GASPARINI, S. THEMISTOCLAKIS, A. BONSO AND A. CORRADO

Background

Vasovagal events, like many other autonomic nervous system disturbances, have a cyclic and unpredictable course with usually brief periods of symptom recrudescence (so-called "clusters") alternating with sometimes very long periods of quiescence and asymptomatic status [1, 2]. Thus, chronic therapy with drugs does not appear indicated in the majority of cases and is often associated with serious or intolerable side effects as well as poor patient compliance, especially in young people [3]. Moreover, when events occur, prevention of vasovagal reaction usually requires high drug plasma levels which are difficult to attain through chronic oral administration [4]. Indeed, only occasionally have oral drugs proved to be effective in the few double-blind, randomized, placebo-controlled trials performed to date [5-9]. It is also noteworthy that electrical treatment with a pacemaker, even when useful, rarely leads to complete elimination of symptoms [10, 11], because of the hypotensive effects of the vasodepressor reflex that is practically present in all subjects, generally precedes cardioinhibition and bradycardia [12] and is not amenable to correction or reversal by cardiac pacing. For all these reasons, it seems logical and desirable to develop an implantable drug delivery system for treatment of vasovagal syncope [3]. Such a device would allow the automatic "on demand" delivery of a bolus of a vasoactive or a cardioactive drug, previously recognized to be effective and safe in preventing tilt-induced syncope, possibly together with the activation of sequential cardiac pacing.

Key-Issues for the Development of a Fully Automatic Drug Delivery System

There are a number of key issues to be addressed prior to implementation of a fully automatic drug pump for treatment of vasovagal syncope. They include:
- The search for the most appropriate drug to be used for this purpose

Divisione di Cardiologia, Ospedale Umberto I, Mestre, Venice, Italy

- The choice of a reliable marker for an imminent vasovagal faint
- Conception and building of the device

At the present, the latter two problems are difficult to overcome.

Rationale for a Patient-Activated Drug Delivery System

However, besides a fully automatic pump, there is also the possibility of using a patient-activated drug delivery system. Indeed, about 70% of patients with frequently recurrent vasovagal syncope have prodromes for a sufficiently long period of time to allow the patient to activate the device manually [13] and interrupt the vasovagal reaction before syncope occurs. Moreover, it is easy to modify some already commercially available patient-activated pumps, such as Algomed (Medtronic Inc., Minneapolis, USA) currently used for delivery of pain-relieving drugs into the spinal area in patients with cancer or other painful diseases, and render them suitable for delivery of a vasoactive or a cardioactive drug directly into circulation (preferably into the right cardiac chambers) in patients with vasovagal syncope (Fig. 1). Thus, the main problem that nowadays remains to be solved for a patient-activated drug delivery system for treating vasovagal syncope is the choice of an appropriate drug.

Ideal Drug for a Patient-Activated Drug Delivery System

The ideal drug for a patient-activated pump should have the following properties: it should be fast-acting, to minimize the intervention delay in order to achieve the

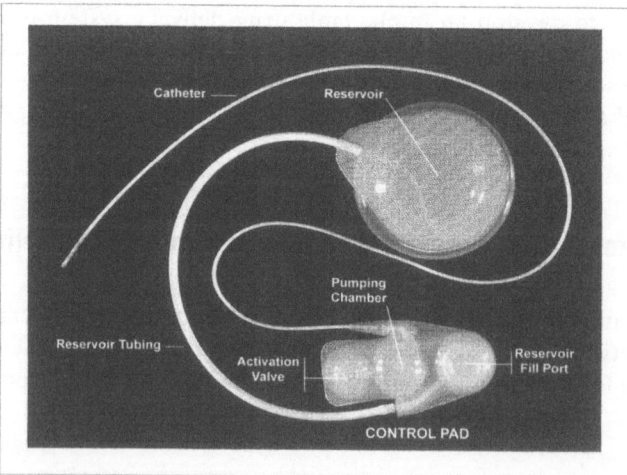

Fig. 1. Prototype of patient-activated drug delivery system for treatment of vasovagal syncope derived from the Algomed system (Medtronic Inc., Minneapolis, USA)

goal of aborting syncope; it should have a short duration of action, to eliminate or reduce side effects and to permit repeated drug infusions, if necessary [12, 14]; and, finally, it should be stable over time at body temperature and its effective dose should be contained in a small volume, to prevent frequent refilling of the drug reservoir [12, 14].

Evaluation of Phenylephrine as Pharmacological Agent for a Patient-Activated Drug Delivery System

Among the theoretically potential candidates, phenylephrine, an alpha-agonist agent with potent vasoconstrictor effect, currently used to treat hypotensive crises in the operating room and to asses baroreflex sensitivity after myocardial infarction [15], is probably the most appropriate drug for this application. Its action is almost immediate [16], the half-life is 5 min [17] and the drug is safe and well tolerated at a recommended dosage of 0.5-1.0 mg (as bolus) [16, 18, 19]. Finally, in sterile water for injection phenylephrine is stable for a long time (up to 84 days at 60°) [20] and the effective dose is concentrated in a small volume (1 ml of the drug preparation contains 10 mg of the active principle).

Pilot Study with Phenylephrine

In order to establish the value of phenylephrine as pharmacological agent for a drug delivery system for treatment of vasovagal syncope, we performed in our institution a pilot study [21] in which the efficacy and safety of phenylephrine in aborting tilt-induced syncope were tested.

Patients and Methods

Ten patients (nine women and one man, mean age 44 ± 18 years, range 21-73) were studied. All had frequent episodes of vasovagal syncope (median number 18, range 6-100) before entry into the study and all had been non-responder to at least two drugs chronically administered per os. In all cases baseline head-up tilt testing was reproducibly positive. The type of response during tilt-induced syncope was mixed in six patients, cardioinhibitory in three and vasodepressor in one. We used a shortened version of sublingual nitroglycerin head-up tilt testing as tilt protocol: initially, patients were tilted up at 60° for 20 min without medication; if syncope did not occur, patients were given 300 μg nitroglycerin sublingually and continued to be tilted up at the same angle for another 20 min or until syncope occurred [22, 23]. After baseline evaluation, each patient underwent two further tilt tests with the same protocol; in one a bolus of phenylephrine (1 mg in 3 ml of saline solution) was injected into the right atrium, through a catheter introduced via the right internal jugular vein, at the time the patient became symptomatic and blood pressure suddenly decreased to less than 50% of basal values; in the other the same volume of placebo (saline solution) was administered at the same time. Both tests were performed on the same day in a randomized sequence, one shortly after the other.

Results

The main results may be summarized as follows. All patients experienced a vasovagal reaction during both head-up tilt tests, with phenylephrine and placebo injection. The administration of phenylephrine caused a significant and immediate rise in blood pressure capable of aborting syncope in six patients and restoring consciousness in three patients within a few seconds after injection, although the subjects continued to be tilted up at the same angle. Only one patient who had severe cardioinhibitory reflex, failed to respond to the drug. In contrast, the administration of placebo was never successful in avoiding syncope. Phenylephrine was well tolerated in every case. The efficacy of phenylephrine was significantly higher than that of placebo (90% vs 0%, $p < 0.001$).

In Table 1 the mean values of systolic blood pressure, diastolic blood pressure and heart rate are reported at different times during the two head-up tilt tests performed with phenylephrine and placebo injection, respectively. The mean values of these parameters did not significantly differ with the patient in supine position before tilt, just after tilting started, at the onset of symptoms and at the time of phenylephrine and placebo injection. This suggests a similar extent of the vasovagal reaction in both tests. It is important to note that, when phenylephrine and placebo were administered, the mean value of systolic blood pressure was < 60 mmHg and that of heart rate around 65-75 beats per minute. Following phenylephrine injection, heart rate continued to decrease (from 65 to 48 beats per minute) as an expression of the baroreceptor reflex activated by the drug-induced increase in blood pressure. The maximum values of systolic and diastolic blood pressure after phenylephrine injection were 163 mmHg and 96 mmHg, respectively.

Table 2 shows that the time between the onset of symptoms and the injection of phenylephrine or placebo was similar (43 s and 60 s, respectively). Following phenylephrine injection, the first effect of the drug was observed

Table 1. Blood pressure (BP) and heart rate during head-up tilt testing with placebo and phenylephrine injections in the studied patients (mean ± SD)

	Systolic BP (mmHg)			Diastolic BP (mmHg)			Heart rate (bpm)		
	placebo	phenyl	p	placebo	phenyl	p	placebo	phenyl	p
Supine	121 ± 24	134 ± 23	ns	65 ± 17	77 ± 15	ns	72 ± 9	75 ± 16	ns
60° tilt	117 ± 20	133 ± 33	ns	72 ± 17	81 ± 20	ns	88 ± 16	79 ± 13	ns
Onset od symptoms	81 ± 23	90 ± 27	ns	53 ± 17	60 ± 18	ns	90 ± 17	94 ± 24	ns
Injection	52 ± 15	56 ± 18	ns	37 ± 13	39 ± 13	ns	74 ± 14	65 ± 17	ns
End point	43 ± 16	66 ± 16	< 0.05	31 ± 12	45 ± 20	< 0.05	64 ± 17	50 ± 15	ns
Maximum effect	-	169 ± 54		-	96 ± 28		-	48 ± 11	

End point, syncope or restoration of consciousness; BP, blood pressure; phenyl, phenylphrine

Table 2. Timing of the effects of placebo and phenylephrine injections during head-up tilt testing in the studied patients (mean ± SD)

	Time (s)		
	Placebo	Phenylephrine	p
Onset of symptoms to injection	43 ± 22	60 ± 38	ns
Injection to onset of effect	-	9.4 ± 7.2	
Injection to end point	45 ± 29	14 ± 7	< 0.01
Injection to tilt-down	54 ± 27	-	
Injection to maximum effect	-	72 ± 19	
Injection to baseline values	-	490 ± 222	

End point, syncope or restoration of consciousness

within a mean time of 9.4 ± 7.2 s and all patients who recovered consciousness did so within 14 ± 7 s. The maximum effect of phenylephrine was observed after 72 ± 19 s. Blood pressure and heart rate took about 8 minutes to return to baseline values, after wich patients were returned to the supine position. Following placebo injection, syncope developed after a mean time of 45 ± 29 s and patients were returned to the supine position within 54 ± 27 s.

Figures 2 and 3 represent the time-course of heart rate and blood pressure during head-up tilt testing with phenylephrine and placebo injection, respectively, in one of the patients studied.

Conclusions

The above-described results, together with some literature data [24, 25], clearly indicate that phenylephrine is effective and safe in aborting tilt-induced syncope. They also suggest that the drug may be appropriately used in an implantable drug pump for treatment of vasovagal syncope. However, further studies are needed to verify this possibility.

Future Studies

In cooperation with Medtronic Europe, we have designed and built a prototype of a patient-activated drug delivery system for the treatment of vasovagal syncope, consisting of a modification of the already existing drug pump called Algomed (Medtronic Inc., Minneapolis, USA) (Fig. 1). We are starting clinical evaluation of this prototype in our institution. The study will involve two phases, an acute phase and a chronic phase. In the acute phase we will assess the functioning of the system during head-up tilt testing without implanting it, while in the chronic phase we will assess the efficacy and safety of the implanted system during patient lifetime. In both phases phenylephrine will be used as the active drug. The results of this study will be available by the year 2000.

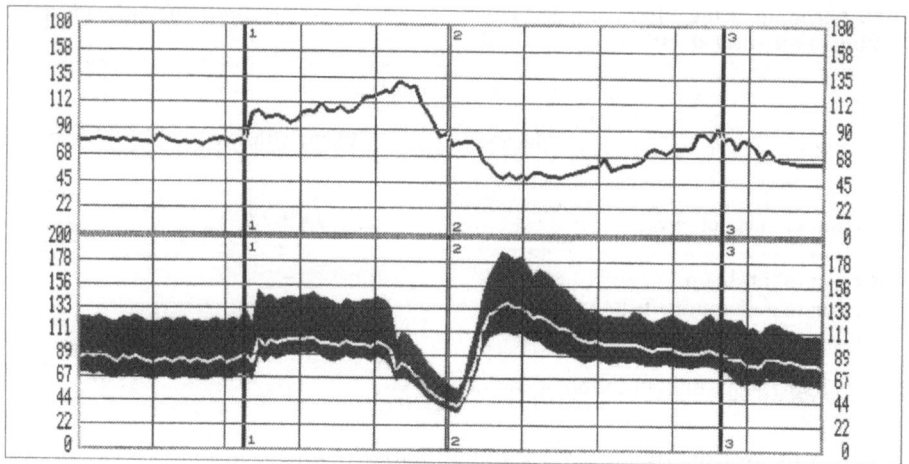

Fig. 2. Graph representing the time-course of heart rate (*upper panel*) and blood pressure (*lower panel*) during head-up tilt testing with phenylephrine injection in one of our patients. The drug was injected in coincidence with the vertical bar *2*, when blood pressure and heart rate suddenly decreased and the patient become syncopal. Phenylephrine was able to significantly increase blood pressure and restore consciousness although the patient continued to be tilted up. Note the further decrease in heart rate secondary to the increase in blood pressure, as expression of the activation of the baroreceptor reflex. Vertical bar *1* indicates onset of tilting; vertical bar *3* indicates termination of tilting with return of the patient to supine position. Heart rate values are expressed in beats/minute and blood pressure values in mmHg

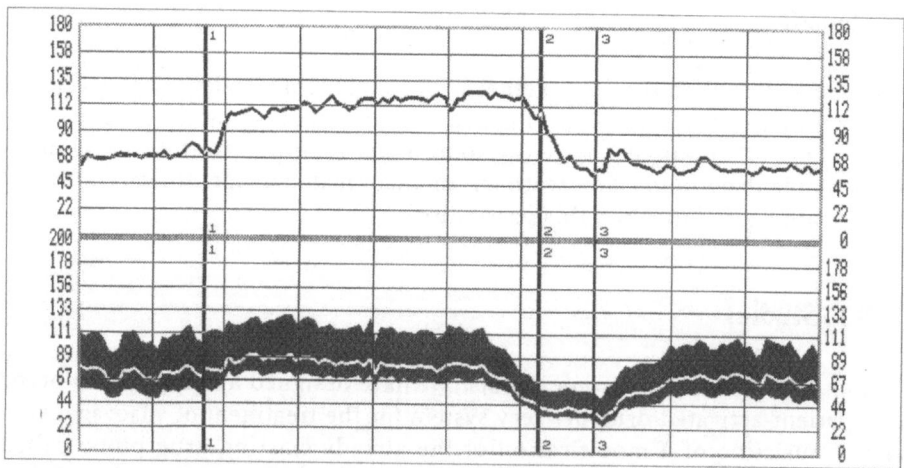

Fig. 3. Graph representing the time-course of heart rate (*upper panel*) and blood pressure (*lower panel*) during head-up tilt testing with placebo injection in the same patient as in Fig. 2. The placebo was injected at the same time as phenylephrine (vertical bar *2*) but did not prevent syncope; blood pressure and heart rate continued to decrease and patient had to be returned to supine position (vertical bar *3*) to restore consciousness. Vertical bar *1* indicates onset of tilting. Heart rate values are expressed in beats/minute and blood pressure values in mmHg

References

1. Sheldon R, Rose S, Flanagan P et al (1996) Risk factors for syncope recurrence after a positive tilt table test in patients with syncope. Circulation 93:973-981
2. Raviele A, Themistoclakis S, Gasparini G (1996) Drug treatment of vasovagal syncope. In: Blanc JJ, Benditt D, Sutton R (eds) Neurally mediated syncope: pathophysiology, investigations and treatment. Futura, Armonk, NY, pp 113-117
3. Raviele A, Brignole M, Menozzi C, Giada F (1997) Development of an implantable drug delivery system for the treatment of vasovagal syncope: a dream or a real prospect? In: Raviele A (ed) Cardiac Arrhythmias 1997. Springer-Verlag Italia, Milan, pp 422-427
4. Kelly PA, Mann DE, Adler SW et al (1994) Low dose disopyramide often fails to prevent neurogenic syncope during head-up tilt testing. PACE 11:1202-1206
5. Fitzpatrick AP, Ahmed R, William S, Sutton R (1991) A randomized trial of medical therapy in "malignant vasovagal syndrome" or neurally-mediated bradycardia/hypotension syndrome. Eur J Cardiac Pacing Electrophysiol 2:99-102
6. Brignole M, Menozzi C, Gianfranchi L et al (1992) A controlled trial of acute and long-term medical therapy in tilt-induced neurally mediated syncope. Am J Cardiol 70:339-342
7. Morillo CA, Leitch JW, Yee R, Klein GJ (1993) A placebo-controlled trial of intravenous and oral disopyramide for prevention of neurally mediated syncope induced by head-up tilt. J Am Coll Cardiol 22:1843-1848
8. Raviele A, Brignole M, Sutton R et al (1999) Effect of etilefrine in preventing syncopal recurrence in patients with vasovagal syncope. A double-blind, randomized, placebo-controlled trial. Circulation 99:1452-1457
9. Di Girolamo E, Di Iorio C, Sabatini P et al (1999) Effects of paroxetine hydrochloride, a selective serotonin reuptake inhibitor, on refractory vasovagal syncope: a randomized, double-blind, placebo-controlled study. J Am Coll Cardiol 33:1227-1230
10. Petersen MEV, Chamberlain-Webber R, Fitzpatrick AP, Ingram A, Williams T, Sutton R (1994) Permanent pacing for cardioinhibitory malignant vasovagal syndrome. Br Heart J 71:274-281
11. Connolly SJ, Sheldon R, Roberts RS, Gent M (1999) The North American Vasovagal Pacemaker Study (VPS). A randomized trial of permanent cardiac pacing for the prevention of vasovagal syncope. J Am Coll Cardiol 33:16-20
12. Raviele A, Gasparini G, Di Pede F, Delise P, Bonso A, Piccolo E (1990) Usefulness of head-up tilt test in evaluating patients with syncope of unknown origin and negative electrophysiologic study. Am J Cardiol 65:1322-1327
13. Brignole M, Menozzi C, Corbucci G, Garberoglio B, Plicchi G (1997) Detecting incipient vasovagal reaction: intraventricular acceleration. PACE 20(Pt.II):801-805
14. Nappolz T (1994) Combination of drug delivery systems and implantable cardioverter-defibrillators: is there a possible marriage? In: Singor I (ed) Implantable cardioverter-defibrillator. Futura, Armonk, NY, pp 731-749
15. La Rovere MT, Specchia G, Mortara A, Schwartz PJ (1988) Baroreflex sensitivity, clinical correlates, and cardiovascular mortality among patients with a first myocardial infarction. A prospective study. Circulation 78:816-824
16. Arky R (1996) Physicians' Desk Reference. Medical Economic Company, Montvale, NY
17. Hengstmann JH, Goronzy J (1982) Pharmacokinetics of 3H phenylephrine in man. Eur J Clin Pharmacol 21:335-341

18. USPDI (1996) Drug information for the health care professional, 16th ed. US Pharmaceutical Convention, Rockville, Md

19. Reynolds JEF (1993) Martindale: The Extra Pharmacopoeia. The Pharmaceutical Press, London

20. Weber JC, Gupta VD (1970) Stability of phenylephrine HCl in intravenous solutions. Am J Hosp Pharm 28:200

21. Giada F, Raviele A, Giardiello G, De Seta F (1999) Evaluation of efficacy of phenylephrine to abort syncope during tilt table testing: the first step for the development of an implantable drug delivery system for treatment of vasovagal syncope. PACE 22:756 (abstr)

22. Raviele A, Menozzi C, Brignole M et al (1995) Value of head-up tilt testing potentiated with sublingual nitroglycerin to assess the origin of unexplained syncope. Am J Cardiol 76:267-272

23. Giada F, Themistoclakis S, Brignole M et al (1997) Short-duration pharmacological head-up tilt test: low-dose isoproterenol or nitroglycerin? J Am Coll Cardiol 29:468A (abstr)

24. Strieper MJ, Campbell RM (1993) Efficacy of alpha-adrenergic agonist therapy for prevention of pediatric neurocardiogenic syncope. J Am Coll Cardiol 22:594-597

25. Mangru NN, Young ML, Mas MD, Chandar JS, Pearse LA, Wolff GS (1996) Usefulness of tilt test with normal saline solution infusion in management of neurocardiac syncope in children. Am Heart J 131:953-955

PACEMAKER

Lead Extraction: How Easy and Safe Is It Today?

M.G. Bongiorni, G. Arena, E. Soldati, G. Gherarducci and M. Mariani

The introduction of the techniques for transvenous lead removal in clinical practice have changed the management of infected or abandoned implanted cardiac
devices. Retention of functionless pacing leads is becoming relatively common
because the performance of implanted leads decreases over time [1, 2]. Moreover,
although the structural complexity of last-generation pacing leads (bipolar leads,
preshaped leads, J-retention wire leads, etc.) allows better pacing therapy, it also
exposes the patients to new and old complications such as crashes, insulation failures, cardiac chamber perforations, and venous occupation. Infection is another
complication of the pacing systems; it is reported to occur in 0%-19% of patients
[3, 4].

Implantable cardioverter defibrillators (ICD) have many features in common
with implanted pacemakers. Both systems consist of electrodes and a pulse generator, and are manufactured using the same materials. The endocardial defibrillating leads seem to produce the same complications as occur with transvenous
pacing leads. Thus, conductor fractures at the sites of stress or of the binding
sutures are possible, as well as insulation failures due to mechanical stress or
enzymatic degradation of polyurethane. Infections occurring after implantation
of an ICD are a very dangerous condition, with a reported incidence of 2%-7%.

Indications for Lead Removal

The indications for pacing and ICD lead removal are today divided into the categories mandatory, necessary, and discretionary [5].

Mandatory conditions are typically life-threatening conditions such as sep-
ticemia, endocarditis, or myocarditis, or the presence of a fragmented lead with
the possibility of lead migration and ventricular tachyarrhythmias. Obliteration
of all the usable veins is another mandatory indication, because reimplantation is
then possible only after removal of the old lead. Documented device interferences

Unità di Aritmologia Interventistica, Dipartimento Cardiovascolare e Polmonare,
Ospedale Cisanello, Pisa, Italy

caused by multiple leads, particularly in ICD patients at risk of inappropriate shocks, are an indication for their removal. Recurrent fever despite antibiotic therapy in patients with an implanted pacemaker or defibrillator is another indication for removal of the hardware system, if all other causes of infection can be clearly excluded.

Necessary conditions are those which may later become life-threatening. Some examples are pocket infection, chronic draining sinus, and pacing system erosion with partial exposure of the pacemaker and/or the leads. It is well known that too many leads in the venous system can produce a fibrous reaction with vein obliteration and, possibly, superior vena cava syndrome when the leads come from opposite sides; therefore, in the presence of a lead failure and if a third lead or more leads are needed, extraction of the functionless ones may be necessary. The possibility of device interferences caused by multiple leads, particularly in ICD patients at risk of inappropriate shocks, should be an indication for their removal.

Discretionary conditions are all cases of noninfected functionless or abandoned pacing leads. This is a controversial indication for lead removal: although abandoned leads do not cause any symptomatic abnormalities for many years, the incidence of asymptomatic thrombosis has been reported to be as high as 44%; moreover, the difficulty of removing the leads increases over time. Discretionary conditions are probably influenced by other variables like the patient's age and his/her clinical conditions, or the implant duration of the leads.

The indications for removal of particular leads (Telectronics, Accufix, and Encor leads) depend mainly on the lesions of the J-retention wire, with other factors such as patient age and life-style being taken into consideration.

Factors Affecting the Feasibility and Safety of Lead Removal

Many factors and conditions can play an important role in transvenous removal procedures. These factors may affect: (1) the feasibility of the removal, (2) the complexity and duration of the procedure, (3) the outcome of the attempt, and (4) the complications. Some can be predicted before the procedure, while others can only be observed once the removal procedure has started.

The factors making a lead extraction procedure difficult can be divided into technical and clinical.

Technical factors relate to various physical aspects of pacing and defibrillating leads.

- *Fixation mechanism.* In the literature [6], pacing leads provided with an active fixation mechanism are reported to be extracted with a higher success rate than other fixation mechanisms. This may be related to the different way in which the tip adheres to the myocardial wall, because detachment of the tip is easier once the screw has been retracted or unscrewed. On the other hand, removal of an unscrewed lead is more difficult than that of a tined lead. It must be pointed out that some fixation mechanisms that cannot be unscrewed, such as the helix of the Vitatron Helifix, make the procedure carry a very high risk of myocardial perforation and cardiac tamponade.

- *Lead polarity.* Bipolar leads usually require more complex and time-consuming procedures. The complexity of a bipolar lead results in increased fragility of the lead; traction can result in detachment of the inner coil and insulation from the outer coil, leading to a partial removal of the lead. In addition, the presence of a proximal electrode is often associated with a variation of the diameter of the lead; this can be responsible for more frequent adherences, greater difficultty in retrieving the lead from the vein of insertion, and, finally, greater difficulty in dilating the adherences.
- *Lead insulation.* Polyurethane is more fragile than silicon insulation, whether used as outer insulation for the lead or as insulation between the inner and the outer coils. As a consequence, the removal of a polyurethane lead must be performed with delicacy and is time-consuming. In the absence of insulation failures, no differences in the outcome of the procedures were found between silicon and polyurethane leads.
- *Lead shape and diameter.* As already said about the lead polarity, a completely cylindrical lead shape, i.e. one that is isodiametric from the connector to the tip, allows easier retraction of the lead once the tip is free. Moreover, dilation of adherences is facilitated by a uniform diameter. With very thin leads dilation is usually more difficult and requires care; this is due both to the difference between the lead shape and the size of the dilator sheath, and to the softness of the lead body, increasing the risk of lead fracture or venous tears.
- *Defibrillating leads.* In case of defibrillating leads all the above-mentioned features must be considered. In addition, these leads are provided with large exposed defibrillating coil electrodes; their particular design can lead to very extensive and tenacious adherences, requiring more complex removal procedures.
- *Intravascular leads.* The removal of intravascular leads is always a more complex procedure. When no part of the lead can be approached outside the vessels, the first problem is to catch the lead. This manoeuvre requires use of the transfemoral workstation. Furthermore, the lead must be accessible and one end of the lead must be free or made free. If using the transvenous approach can expose the proximal end of the lead, a standard procedure can be performed. Otherwise, traction, dilation and countertraction must be performed by the transvenous workstation; in this case, traction is usually more difficult, and dilation and countertraction are often impossible.
- *Fractured coil.* Fracture of the coil usually prevents the operator from advancing the locking stylet up to the tip of the lead, making internal traction impossible. Traction on the insulation sheath usually produces a fracture of the insulation, leading to a completely intravascular coil.
- *Insulation failure.* Damage to the insulation adversely affects the removal procedure. The damage to the lead insulation increases adherences to the venous wall and causes infiltration of the coil lumen, thus preventing the possibility of advancing the stylet up to the tip of the lead. Extensive deterioration of the lead

insulation can result in complete adherence of the lead to the vessels and epithelialization, making both transvenous and surgical removal very difficult.

- *J-retention wire fracture*. These fractures involve the Telectronics Accufix and Encor leads. The procedures for removing these complicated leads must be planned case by case depending on the fracture site, partial migration of a part of the wire, or the presence of multiple fractures. Generally the procedure is at high risk of complication because the fractured wire can perforate the heart or migrate during the attempt to remove it. Other tools, like catchers and lassos, are necessary to remove the J-wire before extracting the lead, strictly with a cardiosurgical standby.

- *Lead damage caused by previous unsuccessful removal attempts*. Often leads are seriously damaged by previous unsuccessful attempts at removal. The most frequent damage is straightening of the coil, with consequent irregular reduction of the coil lumen width, which make use of the locking stylet impossible. Other possible kinds of damage are coil fracture and insulation fractures, with the consequences described above.

- *Impervious coil lumen*. In various circumstances the locking stylet cannot be inserted or advanced inside the lead, because the coil lumen is not pervious. This is observed where there is a narrow bend of the coil (sometimes performed at the implant time), in the presence of various materials inside the coil (blood, inflammatory tissue, pieces of stylet) or infiltration following an insulation defect. This factor strongly affects the feasibility of the removal procedure, making the traction impossible. Sometimes countertraction can be performed using the lead without the stylet, while applying the external traction on its proximal end.

The *clinical factors* are:

- *Implant duration*. This is one of the most important factors affecting the difficulty, complexity and outcome of the removal procedure, and it is directly related to the presence and tightness of scar tissue. Often the removal procedure is easily performed by manual traction on the proximal end of the lead, if the latter has been implanted for less than 6 months. The complexity of the procedure increases the longer the lead has been implanted.

- *Number of leads*. In the presence of multiple leads, the procedures are more difficult and complex, and sometimes, if no further progress can be made on the first lead, switching attention to the next one may help, since removal of the first lead may be easier after the second is extracted. Multiple leads are often fibrosed all together.

- *Atrial or ventricular leads*. Ventricular leads are more difficult to extract than atrial leads, because of their adherences to the tricuspid valve and ventricular wall.

- *Calcified scar tissue*. The presence of scar tissue [7] is the primary reason for partial or failed removal of a lead; most complications are related to difficulties in freeing leads from these adherences. Scar tissue is usually present in multiple locations; the most frequent sites are the venous entry/subclavian area (66%) and the ventricle (72%). Older leads tend to be associated with more severe scarring and often calcifications are present. The presence of calcium around the lead, often visible at fluoroscopy, makes the extraction procedure nearly impossible; moreover, tears on the venous systems are often produced while performing dilation of these particular adherences.

Transvenous Techniques for Lead Removal

Transvenous techniques for lead removal are continuously evolving; to date the most extensive experience has been gained using mechanical sheath dissection/countertraction and excimer lase-assisted extraction.

Table 1 shows the findings of two great multicentre registries on mechanical sheath dissection. In the USA Registry the system provided by Cook Vascular was used. This system is provided with locking stylets and dilator sheaths [8-11]; they are used as a first choice when the proximal end of the lead is exposed (superior approach). A transvenous workstation with a tip deflecting wire, Dormier basket and loop retriever is the tool of choice in the case of totally intravascular leads (inferior approach). A similar system has been developed by VascoMed [12], and this was used in the Europe Registry. The VascoExtor system consists of a locking stylet provided with a remote control anchoring mechanism at the tip. A rotating motor can be applied to the stylet in order to facilitate advancement or withdrawal of the stylet. This system can be used on a wide range of coil lumen dimensions; one possible advantage is the possibility of withdrawal in the case of an unsuccessful attempt. A dilator sheath and a transfemoral workstation provided with a snare-loop catheter for intravascular lead extraction are also available. As shown in Table 1, the results of the two systems were quite similar.

Table 2 shows the results of two multicentre studies, PLEXES [13] and PLESSE [14], performed in recent years using excimer laser assisted techniques. Although results are similar to those of mechanical sheath techniques, the duration of procedures and, consequently, the radiation exposure are shorter; on the other hand, using laser techniques is more expensive. In the near future the cost/benefit ratios of mechanical and laser techniques must be carefully evaluated; probably most procedures can be performed by mechanical techniques, reserving laser techniques for difficult cases.

Table 1. Results of lead removal with mechanical sheath dissection

	USA Registry	Europe Registry
Years recorded	1988-1994	1990-1994
Total number of leads	2495	150
Number of leads per centre	11.4	21.4
System used	Cook Vascular	Vascomed
Success rate:		
Total success (%)	86.8	81
Partial success (%)	7.5	12
Failure (%)	5.7	7
Major complications (%)	2.5	0
Deaths (%)	0.9	0

Table 2. Results of lead removal with excimer laser-assisted techniques

	PLEXES [13]	PLESSE [14]
Years recorded	95-97	96-97
Total number of leads	1285	113
System used	Spectranetics	Spectranetics
Success rate:		
Total success (%)	90	92
Partial success (%)	3	4
Failure (%)	7	4
Major complications (%)	2.7	1.1
Deaths (%)	0.4	0
Median extraction time (min)	n.r.	12 (range 1-180)

n.r., not recorded

Electrodissection using radiofrequency, by Cook Vascular Inc., is another new technique for transvenous lead removal; it is based on the use of dilation sheaths connected to a radiofrequency generator able to induce a thermal effect at their distal end and allow cutting of the adherences. This technique is at present under clinical evaluation in the USA.

Personal Experience of Transvenous Lead Removal

From December 1989 to March 1999 we managed a total of 380 patients (275 men and 105 women, mean age 67 years, age range 17-93 years), with indications for the extraction of 593 leads that had been implanted for a mean period of 63 months (range 1-276 months). There were 562 pacemaker leads and 31 ICD leads; 390 were ventricular leads, 196 were atrial leads and the other 7 leads were implanted in the superior vena cava (ICD leads). The indications for extraction were mandatory in 36.3% of the leads, necessary in 54.2% and discretionary in 9.5%. The numbers of procedures have increased particularly in the last 3 years, as shown in Fig. 1, which reports the number of attempted lead extractions per year.

In our experience 91.6% of leads were removed; partial removal that did not solve the clinical problem was considered as failure. Major complications were observed in five patients (1.3%): in two cases cardiac tamponade, in two pulmonary embolism, and in one unitended dislodgement of another pacing lead. No deaths were observed during the procedures. However, three deaths (0.76%) occurred perioperatively because of: (1) ventricular fibrillation 10 days after extraction in a patient with long-standing systemic infection and myocarditis; (2) acute right ventricular failure 41 h after extraction in a patient with Down syndrome and Eisenmenger syndrome; at autopsy no lesion related to the procedure was found; (3) cardiac tamponade 12 h after extraction performed by gentle manual traction; the patient had in the past suffered pulmonary embolism and, because of sudden dyspnoea, was treated with intravenous heparina.

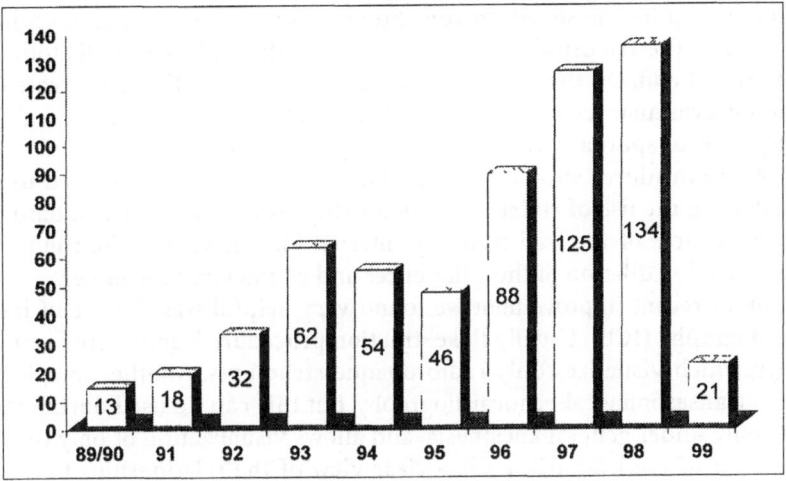

Fig. 1. Number of lead extraction procedures per year

The success rate has increased with growing experience; as shown in Fig. 2, it was about 70% in the first 2 years and about 98.5% in the last 2 years.

These results outline the importance of improvements of both materials and techniques to enhance the effectiveness of extraction procedures, and to reduce time and the risk of complications. The presence of adherences is in our experience a key reason for partial or failed removal of a lead; most complications are related to difficulties in freeing leads from these adherences. Dilation of adherences by sheaths is often highly symptomatic, inducing severe parasympathetic stimulation. Another relevant problem is the removal of intravascular leads; using the standard femoral approach, dilation of endoventricular adherences and coun-

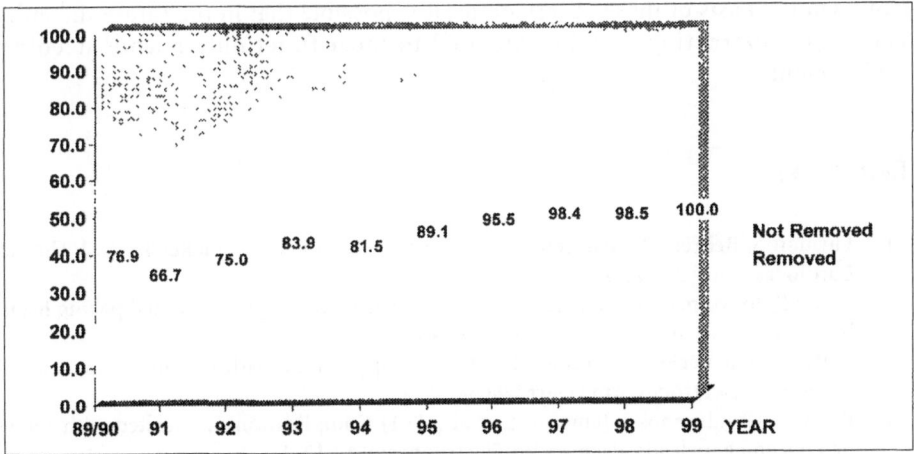

Fig. 2. Percentage of leads successfully removed per year

tertraction require the sheath to run through the inferior vena cava up into the right atrium, the tricuspid valve, and then into the right ventricle, following a very narrow bend. On the basis of these observations, for the last 3 years (in the case of intravascular leads and strong adherences) we have found the right internal jugular vein approach very useful. After percutaneous puncture and advancement of an introducer sheath into the vein, the leads could be exposed from this vein, allowing the use of stylets and dilator sheaths to perform a standard procedure. The course of the lead from the internal jugular vein to the right heart is straight, making dilation of the adherences and countertraction easier.

Another recent improvement we found very helpful was the use of intracardiac echography (ICE). Usually the extraction procedure is monitored using fluoroscopy, which visualizes only radio-opaque structures. Another imaging technique is transesophageal echocardiography, but this can be used during the procedure only under general anesthesia, and allows visualization of only the intracardiac tract of the lead. ICE gives a clear view of the relationships between the leads and most anatomical structures as well as of pathological findings. However, because of the costs and the need for an additional venous puncture and a dedicated operator, it is likealy that ICE will be of great utility only in selected cases: difficult cases or cases where there are multiple leads, suspicion of vegetation, old leads, intravascular leads, and so on.

Conclusions

Today transvenous removal of pacing and defibrillating leads is feasible with a high success rate and few complications. The experience of the team is a major factor influencing the outcome of the procedures. New techniques (laser, radiofrequency) may be very useful especially in reducing the duration of the procedures, while the use of new monitoring systems (ICE) may reduce the risks of complications. On the basis of these observations, it is possible that in the future the indications for extraction may be extended to most functionless leads needing replacement.

References

1. Furman S, Behrens M, Andrews C et al (1987) Retained pacemaker leads. J Thorac Cardiovasc Surg 94:770-772
2. Zerbe P, Ponizynski A, Dyszkiewicz W et al (1985) Functionless retained pacing leads in the cardiovascular system. Br Heart J 54:76-79
3. Rettig G, Doenecke P, Sen S et al (1979) Complications with retained transvenous pacemaker electrodes. Am Heart J 98:587-594
4. Parry G, Goudevenos J, Jameson S et al (1991) Complications associated with retained pacemakers leads. Pacing Clin Electrophysiol 14:1251-1257
5. Byrd CL, Schwartz SJ, Hedin NB (1992) Lead extraction: indications and techniques. Cardiol Clin 10:735-748

6. Heidi JM, Neal EF, Byrd CL, Wilkoff BL et al (1994) Five-years experience with intravascular lead extraction. Pacing Clin Electrophysiol 17:2016-2020

7. Robboy SJ, Harthorne JW, Leinbach RC et al (1969) Autopsy findings with permanent pervenous pacemakers. Circulation 39:495-501

8. Byrd CL, Schwartz SJ, Hedin NB et al (1990) Intravascular lead extraction using locking stylets and sheaths. Pacing Clin Electrophysiol 13:1871-1875

9. Byrd CL, Schwartz SJ, Hedin NB (1991) Intravascular techniques for extraction of permanent pacemakers leads. J Thorac Cardiovasc Surg 101:989-997

10. Bongiorni MG, Petz E, Levorato D et al (1991) Removal of chronic leads for permanent pacing. Clinical experience with transvenous extractors. In: Antonioli GE (ed) Pacemaker leads. Elsevier Science, Amsterdam, pp 289-294

11. Bongiorni MG, Arena G, Soldati E, De Simone L (1994) A "step by step" protocol for lead extraction procedures: relation with success rate and complications. Pacing Clin Electrophysiol 17, 4 (II): 786 (abstr)

12. Reinhardt J, Alt E, Neuzner J et al (1993) Clinic pacemaker lead removal using a new method in 38 patients with 61 implanted leads. Multicenter experience. Pacing Clin Electrophysiol 16:1175 (abstr)

13. Byrd C, Wilkoff B, Love C et al (1997) Clinical study of the laser sheath: results of the PLEXES trial. Pacing Clin Electrophysiol 20, 4 (II): 1053 (abstr)

14. Kennergren C (1997) Initial European experience with excimer laser assisted extraction of permanent pacemaker leads. Pacing Clin Electrophysiol 20, 4 (II): 1111 (abstr)

Pacemaker/ICD Patients: To Anticoagulate or Not To Anticoagulate?

M. Santomauro, A. Costanzo, L. Ottaviano, R. Cresta, S. Minichiello, M. Prastaro and M. Chiariello

Patients with atherosclerosis, valvular, ischemic, and dilatative cardiomyopathies, or atrial fibrillation, and those with a cardiac valvular prothesis, by-pass, pacemaker, or ICD, may be subject to thrombotic or thromboembolic events (TEEs). TEEs associated with the implantation or chronic presence of permanent pacing leads have been described in many case reports but are actually considered a relatively uncommon complication of cardiac pacing [1]. TEEs have traditionally been reported as a late problem (more than 1 month after implantation of a pacemaker or ICD), and embolic complications have been reported as occurring at any time following implantation. However, venous obstruction can also occurr soon after implantation [2, 3]. Venous stenosis and thrombosis after permanent cardiac pacing are probably more common than previously thought because most patients remain asymptomatic and the condition remains undetected. An understanding of the thromboembolic complications of transvenous cardiac pacing is important because prompt diagnosis and therapy may diminish the potential for morbidity and mortality. The pathogenesis of venous thrombosis after implantation of a permanent transvenous pacemaker or ICD has not been clearly determined. Possible causes of early thrombosis include the following:

1. Extrusion of thrombus from the ligated vein (especially with the cephalic vein approach)
2. Lead entry site
3. Lead-induced endothelial trauma, which causes local release of coagulation factors
4. Hypercoagulability induced by the surgical procedure
5. Atrioventricular asynchronism that causes numerous atrial contractions against closed atroventricular valves (this mechanism is even more significant in patients with 1:1 ventricular retrograde conduction)
6. Presence of the lead in the right ventricle
7. Old age in patients with pacemaker or ICD
8. Interventricular and intraventricular asynchronism of contraction.
   Venous thrombosis that occurs more than 1 year after implantation of a per-

Dipartimento di Cardiologia e Cardiochirurgia, Università Federico II, Naples, Italy

manent transvenous pacemaker is usually associated with underlying venous stenosis, which may result from fibrosis of preexistent venous thrombi. The long-term residence of a permanent lead in the venous system may also act a continuing nidus for formation of a thrombus [4-6]. The presence of multiple transvenous pacemaker leads, especially if one is severed, also increases the risk of thrombosis [7, 8]. In addition, the pacing lead may produce a foreign-body type of reaction and subsequent inflammation and fibrosis along the course of the lead. In some reports on the evaluation of antiplatelet therapy and platelet aggregability in patients with pacing [9, 10], Fazio et al. have shown an increase of TEEs (fatal and nonfatal stroke, fatal and nonfatal myocardial infarction, inferior limb thromboembolism) in patients treated with antiplatelet therapy compared to those not so treated ($p < 0.05$) [9]; they have shown a significant increase of β-Tromboglobulin (β-Tg) in paced patients with respect to controls. Even if their data do not conclusively demonstrate a precise causal relationship between platelet activation and increase of TEEs in patients with pacemakers or ICDs, they strongly suggest that antiplatelet drugs could represent a pathogenic treatment in these patients.

Symptomatic thrombosis of the upper extremities and central veins attributed to permanent transvenous leads is uncommon; it affects 0.3%-3% of patients with permanent transvenous leads [5, 11]. Most patients with chronic deep venous thrombosis remain asymptomatic because the gradual formation of a thrombus facilitates the development of an adequate venous collateral circulation. Symptomatic lead-induced deep venous thrombosis of the upper extremities or central veins generally implies either acute venous thrombosis or extension of a previously localized thrombus that occludes venous collaterals.

In the past, venous thrombosis has frequently been described in association with implantation of a permanent transvenous lead [11, 12]. The reported incidence of partial venous obstruction in association with permanent transvenous leads varies from 31% to 50%, and up to one-third of the patients have venous occlusion [11, 13-15]. Venous thrombosis, either partial obstruction or occlusion attributed to long-term residence of a transvenous pacing lead, most commonly involves the axillary or subclavian vein or the superior vena cava. At the time these reports were published, the insulation material used was polyethylene, which is rare in leads today – nowadays silicon or polyurethane leads are used. It has been demonstrated that venous thrombosis can occurr early after placement of a permanent transvenous lead [2]. The 23% incidence of partial or complete venous obstruction after short-term implantation of a permanent transvenous lead approximates that described in other series after long-term cardiac pacing [11].

Antonelli et al. described a prospective study of 40 consecutive patients who underwent transvenous cardiac pacing and had serial venography at 1-18 months [2]. The group was analyzed in regard to the number of leads, type of lead insulation, and venous approach used for implantation of the pacing lead. At 1-6 months, 31 patients had normal findings on venography, 6 had partial venous obstruction, and 3 had venous occlusion. The most common site of venous obstruction was the subclavian vein, proximal to the junction with the cephalic vein; 2 patients had obstruction of the innominate vein. At 6-12 months, 5 of these patients with previously normal venographic findings showed progression to partial venous obstruction. Of the patients who initially had partial venous obstruction, none showed progression to occlusion during the rest of the study.

No statistically significant difference in venographic findings was noted between the cephalic and the subclavian vein approaches. It had been demonstrated by an earlier study that venous stenosis tended to develop in patients with more than one transvenous lead because of irritation of the vein wall where the leads intersected [16].

Fazio et al. studied the efficacy of ticlopidine in the prevention of TEEs in patients with pacemakers [9]. One hundred eleven patients with a pacemaker were randomized between two groups. Group A was treated with ticlopidine 250 mg/day. Group B was not treated and was used as control group. The analysis of the efficacy of the treatment was based on the incidence of TEEs and of total cardiovascular and cerebrovascular deaths. The results show that in group A there was a significant reduction of total TEEs ($p < 0.05$). Moreover, there was a decrease in total cardiovascular and cerebrovascular mortality ($p = 0.05$). Three stroke deaths and five fatal myocardial infarctions occurred in the group of patients treated with ticlopidine as compared to ten stroke deaths and eight fatal myocardial infarctions in the control group. The results of this study demonstrate that long-term treatment with ticlopidine produces a significant reduction of TEEs. These data thus confirm earlier results obtained with warfarin and indicate that serious prevention of TEEs episodes in patients with pacing may be achieved with more manageable drugs like ticlopidine. In a case from among our own patients, apical four chamber echocardiography 2 weeks after implantation of a VVI pacemaker shows the presence of a frail formation (thrombus) in the right ventricle on the middle one-third of the transvenous lead (Fig. 1), followed by partial resolution after only 1 week of anticoagulant treatment with warfarin sodium 5 mg (INR 3.2) (Fig. 2) and its total resolution after 2 weeks of treatment.

Transvenous placement of defibrillator leads provides another potential source of catheter-related thrombotic complications. Schwartzman et al. described complications that occurred in a group of 170 patients with ICDs [17]. They identified subclavian vein thrombosis in three patients (1.8%), diagnosed 2-50 days after implantation. Of the two patients in whom thrombotic complications were noted early, i.e., before hospital discharge, the leads had been placed via the cephalic vein in one and subclavian vein in the other. Thrombotic complications were recognized at day 60 in a third patient in whom the leads had been placed via subclavian puncture. All three patients received anticoagulant treatment with resolution of the swelling.

Benedini et al. [18] described TEEs as possible complications at implantation or during follow-up in ICD patients. They evaluated the clinical characteristics of the patients, the circumstances in which TEEs occurred, and possible

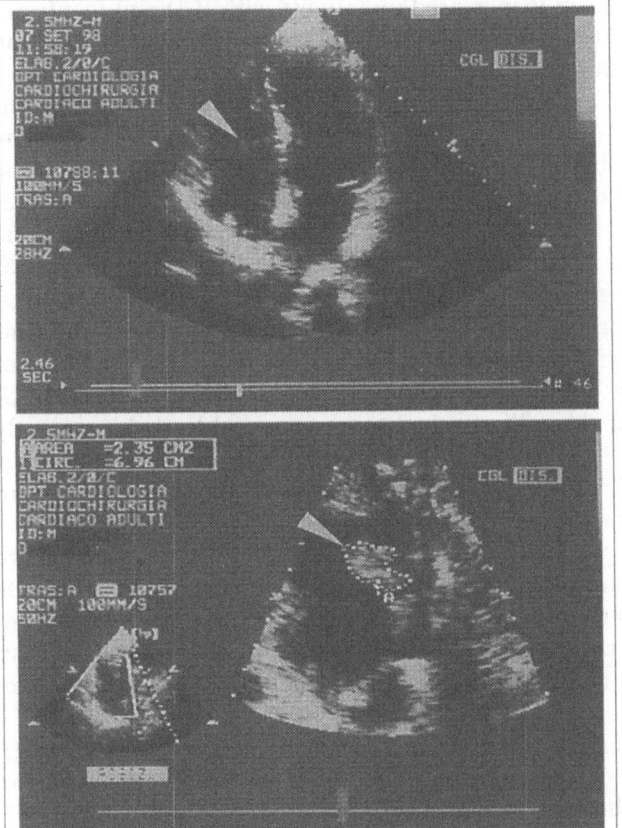

a

b

Fig. 1a,b. Apical four-chamber echocardiography showing frail thrombus formation (*arrow head*) in the right ventricle in a patient 2 weeks after implantation of a VVI pacemaker. In **b** (modified parasternal view) the thrombus can be seen to be located on the middle third of the transvenous lead

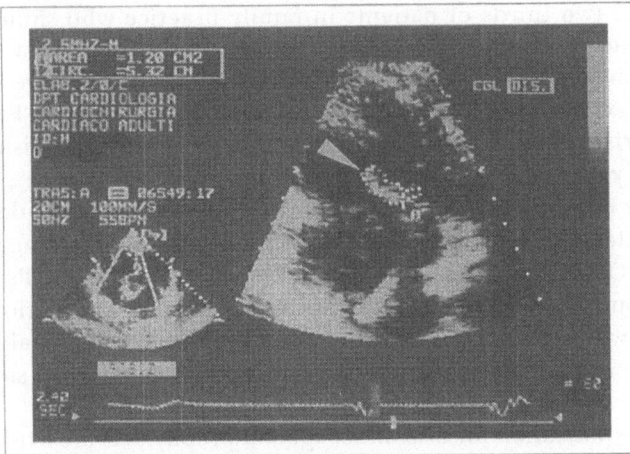

Fig. 2. Apical four-chamber echocardiography: partial resolution of the frail formation after 1 week of anticoagulant treatment with warfarin sodium

risk factors. Risk of embolism is increased in patients with ICD and to a lesser extent in patients with chronic left ventricular aneurysm. Cardiac dysfunction and heart disease predispose to stroke by impairing pump function and are a possible source of emboli. Low-intensity anticoagulant therapy has been recommended in such patients even in the absence of evident clots [19-21]. Despite the recent observation that atrial pathology is considered to have embolic potential, and that atrial clots are frequent in patients with unexplained cerebral ischemia and can be better demonstrated using transesophageal echocardiography (TEECHO) [22], their patients underwent only conventional echocardiography, which did not demonstrate gross left atrial pathology or clots. For this reason they imagined other possible explanations for TEEs. The simplest is that atrial or ventricular clots of a size below the resolution capability of TEECHO may have been detached anywhere as a consequence of ICD shock delivery. The presence of thrombi attached to endocardial leads has recently been demonstrated with TEECHO [23]. The clinical relevance of these findings remains to be established, but they might explain some reported case of TEEs in the absence of clear cardiac sources of embolism.

TEEs may complicate pacemaker and ICD implantation in the postoperative period or may arise during the follow-up. Patients with pacemakers and ICDs are often at risk for TEEs from their own heart disease, and in some cases from the pacemaker or ICD therapy itself. In patients with chronic atrial fibrillation judged to be at high risk of TEEs, chronic anticoagulant therapy might be recommended.

The encouraging results derived from clinical trials involving warfarin appear to be variably received. A recent study at a teaching hospital in the United States indicated that only 44% of the patients who were suitable candidates for warfarin treatment were prescribed this drug. Other studies suggest that warfarin is underused in both hospital and chronic care settings, and that approximately two thirds of patients in family practice who should be given warfarin do not receive it [24-27]. These findings strongly suggest that clinical trial data regarding the usefulness of warfarin therapy either have not reached all physician or have not been fully accepted by them, or both. Perhaps concerns about risks related to the use of warfarin, including the risk of hemorrhage, partly explain its lack of use among primary care physicians. Furthermore domiciliary self-determination of oral anticoagulant therapy ensures a better quality of treatment than traditional monitoring systems. In the trial's SPOG (Schulungs- und Behandlungsprogramm für Patienten mit oraler Gerinnungshemmung) with CoaguChek (Check of coagulation's parameters) results (which allows self-determination of INR, international normalized ratio) not one of 179 monitored patients had TEEs. Ten have had slight hemorrhage.

Finally, the indication for oral anticoagulant prophylaxis are expanding, particularly in pacemaker and ICD patients, and are now much less empirical than in the past. Our study confirms the incidence of TEEs in patients with pacemakers and ICDs and shows the efficacy of anticoagulant therapy in preventing TEEs in the long term.

References

1. Spittell PC, Hayes DL (1992) Venous complications after insertion of a transvenous pacemaker. Mayo Clin Proc 67:258-265
2. Antonelli D, Turgeman Y, Kaveh Z et al (1989) Short-term thrombosis after transvenous permanent pacemaker insertion. Pacing Clin Electrophysiol 12:280-282
3. Mazzetti H, Dussaut A, Tentori C et al (1993) Superior vena cava occlusion and/or syndrome related to pacemaker leads. Am Heart J 125:831-837
4. Fritz T et al (1983) Venous obstruction: a potential complication of transvenous pacemaker electrodes. Chest 83:534-539
5. Crook BRM et al (1977) Occlusion of the subclavian vein associated with cephalic vein pacemaker electrodes. Br J Surg 64:329-331
6. Friedman SA et al (1973) Venous thrombosis and permanent cardiac pacing. Am Heart J 85:531-533
7. Krug H, Zerbe F (1980) Major venous thrombosis: a complication of transvenous pacemaker electrodes. Br Heart J 44:158-161
8. Fruman S et al (1987) Retained pacemaker leads. J Thorac Cardiovasc Surg 94:770-778
9. Fazio S, Santomauro M, Cittadini A et al (1991) Efficacy of triclopidine in the prevention of thromboembolic events in patients with Vvi pacemakers. Pacing Clin Electrophysiol 14(I):168-173
10. Fazio S, Cittadini A, Sabatini D et al (1993) Platelet aggregability in patients with a VVI pacemaker. Pacing Clin Electrophysiol 16:254-256
11. Stoney WS, Addlestone RB, Alford WC Jr et al (1976) The incidence of venous thrombosis following long-term transvenous pacing. Ann Thorac Surg 22:166-170
12. Youngson GG, McKenzie FN, Nichol PM (1980) Superior vena cava syndrome. Case report: a complication of permanent transvenous endocardial cardiac pacing requiring surgical correction. Am Heart J 99:503-505
13. Wertheimer M, Hughes RK, Castle CH (1973) Superior vena cava syndrome: complication of permanent transvenous endocardial cardiac pacing. JAMA 224:1172-1173
14. Marx E, Schulte HD, Balau J et al (1972) Phebographische und klinsche FrYh-und SpSt-Befunde bei transvenös implantierten Schrittmacherelektroden. Z Kreislaufforsch 61:115-123
15. Balau J, Buysch KH, Marx E et al (1971) Thrombose der Vena subclavia nach transvenöser Schrittmacherimplantation. Radiologe 11:50-53
16. Pauletti M, Pingitore E, Contini C (1979) Superior vena cava stenosis at site of intersection of two pacing electrodes. Br Heart J 42:487-489
17. Schwartzman D et al (1995) Postoperative lead related complications in patients with nonthoracotomy defibrillation lead systems. J Am Coll Cardiol 26:776-786
18. Benedini G et al (1995) Implantable defibrillation and thromboembolic events. Pacing Clin Electrophysiol 18:199-202
19. Wolf PA (1993) Contributions of epidemiology to the prevention, of stroke. Circulation 88:22471-22478
20. Meltzer RS et al (1986) Intracardiac thrombi and systemic embolization. Ann Intern Med 104:689-698

21. Hirsh J, Fuster V (1994) Guide to anticoagulant therapy. Part II: Oral anticoaglants. Circulation 898:1469-1480
22. Labovitz AJ, Camp A, Castello R et al (1993) Usefulness of transesophageal echocardiography in unexplained cerebral ischemia. Am J Cardiol 72:1448-1452
23. Febske W, Jung W et al (1993) Multiplane transesophageal echocardiographic evaluation of transvenous defibrillation leads. Xvth Congress of the European Society of Cardiology. Eur Heart J 14:67 (abstr)

How Risky Are Cellular Telephones for Patients Implanted with a Pacemaker or ICD?

M. Gulizia[1], M. Santomauro[2] and S. Mangiameli[1]

Mobile telephones are today the most universal means of communication that has ever existed, with widespread distribution and use of these devices. Problems relating to electromagnetic interference from mobile telephones in permanently paced patients or those with ICDs implanted are very much under discussion at present and the subject arouses strong interest not only among physicians but also among the public.

In 1968 Furman and coworkers [1] called attention to electromagnetic interference (EMI), although without any reports of severe side effects on pacing or on clinical conditions. The issue of EMI with pacemakers was emphasized in 1994 when the results of three studies (both in vitro and in vivo experiments) presented at the annual Bioelectromagnetic Society scientific conference demonstrated that interference could occur when the cellular telephone was held very close to the pacemaker [2-4]. Most of the interferences resulted in pacemaker tracking, inhibition, or conversion to noise mode [5-7].

EMI and Pacemakers

As specified by Irnich in a guest editorial [8], the physical interaction of the telephone-generated electromagnetic field and the pacemaker system is clear: a field of sufficient strength penetrates the body, but it is exponentially attenuated by the conductive tissue according to its "penetration depth" (50 mm at 450 MHz, 22 mm at 2000 MHz) and to the thickness of the tissue layer covering the lead. The signal is electrically coupled to the lead conductor, but this signal is largely damped by the surrounding conductive tissue. Only the last 5-10 cm, and especially the nonshielded connector, contributes to a signal at the input of the pacemaker or defibrillator that can be greater than 10 V. If not rejected by a feedthrough capacitor or an equivalent short-circuiting capacitor at the entrance into

[1]Cardiologia con UTIC, Az. Ospedaliera di Rilievo Nazionale "G. Garibaldi", Catania, Italy;
[2]Reparto di Cardiologia e Cardiochirurgia, Università Federico II, Naples, Italy

the shielding case, the signal is demodulated or rectified by nonlinear components such as Zener diodes or transistors and produces a low-frequency signal.

If this signal contains components with a repetition rate of 1-3 Hz, a pacemaker may respond with inhibition, or triggering in dual-chamber systems. A repetition rate of 5 Hz or more may cause pacemaker reversion to the interference mode, and a rate of 3 Hz or more can provoke defibrillator discharge if the interference duration is longer than some 5 s, depending on the detection algorithm (defibrillators are not capable of noise reversion).

However, considering the coupling mechanism, the possibilities of mobile phone interference are different in Europe and North America and even more different between analog and digital transmission.

The Total Access Communications Standard (TACS) protocol operates on an analog basis: the carrier frequency (450 or 900 MHz) modulates within 25 kHz according to the voice signal. Both carrier and modulation frequencies are totally outside the spectrum of cardiac signals recognized by a pacemaker, but modulation may occur at a repetition rate comparable to such signals, both at the beginning and at the end of a call, when the carrier frequency is switched on or off.

The GSM (Global System for Mobile telecommunications) protocol is based on digital techniques: the voice signal is digitized and then transmitted from the phone to the nearest base station. The digital code is sent at fixed intervals. The phone uses radiofrequency carriers in the 890-960 MHz range modulated by pulses at a repetition rate of 217 Hz. The protocol employs a transmission phase, called DTX, for "energy saving" purposes. During this phase all data are sent within short time slots of 0.5 ms at periods of 4 ms or shorter when there is no answer. The DTX consists of two separate components: the Silence Descriptor (SID), at 2.08 Hz, and the Slow Associated Control Channel (SACCH), operating with a repetition frequency of 8.33 Hz. These two last frequencies are compatible with the band-pass of the pacemaker sensing amplifiers [9-11].

Barbaro et al. [12] tested two European GSM telephones of 2 W power in an in vivo trial on 101 pacemaker-implanted outpatients demonstrating interferences such as pulse inhibition, ventricular triggering, or asynchronous pacing, with a minimum effect duration of ca. 3 s but in some cases with prolongation until an interfering GSM signal was on. These described interferences occurred within a maximum distance of 10 cm between the telephone's antenna and the patient's chest.

Barbaro et al. [13] also studied analog telephone (TACS) in vitro with a human trunk simulator reproducing an actual pacemaker implant. The results demonstrated that when the telephone antenna was in close proximity to the pacemaker head (≤ 13 cm) it was possible to detect (at the moment of an incoming call and throughout ringing) pacemaker desensitizing and sensitizing and pulse inhibition (in the worst case the pacemaker skipped three non-consecutive beats and then resumed its normal pacing) in a large number of the devices tested (10/25). A large study using an in vitro measuring setup was performed by Irnich et al. [10]. These authors tested 231 pacemaker models from 20 manufacturers during the use of the three nets existing in Germany or in Europe: the C-net (450 MHz, analog), the D-net (900 MHz, digital pulsed) and the E-net (1,800 MHz, digital pulsed). Results demonstrated that 30.7% and 34.2% of models were influenced by the C- or D-net, respectively. All models were resistant to the E-net. Considering that many of the models tested were explanted from deceased patients before cremation, and so some of these were "old models," the susceptible models may be taken to represent about 27% of today's living patients. No differences were found between bipolar vs unipolar pacemakers in relation to EMI. However, possible interference with pacemakers is excluded if the minimum distance between pacemaker and a 2-W handy phone is 20 cm or more, or 40 cm between pacemaker and a portable 8-W device.

In view of the fact that patients with a single-lead VDD pacemaker could be at high risk of EMI causing malfunctioning of the device (often programmed to low levels owing to the underlying high-degree AV block and the atrial sensitivity). Nowak and colleagues [14] evaluated 31 patients with three types of single-lead VDD during cellular mobile phone (D-net) use. No interference was detected when a phase of multiple telephone calls was performed, although the authors admit that their study design does not allow complete exclusion of the possibility of interference from a mobile phone.

Sparks and colleagues [15] studied the possibility of EMI due to simulated GSM transmissions (900 MHz, repetition rate 217 Hz with a pulse width of 0.6 ms) in 16 patients implanted with a rate-adaptive pacemaker. They demonstrated: (1) no changes in minute ventilation rate adaptive pacing and (2) rare single- beat ventricular triggering in only one device with pulse generators programmed to more routine sensitivities.

Wilke and colleagues [16] also tested 50 patients with permanent pacemakers (all in unipolar sensing mode) after routine pacemaker check during short calls using a D-net cellular phone (European GSM Standard). Results showed only two cases (4% of the study population) of repeated intermittent pacemaker inhibition during cellular phone calls.

Recently, Altamura and colleagues [17] studied effects of EMI produced by TACS or GSM phone calls in over 200 permanently paced patients with a multi-programmable device, in a right pectoral location and almost all cases (199/200) connected to unipolar leads. Results showed protracted pacing inhibition (> 4 s) 15 times during GSM phone tests and only once during the TACS one. Fifty-two cases of interference were observed during the ringing phase versus 16 during the on/off phase ($p < 0.0001$). The GSM system proved to be associated with a higher number of events than the TACS system ($p < 0.005$).

However, it is not only cellular phone calls that can cause EMI and possible pacemaker malfunction. Santomauro and colleagues [18] demonstrated the possible negative effects on pacemakers of environmental electromagnetic radiation due to electrical lines or cable and electrostatic induction. Data obtained from the two different test objects of the study (pacemakers lodged inside and outside a trolley-bus equipped with an electrical operating device of medium power with interference also produced by a walkie-talkie used as communication system) showed temporary malfunction of all four pacemakers tested, with V00 setting at the programmed rate and with temporary pacing inhibition in two devices. Moreover, results confirmed that pacemakers with unshielded and untwisted leads are much more heavily affected by EMI than pacemakers with twisted leads and a grounded shield.

Antonioli and colleagues [9] also described EMI with pacemakers during cellular calling by TACS and GSM phones as already described: intermittent inhibition of the ventricular channel and/or constant inhibition of the atrial one, with ventricular rate tracking at the upper limit and asynchronous pacing. Moreover, these authors found a more complex behavior in seven patients in which it was possible to record an arrhythmic high rate sometimes anticipated by a long period (> 3 s) of total inhibition and where it was necessary to stop the anomalous rate by using a magnet or, in two cases, reprogramming the device.

EMI and Implantable Cardioverter-Defibrillators

With the ultimate goal of allowing patients to return to work, Fetter et al. [19] tested whether an electrically hostile work site could determine the susceptibility of an implanted cardioverter-defibrillator (ICD) to EMI in a small cohort of patients tending welding equipment or motor-generator systems. The results demonstrated that even if the EMI produced two sources of potential interference on the sensing circuit or reed switch operation, none of the implanted ICDs tested (Medtronic models 7217 and 7219) were affected by oversensing of the electric field as verified by telemetry from the detection circuits.

McIvor [20] described a case of an ICD-implanted patient (PRx ICD model 1705) who experienced an inappropriate firing while in close proximity to an electronic article surveillance (EAS) device. Subsequent tests revealed that the ICD was able to detect high-frequency noise when close to the EAS device.

In a more recent paper, Fetter and colleagues [21] demonstrated that the static magnetic field generated by a cellular phone placed over an ICD at a distance of 0.5 cm or less activates the internal reed switch, resulting in temporary suspension of ventricular tachycardia and fibrillation detection, even though none of the 41 ICD patients tested were affected by oversensing of the EMI field by the cellular phones during the in vivo study.

Using two different types of North American digital phones (TDMA-11 Hz and TDMA-50 Hz) and one analog cellular phone operating at their maximum power, Bassen and colleagues [22] studied potential interferences on ICDs in vitro. EMI was observed in ICDs in the form of pacer output inhibition, high voltage firings (with the TDMA-11 Hz phone placed within 2.3 cm of the ICD) and inhibition followed by firing (with the TDMA-50 Hz phone placed within 2.3 cm of the ICD).

Occhetta and colleagues [23] did not find any false arrhythmia detection by tested devices during TACS or GSM cellular phone use in a study group of 25 ICD patients. However, these authors demonstrated, in all evaluated models, significant noise in the telemetric transmission when the cellular phones were located near the ICD and the programming head, thus causing loss of telemetry in most cases, particularly during call and reception.

Electromagnetic Field Absorber

From the beginning of this year a little ladybird increased its presence on the cellular phone models of most diligent persons. This device, in Italy called "Zeropa", is a product which absorbs electromagnetic waves [24]. Just as the ladybird eliminates insects which are damaging to plants, Zeropa absorbs the electromagnetic waves which are a potential risk to the human body. The product is capable of absorbing almost all electromagnetic waves and protects us from harmful wavelengths. It consists of a combination of absorptive and conductive materials which form a molecular structure with a high plasticity yield temperature of above 1600 °C. This material absorbs the potentially noxious long electromagnetic waves (electric field and magnetic field); some of these are extinguished and some are modified and radiated as 2.5- to 25-μm original infrared rays, which represent a source of useful bionic energy for the human body. The quantity of irradiated energy is equal to the quantity of energy absorbed. Zeropa is a semipermanent product which repeats resonance. Just as radiated infrared rays facilitate animal and plant growth and blood circulation, it neutralizes the potential risk to the human body, activates our bionics, and absorbs the harmful electromagnetic waves [24]. Recently, a new, larger model of this device showed specific absorption rate (SAR) reductions of 27% when placed on the side of the antenna facing the phantom head and a larger reduction of 34% when it was attached to the stub of the antenna [25].

Since these new data were published we have started evaluation of patients with various pacemakers and ICDs while using TACS and GSM cellular phones to investigate whether using Zeropa can reduce EMI-related pacemaker and ICD malfunctioning.

Conclusions and Recommendations

It is really difficult to furnish standard guidelines for patients with permanently implanted pacemakers or ICDs, because of the large variety of cardiac devices used, the ever-increasing numbers of cellular phone models and systems, and the variations in their use; for instance, some people use them daily at work, others only occasionally.

However, on the basis of the studies mentioned above, we can suggest the following:

Patients with Pacemakers

1. Patients with pacemakers could be safer using analog cellular than digital phones.

2. Only the digital 1.8-GHz mobile phone system (E-net) did not influence any pacemaker [10].
3. It is sensible to avoid carrying an activated cellular phone in any clothes pocket overlying the pacemaker.
4. Programming pacemaker sensing at or near the maximum value should be avoided.
5. Cellular phone should not be used within 20 cm (handy models) or 40 cm (portable devices) from the pacemaker pocket. Never place the phone antenna upon the pulse generator. Remember to use the phone with the ear that is contralateral to the inserted pacemaker.
6. Patients can ask their physician to test for possible EMI between their pacemaker and their cellular phone.

Patients with ICDs

In these patients the same considerations are valid as for pacemaker subjects, with some possible reservations related to the implantation techniques [8]. "Old" implanted models (abdominal site) are not susceptible to EMI from cellular phones during conversation, but could be affected if the phone is switched on (i.e., ringing or vibration phase) when kept on the belt.

Implantation of the new devices deep to the pectoralis major muscle (as compared to the usual pacemaker implantation in a subcutaneous pocket with only a small sheet of damping) can reduce the penetration interference of most cellular phone systems but is not enough to avoid interference or inappropriate firing in the case of a high field of EMI [19, 20].

Patients with ICDs should *avoid*:
1. Using a cellular phone too near to the device or at close range in receiving and conversation mode and on the ear that is ipsilateral to ICD implantation.
2. Keeping the telephone "on" during an ICD check or during any telemetric interrogation.
3. Operating electrical equipments without wearing insulated gloves.
4. Being in close contact with electronic article surveillance devices.
5. Panicking. No definitive information exists at present about cellular phone use and ICD or pacemaker malfunctioning.

The upshot is: pacemaker-dependent patients should avoid using cellular phones or should take special precautions until more definitive information becomes available.

References

1. Furman S, Parker B, Krauthammer J et al (1968) The influence of electromagnetic environment on the performance of artificial cardiac pacemakers. Ann Thorac Surg 6:90-95
2. Barbaro V, Bartolini P, Donato A et al (1994) GSM cellular phones interference with

implantable pacemakers: in vitro and in vivo observations. Presented at the 1994 Bioelectromagnetic Society conference. Copenhagen, June 1994

3. Joiner KH, Anderson V, Wood MP (1994) Interference and energy deposition rates from digital mobile phones. Proceedings of the Bioelectromagnetic Society Copenhagen, June 1994, p 67

4. Eicher B, Ryser H, Knsfl U et al (1994) Effects of TDMA-modulated hand-held telephones on pacemakers. In: Proceedings of the Biochectromagnetic Society Copenhagen, June 1994, p 67

5. Carrillo R, Saunkeah B, Pickels M et al (1995) Preliminary observations on cellular telephones and pacemakers. Pacing Clin Electrophysiol 18:863 (abstr)

6. Hayes DL, VonFeldt L, Neubauer S et al (1995) Effect of digital cellular phones on permanent pacemakers. Pacing Clin Electrophysiol 18:863 (abstr)

7. Ehlers C, Andresen D, Brüggemann T et al (1995) Functional pacemaker interference by mobile phones. Eur Heart J 16:5 (abstr)

8. Irnich W (1996) Mobile telephones and pacemakers. [Guest editorial] Pacing Clin Electrophysiol 19:1407-1409

9. Antonioli GE, Guardigli G, Holzl A et al (1998) Unusual pro-arrhythmic effects in implantable cardiac pacemakers induced by mobile phones interference. Proceedings of the 13th International Congress: The "New Frontiers" of Arrhythmias. G Ital Cardiol 28 [Suppl 1]:193-195

10. Irnich W, Lothar B, Müller R et al (1996) Electromagnetic interference of pacemakers by mobile phones. Pacing Clin Electrophysiol 19:1431-1446

11. Hayes DL, Carrillo RG, Gretchen KF et al (1996) State of the science: pacemaker and defibrillator interference from wireless communication devices. Pacing Clin Electrophysiol 19:1419-1430

12. Barbaro V, Bartolini P, Donato A et al (1995) Do European GSM mobile cellular phones pose a potential risk to pacemaker patients? Pacing Clin Electrophysiol 18:1218-1224

13. Barbaro V, Bartolini P, Donato A et al (1996) Electromagnetic interference of analog cellular telephones with pacemakers. Pacing Clin Electrophysiol 19:1410-1418

14. Nowak B, Rosocha S, Zellerhoff C et al (1996) Is there a risk for interaction between mobile phones and single lead VDD pacemakers? Pacing Clin Electrophysiol 19:1447-1450

15. Sparks PB, Mond HG, Joyner KH et al (1996) The safety of digital mobile cellular telephones with minute ventilation rate adaptive pacemakers. Pacing Clin Electrophysiol 19:1451-1455

16. Wilke A, Grimm W, Funck R et al (1996) Influence of D-Net (European GSM-Standard) cellular phones on pacemaker function in 50 patients with permanent pacemakers. Pacing Clin Electrophysiol 19:1456-1458

17. Altamura G, Gentilucci G, Pandozi C et al (1998) Electromagnetic or myopotential interferences: how to abolish them? In: Proceedings of the International Symposium "Progress in Clinical Pacing". Futura, Armonk, NY, pp 345-350

18. Santomauro M, Amendolara A, Costanzo A et al (1997) Cellular phones and pacemakers: how do they interact? In: Raviele A (ed) Cardiac Arrhythmias. Springer, Milan, pp 514-521

19. Fetter JG, Benditt DG, Stanton MS (1996) Electromagnetic interference from welding and motors on implantable cardioverter-defibrillators as tested in the electrically hostile work site. J Am Coll Cardiol 28:423-427

20. McIvor ME (1995) Environmental electromagnetic interference from electronic article surveillance devices: interactions with an ICD. Pacing Clin Electrophysiol 18:2229-2230

21. Fetter JG, Ivans V, Benditt DG et al (1998) Digital cellular telephone interaction with implantable cardioverter-defibrillators. J Am Coll Cardiol 31:623-628
22. Bassen H, Moore HJ, Ruggera PS (1998) Cellular phone interference testing of implantable cardiac defibrillators in-vitro. Pacing Clin Electrophysiol 21:1709-1715
23. Occhetta E, Plebani L, Sacchetti G et al (1998) Evaluation of cellular phones electro-magnetic interferences on implantable cardioverter defibrillators functioning. Proceedings of the 13th International Congress: The "New Frontiers" of Arrhythmias. G Ital Cardiol 28 [Suppl 1]:195-199
24. Anonymous (1998) Zeropa Handbook and technical features. Harvest Lodge Limited, London
25. Manning MI (1999) SAR and efficiency tests of "Zeropa" devices using three different mobile telephones. SARTest Report 64/99, SARTEST Ltd, Newdigate, UK

What Are the Risks for Pacemaker/ICD Patients Undergoing Magnetic Resonance Imaging or Other Medical Procedures?

E. Adinolfi and P. Dini

In the medical environment there are several sources of possible magnetic interference, such as magnetic resonance imaging (MRI), clinical radiation therapy, electrocautery, and lithotripsy. Certain types of electrical equipment may interfere with automatic implantable cardioverter defibrillator (AICD) and/or pacemaker performance. The reason why this occurs is that AICDs and pacemakers are designed to sense the electrical activity of the heart. In the event a particular piece of equipment should mimic the activity of the heart, the pulse generator may be affected.

Magnetic Resonance Imaging

In the case of MRI the interfering forces consist of a static magnetic field which aligns the hydrogen nuclei, a gradient magnetic field that allows selection of the imaging volume, and a pulse radiofrequency (RF) field that reorients specific hydrogen nuclei for imaging. The static magnetic field can exert a torque effect on the pulse generator and lead to displacement of the pacemaker from the overlying tissue [1]. It may also result in spontaneous closure of the reed switch and asynchronous pacing at the programmed rate [1]. The gradient magnetic field may generate sufficient voltage and electromagnetic interference to result in inhibition of a pacemaker programmed to the demand mode [1]. The pulsed RF field may produce sufficient electrical current within the pacing system to result in rapid cardiac pacing [2]. Reed switch malfunction, thermal injury to patients, a change in the programming mode and ventricular fibrillation are all potential complications of this imaging modality [2-4]. Animal and in vitro studies have demonstrated that rapid cardiac pacing was related to the RF pulse delivered during MRI, and there have been documented cases in patients [4-7]. Unexpected death in patients undergoing MRI has been reported, but without documentation of any cardiac arrhythmias [8].

Dipartimento di Cardiologia, Ospedale S. Camillo, Rome, Italy

Static Magnetic Field

The static magnetic field can exert forces of up to 5 N (about tenfold the pacemaker's weight) on pacemakers containing ferromagnetic materials [2]. In the study by Tobisch et al. [9] only two pacemakers were moved when positioned freely on the MRI examination bed. The danger of dislocation can be ruled out for the other models when implanted in a patient. Furthermore, the static magnetic field usually operates the pacemaker's reed switch causing asynchronous pacing, which seems to be the safest pacing mode during MRI.

However, it is theoretically possible that the reed switch may not be activated if the MRI static magnetic field is oriented perpendicularly to the switch's axis [9, 10]. In this case, the effects of inhibition or triggering that have been observed during pacing in VVI and DDD pacing modes may constitute a danger to the patient. Moreover, the operation of the reed switch itself and consequent asynchronous pacing have been reported to be the cause of ventricular fibrillation in a patient [2]. For this reason, no patient with a pacemaker should approach an MRI unit unless a defibrillator is available.

Gradient Magnetic Field and Radiofrequency Field

The effect of rapidly changing electromagnetic fields on electrodes has been investigated systematically for the first time in the Achenbach [11] study. In these phantom experiments, exposing isolated pacemaker leads to MRI caused significant heating of the electrodes. The heating was caused by the induction of currents in the electrodes, which act as antennae for the electromagnetic fields. It must also be kept in mind that patients carry isolated pacemaker leads left in place after pacemaker removal. One increase in the temperature measured at the electrode tip exceeded 15°C.

The average temperature increase of the electrodes at the electrodes tip tended to be less pronounced when the electrodes were connected to a pacemaker and was further attenuated when both the pacemaker and the electrodes were submersed in a tank filled with saline solution. In general, heating of unipolar electrodes was stronger than that of bipolar electrodes.

Interaction with metallic implants such as cardiac pacemakers could lead to several adverse effects: the static magnetic field could cause dislocation of the pacemaker and electrodes if they contain ferromagnetic material. Because of the electromagnetic field, pacemaker electronics could be destroyed or the programmed settings could be altered, while induction of currents in the electrodes could result in sensing and triggering, with consequent inhibition or rapid pacing, as well as heating of metallic components.

Although the general policy of never exposing a patient with a pacemaker to MRI should not be revised, we think that if the imaging is considered essential, it could be safely performed in certain carefully selected patients.

Further studies are needed to understand the mechanism of rapid cardiac pacing and arrhythmogenesis occurring in patients undergoing MRI evaluation.

Clinical Radiation Therapy

Studies have shown that clinical radiation therapy doses of an accumulated 70 Gy may produce malfunction of most pulse generators currently available. These anomalies would appear to be isolated to the newer CMOS (complementary metal-oxide semiconductor) technology, since the same study showed less effect on older demand-type pulse generators. Opinion seems to vary as to the actual pulse generator damage caused by therapeutic radiation, and therefore all manufacturers make the following suggestions. If the pulse generator is directly in the beam of radiation, a CT scan should be done prior to the therapy in an attempt to locate an alternate port of entry which would not transect the pulse generator. If the pulse generator is directly over the radiation target and no other entry port is available, consideration should be given to moving the pulse generator to a different site rather than irradiating through it. If the pulse generator is only in the general area of the tumor and not directly in the radiation beam, it may be possible to shield the pulse generator with some radiation-resistant material. Generally, scatter radiation or accumulations of less than 10 Gy are safe amounts of radiation exposure for pulse generator CMOS technology.

Another concern regarding radiation therapy would include the large magnetic fields commonly developed by the therapy equipment. Betatrons and linear accelerators are capable of producing large magnetic fields. A magnetic field of 10 G or stronger at the surface of the pulse generator may cause reed switch closure, resulting in intermittent beeping tones from the AICD or pacing at the magnetic rate in the pacemaker. While uncommon, this possibility leads manufacturers to recommend monitoring the patient's heart rate and generator operation during therapy sessions.

To ensure that the device is operating correctly, it is advisable to interrogate the device after the first treatment and then perform a complete follow-up.

Electrocautery

In the AICD system the electromagnetic signal produced by electrocautery may mimic an R wave in both frequency and amplitude. The high frequency energy of electrocautery may be interpreted as an arrhythmia by the AICD, resulting in an unwanted shock. The AICD should be deactivated prior to any surgery where the use of electrocautery is possible. Following the surgical procedure, the AICD may be reactivated.

A pacemaker detecting the electromagnetic signal given off by electrocautery may respond in one of two different ways. A pulse generator sensing a continuous high-frequency burst of such signals would identify them as "noise" and revert to asynchronous pacing at the programmed rate. If electrocautery is applied in short bursts the pulse generator may sense the signal as an R wave and pacing may be inhibited. This inhibition will cease once the electrocautery is turned off. Electrocautery may also cause a triggered mode of operation.

When using electrocautery, manufacturers suggest following these guidelines:
1. The current path (electrode tip to ground plate) should be kept as far away as possible from the pulse generator.
2. The electrocautery should be set at the lowest possible clinically effective setting.
3. Electrocautery should not be applied directly on or over the pulse generator.
4. Electrocautery on or near the lead tip may cause burning of the lead-tissue interface.
5. If the pulse generator is continually inhibited by frequent bursts of electrocautery, a magnet may be placed on the pulse generator, which will result in asynchronous pacing.

Lithotripsy

The published literature regarding pacemaker/lithotripsy interactions contains reports that extracorporeal shock-wave lithotripsy (ESWL) can be performed safely in most patients with implanted pacemakers. These studies involved in-vitro testing of pulse generators using worst-case scenarios. Pulse generators were implanted in the abdomen and exposed to the focused shock waves. The following are some of the guidelines resulting from these studies:
1. Patients should be monitored by ECG to continually assess pacemaker function. All of the authors in the studies make this point. The authors of a German study go so far as to recommend inserting a temporary pacing electrode in a patient who is pacemaker-dependent and having a cardiologist present during the procedure.
2. The lithotriptor should be programmed to deliver its shock wave synchronously with the R waves of the ECG. This should prevent any spark-gap-induced elctromagnetic interference (EMI) from inhibiting the pulse generator, since the spark and the resultant shock wave would occur during the ventricular refractory period of the pacemaker.
3. Following the procedure, the pulse generator should be interrogated and the programmed parameters verified. None of the studies reported spontaneous reprogramming or permanent pulse generator damage from the therapy under the study conditions.
4. According to these reports, dual-chamber pulse generators may need to be programmed to VVI mode during the procedure. In the DDD mode, an atrial pacing spike could trigger the lithotriptor. If this occurs, the ventricular sensing channel could sense the resultant spark gap and inhibit ventricular output. A Cleveland Clinic study recommends routinely reprogramming a DDD pacemaker to the VVI mode whenever there is any atrial pacing.

With respect to AICDs, very little has been published. One study of ten patients with implanted AICDs suggests that contralateral ESWL may be performed safely in patients with AICDs. The authors recommend programming the AICD to the inactive mode to avoid false detection, particularly if the generator is less than 10 cm from the focal point of the shock wave. The patients should then undergo testing after the ESWL to ensure appropriate function of the AICD. Ipsilateral ESWL is contraindicated due to the potential for causing a spurious shock from the AICD.

Conclusions

Although the general policy not to expose a patient with a pacemaker or AICD to MRI or other medical procedures should not be revised, we think that if the imaging or therapy is considered essential, it may be safely used in certain carefully selected patients.

Further studies are needed to understand the possible interaction between pacemaker/AICD and systems generating magnetic interference.

References

1. Pavlicek W, Gensiger M, Castle L et al (1983) The effects of nuclear magnetic resonance on patients with cardiac pacemakers. Radiology 147:149-153
2. Fetter J, Aram G, Holmes DR et al (1994) The effects of nuclear magnetic resonance imagers on external and implantable pulse generators. Pacing Clin Electrophysiol 7:720-727
3. Peden CJ, Collins AG, Butson PC et al (1993) Induction of microcurrents in critically ill patients in magnetic resonance system. Crit Care Med 21:1923-1928
4. Erlebacher JA, Cahill PT, Panizzo F et al (1986) Effect of magnetic resonance imaging on DDD pacemakers. Am J Cardiol 57:437-440
5. Shellock FG, Kanal E (1992) SMRI report: policies, guidelines, and recommendations for MR imaging safety and patient management. J Magn Reson Imaging 2:247-248
6. Pohost GM, Blackwell GG, Shellock FG (1992) Safety of patients with medical devices during applications of magnetic resonance method. Ann N Y Acad Sci 649:302-312
7. US Food and Drug Administration Center for Devices and Radiological Health (1996) MR products reporting program and medical device report program. Microfiche MDR # 175218 # 353516, # 125938. Obtainable through Freedom of Information request
8. Avery JE (1988) Loos prevention case of the month. Not my responsibility! J Tenn Med Assoc 81:53
9. Tobisch RJ, Inrich W, Bachmann J, Batz L (1993) Elektromagnetische Auswirkungen des Kerrnspintomographen auf den Herzschrittmacherpatienten. Biomed Tech (Berl) 38[Suppl]:435-437
10. Seipel L, Bud E, Driwas S (1975) Kammerflimmern bei Funktionsprüfung eines Demand-Schrittmachers. Dtsch Med Wochenschr 100:2439-2444
11. Achenbach S (1997) Effect of magnetic resonance imaging on cardiac pacemaker and electrodes. Am J Cardiol 134:467-473

Pacemaker Treatment for Hypertrophic Obstructive Cardiomyopathy: Are Long-Term Results as Good as Short-Term Ones?

L.J. Kappenberger, N. Aebischer and X. Jeanrenaud

Introduction

Hypertrophic cardiomyopathy (HCM) is a complex disease of multiple genetic origins. It is usually a familial cardiac disorder, recognised to be of heterogeneous expression with diverse clinical manifestations and outcome. This structural and functional abnormality of the myocardium is the phenotype of many genetic disorders of encoding proteins of the sarcomere. The diagnostic disorder is a thickened and non-dilated left ventricle in the absence of an associated condition that could explain the hypertrophy.

Echocardiography is the main diagnostic tool for identification of the hypertrophy. The prevalence in the general population is estimated as high as 0.2% and about 25% of those might present with septal hypertrophy leading to dynamic obstruction of the left-ventricular outflow tract [1-3]. Since many patients have additional malformations of the mitral valve apparatus with enlargement of leaflets or anomalous insertion of the papillary muscle, the systolic movement of this valve may be modified and anterior displacement can further contribute to the dynamic subaortic obstruction and mitral incompetence. The symptoms are multifactorial and partially explainable through the anatomic abnormalities. Dyspnea is a consequence of diminished compliance of the left ventricle and to mitral incompetence. Chest pain, which may be typical of angina, reflects increased oxygen consumption of the thickened myocardium but is also a consequence of changes in the small vessels typical for HCM [4, 5]. Impaired consciousness, palpitations, syncope and sudden death may reflect the hemodynamic consequence of severe obstruction, inadequate autonomic balance arrhythmias such as atrial fibrillation and ventricular tachycardias [6, 7]. Prognosis in most asymptomatic patients seems good but the condition might be invalidating and

Division of Cardiology, Centre Hospitalier Universitaire Vaudois (CHUV), Lausanne, Switzerland

need treatment [8, 9]. In order to reduce the hyperdynamic contraction of the left ventricle, beta-blockers, calcium-antagonists and disopyramide have been prescribed with success but no appropriate evaluation of the benefit of these treatments has been made [10-12]. As the septal hypertrophy and systolic anterior movement of the mitral valve cause mechanical obstruction, myotomy and myectomy as well as mitral valve replacement have been proposed in extremely severe and symptomatic cases, with acceptable (0%-2%) operative mortality and favorable outcome in the long term [13, 14]. Transcoronary alcoholization of the septum to create a localized infarct and septal shrinking, therefore reduction of obstruction, has recently been proposed and extensive clinical experience of this procedure shows promising results [15]. As with any of the proposed treatments so far, no causal approach to the disease could be offered; therefore, our goal must be to improve symptoms in symptomatic patients. As reduction of obstruction is the only objective parameter that can acutely tell us how treatment is influencing the phenotype, this is the first parameter to understand the mechanisms by which improvement can be achieved.

Pacing has been recognised for over 20 years to reduce left ventricular outflow tract (LVOT) pressure gradient in patients with HOCM [16, 17]. As the atrial contribution to ventricular filling in the noncompliant hypertrophied heart is critical, only reliable dual-chamber pacing with full ventricular capture, which needs often a short paced A-V interval, allowed pacemaker therapy to be considered on long-term basis. There are several single-center experiences published showing reduction of subaortic gradients and relief of symptoms [9, 18, 19]. The theoretical background of beneficial effects of pacing again seems multifactorial, from reduced contractility [20] to modification of activation sequence [21]. Three randomized blinded cross-over studies showed less impressive improvement of quality of life and Doppler assessed dynamic obstruction, but in comparison to surgical series the follow up was short. We therefore analyze in this chapter our experience in acute and long-term pacing for HOCM and compare to recent publications in the field.

Methods

The European multicentre study for evaluation of pacemaker treatment in HOCM investigated the effect of adding cardiac pacing to conventional medical treatment in patients with HOCM. The study objective was to test the hypothesis that dual-chamber pacing for HOCM was safe and improved quality of live in optimal dual-chamber mode (ON) or pacemaker in atria inhibited mode (OFF) for a 3-month period following which they were crossed over to the alternative phase as published elsewhere [22]. Thereafter, all patients were further followed up in an open phase in the mode they preferred with repetitive clinical and Doppler-echocardiographic evaluation for 36 months.

The study was based on the guidelines of the European Standard EN 540, the

European norm for Clinical Evaluation of Medical Devices, which includes compliance to the Declaration of Helsinki.

Patients included fulfilled the following inclusion criteria:

1. typical subaortic muscular obstruction with septal thickness of more than 11 mm,
2. LVOT with systolic gradient at rest, of at least 30 mmHg or more as measured by Doppler or catheter technique, while on usual medical treatment,
3. symptoms refractory to drugs or intolerance to drug therapy,
4. NYHA class II or III,
5. age over 18 years.

Patients were excluded from pacemaker therapy, if they had:

1. acute deterioration of hemodynamics with an acute pacing test,
2. chronic atrial fibrillation,
3. other indications for pacemaker treatment,
4. severe valvular heart disease not related to HOCM,
5. systemic hypertension refractory to treatment,
6. recent myocardial infarction or symptomatic coronary artery disease.

Pacemaker implant was performed under local anesthesia with transvenous electrode placement in the right atrium and right ventricle. Attention had to be given to placement of the RV-electrode in the most apical position possible. Selection of the brand and type of the pacemaker could be determined by the individual investigator. However, the pacemaker should be a DDD device with separately programmable paced and sensed A-V delays. After pacemaker implantation and optimization of the A-V-interval, i.e., lowest gradient without fall in aortic pressure or diastolic mitral flow, patients were randomized into one of the two branches with defined sequence of therapy as mentioned. Thus, the patient left hospital with the pacing mode as stipulated by randomization. Patients were reassessed according to schedule or at their discretion. Medication had to be kept unchanged during the crossover phase. After 12 months investigators were free to treat the patients with whatever they considered appropriate but tracking the cases for this report was requested.

Holter recordings were performed in each phase to confirm appropriate functioning of the pacemaker; they were analyzed in a central laboratory and no information was given immediately to the investigator. Exercise testing followed a symptom limited modified Bruce protocol.

The influence on symptoms was evaluated according to NYHA classification for dyspnea and angina interpreting anamnestic data of the patient during the follow-up visits. In addition, a specific quality of life assessment questionnaire was applied. Details on this QOL questionnaire have been described elsewhere [23, 24]. It has been specially designed and validated for patients under pacing as well as those with ischemic heart disease. Translations of this document were validated against the original. The patients filled out the QOL-document after instruction by a nurse otherwise not involved in the study and not informed of the status of the patient.

The key analysis of the crossover phase consisted of intrapatient comparison. The patient status in pacemaker OFF was compared with the status of the same patient in pacemaker ON using paired tests as published earlier, while data obtained after 1 year can be compared with screening of the pacemaker OFF and ON period. Evaluation over time was realized by comparing the results of the different follow-up examinations in chronological order. The long-term therapeutic effect was tested by comparing the results after 1 year with the baseline.

Results

For the PIC-Study, 83 patients were randomized for the cross-over phase without bias as the two patient groups were comparable in all standard parameters. Of the whole study population, one patient died in hospital due to perforation of the right ventricle with the pacemaker electrode followed by tamponnade and irreversible shock, 79 patients could be investigated at the 1-year follow-up examination, and 82 patients were tracked after a mean follow-up period of 36 months (22-46 months).

Compared to screening, all patients had lower gradients in the follow-up examinations. There was a spontaneous slight but significant reduction of the LVOT-gradient after implantation of the pacemaker even if the device was not activated (OFF). With dual-chamber pacing however, an important reduction of the obstruction could be documented in all patients with acute response (72±35 mmHg to 28±24 mmHg) at 3 months. At 1 year, the favorable hemodynamic effect remained unchanged and significantly lower gradient compared to baseline or pacemaker OFF phase (28±21 mmHg) [25] was measured. Symptoms of angina and dyspnea were significantly and long-lastingly improved with an overall 30 % placebo-effect related to the pacemaker implantation.

Syncopes were reported by ten PIC patients to have occurred before entering the study. During the whole observation only four syncopal events were reported and no death occurred within 36 months. These studies were, however, not designed to investigate the rhythmic complications of HOCM.

Discussion

Today, three randomized double-blind studies showed that pacing reduces gradients in HOCM over long periods of time. The PIC-Study and two additional studies with similar design have recently been published [25-27]. Nishimura et al [26] investigated 21 patients but could only follow up 14 in the crossover phase. The M-Pathy-study included 48 patients but only in 23 was full comparison possible throughout the study period. Patients with hypertrophic obstructive cardiomyopathy and a resting gradient over 30 mmHg despite maximal conventional drug treatment and well-tolerated acute testing, especially those above 50 years of age, may benefit most [27]. This effect persists in PIC-trial in 75 of 83 patients beyond 1 year (Table 1). These observations have to be validated in comparison to so-called established therapies for HOCM. The benefit of beta-

Table 1. Comparison of PM in hypertrophic obstructive cardiomyopathy (HOCM) trials

Ref.	Randomization duration (months)	n-patients PM off	Complete follow-up PM on	Pressure gradient PM off	PM on	NYHA	NYHA
[18]	No	84	28	96 ± 41	27 ± 31*	3.2	1.6*
[17]	No	12	44	82 ± 42	47 ± 34*	2.8	1.3*
[19]	Yes	21	06	76 ± 61	55 ± 38*	2.4	2.6
[30]	Yes	83	36	72 ± 35	28 ± 24*	2.4	1.4*
[27]	Yes	48	12	82 ± 32	48 ± 32*	—	—

*Significant difference at $p < 0.05$

blockers, Ca-antagonists and recently class 1 antiarrhythmics is well accepted but has never been evaluated in a study of scientific rigor, as should be mandatory today. All drug therapies are aimed at reduction of hypercontractility of the ventricular myocardium in symptomatic patients, while prophylactic benefit has never been documented for any of these treatments. In the different HOCM-pacing studies, a randomized and blinded assignment to inactive or active pacing was the first step. This proved the superiority of active pacing to sham-intervention. This result is even more surprising as the results were obtained in multicenter designs. Despite the absence of symptomatic benefit in the whole group studied by Nishimura et al. [26], several patients clearly deteriorated while on pacing. In contrast, the studies of PIC-group [26], as well as Maron et al. [27], show similar observations. An important difference, however, might be found in the patient selection. In PIC only, patients with well-tolerated temporary pacing, significantly reduced gradient and stable cardiac output, were included. In both other trials, a pacemaker was implanted without taking into consideration hemodynamic testing. In none of the three studies was the acute gradient-reduction predictive of long-term benefit, but it can be concluded that those who do not improve in the short term will also not improve in the long term.

Therefore, the more selective approach in PIC might account for the significant difference which after all is also due to a much greater study population. This leads to the importance of gradient reduction in HOCM. Clearly the symptoms in HOCM are multifactorial including left ventricular diastolic dysfunction, impaired coronary vasodilator reserve and myocardial ischemia. The contribution of these factors to symptoms varies amongst patients and a direct one-to-one correlation with any particular pathophysiological mechanism seems not to be evident, not even with the subaortic gradient. However, the perceived benefits of surgery on symptoms are reported to be largely the consequence of reduction of the outflow gradient [14, 28]. The studies discussed here demonstrate a similar finding. As we included only patients with significant gradients, we cannot discuss how pacing might act in nonobstructive forms or in patients with no gradient reduction at all. We can however conclude, in accordance with careful observations in HOCM patients, that the amount of initial gradient reduction is not predictive of symptoms, nor are symptoms predictive of relief with pacing, but in comparison with other studies, we believe that the fact that there is no gradient reduction does not justify a pacemaker implantation. Clearly pacing influences the ventricular contraction in different ways. In HOCM not only is the inverted septal activation of importance, but also the redistribution of wall-stress probably leading to modification of coronary flow, as documented in animal experiments and human studies [20, 30].

In contrast to this subjective improvement and objective gradient reduction, a limitation of this study is that no improvement of exercise tolerance or structural changes could be documented so far.

In any randomized study, the variable symptom-appearance, the fluctuation of the obstruction and the relatively good basic exercise tolerance made it difficult to show improvements. In fact, most of the patients in all three studies had come over stage 3 of the Bruce protocol.

In conclusion, the pacemaker treatment in HOCM can lead to reduction of the obstruction in some cases with no deterioration in systemic hemodynamics. This can be considered as a basis for permanent PM implantation in drug-refractory patients, especially those who suffer from angina and are over 50 years of age or opposed to surgery. It should be noted that pacemaker treatment does not exclude alcohol ablation of the septum [29] or myectomy should the pacing improvement not satisfy the patient.

Acknowledgements. This work was supported by the Swiss National Foundation for Scientific Research and Medtronic, Bakken Research Center.

References

1. Maron BJ, Bonow RO, Cannon RO, Leon MB, Epstein SE (1987) Hypertrophic cardiomyopathy: interrelations of clinical manifestations, pathophysiology and therapy. N Engl J Med 316:780-789, 844-852
2. Wigle ED, Sasson Z, Henderson MA et al (1985) Hypertrophic cardiomyopathy: the importance of the site and extent of hypertrophy: a review. Progr Cardiovasc Dis 28:1-83
3. Maron B, Gardin J, Flack J, Gidding S, Bild D (1995) Assessment of the prevalence of hypertrophic cardiomyopathy in a general population of young adults: echocardiographic analysis of 4111 subjects in the CARDIA study. Circulation 92:785-789
4. Maron BJ, Wolfson JK, Epstein SE, Roberts WC (1986) Intramural «small vessel» coronary artery disease in hypertrophic cardiomyopathy. J Am Coll Cardiol 8:545-557
5. Posma J, Blanksma P, Van der Wall E, Vaalburg W, Crijns H, Lie K (1996) Effects of permanent dual chamber pacing on myocardial perfusion in symptomatic hypertrophic cardiomyopathy. Heart 76:358-362
6. Frenneaux MP, Counihan PJ, Caforio ALP, Chimakori T, McKenna WJ (1990) Abnormal blood pressure response during exercise in hypertrophic cardiomyopathy. Circulation 82:1995-2002
7. McKenna W, Camm J (1989) Sudden death in hypertrophic cardiomyopathy. Assessment of patients at high risk. Circulation 80:1489-1492
8. Cecchi F, Olivotto I, Montereggi A, Santoro G, Dolara A, Maron BJ (1995) Hypertrophic cardiomyopathy in Tuscany: clinical course and outcome in an unselected regional population. J Am Coll Cardiol 26:1529-1536
9. Fananapazir L, Chang A, Epstein S, McAreavy D (1992) Prognostic determinants in

hypertrophic cardiomyopathy: prospective evaluation of a therapeutic strategy based on clinical, Holter, hemodynamic and electrophysiologic findings. Circulation 85:2149-2161

10. Harrison DC, Braunwald E, Glick G, Mason DT, Chidsey CA, Ross J Jr (1964) Effects of beta-adrenergic blockade on the circulation, with particular references to observations in patients with hypertrophic subaortic stenosis. Circulation 29:84-98

11. Hopf R, Kaltenbach M (1987) 10-year results and survival of patients hypertrophic cardiomyopathy treated with calcium-antagonists. Z Kardiol 76[Suppl 3]:137-144

12. Sherrid M, Delia E, Dwyer ED (1988) Oral disopyramid therapy for obstructive hypertrophic cardiomyopathy. Am J Cardiol 62:1085-1088

13. Ten Berg JM, Suttorp MJ, Knaepen PJ, Ernst S, Vermeulen FEE, Jaarsma W (1994) Hypertrophic obstructive cardiomyopathy: initial results and long-term follow up after narrow septal myectomy. Circulation 90:1781-1785

14. Seiler C, Hess OM, Schoenbeck M et al (1991) Long-term follow up of medical versus surgical therapy for hypertrophic cardiomyopathy: a retrospective study. J Am Coll Cardiol 17:634-642

15. Sigwart U (1995) Non-surgical myocardial reduction for hypertrophic obstructive cardiomyopathy. Lancet 346:211-213

16. Hassenstein P, Wolter HH (1967) Therapeutische Beherrschung einer bedrohlichen Situation bei der idiopathischen hypertrophischen Subaortenstenose. Verh Dtsch Ges Kreisl 33:242-246

17. Page A, Boudaut R, Bemurat M, Clementy J, Levy S, Besse P (1979) Importance of sequential atrioventricular pacing in obstructive myocardiopathy with atrioventricular block. Arch Mal Coeur 72:1253-1258

18. Jeanrenaud X, Goy JJ, Kappenberger L (1992) Effects of dual-chamber pacing in hypertrophic obstructive cardiomyopathy. Lancet 339:1318-1323

19. Fananapazir L, Epstein ND, Curiel RV et al (1994) Longterm results of dual-chamber (DDD) pacing in obstructive hypertrophic cardiomyopathy. Evidence for progressive symptomatic and hemodynamic improvement and reduction of left ventricular hypertrophy. Circulation 90:2731-2742

20. Prinzen FW, Augustijn CH, Arts T, Allessi MA, Reneman RS (1990) Redistribution of myocardial fiber strain and blood flow by asynchronous activation. Am J Physiol 258:H300-H308

21. Kappenberger L , Grobéty M , Jeanrenaud X (1998) The features of a paced heart beat. In: Vardas PE (ed) Cardiac arrhythmias, pacing and electrophysiology. Kluwer, UK, pp 331-336

22. Kappenberger L, Linde C, Daubert C, McKenna W, Meisel E, Sadoul N, Chojinowska L, Guize L, Gras D, Jeanrenaud X, Ryden L (1997) Pacing in hypertrophic obstructive cardiomyopathy, the PIC trial. Eur Heart J 21:1249-1256

23. Undén A, Schenck-Gustavsson K, Axelson P (1993) Positive effects of increased nurse support for male patients after acute myocardial infarction. Qual Life Res 2:121-127

24. Gadler F, Linde C, Juhlin-Dannfelt A, Ribeiro A, Ryden L (1997) Longterm effects of pacing in patients with hypertrophic cardiomyopathy without outflow tract obstruction at rest. Eur Heart J 18:636-642

25. Kappenberger LJ, Linde C, Jeanreanud X, Daubert C, McKenna W, Meisel E, Sadoul N, Chojnowska L, Guize L, Gras D, Aebischer N, Gadler F, Rydén L, and the Pacing in Cardiomyopathy (PIC) Study Group (1999) Clinical progress after randomized on/off pacemaker treatment for hypertrophic obstructive cardiomyopathy. Europace 1999; 1:77-84

26. Nishimura RA, Trusty JM, Hayes DL et al (1997) Dual-chamber pacing for patients

with hypertrophic cardiomyopathy: a prospective randomized double-blind crossover trial (abstract). J Am Coll Cardiol 29:435-441

27. Maron B, Nishimura R, McKenna W (1999) The M-Pathy study investigators assessment of permanent dual-chamber pacing as a treatment for drug-refractory symptomatic patients with obstructive hypertrophic cardiomyopathy. Circulation 99:2927-2933

28. Wigle ED, Rakowsky H, Kimball BP, Williams WG (1995) Hypertrophic cardiomyopathy, clinical spectrum and treatment. Circulation 92:1680-1692

29. Knight C, Kurbaan A, Seggewiss H, Henein M, Gunning M, Harrington D, Fassbender D, Gleichmann U, Sigwart U (1997) Nonsurgical septal reduction for hypertrophic obstructive cardiomyopathy. Circulation 95:2075-2081

30. Prinzen FW, Augustijn CH, Allessie MA et al (1992) The time sequence of electrical and mechanical activation during spontaneous beating and ectopic stimulation. Eur Heart J 13:535-543

Theophylline for Treatment of Bradyarrhythmias: When Is it Indicated?

N. Paparella and P. Alboni

Theophylline is a methylated xanthine which exerts several pharmacological actions of therapeutic interest. It stimulates the central nervous system, acts on the kidney to produce diuresis, stimulates cardiac muscle and relaxes smooth muscles, notably bronchial muscles. Moreover, the drug exerts positive chronotropic and dromotropic action. In fact at therapeutic plasma concentrations, theophylline produces a modest increase in sinus rate in normal individuals [1]. An improvement in sinus node (SN) function and in atrioventricular (AV) nodal conduction has been reported after both intravenous and oral administration of the drug [2-4]. There are several mechanisms by which theophylline might exert positive chronotropic and dromotropic action; however, several observations suggest that the primary action of theophylline at therapeutic concentrations is blockade of adenosine receptors [5]. Adenosine has been shown to slow sinus rate and depress AV nodal conduction in laboratory animals and in humans. Theophylline antagonizes the negative chronotropic and dromotropic action of adenosine by blocking extracellular adenosine receptors [5]. Clinical studies have shown that oral theophylline can be efficacious in the treatment of symptomatic sick sinus syndrome (SSS) [2, 6-9] and of atrial fibrillation (AF) with a slow ventricular response [10, 11].

Patients with Sick Sinus Syndrome

At present the natural history of SSS in largely unknown. Patients with this disease are generally old and frequently have a concomitant heart disease. Various symptoms presumably related to SN dysfunction may be superimposed; in addition, syncope generally comes unexpectedly and unpredictably [12, 13]. Permanent pacing is currently being used as the elective therapy to relieve symptoms in patients with SSS; however, controlled studies assessing the impact of this therapy on the natural course of the disease are lacking.

In unpaced patients with SSS, dizziness and syncope did not evidence prog-

Divisione di Cardiologia, Ospedale Civile, Cento (FE), Italy

nostic implications; total mortality and sudden death did not seem to be higher than in the general population; moreover, ventricular pacing did not seem to reduce mortality [14]. These observations provided the rationale to test oral theophylline as an alternative to pacemaker therapy. Benditt et al. [2] observed a reduction in symptoms during long-term treatment with oral theophylline in ten young subjects with paroxysmal sinsus bradyarrhythmias or AV block. The drug diminished the frequency and severity of bradycardia in newborn infants with spells of apnea-bradycardia [6, 7]. We carried out a study [8] on the effects of slow-release theophylline (700 mg daily) in 17 patients with symptomatic sinus bradycardia. The drug increased resting sinus rate (46 ± 7 versus 62 ± 18 beats/min, $p < 0.01$), mean 24-h heart rate (51 ± 6 versus 64 ± 16 beats/min, $p < 0.01$) and minimal 24-h heart rate (36 ± 6 versus 43 ± 10 beats/min). Cardiac pauses > 2500 ms were present in 4 patients during control recording and disappeared after theophylline. The daily number of premature supraventricular and ventricular beats increased slightly after the drug. Exercise sinus rate was higher after theophylline than during the control test ($p < 0.01$). Thirteen patients were followed for a period of 17 ± 3 months. Suppression of symptoms was achieved in 12 patients. Asthenia and easy fatigue were reduced markedly by the drug. During long-term therapy, the sinus rate was similar to that observed at the steady-state. In 3 of the 17 patients (17%) theophylline had to be discontinued because of gastric intolerance. These data suggest that oral theophylline can represent an effective therapy in patients with symptomatic sinus bradycardia. However, like pacemaker therapy, the drug has not been investigated in controlled studies.

Results of the THEOPACE Study

We performed a randomized, controlled trial to assess the effects of oral theophylline and of permanent pacemaker on the symptoms and complications of SSS (THEOPACE study) [15]. Patients who met the entry criteria were randomized to one of the following arms: (1) no treatment (control group), (2) oral theophylline at the dosage of 550 mg/day, and (3) permanent pacemaker (DDDR).

Patients were evaluated for randomization if they met all of the following criteria: (1) age ≥ 45 years; (2) mean resting sinus rate < 50 beats/min, and/or intermittent sinoatrial block in more than one standard electrocardiogram recorded during diurnal hours on different days, and (3) symptoms attributable to SN dysfunction, such as syncope or dizziness and/or easy fatigue or effort dyspnea.

Criteria for exclusion included the following: very severe SSS, namely, symptomatic resting sinus rate < 30 beats/min or sinus pauses > 3 s in standard electrocardiograms recorded during diurnal hours or heart failure refractory to treatment with ACE-inhibitors and diuretics; recent myocardial infarction or stroke or other acute disease; very severe general disease, likely to be fatal in < 2 years; significant renal or hepatic diseases; history of documented sustained ventricular tachyarrhythmias; bradycardia secondary to transient causes (effect of drugs, etc); a need for β-blockers or calcium antagonists (verapamil or diltiazem); other definite or potential causes of syncope in patients complaining of syncopal attacks.

During the recruitment period, 162 patients were evaluated for inclusion. Of these, 12 (7%) were not enrolled because of very severe SSS and 43 for one or more of the other exclusion criteria. Therefore, 107 patients met the inclusion criteria and underwent randomization.

The following parameters served as *end point*: occurrence of the first episode of syncope, development of overt heart failure, thromboembolic events (stroke and peripheral embolus), development of permanent AF, and symptom scores as assessed by a self-administered questionnaire. In case of development of permanent AF, the patients were still followed-up, but the heart rate and other variables of the Holter recording were not reported for analysis. The patients were enrolled in a long-term study and were seen at the outpatient clinic every 3 months. During follow-up, the patients were withdrawn from the control or the theophylline arm if they developed syncope, overt heart failure, poorly tolerated episodes of sustained paroxysmal tachyarrhythmia that were drug refractory or not manageable with antiarrhythmic drugs, or any other event (e.g., myocardial infarction) requiring reevaluation of the therapy. In case of thromboembolism, the decision on whether to leave the patient in the assigned arm was left to the investigator's best judgment. Owing to the permanent nature of pacemaker treatment, patient withdrawal from the pacemaker arm was not possible.

The three groups were similar with regard to the clinical, electrocardiographical and electrophysiologic variables. The clinical events during the follow-up are reported in Table 1.

Syncope

Eight patients (23%) in the control arm, six (17%) in the theophylline arm, and two (6%) in the pacemaker arm had syncope during the follow-up. In patients assigned to pacemaker therapy, the incidence of syncope was lower than in control patients ($p = 0.02$) and tended to be lower than in those assigned to theophylline ($p = 0.07$).

Development of Overt Heart Failure

Six patients (17%) in the control arm, one (3%) in the theophylline arm, and one (3%) in the pacemaker arm developed overt heart failure during follow-up. The

Table 1. Clinical end points observed during follow-up in the three groups of patients

	No treatment	Theophylline	Pacemaker
Follow-up, months	18 ± 15	16 ± 13	23 ± 13
Episodes of syncope, n (%)	8 (23)	6 (17)	2 (6)[1]
Development of overt heart failure, n (%)	6 (17)	1 (3)[2]	1 (3)[3]
Development of chronic atrial fibrillation, n (%)	4 (11)	2 (6)	3 (9)
Episodes of paroxysmal tachyarrhythmia, n (%)	9 (26)	10 (28)	10 (28)
Thromboembolism, n (%)	1 (3)	3 (9)	3 (9)

[1] $p = 0.02$, pacemaker group vs no-treatment group
[2] $p = 0.05$, theophylline group vs no-treatment group
[3] $p = 0.05$, pacemaker group vs no-treatment group

incidence of overt heart failure was significantly lower in the theophylline arm and in the pacemaker arm than in the control arm ($p = 0.05$).

Paroxysmal Tachyarrhythmias and Permanent Atrial Fibrillation

All patients were in sinus rhythm at the time of randomization. Nine patients (26%) in the control arm, ten (28%) in the theophylline arm, and ten (28%) in the pacemaker arm complained of sustained paroxysmal tachyarrhythmia during follow-up (p = NS).

Four patients (11%) in the control arm, two (6%) in the theophylline arm, and three (9%) in the pacemaker arm developed permanent AF during follow-up (p = NS).

Thromboembolism

Thromboembolic events occurred in one patient (3%) in the control arm, three (9%) in the theophylline arm, and three (9%) in the pacemaker arm (p = NS). Of the seven patients who had thromboembolic events during follow-up, three already had bradycardia-tachycardia syndrome at the time of randomization, and one of these had developed permanent AF before the event.

Symptoms

There were no significant differences in the NYHA class score or in the fatigue, dizziness and palpitation scores among the three groups of patients at the time of randomization and after 3 months.

Heart Rates

At the time of randomization, there were no significant differences among the three groups in resting sinus rate evaluated by standard electrocardiogram, maximum exercise sinus rate and minimum, mean and maximum heart rate evaluated by 24-h Holter recording. During follow-up, resting sinus rate was always higher in the theophylline group than in the control group. Heart rates evaluated by 24-h Holter recording also showed a trend toward higher values in the theophylline group than in the control group. The number of premature supraventricular and ventricular beats and the number of patients with cardiac pauses > 2.5 s did not show significant differences among the three groups.

The main finding of the present study is that in patients with symptomatic SSS, pacemaker therapy reduces the incidence of syncope and overt heart failure and oral theophylline reduces the incidence of overt heart failure. The increase in sinus rate and a slight inotropic action may account for this drug effect in patients with SSS. On the contrary, neither pacemaker nor theophylline reduces the incidence of thromboembolism, paroxysmal tachyarrhythmias and evolution toward permanent AF.

The effects of both theophylline and pacemaker appear particularly interesting on minor symptoms, such as easy fatigue and dizziness. Both treatments reduced these symptoms, as previously reported in noncontrolled studies. However, the same reduction was observed after 3 months in the non-treated patients and, consequently, there were no significant differences in the fatigue and dizziness scores among the three groups of patients at the time of randomization and after 3 months. This means that the benefits of pacemaker and theophylline on minor symptoms are actually due, at least in part, to a spontaneous improvement of the patient's clinical picture. These fluctuations of clinical pattern and of sinus rate in patients with SSS have no obvious explanation; the autonomic nervous system likely plays a major role.

In conclusion, the results of the present study suggest that oral thophylline is indicated in SSS patients with episodes of overt heart failure or with only minor symptoms such as easy fatigue and dizziness (Table 2). On the basis of our experience, the serum theophylline level should be between 5 ng/mL and 15 ng/mL [8, 11]. On the contrary, when syncope represents a relevant clinical problem, pacemaker implantation is the first-choice treatment.

Patients with Sinus Node Dysfunction Following Cardiac Transplantation

A high incidence (about 50%) of symptomatic bradycardia is observed after orthotopic heart transplantation. This SN failure is transient in most patients or at least reverts to a latent, asymptomatic form of SN dysfunction [16]. Pacemaker implantation has been widely used in the treatment of this bradyarrhythmia; however, due to the transient nature of severe SN dysfunction after cardiac transplantation, this treatment does not appear particularly useful during the long-term period. It has been observed that oral thophylline improves SN function and increases donor sinus rate by about 50%, avoiding the need for pacemaker implantation [17, 18]. At present, theophylline seems to represent the first-choice treatment in patients with symptomatic sinus bradycardia following cardiac transplantation (Table 2). When it is not efficacious or causes undesirable side effects, it does not prevent any pacemaker implantation.

Patients with AF and a Slow Ventricular Response

At present we have no epidemiological and prognostic data on patients with AF and a slow ventricular response; in particular we do not know whether prognosis is different from that of patients with AF and a normal resting heart rate. The

Table 2. Indications to oral theophylline in patients with bradyarrhythmias

---

1. Sick sinus syndrome patients with episodes of overt heart failure or with "minor" symptoms (easy fatigue, dizziness)

2. Cardiac transplant patients with symptomatic sinus node dysfunction

3. Patients with atrial fibrillation and symptomatic slow ventricular response

---

current therapy for symptomatic slow response AF is based on permanent stimulation; however, in the literature these is no evidence that pacemakers prolong survival in these patients. Theophylline has been shown to enhance AV nodal conduction; it shortens both the AF interval and the cycle length of the fastest 1:1 AV conduction [3]. This observation provides the rationale to test this drug as an alternative to pacemaker therapy in patients with persistent AF and a slow ventricular response. In a short-term study we investigated the effects of slow-release theophylline (700 mg daily) at the steady-state in these patients [10]. The drug increased mean resting heart rate (51 ± 6 vs 67 ± 13 beats/min, $p < 0.01$), mean 24-h rate (51 ± 6 vs 68 ± 14 beats/min, $p < 0.01$) and minimum 24-h heart rate (32 ± 6 vs 42 ± 11 beats/min, $p < 0.01$). Cardiac pauses > 2500 ms were present in 13 patients during control recording; after theophylline they disappeared in 11 and decreased in the remaining 2. The daily number of wide QRS complexes increased (428 ± 752 vs 1146 ± 1464, $p < 0.01$). Exercise heart rate, evaluated at the end of first and second stage (Bruce protocol), was higher after theophylline than during control test ($p < 0.01$).

Subsequently we carried out a long-term study in 17 patients with AF and a slow ventricular response not related to drugs [11]. Criteria for inclusion were the following: (1) mean resting heart rate < 60 beats/min constantly present for some days during several resting electrocardiograms; (2) symptoms attributable to slow heart rate. The exclusion criteria were the following: (1) presence of bundle branch block; (2) recent myocardial infarction or acute disease of any type; (3) significant renal or hepatic disease; (4) New York Heart Association class IV. The mean age was 78 ± 9 years. Fourteen patients had heart disease. Sixteen patients were in New York Heart Association class I-II and one in class III. Twelve patients complained of syncope or presyncope before the hospitalization; four complained of easy fatigue and one of dyspnea after slight effort.

The mean follow-up was 20 ± 18 months. Long-term therapy was initiated at a dosage of 400-600 mg daily. During the follow-up, seven patients died after 15 ± 14 months of treatment. One patient died of heart failure, two of arterial embolism and four of noncardiovascular disease. This high mortality rate appears mainly related to the high age (about 80 years) and to the presence of heart disease. However, in no patient was death attributable to the AV conduction disturbance, since none of them died suddenly. We did not include patients with bundle branch block in which the slow ventricular response could be an expression of a conduction disturbance within the His-Purkinje system, where theophylline does not appear effective. Theophylline markedly reduced easy fatigue in the patients complaining of this symptom. Only one patient complained of syncope during the follow-up. Our results, therefore, suggest a reduction in bradycardia-related symptoms in patients with AF and a slow ventricular response treated with oral theophylline; this observation seems to be strengthened by the marked reduction in the frequency of cardiac pauses. However, the natural history of AF with a slow ventricular response is unknown; in particular, we do not know whether in this type of arrhythmia the course of neurological symptoms is variable from patient to patient with spontaneous remissions as in SSS patients. To this regard, a very high incidence of spontaneous remission of syncope has been observed since 89% of nonpaced patients with AF and cardiac pauses reported resolution of their cerebral symptoms during a mean follow-up period of 2 years [19].

The effects of theophylline that we reported cannot be considered conclusive since a controlled study is required. However, like theophylline, pacemaker therapy has not been investigated by controlled studies in patients with AF and a slow ventricular response and, therefore, at present oral theophylline appears indicated in the treatment of these patients (Table 2).

References

1. Ogilvie RI, Fernandez PG, Winsberg F (1977) Cardiovascular response to increasing theophylline concentrations. Eur J Clin Pharmacol 12:409-414
2. Benditt DG, Benson W Jr, Kreitt J, Dunningan A, Pritzker MR, Crouse L, Scheinman MM (1983) Electrophysiologic effects of theophylline in young patients with recurrent symptomatic bradyarrhythmias. Am J Cardiol 52:1223-1229
3. Eiriksson CE, Writer SL, Vestal RE (1987) Theophylline-induced alterations in cardiac electrophysiology in patients with chronic obstructive pulmonary disease. Am Rev Respir Dis 135:322-326
4. Alboni P, Rossi P, Ratto B, Pedroni P, Gatto E, Antonioli GE (1990) Electrophysiologic effects of oral theophylline in sinus bradycardia. Am J Cardiol 65:1037-1039
5. Belardinelli L, Fenton R, West A, Linden J, Althaus J, Berne RM (1982) Extracellular action of adenosine and the antagonism by aminophylline on the atrioventricular conduction in isolated perfused guinea pig and rat hearts. Circ Res 51:569-579
6. Shannon DC, Gotay F, Stein IM, Roger MC, Todras ID, Moylan FMB (1975) Prevention of apnea and bradycardia in low-birthweight infants. Pediatrics 55:583-594
7. Meyers TF, Milsap RL, Krauss AN, Adult PAM, Reindenberg MM (1980) Low-dose theophylline therapy in idiopathic apnea of prematurity. J Pediatr 96:99-103
8. Alboni P, Ratto B, Cappato R, Rossi P, Gatto E, Antonioli GE (1991) Clinical effects of oral theophylline in sick sinus syndrome. Am Heart J 122:1361-1367
9. Saito D, Matsubara K, Yamanari H, Obayashi N, Uchida S, Maekawa K, Sato T, Mizuo K, Kobayashi H, Haraokaj S (1993) Effects of oral theophylline on sick sinus syndrome. J Am Coll Cardiol 21:1199-1204
10. Alboni P, Ratto B, Scarfò S, Rossi P, Cappato R, Paparella N (1991) Dromotropic effects of oral theophylline in patients with atrial fibrillation and a slow ventricular response. Eur Heart J 12:630-634
11. Alboni P, Paparella N, Cappato R, Pirani R, Yiannacopulu P, Antonioli GE (1993) Long-term effects of theophylline in atrial fibrillation with a slow ventricular response. Am J Cardiol 72:1142-1145
12. Gann D, Tolentino A, Samet P (1979) Electrophysiologic evaluation of elderly patients with sinus bradycardia: a long term follow-up study. Ann Intern Med 90:24-29
13. Sasaki Y, Shimotori M, Akahane K, Yonekura H, Hirono K, Endoh R, Koike S, Kawa S, Furuta S, Homma T (1988) Long-term follow-up of patients with sick sinus syndrome: a comparison of clinical aspects among unpaced, ventricular inhibited paced, and physiologically paced groups. Pacing Clin Electrophysiol 11:1575-1583
14. Shaw DB, Holman RR, Gowers JI (1980) Survival in sino-atrial disorder (sick sinus syndrome). Brit Med J 280:139-141
15. Alboni P, Menozzi C, Brignole M, Paparella N, Gaggioli G, Lolli G, Cappato R (1997)

Effects of permanent pacemaker and oral theophylline in sick sinus syndrome. Circulation 96:260-266

16. Kratochwill C, Schmid S, Koller-Strametz J, Kreiner G, Grabenwöger M, Grimm M, Laufer G, Heinz G (1996) Decrease in pacemaker incidence after orthotopic heart transplantation. Am J Cardiol 77:779-783

17. Ellenbogen KA, Szentpetery S, Katz MR (1988) Reversibility of prolonged chronotropic dysfunction with theophylline following orthotopic cardiac transplantation. Am Heart J 110:202-206

18. Heinz G, Kratochwill C, Buxbaum P, Laufer G, Kreiner G, Siostrzonek P, Slobodan G, Derfler K, Gössinger H (1993) Immediate normalization of profound sinus node dysfunction by aminophylline after cardiac transplantation. Am J Cardiol 71:346-349

19. Saxon L, Albert BH, Uretz EF, Denes P (1990) Permanent pacemaker placement in chronic atrial fibrillation associated with intermittent AV block and cerebral symptoms. PACE 13:724-729

SSS Patients: Atrial or Dual-Chamber Pacing?

P. Dini, E. Adinolfi, A. Avella, F. Laurenzi and A. Pappalardo

Symptomatic patients with sick sinus syndrome (SSS) are candidates for permanent pacemaker implantation. Single-chamber atrial (AAI) or dual-chamber (DDD) pacing rather than single-chamber ventricular (VVI) pacing is the recommended pacing mode, with rate response (-R) if appropriate [1]. Most retrospective studies have demonstrated that mortality is greater in VVI paced patients and that atrial-based pacing is hemodynamically superior and associated with a lower rate of atrial fibrillation (AF) and thromboembolic complications [2-6]. Other observational studies comparing physiological (AAI or DDD) with VVI pacing, while they confirmed that VVI pacing was an independent predictor of AF and stroke, did not identify any difference in mortality and heart failure incidence between the two groups [7-9].

Recently Andersen et al., in a prospective randomized study, demonstrated that AAI pacing is superior to VVI pacing in patients with SSS. Compared to VVI-paced patients, AAI-paced patients showed a reduction in the incidence of AF and arterial thromboembolism after 3 years of follow-up; a reduction in mortality and in the incidence of heart failure was statistically significant after 5 years [10-11]. This is in keeping with those studies providing evidence that apical ventricular pacing adversely affects ventricular contraction and results in an increase in the end-systolic dimension of the ventricle and gradual deterioration of its function [3].

By contrast, a prospective randomized study (PASE) comparing the outcome of single- (VVI-R) versus dual-chamber (DDD-R) pacing in patients 65 years of age or older showed a non-significant reduction in mortality (12% vs 6%), stroke (4% vs 2%), and all cardiac events (19% vs 10%) at 1 year of follow-up [12]. The lower than expected benefit with dual-chamber pacing might be attributable to the very short follow-up, which did not permit any final conclusions regarding possible differences in clinical outcome. It is interesting to note that in the study of Andersen et al. too, the differences between AAI and VVI pacing with regard to cardiovascular morbidity and mortality reached significance only after 3 years of follow-up.

Dipartimento di Scienze Cardiologiche, Ospedale S.Camillo, Rome, Italy

Other ongoing randomized studies (Systematic Trial of Pacing to prevent Atrial Fibrillation [STOP-AF study [13]], Canadian Trial of Physiologic Pacing (CTOPP), Mode Selection Trial in Sinus Node Dysfunction (MOST), United Kingdom Pacing and Cardiovascular Events Trial (UK-PACE)], designed to enroll at least 2000 patients in order to have enough statistical power to detect a difference in clinical endpoints, should offer a definitive answer to the question of pacemaker selection in SSS [14].

Data concerning pacemaker implants show that sinus node disease without atrioventricular (AV) block represents approximately 20%-30% of the overall indications. Despite the fact that there is now good evidence to support it, single-chamber atrial pacing is still underused in many countries. The UK National Pacemaker Database shows that in 1995, 44% of such patients were treated with a VVI, 45% with a DDD, and only 11% received an AAI pacemaker [15]. The Italian Pacemaker Registry reports that in 1997 only 4.3% of SSS patients underwent an AAI-R pacemaker implant, while 33.5% received a VVI-R and 62.2% were treated with a DDD-R [16].

The main reason for the underuse of the AAI pacemaker is concern about progression to a high grade symptomatic AV block due to degeneration of the specific conduction system. This would require a further procedure with an implant of a new ventricular lead and a DDD pacemaker. The risk of developing AV block, reported in the literature by some retrospective analyses, gave rise to the opinion that a ventricular lead should also be implanted in these patients [17-20]. However, the annual risk for a second- or third-degree AV block seems to be small during AAI pacing. In a review of 28 studies, Rosenqvist et al. estimated the risk of AV block during AAI pacing to be 0.6% per year (range 0%-4.5%) in SSS patients [21]. In a retrospective follow-up study, Clark et al. observed progression of the conduction disease, requiring a pacemaker upgrade from atrial to dual-chamber, in 5.8% (1% per year) [22]. Other authors, reporting a higher incidence of 1.8% per year, subsequently showed that the AV block could be predicted by a pre-existing bundle-branch block [23], so the real incidence of progression in patients with normal AV conduction at the time of implant seems to be much lower.

In a prospective trial of patients with SSS and intact AV conduction treated with an AAI pacemaker, Andersen et al. [24] observed the occurrence of a second- to third-degree AV block during 5.5 ± 2.4 years of follow-up only in four of 110 patients, with an annual incidence of 0.6%. Two of these four patients had right bundle-branch block before pacemaker implantation. The study excluded patients with: a PQ interval > 0.22 s if up to 70 years old and > 0.26 s if over 70 years old, grade 2 or 3 AV block, bifascicular or complete left bundle-branch block and Wenckebach block point < 100 bpm. Thus, this prospective trial has for the first time demonstrated that a strategy with single-chamber atrial pacing is safe and can be recommended for patients with SSS without bundle-branch block, when additional criteria for normal AV conduction are considered.

The cost of a pacemaker increases with its grade of complexity, both in hardware and in yearly cost of follow-up. At this time there are no prospective data about the cost-effectiveness of a dual-chamber pacemaker. Clarke et al. [22] estimated any cost savings that could be made by implanting atrial rather than dual-chamber pacemaker when appropriate. The cost of upgrading the pacing systems to dual-chamber pacing was added. They concluded that single-chamber atrial pacing is both safe and cost-effective, and that it must be the pacing mode of choice in patients with sinus node disease. According to the American College of Cardiology/American Heart Association guidelines [1] this indication applies to patients with sinus node dysfunction and documented symptomatic bradycardia, including frequent sinus pauses that produce symptoms. Even if atrial pacing alone, in selected patients with brady-tachy syndrome, may be effective in reducing the frequency of recurrences of bradycardia-dependent AF, dual-chamber pacing seems to offer a better choice. In such cases drugs that may affect AV conduction are often used or, in highly symptomatic and drug-refractory patients, AV ablation may be performed.

In conclusion, although a dual-chamber pacemaker protects the patients in case of AV block or AF with bradycardia, the low annual incidence rate of these events, the clinical benefit, and the saving costs recommend more widespread use of single-chamber atrial pacing in SSS. In order to minimize the need for upgrades, the indication for AAI pacing should be dictated by evidence of normal AV conduction, excluding patients with paroxysmal AF or other atrial tachy-arrhythmias.

References

1. Gregoratos G, Cheitlin MD, Conill AE et al (1998) ACC/AHA guidelines for implantation of cardiac pacemakers and antiarrhythmia devices: executive summary. Circulation 97:1325-1335
2. Hesselson AB, Parsonet V, Bernstein A et al (1992) Deleterious effects of long-term single-chamber ventricular pacing in patients with sick sinus syndrome: the hidden benefits of dual chamber pacing. J Am Coll Cardiol 19:1542-1549
3. Paxinos G, Kastritis D, Kakouros S et al (1998) Long term effect of VVI pacing on atrial and ventricular function in patients with sick sinus syndrome. Pacing Clin Electrophysiol 21:728-734
4. Rosenqvist M, Brandt J, Schuller H (1988) Long term pacing in sinus node disease: effects of stimulation mode on cardiovascular morbidity and mortality. Am Heart J 116:16-22
5. Stangl K, Seitz K, Wirtzfeld A et al (1990) Differences between atrial single chamber pacing (AAI) and ventricular single chamber pacing (VVI) with respect to prognosis and antiarrhythmic effect in patients with sick sinus syndrome. Pacing Clin Electrophysiol 13:2080-2085
6. Santini M, Alexidou G, Ansalone G et al (1990) Relation of prognosis in sick sinus syndrome to age, conduction defects and modes of permanent cardiac pacing. Am J Cardiol 65:729-735
7. Sgarbossa EB, Pinski SL, Maloney JD et al (1993) Chronic atrial fibrillation and stroke in paced patients with sick sinus syndrome. Relevance of clinical characteristics and pacing modalities. Circulation 88:1045-1053
8. Sgarbossa EB, Pinski SL, Maloney JD (1993) The role of pacing modality in determining long-term survival in the sick sinus syndrome. Ann Intern Med 119:359-365

9. Sgarbossa EB, Pinski SL, Trohman RG et al (1994) Single-chamber ventricular pacing is not associated with worsening heart failure in sick sinus syndrome. Am J Cardiol 73:693-697
10. Andersen HR, Thuesen L, Bagger JP et al (1994) Prospective randomized trial of atrial versus ventricular pacing in sick sinus syndrome. Lancet 344:1523-1528
11. Andersen HR, Nielsen JC, Thomsen PEB et al (1997) Long term follow-up of patients from a randomized trial of atrial versus ventricular pacing for sick sinus syndrome. Lancet 350:1210-1216
12. Lamas GA, Orav EJ, Stambler BS et al (1998) Quality of life and clinical outcomes in elderly patients treated with ventricular pacing as compared with dual-chamber pacing. N Engl J Med 338:1097-1104
13. Charles RG, McComb JM (1997) Systematic trial of pacing to prevent atrial fibrillation. Heart 78:224-225
14. Lamas GA (1997) Pacemaker mode selection and survival. A plea to apply the priciples of evidence based medicine to cardiac pacing practice. Heart 78:218-220
15. Marshall HJ, Gammage MD, Griffith MJ (1998) AAI pacing for sick sinus syndrome: first choice on all counts. Heart 80:315-316
16. AIAC Associazione Italiana di Aritmologia e Cardiostimolazione (1997) Registro Italiano Pacemaker e Defibrillatori. Associazione Italiana di Aritmologia e Cardiostimolazione, Roma, Bollettino periodico: registrazioni pacemaker gennaio-dicembre
17. Rosen KM, Loeb HS, Sinno MZ et al (1971) Cardiac conduction in patients with symptomatic sinus node disease. Circulation 43:836-851
18. Sutton R, Kenny RA (1986) The natural history of sick sinus syndrome. Pacing Clin Electrophysiol 9:1110-1114
19. Bertholet M, Demoulin JC, Fourny J et al (1983) Natural evolution of atrioventricular conduction in patients with sick sinus syndrome treated by atrial demand pacing: a study of 26 cases. Acta Cardiol 38:227-232
20. Haywood GA, Ward J, Ward DE et al (1990) Atrioventricular Wenckebach point and progression to atrioventricular block in sinoatrial disease. Pacing Clin Electrophysiol 13:2054-2058
21. Rosenqvist M, Obel IWP (1989) Atrial pacing and the risk for AV block: is there a time for change in attitude? Pacing Clin Electrophysiol 12:97-101
22. Clarke KW, Connelly DT, Charles RG (1998) Single chamber atrial pacing: an underused and cost-effective pacing modality in sinus node disease. Heart 80:387-389
23. Brandt J, Anderson H, Fahraeus T et al (1992) Natural history of sinus node disease treated with atrial pacing in 213 patients: implication for selection of stimulation mode. J Am Coll Cardiol 20:633-639
24. Andersen HR, Nielsen JC, Thomsen PE et al (1998) Atriventricular conduction during long-term follow-up of patients with sick sinus syndrome. Circulation 98:1315-1321

Mobitz I AV Block: Why and When to Pace?

R. CAZZIN, P. GOLIA AND G. DI FONZO

The presence of symptoms related to bradyarrhythmia is one of the basic conditions in which there is general agreement in favor of permanent cardiac pacemaker implantation. In patients with Mobitz I atrioventricular (AV) block, clinical manifestations such as transient dizziness, light-headedness, near-syncope, or more generalized symptoms related to exercise tolerance or congestive heart failure, are considered a class I indication for permanent pacing in the guidelines of 1991 ACC/AHA Task Force [1]. In the same guidelines, pacing in asymptomatic subjects with Mobitz type I AV block is indicated, with some divergence of opinion (class II condition), only if an intra- or infra-His bundle block is demonstrated, while there is no indication (class III condition) when the block is at nodal level. In these guidelines relief of symptoms is the only therapeutic goal of pacing, while other aims, such as improved outcome, are not considered since the prognostic role of pacing in the Mobitz I AV block has not yet been fully assessed.

The decision to indicate permanent pacing in asymptomatic patients requires a knowledge of the pathophysiology and natural history of the AV block. The Mobitz I block is generally located in the AV node (> 90%); its presence in the His bundle system is uncommon when the QRS is narrow. In the chronic bundle branch block associated with Mobitz type I, the site of block lies in the His Purkinje system in about 30% of cases [2, 3]. The presence of Mobitz I AV block in the healthy population has been estimated at 0.003% [4]. In a group of 453 elderly subjects, 5.5% of whom had pacemakers implanted, in a long-term follow-up the prevalence of second degree AV block in the patients without implanted pacemakers was 1.5% [5].

Two main studies considered as supporting ACC/AHA recommendations in regard to the asymptomatic Mobitz I AV block [6, 7] were not pertinent or were based on a very small number of cases. The third study, reported by Strasberg and colleagues [8], is more interesting. It relates to a long follow-up of 56 patients with chronic second-degree AV block proximal to the His bundle, 37 of whom had structural heart disease. Of the patients with heart disease, 10 required a

Unità Operativa Cardiologica, Ospedale di Portogruaro, Venice, Italy

pacemaker for heart failure or syncope and 16 patients died during a 4-year follow-up. The authors concluded that chronic Mobitz I nodal block is usually benign and pacing is not necessary in the absence of structural heart disease. When heart disease is present the clinical course seems to have a more malignant trend, but the authors did not suggest prophylactic pacing in these cases. By contrast, the Working Party of the British Pacing and Electrophysiology Group (BPEG) [9], according to the observations of Shaw et al. [10], recommended permanent pacing in many asymptomatic patients with Mobitz I AV block. In the study by Shaw and colleagues [10], 214 subjects with second-degree AV block were followed between 1968 and 1982. The patients were divided into three groups: 77 patients with type I block, 86 with type II, and 51 patients with advanced block (2:1, 3:1). The 5-year survival was similar in all groups, without any influence on prognosis by the presence or absence of bundle branch block, and it was 78% for paced subjects, compared to 42% for unpaced subjects. The authors concluded that these results change the benign reputation of chronic Mobitz type I AV block and suggested that these patients should be considered for pacing even in the absence of symptoms, with the same criteria adopted for higher degree blocks.

The study by Shaw et al. had some limitations, and it was published 12 years ago, but no other study can be found in the literature to confirm or to disconfirm these conclusions.

The BPEG [9], referring to these observations, indicates that "asymptomatic patients with either Wenckebach (type I) or Mobitz II second-degree AV block occurring during most of the day and night would qualify for pacemaker implantation, as would patients with asymptomatic complete heart block".

Connelly and Steinhaus [11], considering the different opinions reached by the two national committees, proposed an ACC/AHA Task Force class II indication for pacing and recommended "permanent pacemaker implantation in patients with asymptomatic Mobitz type I AV block, especially in older patients with structural heart disease". Barold [12], more prudently, advised conservative therapy in asymptomatic patients with Mobitz I AV block and a narrow QRS and, agreeing with others [2, 13, 14], proposed that these patients should be followed carefully. The presence and severity of underlying heart disease rather than the status of the conduction system should be considered the most important prognostic factor when recommending permanent pacing in patients with asymptomatic Mobitz I AV block [3, 11, 15].

Many cardiac pathologies are influenced by the negative hemodynamic effects of a variable AV interval and of inappropriate timing of atrial systole during the diastolic filling period [2, 16, 17]. In patients with these pathologies the duration of AV interval and the number of Wenckebach episodes are often aggravated by the introduction of drugs that interfere with AV nodal conduction. A dual-chamber pacemaker programmed with an optimal AV interval favors hemodynamic stability and makes the pharmacological choice possible in patients with Mobitz I AV block and with underlying heart disease.

References

1. Dreifus LS, Gillette PC, Fisch C et al (1991) Guidelines for implantation of cardiac pacemakers and anti-arrhythmia devices: a report of the American College of Cardiology/American Heart Association Task Force on Assessment of Diagnostic and Terapeutic Cardiovascular Procedures (Committee on Pacemaker Implantation). J Am Coll Cardiol 18:1-13
2. Warton JM, Ellenbogen KA (1995) Atrioventricular conduction system disease. In: Ellenbogen KA, Kay GH, Wilkoff BL (eds) Clinical cardiac pacing. Saunders, Philadelphia, pp 691-703
3. Denes P (1987) Atrioventricular and intraventricular block. Circulation 75[Suppl III]:19-25
4. Hiss RG, Lamb LE (1962) Electrocardiography findings in 122,043 individuals. Circulation 25:947
5. Aronow WS, Epstein S, Swartz KS et al (1987) Prevalence of arrhythmias detected by ambulatory electrocardiographic monitoring and of abnormal left ventricular ejection fraction in person older than 62 years in a long-term health care facility. Am J Cardiol 59:368-369
6. Donoso E, Adler NL, Friedberg CK (1964) Unusual forms of second degree atrioventricular block, associated with Morgagni-Adams-Stokes syndrome. Am Heart J 67:150-157
7. Dhingra RC, Denes P, Wu D et al (1974) The significance of second degree atrioventricular block and bundle branch blok. Observation regarding site and type of block. Circulation 49:638-646
8. Strasberg B, Amat-y-Leon F, Dhingra RC et al (1981) Natural history of chronic second degree atrioventricular nodal block. Circulation 63:1043-1049
9. Clarke M, Sutton R, Ward D et al (1991) Recommendations for pacemaker prescription for symtomatic bradycardia. Report of a working party of the British Pacing and Electrophysiology Group. Br Heart J 66:185-191
10. Shaw DB, Kekwick C, Veale D et al (1985) Survival in second degree atrioventricular block. Br Heart J 53:587-593
11. Connelly DT, Steinhaus DM (1996) Mobitz type I atrioventricular block: an indication for permanent pacing? Pacing Clin Electrophysiol 19:261-264
12. Barold SS (1998) Indication for pacing in acquired atrioventricular block: the 1991 ACC/AHA guidelines should be revised. In: Barold SS, Mugica J (eds) Recent advances in cardiac pacing: goals for the 21st century. Futura, Armonk, NY, pp 115-121
13. Rardon DP, Miles WM, Mitrani RD et al (1995) Atrioventricular block and dissociation. In: Zipes DP, Jalife J (eds) Cardiac electrophysiolgy: from cells to bedside. Saunders, Philadelphia, pp 935-942
14. Kastor JA (1994) Atrioventricular block. In: Kastor JA (ed) Arrhythmias. Saunders, Philadelphia, pp 145-200
15. Schoeller R, Andersen D, Buttner P et al (1993) First or second degree atrioventricular block as a risk factor in idiopathic dilated cardiomyopathy. Am J Cardiol 71:720-726
16. Skinner NS Jr, Mitchell JH, Wallace AG et al (1963) Hemodynamic effects of altering the timing of atrial systole. Am J Physiol 205:499-503
17. Ishikawa T, Kimura K, Miyazaki N et al (1992) Diastolic mitral regurgitation in patients with first degree atrioventricular block. Pacing Clin Electrophysiol 15:1927-1931

Patients Implanted for AV Block: How Many Subsequently Develop Sinus Node Dysfunction?

M. Di Biase, M. Grimaldi, C. Forleo, G. Mavilio and M.V. Pitzalis

Dual-chamber atrio-ventricular synchronous pacing (DDD) has been shown in many studies to provide better hemodynamic parameter [1, 2] and quality of life [3, 4] than VVI pacing in patients with A-V block. The complexity of implant procedures, the unreliability of some atrial leads, the extra time required for atrial lead fixation, the complexity of follow-up, the cost and the need for some patients to be programmed out of DDD created reluctance to implant dual-chamber pacemakers, and VVI pacing has been recommended as an acceptable treatment in the absence of retrograde conduction [5]. In order to avoid problems related to atrial leads, in patients with normal sinus node function and A-V block, newer single-lead systems with atrial dipoles have been shown to provide reliable atrial sensing and to ensure reliable AV synchrony in VDD mode [6, 7]. In patients implanted with this type of pacemaker it is important to know the real incidence of sinus node dysfunction over time. A low incidence would favor single-lead VDD systems, whereas a high incidence would make DDD or DDDR pacemaker systems more effective.

The natural history of sinus node dysfunction in patients with isolated A-V block and submitted to pacemaker implantation is not very well known since only few data are available in the literature, mainly because of problems regarding the diagnosis of sinus node dysfunction. Indeed, there is no agreement on this subject.

In some studies sinus bradycardia on electrocardiography is the only criterion utilized, in others sinus rate at Holter monitoring is stressed, while in a few studies complex criteria, both clinical and electrophysiological, are utilized.

It is our opinion that the following criteria for the diagnosis of sinus node dysfunction in patients with A-V block could be suggested:

At implantation:
- Previous history of sinus node dysfunction
- Inability to complete the modified exercise test (6-min walk)
- Sinus bradycardia (sinus rate < 60 beats/m') most of the time during Holter monitoring associated with A-V block

Reparto di Cardiologia, Università di Bari e Foggia, Italy

- Presence of sinus bradycardia associated with spots of atrial tachyarrhythmias at ECG or during Holter monitoring

  At follow-up:
- Development of stable sinus bradycardia (< 60 beats/min) or sinus pauses (more than two sinus cycle lengths)
- Inability to reach a sinus rate > 100 beats/min on modified exercise test and/or during usual daily activity
- Development of stable atrial fibrillation

Data from the literature show that the development of sinus bradycardia in patients with A-V block is infrequent. No patient developed this complication in a group of 49 with normal sinus function reported by Morsi et al. [8] during a follow-up period of 30.4 months, while in the study of Hunziker et al. [9] 2 out of 86 patients (2.2%) with normal sinus node function and A-V block developed sinus bradycardia during a follow-up period of 10 ± 10 months. In a similar study Ben Ameur [10] reported the development of sinus node bradycardia in 1 patient out of 44 (2.3%) during a follow-up period of 14.5 ± 7 months.

On the other hand, many data are reported in the literature on this topic when the occurrence of atrial fibrillation is one of the diagnostic criteria utilized for the diagnosis of sinus node dysfunction. The main data are given in Table 1.

Other information is available regarding the time of occurrence of atrial fibrillation after pacemaker implantation and the influence of pacing modalities.

Regarding the time of occurrence of atrial fibrillation, Mattioli et al. [14], in a group of 100 patients followed for 5 years, reported an incidence of 10% at 1 year, 11% at 2 years, 23% at 3 years and 31% at 5 years. No statistically significant difference was found between patients with A-V block and patients with sick sinus syndrome.

Regarding the influence of the pacing modalities in the occurrence of atrial fibrillation, Folino et al. reported the following figures on 169 patients followed for 5.5 years: VVI mode 27%, VDD mode 9% and DDD mode 25% [12]. No difference was found if the presence or the absence of retrograde conduction was considered.

Mattioli et al. reported a statistically significantly higher rate of arrhythmia in

Table 1. Reports relating the development of atrial fibrillation after pacemaker implantation in patients with A-V block and normal sinus node function

Author	Reference	Year	Follow-up	Patients	Incidence %
Folino	12	1994	44 m	85	8.2
Ibrahim	11	1995	32 m	180	10
Ben Ameur	10	1997	14.5 m	65	7
Folino	13	1988	5.5 y	169	18.3
Mattioli	14	1988	5 y	100	18.7
Hunziker	9	1998	10 m	86	3.5
Morsi	8	1998	30.4 m	49	2.5
Rey	15	1998	24 m	150	5

y, years; m, months

patients receiving ventricular pacing than in those who received physiological pacing [14].

Conclusions

Very few data are available in the literature regarding the occurrence over time of sinus node dysfunction in patients submitted to pacemaker implantation because of A-V block. Difficulties in completing this kind of research are mainly due to the absence of diagnostic criteria for sinus node dysfunction in these patients, since most of the time they are based on clinical criteria [10, 12]; only in the paper of Morsi et al. [8] have acceptable clinical and electrophysiological criteria been utilized.

If the occurrence of sinus bradycardia or sino-atrial block is considered, sinus node dysfunction after pacemaker implantation for A-V block is infrequent (less than 2% per year). These data would argue that the utilization of a simple single pass VDD system in subjects with normal sinus node function is safe and should be increased. On the other hand, if the occurrence of atrial fibrillation is considered, the incidence of sinus dysfunction is higher, since at 5 years it is between 25% and 35%. This could imply a limitation in the utilization of VDD mode and an extensive utilization of DDD mode with automatic mode switching to face the occurrence of paroxysmal or chronic atrial fibrillation.

References

1. Lau CP, Tai YT, Li JP et al (1992) Initial clinical experience with a single pass VDDR pacing system. PACE 15:1894-1900
2. Leclercq C, Gras D, LeHelloco A et al (1995) Hemodynamic importance of preserving the normal sequence of ventricular activation in permanent cardiac pacing. Am Heart J 129:1133-1141
3. Lau CP, Tai YT, Lee PWH et al (1994) Quality of life in DDDR pacing: atrioventricular synchrony or rate adaptation? PACE 17:1838-1843
4. Lukl J, Doupal V, Heinc P et al (1994) Quality of life during DDD and dual sensor VVIR pacing. PACE 17:1844-1848
5. Petch MC (1993) Who needs dual chamber pacing? BMJ 307:215-216
6. Antonioli GE (1994) Single lead atrial synchronous ventricular pacing: a dream come true. PACE 17:1531-1547
7. Pitts Crick JC (1991) European multicenter prospective follow-up study of 1,002 implants of a single lead VDD pacing system. PACE 14:1742-1744
8. Morsi A, Lau C, Nishimura S et al (1998) The development of sinoatrial dysfunction in pacemaker patients with isolated atrioventricular block. PACE 21:1430-1434
9. Hunziker P, Buser P, Pfisterer M et al (1998) Predictors of loss of atrioventricular synchrony in single lead VDD pacing. Heart 80:390-392.
10. Ben Ameur Y, Martin E, Jarwe M et al (1997) VDD mode single electrode cardiac stimulation: indications, results and limitations of the method. Ann Cardiol Angeiol 46:585-591

11. Ibrahim B, Sanderson JE, Wright B et al (1995) Dual chamber pacing: how many patients remain in DDD mode over the long term? Br Heart J 74:76-79

12. Folino AF, Buja G, Ruzza L et al (1994) Long-term follow-up of patients with single-lead VDD stimulation. PACE 17:1854

13. Folino AF, Buja G, Dal Corso L et al (1998) Incidence of atrial fibrillation in patients with different mode of pacing. Long term follow-up. PACE 21:260-263

14. Mattioli AV, Vivoli D, Mattioli G (1998) Influence of pacing modalities on the incidence of atrial fibrillation in patients without prior atrial fibrillation. A prospective study. Eur Heart J 19:282-286

15. Rey JL, Tribouilloy C, Elghelbazouri F et al (1998) Single-lead VDD pacing: long-term experience with four different systems. Am Heart J 135:1036-1039

16. Mattioli AV, Tarabini Castellani E, Vivoli D et al (1998) Prevalence of atrial fibrillation and stroke in paced patients without prior atrial fibrillation: a prospective study. Clin Cardiol 21:117-122

Optimizing the AV Delay in DDD Pacemakers: How Useful Is it?

S. Sermasi, M. Marconi and M. Mezzetti

Atrial systole contributes to end-systolic ventricular filling, optimizing the filling pressure as well as ensuring closure of the atrioventricular (AV) valve. It also contributes to the regulation of neurohumoral reflexes and the production of atrial natriuretic peptide (ANP) as well as to adjusting preload and afterload, to increasing inotropy, and to ventricular relaxation and myocardial oxygen consumption. The deleterious hemodynamic effects of loss of AV synchrony are well proven [1]. The atrial contribution to ventricular filling declines, and when sustained 1:1 retrograde atrial activation is maintained by ventricular pacing, atrial systole occurs against closed AV valves. The hemodynamic result is a retrograde direction of the hematic flux into pulmonary and systemic veins. Consequently, the mean right atrial and pulmonary wedge pressure increase significantly while the atrial contribution to left ventricular end-diastolic volume during each cardiac cycle is lacking [1, 2].

The increased release of ANP due to both atrial stretching and the increase in atrial pressure causes vasodilatation, which can intensify hypotension [3-5]. These problems are the basis of the so-called pacemaker syndrome, which occurs in ventricularly paced patients when an inappropriately timed native o retrogradely induced atrial activity is present. Symptoms related to pacemaker syndrome are often light and temporary, but occasionally they may be severe and dramatic, including weakness, rapid fatigue, dyspnea, peripheral edema – all due to congestive phenomena and low cardiac output. They may be associated with palpitations, recurrent pulsation in the neck or abdomen, coughing, headache, confusion, fainting, dizzy spells, hypotension, and even syncope [1, 6-8]. The irregular appearance of this variety of clinical manifestations makes the diagnosis of pacemaker syndrome very difficult.

However, in unpaced patients with a very prolonged anterograde AV conduction as well, atrial contraction so close to the preceding ventricular systole causes similar consequences, as when sustained retrograde ventriculoatrial conduction occurs [9, 10]. Symptoms and signs associated with this are very similar to those

Dipartimento di Medicina, Unità Operativa di Cardiologia, Ospedale Infermi, AUSL Rimini, Italy

seen in pacemaker syndrome [11, 12]. When a long PR interval is associated with high diastolic pressure, the diastolic filling period is shortened because the mitral valve closes prematurely [13]. In addition, the ventricular systole following the atrial contraction may be so delayed that the reversed AV pressure gradient, lacking complete mitral valve closure, may cause diastolic mitral regurgitation [14].

AV synchrony may be critical in the aged and when alterations in ventricular filling and compliance or severe left ventricular dysfunction are present. In most cases the atrial contribution to ventricular filling is critical, particularly when atrial function is preserved.

Dual-chamber pacemakers can preserve or restore AV synchrony, allowing selection of the AV delay (AVD). Pacing both the atrium and the ventricle at rest, as proved by echoDoppler techniques, the optimal AVD found was about 150 ms [15], and measuring cardiac output by impedance cardiography the value was decreased to < 120 ms from atrial stimulus to ventricular stimulus [16]. Thus an optimal AVD at rest may be considered to be in the range of 120-150 ms.

However, the AVD in a dual-chamber pacemaker can vary on the basis of four different conditions, all of which can affect hemodynamics: (a) atrium paced and ventricle sensed, (b) atrium paced and ventricle paced, (c) atrium sensed and ventricle paced, (d) atrium sensed and ventricle sensed. Modern pacemakers incorporate the ability to set the proper AVD on this basis. Taking into account interatrial conduction delays, when the atrium is sensed, the AVD should be shortened by 50 ms [17]. A simple approach to AVD programming may be to set an AVD of 150 ms when atrium and ventricle are paced and 100 ms when the atrium is sensed.

The activation sequence of the ventricle is different in normal condition and in right ventricle pacing. In many patients with no AV block or intermittent AV block it is possible to set a long AVD, avoiding the need to pace the ventricle and preserving its normal activation. However, it is still unclear which is more important: an optimal AVD or a normal activation sequence in the ventricle [18-20].

When the heart rate increases, the PR interval decreases in a linear fashion. The aerobic and hemodynamic benefits of an adaptive AVD during exercise have been well proved [21].

These findings seemed to be more manifest at the high rate achieved at peak exercise in a comparison of rate-adaptive AVD to fixed AVD in chronotropic competent patients suffering from complete AV block [22].

The importance of the correct AVD for improving hemodynamics in patients with selected heart diseases has been stressed.

The optimal AVD, able to maximize the stroke volume, seems to be different in patients with left ventricular hypertrophy to that in normal subjects [23].

Physiological cardiac stimulation in the treatment of hypertrophic obstructive cardiomyopathy proved to be capable of reducing the preexisting subaortic pressure gradient so long as a critical AVD was present that was able to ensure the sustained artificial ventricular activation. The data collected are consistent with an altered ventricular activation sequence producing delayed septal activation, which is suspected to be one of the mechanisms leading to outflow tract gradient reduction [24, 25].

Some studies have shown both acute and long-term efficacy of dual-chamber pacing in the treatment of idiopathic dilated cardiomyopathy using short AVD (< 100 ms) [26-28].

In our experience, the higher stroke volume obtained with a given AVD is the true criterion of proper AV coupling, because the stroke volume is the final result of all components affecting the regular working of the heart [29].

In summary, many patients, especially those with organic heart disease, cannot fully benefit from dual-chamber pacing unless the timing between left atrial systole and left ventricular contraction is optimized at all times, both at rest and during exercise. Optimization should be individual, according to the physiological and pathological characteristics of each patient. Many studies have stressed this problem but proposed solutions are limited and an automatic system computing the optimal AVD is a long way off. Some recently available physiological sensors, such as those measuring peak endocardial acceleration and/or cardiac impedance for example, able to give hemodynamic data, should be utilized to automatically select the best AVD on this basis. This possibility is still being examined experimentally.

References

1. Asubel K, Furman S (1985) The pacemaker syndrome. Ann Intern Med 103:420-429
2. Sermasi S, Marconi M (1993) The pacemaker syndrome. G Ital Cardiol 23:485-493
3. Haas M, Fischer TA, Dietz R (1987) Is atrial distension the physiological stimulus for release of atrial natriuretic peptide? Lancet 28:1269-1270
4. Millaire A, Ducloux G, De Groote O et al (1990) Le facteur auriculaire natrurétique. Etat actuel des connaissances et des implications en patologie cardiaque. Informat Cardiol 14:604-610
5. Stangl K, Weil J, Seitz K et al (1988) Influence of AV synchrony on the plasma levels of atrial natriuretic peptide (ANP) in patients with total AV block. Pacing Clin Electrophysiol 11:1176-1181
6. Das G (1984) Pacemaker headache. Pacing Clin Electrophysiol 7:802-805
7. Nishimura RA, Dersh BJ, Holmes DR Jr (1983) Outcome of dual-chamber pacing for the pacemaker syndrome. Mayo Clin Proc 58:452-456
8. Heldman D, Mulvihill D, Messenger J et al (1990) True incidence of pacemaker syndrome. Pacing Clin Electrophysiol 13:1742-1750
9. Barold SS (1996) Indications for permanent cardiac pacing in first-degree AV block: class I, II or III? Pacing Clin Electrophysiol 19:747-751
10. Shuller H, Brandt J (1991) The pacemaker syndrome: old and new causes. Clin Cardiol 14:336-340
11. Wharton JM, Ellenbogen KA (1995) Atrioventricular conduction system disease. In: Ellenbogen KA, Kay GN, Wilkoff BL (eds) Clinical cardiac pacing. Saunders, Philadelphia, pp 304-320
12. Kim YH, O'Nunain S, Trouton T et al (1993) Pseudopacemaker syndrome following inadvertent fast pathway ablation for atrioventricular nodal reentrant tachycardia. J Cardiovasc Electrophysiol 4:178-182
13. Nishimura RA, Hayes DL, Holmes DR et al (1995) Mechanism of hemodynamic improvement by dual-chamber pacing for severe left ventricular dysfunction: an acute Doppler and catheterization hemodynamic study. J Am Coll Cardiol 25:281-288

14. Ishikawa T, Tamura K, Miyzaki N et al (1992) Diastolic mitral regurgitation in patients with first degree atrioventricular block. Pacing Clin Electrophysiol 15:1927-1931
15. Haskel RJ, French WJ (1986) Optimum AV interval in dual-chamber pacemakers. Pacing Clin Electrophysiol 9:670-675
16. Ovsyshcher I, Zimlichman R, Katz A et al (1993) Measurements of cardiac output by impedance cardiography in pacemaker patients at rest: effects of various atrioventricular delays. J Am Coll Cardiol 21:761-767
17. Camous JP, Raybaud F, Dolisi C et al (1993) Interatrial conduction in patients undergoing AV stimulation: effects of increasing right atrial stimulation. Pacing Clin Electrophysiol 16:2082-2086
18. Harper GR, Pina IL, KutaleK SP et al (1991) Intrinsic conduction maximizes cardiopulmonary performance in patients with dual-chamber pacemakers. Pacing Clin Electrophysiol 14:1787-1791
19. Rosenqvist M, Isaaz K, Botvinik EH et al (1991) Relative importance of activation sequence compared to atrioventricular synchrony in left ventricula function. Am J Cardiol 67:148-156
20. Jutzy RV, Feenstra L, Pai R et al (1992) Comparison of intrinsic versus paced ventricular function. Pacing Clin Electrophysiol 15:1919-1922
21. Occhetta E, Rognoni G, Perucca A et al (1993) The functional and hemodynamic benefits of automatic atrioventricular interval delay in permanent atrial synchronized pacing. G Ital Cardiol 23:877-886
22. Sheppard RC, Ren JF, Ross J et al (1993) Doppler echocardiographic assessment of the hemodynamic benefits of rate adaptive AV delay during exercise in paced patients with complete heart block. Pacing Clin Electrophysiol 9:2157-2167
23. Crepaz R, Pitsheider W, Zammarchi A et al (1991) Role of echo-Doppler in programming of sequential pacemakers. Evaluation of optimal atrioventricular delay in patients with normal or hypertrophic left ventricle. G Ital Cardiol 21:975-982
24. Fananapazir L, Cannon RO, Tripodi D et al (1992) Impact of dual-chamber permanent pacing in patients with obstructive cardiomyopathy with symptoms refractory to verapamil and beta-adrenergic blocker therapy. Circulation 85:2149-2161
25. Jeanrenaud X, Goy JJ, Kappenberger L (1992) Effects of dual-chamber pacing in hypertrophic obstructive cardiomyopathy. Lancet 339:1318-1323
26. Hochleitner M, Hortnagl H, Ng CK et al (1990) Usefulness of physiologic dual-chamber pacing in drug-resistant idiopathic dilatec cardiomyopathy. Am J Cardiol 66:198-202
27. Hochleitner M, Hortnagl H, Hortnagl H et al (1992) Long-term efficacy of physiologic dual-chamber pacing in the treatment of end-state idiopathic dilated cardiomyopathy. Am J Cardiol 70:1313-1325
28. Brecker SJD, Xiao H, Sparrow J et al (1992) Effects of dual-chamber pacing with short atrioventricular delay in dilated cardiomyopathy. Lancet 340:1308-1312
29. Sermasi S, Marconi M, Mainardi MA (1993) Stimolazione cardiaca permanente: quanto è importante conservare la normale conduzione AV e sequenza di attivazione ventricolare? In: Piccolo E, Raviele A (eds) Aritmie cardiache. Centro Scientifico Editore, Torino, pp 472-478

What Are the Long-Term Benefits of the Dual-Chamber Rate-Responsive System Driven by Contractility?

J. Clémenty, S. Garrigue, P. Jaïs, D.C. Shah, M. Hocini, M. Haïssaguerre, G. Gaggini and the PEA European Group

Myocardial contractility beat-to-beat evaluation is now possible using an implanted microaccelerometer located on the tip of an endocardial lead in the right ventricle. The signal provided by this device is closely related to right ventricle dp/dt curve. The maximal value of the accelerometer signal, peak of endocardial acceleration (PEA) is correlated with dp/dt max (mm Hg) during dobutamine infusion. Some previous studies have clearly established a direct correlation between right and left ventricle contractility [1-3]. Increased cardiac output during exercise and emotional or psychological stress is mediated by the autonomic nervous system, sympathetic tone increasing myocardial contractility and heart rate [4]. In an individual patient, every PEA value is associated with a heart rate value. These two parameters related by a closed loop algorithm can be used to drive a rate-responsive pacemaker in patients with chronotropic incompetence but normal contractility adaptation during sympathetic stimulation. A DDDR device was provided by Sorin (Italy) Living 1 pacemaker. This works using a specially designed ventricular lead tipped by a microaccelerometer and a standard pacing unipolar electrode. Some studies have demonstrated the efficacy of this pacemaker [5-7]. The aim of this paper is to study the long-term stability of the correlation linking PEA and heart rate variations in implanted patients.

Patients and Methods

A double short-term and long-term study was performed using data from a Multicentric European Study.

Short-Term Study

From December 1995 to January 1997, 105 patients were implanted with a Living 1 DDDR pacemaker. Fifty-four patients in sinus rhythm and normal chronotropic function 1 month after implantation were selected: sixteen females and 38

CHU de Bordeaux, Hôpital Cardiologique du Haut-Lévêque, Bordeaux-Pessac, France

males, mean age 65.6 ± 12.4 years. Pacemaker indications were: high grade AV block in 25 patients and sick sinus syndrome in 29 patients. No cardiac underlying disease had been detected in any patient. A 24-h Holter monitoring was obtained in all patients and 31 patients underwent a cycloergometer exercise test of three 25 watts levels for 3 min (75 watts/9 min). Using a radiotelemetry system recorder, PEA and heart rate values were continuously obtained during the two tests [8]. For every patient, PEA values (expressed in g) and heart rates (in bpm) were correlated using a moving average of four beats, providing a stable correlation coefficient (Fig. 1), and the mean correlation coefficient was calculated.

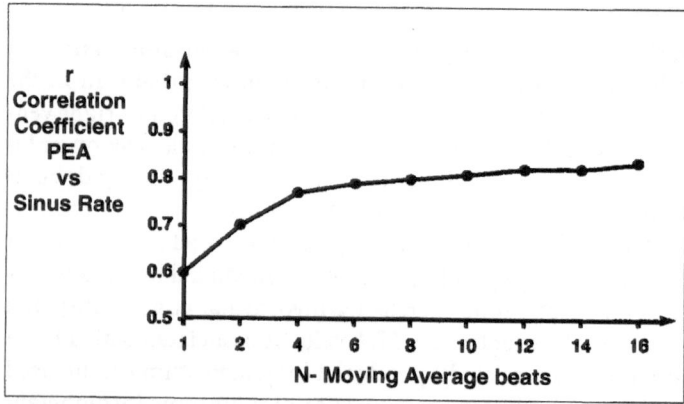

Fig. 1. Correlation coefficient variations using moving average

Long-Term Study

A cohort of 70 patients (54 previously included + 16 newly included patients) was evaluated according to the same method, 1 month and 1 year after pacemaker implantation (28 females and 42 males, mean age 67.2 ± 11.8 years). Pacing indication was AV block in 25 patients, sick sinus syndrome in 39 patients and vasovagal syncope in 6 patients. Good quality Holter monitoring was obtained in 61 patients and exercise tests in 42 patients.

Assessment of Electrical Properties

Assessment of electrical propeties of the specially designed ventricular pacing lead was obtained at implantation and at 1 year: pacing threshold, lead impedance and detected QRS amplitude.

Results

One Month After Implantation

In a bicycle stress test (Fig. 2) PEA values increased from 0.41 ± 0.26 g to 1.63 ± 0.67 g (+ 400%) and heart rate from 73 ± 9 bpm to 123 ± 20 bpm (+ 77%). The correlation coefficient was 0.74 ± 0.15 ($p < 0.005$).

In daily life exercises obtained by Holter recordings, PEA increased from 0.35 ± 0.2 g to 1.44 ± 0.65 g (+ 311%) and heart rate from 66 ± 4 bpm to 109 ± 16 bpm (+ 65%), the correlation coefficient was 0.67 ± 0.15 (p < 0.05).

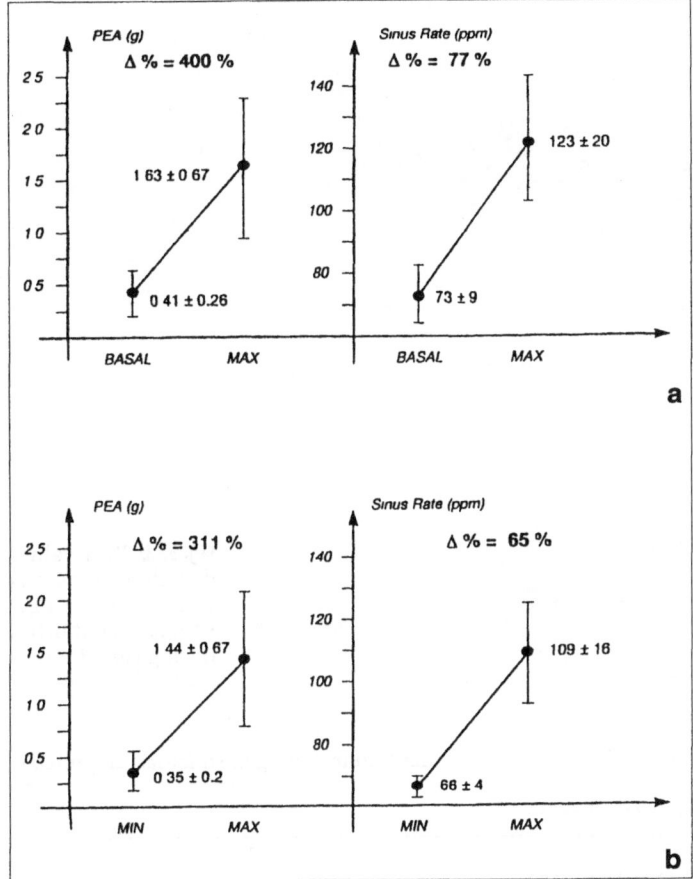

Fig. 2a,b. PEA /heart rate correlations during stress test (a). PEA/heart rate correlations during Holter monitoring (b)

One Year After Implantation

The mean correlation coefficient was 0.65 ± 0.14 (*p* < 0.005) in daily life Holter activities and 0.77 ± 0.11 (*p* < 0.005) in the stress test. No significant difference was observed between late values and short-term values: PEA values distribution were comparable at 1 month and at 1 year (Fig. 3).

Electrical Properties of Ventricular Lead

Electrical properties of ventricular lead (Table 1) show an increase of pacing threshold from 0.49 ± 0.18 V to 1.23 ± 0.42 V (*p* < 0,01) and of the pacing impedance from 598 ± 150 Ohms to 662 ± 98 Ohms (*p* < 0.05).

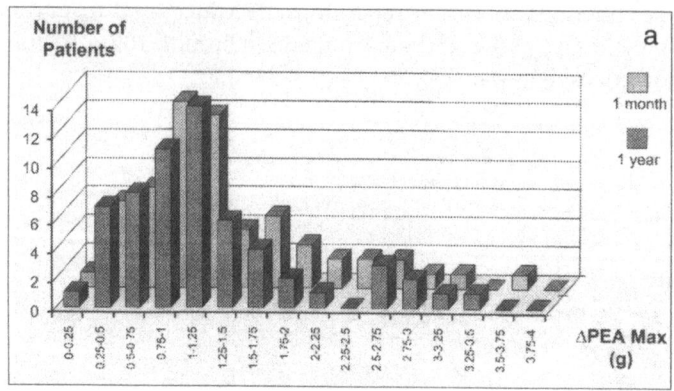

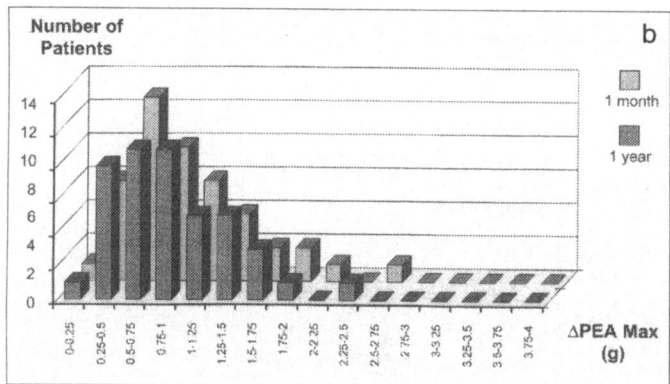

Fig. 3a,b. PEA values distribution during stress test. (a) PEA values distribution during Holter monitoring (b)

Table 1. Electrical properties of the special ventricular lead including the microaccelerometer

Lead sensing and pacing performances

At implant	
• Pacing threshold	0.49 V ± 0.18 V
• Pacing impedance	598 Ω ± 150 Ω
• QRS amplitude	12.6 mV ± 5.0 mV

1 year follow-up	
• Pacing threshold	1.23 V ± 0.42 V
• Pacing impedance	662 Ω ± 98 Ω
• Pacing amplitude	11.8 mV ± 3.1 mV

Discussion

Patients without significant structural heart diseases, assessed by echocardiography, have a parallel evolution of PEA values and heart rate during submaximal exercises. PEA could be safety used as a sensor for chronotropic modulation in patients suffering from chronotropic incompetence. During daily life activities, some of the paced patients performed only submaximal exercises. In these tests myocardial contractility and rate increase both contribute to cardiac output elevation. Whether PEA is a reliable index during stronger efforts remains unestablished. Non-increase of stroke volume during heavy exercise does not mean the contractility is unmodified: pre-load, after load, heart rate are implied together with contractility in stroke volume production [9, 10].

Long-term stability of PEA values in individual patients is assessed by this study. PEA values range between 0.15 and 2.5 g in daily life activities and 0.20 g to 4 g in stress tests. The distribution peak shifts to a lower value in daily life versus stress tests. Probably exercise intensity is greater in the bicycle test than in Holter activities, and individual and time-to-time variations in exercise levels are more important in Holter activities than in stress tests. A wide range of PEA values is obtained during similar standardised exercises in this population of patients with a normal or subnormal heart function. This could be explained by difference in age, in sympathetic tone, in lead tip position against right ventricular endocardium and variable fibrosis reaction to the electrode. No loss of signal at rest and during exercise related to a destruction of the microaccelerometer was observed in any patient.

The device is equipped by an additional sensor: a mercury ball gravitometer system included in the pulse generator providing rate modulation if the microaccelerometer is inoperative. This additional sensor could be used for other functions: cross checking of microaccelerometer signal as a patient position indicator, improvement of rate modulation, amongst other functions.

Finally, electrical properties of this lead do not differ from those of standard ventricular unipolar leads.

Conclusions

The comparison of 1-month and 1-year data demonstrated that PEA is a long-term stable parameter and that it can be used for physiological driving of RR pacemakers. This evaluation also confirms the absence of any adverse long-term effect and the reliability of the sensor-lead. The sensing and pacing performances of the lead remain within the normal range.

References

1. Bongiorni MG, Soldati E, Arena G, Quirino G, Vernazza F, Bernasconi A, Garberoglio B (1996) Is local myocardial contractility related to endocardial acceleration signals detected by a transvenous pacing lead? PACE 19(II):1682-1688
2. Rickards AF, Bombardini T, Corbucci G, Plicchi G (1996) An implantable intracardiac accelerometer for monitoring myocardial contractility. PACE 19:2066-2071
3. Occhetta E, Perucca A, Rognoni G, Corbucci G, Garberoglio B, Liverani L, Plicchi G (1995) Experience with a new myocardial acceleration sensor during Dobutamine infusion and exercise test. Eur J C P E 5:204-209
4. Gleason WL, Braunwald E (1962) Studies on the first derivative of the ventricular pressure pulse in man. J Clin Invest 41:80

5. Sharma A, Sutton R, Bennett T et al (1986) Physiologic pacing based on beat-to-beat measurement of right ventricular dp/dt max: initial feasibility studies in man. J Am Coll Cardiol 7:3A (abstr)

6. Menozzi C, Tomasi C, Brignole M, Lolli G, Bottoni N, Garberoglio B, Corbucci G, Plicchi G (1996) Cardiac contractility: concepts and advances in implantable system application. In: Adornato E (ed) Therapies for cardiac arrhythmias in 1996: where we are going? Luigi Pozzi, Rome, pp 383

7. Ritter Ph, Corbucci G, Plicchi G, Gaggini G, Garberoglio B (1996) Diagnostic applications of a new cardiac contractility sensor. In: Adornato E (ed) Therapies for cardiac arrhythmias in 1996 : where we are going. Luigi Pozzi, Rome, pp 397

8. Parlapiano M, Bizzini A, Corbucci G et al (1994) Implantable radiotelemetry system (I.R.S.) for peak endocardial acceleration (P.E.A.) measurements on free sheep. Eur J C P E 4[Suppl 4]:60 (abstr)

9. Loeppky JA, Greene ER, Hoekenger DE et al (1981) Beat-by-beat stroke volume assessment by pulsed Doppler in upright and supine exercise. J Appl Physiol 50:1173-1182

10. Higginbotham MB, Morris KG, Williams RS et al (1986) Regulation of stroke volume during submaximal and maximal upright exercise in normal man. Circ Res 58:281-291

Haemodynamic Sensors: What is Their Role in Monitoring Heart Function?

L. Padeletti[1], M.C. Porciani[1], A. Colella[1], A. Michelucci[1], A. Costoli[1], P. Pieragnoli[1], P. Ritter[2], H. Luttikhuis[3], J.C. Deharo[4], G. Gaggini[5] and G.F. Gensini[1]

Introduction

For many years implantable devices for cardiac pacing applications have been developed with the main aim of treating AV block and sinus node dysfunction. With the introduction of rate-responsive pacing in 1983, different kinds of sensors have been developed, clinically validated and introduced into the clinical practice for driving rate adaptive pacemakers.

In the last years, pacing indications have noticeably enlarged to include areas like supraventricular tachyarrhythmias, dilatative or hypertrophic cardiomyopathies and vasovagal syncope.

A variety of pacing approaches has been proposed, and has been clinically tried, for the prevention and for the treatment of these pathologies. The intrinsic complexity of these syndromes, largely greater than that of pure rhythm disturbances, underlined the potential role of implantable sensors for long-term monitoring of overall heart function.

Research is in progress, at different stages, to develop sensors able to supply information about important vital parameters, such as blood pressure, oxygen saturation and cardiac output.

However, real use of these sensors for long-term monitoring showed quite severe limitations, particularly because of body tissue reactions adversely affecting their sensitivity and reliability.

As of today, the sole application is a device (Reveal by Medtronic), which is anyway restricted to the monitoring and recording of ECG only.

An Active Lead for Long-Term Contractility Monitoring

In an attempt to overcome the technical limitations and the lack of long-term stability discussed above, SORIN has developed a new sensor (BEST –

[1]Department of Internal Medicine and Cardiology, University of Florence, Italy; [2]InParys, Paris, France; [3]Sophia Hospital, Zwolle, The Netherlands; [4]S. Marguerite Hospital, Marseille, France; [5]Sorin Biomedica Cardio, Saluggia, Italy

Biomechanical Endocardial Sorin Transducer) (Fig. 1), able to detect the cardiac acceleration signal coincident with the isovolumetric contraction phase.

As the myocardium contracts isometrically, it generates vibrations that are transmitted through the heart. These vibrations are, in their audible component, responsible for the first heart sound and can be measured with a microaccelerometer located inside the tip of a standard unipolar pacing lead. The microaccelerometer is hermetically sealed and needs no external reference or calibration. Theoretical and experimental evidence has shown that changes in myocardial contractility are reflected in a change of amplitude of the preejection vibrations [1].

The peak-to-peak value of the endocardial acceleration signal (Fig. 2), measured in a time window containing the isovolumetric contraction phase, was called PEA (peak endocardial acceleration). In vivo preclinical tests on animals and humans were carried out to evaluate the PEA signal for rate responsive pacing. A very high correlation between PEA and dP/dt max both in the right and in the left ventricle during dobutamine test was also discovered. Further analysis showed that although the PEA signal is recorded by a lead placed in the right ventricular apex, it is representative of the function of the whole heart, which is largely dependent on the left ventricle, where most of the muscular mass is found. Recordings obtained during pulmonary artery balloon occlusion in sheep have confirmed this. In this situation the right ventricle is totally full and therefore its dP/dt max increases greatly, while at the same time PEA falls following the LV dP/dt max trend (Fig. 3) [1, 2].

The concept of measuring contractility by an implantable accelerometer was validated through a Multicentric Study on a Rate Responsive pacing system (BEST – Living from SORIN BIOMEDICA), in which 100 units were implanted and followed for 1 year [3].

This study positively demonstrates that measurement of PEA is feasible in the

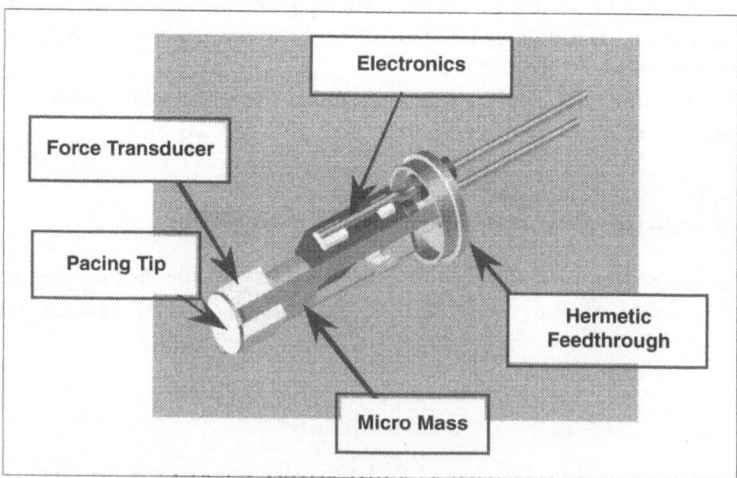

Fig. 1. Contractility Sensor (BEST) structure

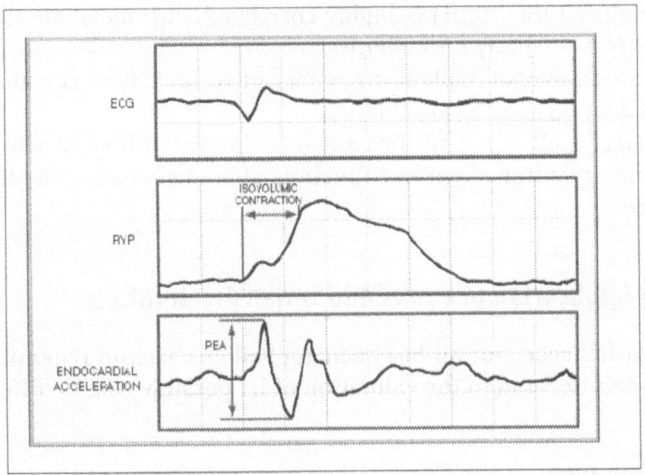

Fig. 2. Peak endocardial acceleration (PEA)

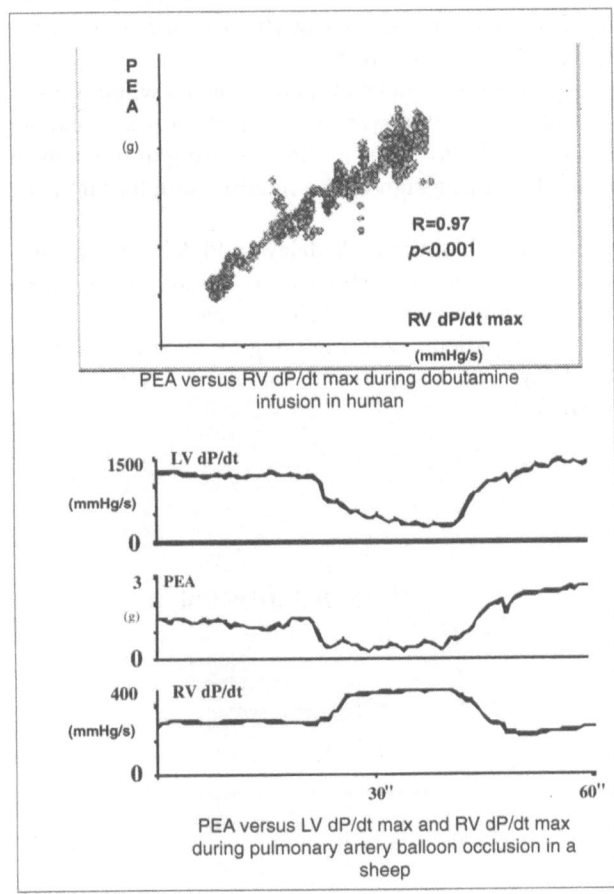

Fig. 3. PEA is a potential overall heart monitor

long-term and that this signal is highly correlated with metabolic demand both during stress test and daily life activities.

Up till now, an overall implant experience of about 850 units with a maximum follow-up of 3.5 years has been achieved.

The results of all these studies suggest the possibility of using PEA as a haemodynamic monitor of cardiac function, able to overcome the limitations of other sensors.

Monitoring Application of Peak Endocardial Acceleration

Peak endocardial acceleration has been applied as a haemodynamic sensor in a series of studies devoted to the validation of its possible role in different clinical areas.

AV Delay Optimization

It is well established that optimization of AV delay is of great importance, from a haemodynamic point of view, in patients with high degree AV block. Current clinical practice uses assessment of optimal AV delay by ECHO; this method is time consuming and possible only with the patient at rest.

PEA, as first heart sound, depends on AV delay; it is maximized when there is competition between atrial and ventricular systole, when it shows a plateau lengthening AV delay (see Fig. 4) [4]. The AV delay at the beginning of the plateau has been identified as the optimal one, as a sign of the natural completion of the atrial systole.

A study has been performed in which optimal AV delay by PEA has been compared with that obtained by ECHO, as the one which corresponds to the maximum LV diastolic filling time, without interruption of the A wave.

The results, in a population of 19 patients with high degree AV block, showed similar values of optimal AV delay, with a significant correlation coefficient as shown in Fig. 5 and Table 1 [5].

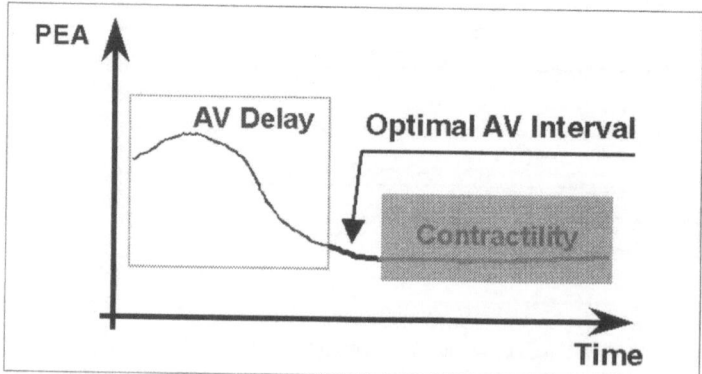

Fig. 4. Optimal AV delay

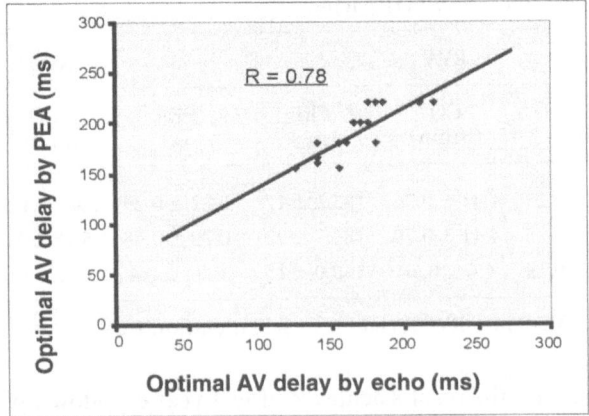

Fig. 5. Correlation between optimal AVDs obtained by Echo and by PEA. AVD, AV delay

Table 1. Comparison between the optimal AVDs obtained with PEA method and the Echo method

	AVD (PEA)		AVD (Echo)
DDD	202 ± 21 ms	< 0.05	179 ± 25 ms
	< 0.001		< 0.001
VDD	145 ± 18 ms	< 0.05	124 ± 18 ms

The conclusions from this study allowed the validation of PEA as a new method for AV delay optimization; optimal AV delay may be obtained directly from an implanted device making it possible to optimize it also under effort.

A multicentric study on this application of PEA as a haemodynamic sensor is in progress. The study focuses on the dependence of optimal AV delay with effort level, in the perspective of developing an automatic AV delay adapting algorithm.

Comparison of Right Ventricular Outflow Tract Pacing Vs Apical Pacing

Comparative studies on haemodynamic effects of right ventricular outflow tract (RVOT) and right ventricular apex (RVA) pacing have not given definitive answers [6, 7].

It was proposed to use PEA in a prospective, randomized and single blind study to evaluate contractility in the long-term follow-up of patients paced in RVOT and RVA.

Thirteen patients with chronic atrial fibrillation, high degree AV block or RF ablated AV node were implanted with a DDDR pacemaker able to measure PEA; the RVOT screw-in lead was connected to the atrial port and the sensor equipped lead was connected to the ventricular port. This configuration allowed pacing of the two sites separately, with simultaneous measurement first of the PEA signal and then of contractility.

Table 2. Comparison of RVA vs RVOT pacing

	RVA			RVOT		
	PEA (g)	CO (l/min)	PEI (ms)	PEA (g)	CO (l/min)	PEI (ms)
Implant	0.48 ± 0.23	4.41 ± 0.76	183.8 ± 17	0.82 ± 0.29	5.41 ± 1.12	157.5 ± 17
6 months	0.43 ± 0.25	4.41 ± 0.70	181.7 ± 23	0.79 ± 0.48	5.78 ± 1.5	167.5 ± 22
1 year	0.46 ± 0.19	4.4 ± 0.50	180.0 ± 15	0.84 ± 0.4	5.74 ± 1.02	156.0 ± 17

RVA, right ventricular apex; RVOT, right ventricular outflow tract

Table 2 reports on the results achieved after 1 year of follow-up which confirm that pacing in RVOT significantly improves left ventricular contractility (PEA and PEI) and haemodynamic indexes (CO) [8].

Also in this context, PEA demonstrates its validity as a parameter for monitoring of the overall heart function.

Contractility Monitoring During Head-Up Tilt-Induced Vasovagal Syncope

Several authors have presented the hypothesis of a role played by mechanoreceptors in vasovagal syncope pathophysiology, but it is still under discussion [9, 10].

A study has been designed to validate this hypothesis, using PEA as a contractility index, during head-up tilt-test (HUT) of patients with a history of vasovagal disorders.

PEA was recorded from a temporarily implanted sensor-lead, simultaneously with surface ECG and non-invasively measured blood pressure, during HUT performed according to the Westminster protocol, in ten consecutive patients.

Table 3 reports on the data obtained which show a statistically significant increase of PEA before syncope and, even more important, an evident time delay between PEA peak and syncope [11].

This last finding suggests that PEA-driven dual-chamber pacing could overcome the limitations of pacing in ameliorating symptoms in vasovagal patients, limitations are often related to the presence of a vasodepressor component, generally preceding the bradycardia in time.

In 1998, the case of a patient with malignant primary depressive vasovagal syncope positively treated by rate-responsive pacing driven by contractility was reported [12].

On the basis of these overall findings, a randomized, crossover and single blind study was started to compare the effects of DDI versus PEA driven rate responsive pacing in the treatment of vasovagal syncope.

First enrolment was performed in March 1999, and the results will be available in the second half of year 2000.

Table 3. Individual PEA values in the supine and tilt position and before syncope

Patient	Baseline PEA (g)	Tilt PEA (g)	Max PEA before syncope (g)	Delay Between Max PEA recording and syncope (min)
1	0.40	0.70	2.56	0.5
2	1.19	1.07	1.24	0.5
3	0.42	0.49	0.48	5
4	0.34	0.22	0.33	0.5
5	0.49	0.51	0.60	5
6	0.85	0.95	1.70	3
7	0.46	0.33	0.52	6.5
8	1.24	1.73	2.57	2.5
9	0.48	0.44	0.49	0.25
10	0.36	0.74	1.48	5
Mean ± SD	0.62 ± 0.34	0.72 ± 0.44	1.19 ± 0.86*	2.8 ± 2.40

* $p = 0.004$ as compared to PEA value during the stable phase of tilt (Wilcoxon Signed tank test)

Future Perspectives

The area of possible applications of PEA for long-term heart function monitoring is wide, particularly bearing in mind the unique ability of this sensor to evaluate left ventricular contractility even if implanted in the right ventricle, with a fully standard procedure.

Among the possible applications, we would like to underline the following, on which preliminary studies are in progress:
- Monitoring of rejection after heart transplantation.

Previous studies (CHARM) have already demonstrated that advanced PM may monitor acute rejection by recording and transmitting the intramyocardial signal. This parameter has proved to be a reliable parameter in excluding rejection.

Thanks to the correlation between acute rejection and contractility and between dP/dt max and PEA, it should be possible to verify the rejection event by monitoring the long-term trend of this signal.
- Evaluation of haemodynamic results in congestive heart failure patients.

Recent studies by different authors, have demonstrated the effectiveness (in the short- and mid-term) of biventricular pacing in heart failure patients with widened QRS. The beneficial haemodynamic effects of this clinical approach were apparent during acute pacing and were sustained during periods of follow-up.

Theoretically, the advantages should be due to the modification in the activation sequence caused by the left ventricular stimulation, which counteracts the effects of RV pacing, decreasing interventricular delay.

In many studies acute haemodynamic evaluation was performed by LV dp/dt max and, also in this case, the already demonstrated correlation of PEA with this important parameter opens the way for its use in the long-term monitoring of heart failure patients.

Conclusions

The possibility of long-term measurement of contractility through an accelerometer, hermetically housed into the tip of a standard pacing lead, has been demonstrated by the good performances obtained with its use for rate-responsive pacing application.

In independent studies performed on different topics, positive results on the possibility of using PEA for the monitoring of overall heart function monitoring have been achieved, confirming that a mechanical sensor is free of the long term effects which constitute the unavoidable limits of other haemodynamic sensors.

Further studies are needed and are in progress to confirm, in different clinical application, the usefulness of this signal as a haemodynamic sensor for monitoring heart function.

References

1. Rickards AF, Bombardini T, Corbucci G, Plicchi G, on behalf of the Multicenter PEA Study Group (1996) An implantable intracardiac accelerometer for monitoring myocardial contractility. PACE 19:2066-2071
2. Occhetta E, Perucca A, Rognoni G, Corbucci G, Garberoglio B, Liverani L, Plicchi G (1995) Experience with a new myocardial acceleration sensor during dobutamine infusion and exercise test. Eur CPR 5:204-209
3. Clementy J, on behalf of the European PEA Clinical Investigation Group (1998) Dual chamber rate responsive pacing system driven by contractility: final assessment after 1-year follow-up. PACE 21:2192-2197
4. Stept ME, Heid CE, Shaver JA, Leon DF, Leonard JJ (1969) Effect of altering P-R interval on the amplitude of the first heart sound in the anaesthetised dog. Circ Res 25:255
5. Ritter P, Padeletti L, Gillio-Meina L, Gaggini G (1999) Determination of the optimal atrioventricular delay in DDD pacing. Comparison between echo and peak endocardial acceleration measurements. Europace 1:126-130
6. Giudici MC, Thornburg GA, Buck DL, Coyne EP, Walton MC, Paul DL, Sutton J (1997) Comparison of right ventricular outflow tract and apical lead permanent pacing on cardiac output. Am J Cardiol 79:209-212
7. Victor F, Leclercq C, Mabo P, Pavin D, Deviller A, de Place C, Pezard P, Victor J, Daubert C (1999) Optimal right ventricular pacing site in chronically implanted patients: a prospective randomised crossover comparison of apical and outflow tract pacing. J Am Coll Cardiol 33:311-316
8. Porciani MC, Padeletti L, Michelucci A, Colella A, Costoli A, Chelucci A, Pieragnoli P, Gensini GF (1999) Left ventricular performance in right ventricular outflow tract pacing. A comparison with right ventricular apex pacing. PACE 22:906
9. Kosinki D, Grubb BP, Temesy-Armos P (1995) Pathological aspects of neurocardiogenic syncope: current concepts and new perspectives. PACE 18:716-724

10. Sra JS, Akhtar M (1995) Cardiac pacing during neurocardiogenic (vasovagal) syncope. J Cardiovasc Electrophysiol 6:751-760
11. Deharo JC, Peyre JP, Ritter PH, Chalvidan T, Berland Y, Djiane P (1998) A sensor-based evaluation of heart contractility in patients with head-up tilt-induced syncope. PACE 21(II):223-226
12. Deharo JC, Peyre JP, Ritter PH, Chalvidan T, Le Tallec L, Djiane P (1998) Treatment of malignant primary vasodrepressive neurocardiogenic syncope with a rate responsive pacemaker driven by heart contractility. PACE 21:2688-2690

What Is the Optimal Site for Right Ventricular Pacing: Outflow Tract or Apex?

P.E. Vardas and E.N. Simantirakis

Although the first permanent transvenous pacing lead was implanted by Furman [1] in the right ventricular outflow tract, the site which came to be the standard for permanent cardiac pacing was the right ventricular apex. This site is easily accessible and ensures low sensing and pacing thresholds, while the chance of lead dislodgement is small. However, in cases where the activation of the ventricular myocardium occurs entirely through pacing – such as in complete atrioventricular block – the initiation of repolarisation from the right ventricular apex leads to desynchronisation of the contraction of the left ventricle and consequent haemodynamic disturbances, to disturbances of myocardial perfusion and innervation, and possibly to structural damage. Apart from the special case of patients with hypertrophic obstructive cardiomyopathy, where apical stimulation leads to a reduction in the obstruction of the left ventricular outflow tract and to an improvement in symptoms, in every other case electrical stimulation at the right ventricular apex is not best for the patient. Thus in recent years, as our understanding of the pathophysiology of the paced heartbeat has grown, new sites have been sought for the implantation of ventricular leads. Among these, the right ventricular outflow tract has been considered suitable, since access to it is relatively easy, it provides satisfactory sensing and pacing thresholds and, more importantly, it restores a more physiological activation sequence. However, there is conflict among the data in the available literature as regards the comparative evaluation of the two pacing sites, while other pacing sites or combinations of sites have been investigated both in patients with normal hearts and in those with heart failure.

Pacing from the Right Ventricular Apex: Pros and Cons

Pacing through the right ventricular apex (RVA) has come under a considerable amount of criticism. Many years ago it was shown that RVA pacing caused a reduction in dP/dT and an asynchronous contraction pattern [2]. Apart from

Cardiology Department, Heraklion University Hospital, Crete, Greece that, more recent studies have led to the conclusion that RVA pacing leads to disturbances of left ventricular systolic and diastolic function [3-5] and have also shown that it may cause disturbances of perfusion and innervation of the left ventricular myocardium [6, 7]. Furthermore, experimental studies indicate that long-term RVA pacing may entail structural damage to the ventricular myocardium [8, 9]. The findings of Prinzen et al. [10], which describe slow propagation of the impulse and a delayed start of systole, are indicative. When the propagation of the impulse to the ventricles is through the normal conduction system, all regions of the left ventricle contract simultaneously and under the same preload. In the case where the impulse originates from the RVA, the region around the electrode starts to contract first, with a low preload, while more distant regions contract later, having already been stretched by the contraction of the early stimulated regions. This means that the distant regions contract under a higher preload and have an increased workload. Finally, the long term redistribution of wall stress may possibly lead to morphological changes and remodelling of the left ventricle [11].

Although these changes caused by the paced beat generally have a negative effect on cardiac performance, they appear to be beneficial to patients with hypertrophic obstructive cardiomyopathy (HOCM) [12-17]. In these patients the preexcitation of the apex and the delayed stimulation of the interventricular septum lead to a reduction in the obstruction of the left ventricular outflow tract, to a delay in the systolic anterior movement of the mitral valve with consequent reduction in mitral regurgitation, and to an improvement in the symptoms of patients with drug-refractory HOCM. It has been found recently that these effects can be produced only by RVA pacing, while other pacing sites, such as the septum [18], are unable to confer a similar benefit.

Pacing from the Right Ventricular Outflow Tract: Is This the Optimal Site for Pacing?

In view of the above, it is reasonable to look for other pacing sites which might ensure rapid and even propagation of the electrical impulse to the ventricular myocardium and, consequently, more uniform ventricular contraction. The right ventricular outflow tract (RVOT) may be one such site, since the ventricular electrode is implanted near the upper part of the His bundle and could thus, at least theoretically, achieve a more physiological propagation of the impulse. Furthermore, this site is easily accessible, while the sensing and pacing thresholds in this area have been found to be comparable with those in the RVA [19].

Several studies in recent years have compared left ventricular function and cardiac performance during pacing from the RVA and RVOT. Guidici et al. [20] measured the cardiac output with transthoracic continuous-wave Doppler ultrasonography in 89 patients at the time of pacemaker implantation. They found that cardiac output was 18.8% higher and cardiac index 21% higher during RVOT compared with RVA pacing. Moreover, patients with a lower baseline cardiac index had a greater percentage improvement with RVOT pacing. Ishikawa et al. [21] studied 13 patients and found that, acutely, cardiac output increased significantly while wedge pressure decreased significantly during RVOT compared with RVA pacing. The same authors found that the improvement resulting from RVOT pacing was not dependent on baseline left ventricular function. De Cock et al. [22] measured the cardiac index in 17 patients using a Doppler ultrasonographic technique during RVA and RVOT pacing at three different rates (85, 100 and 120 bpm). In general, RVOT pacing led to significantly higher values for the cardiac index. Of 51 paired observations, 45 showed an increase in cardiac index during RVOT pacing as compared to apical pacing. However, RVOT pacing at 120 bpm resulted in a lower cardiac index than RVA pacing in patients with significant coronary artery disease and/or impaired left ventricular function (EF $\leq$ 50%). In another haemodynamic and Doppler ultrasonographic acute study by Alboni et al. [23] the authors found that, in patients with normal left ventricular function, DDD pacing from the RVOT does not improve cardiac function in comparison with apical pacing. Buckingham et al. [24] found a trend for pacing in the RVOT, as opposed to the RVA, to improve the cardiac output in patients with normal left ventricular function. The same authors in another study [25] found that in patients with poor left ventricular function there may be a subtle improvement in diastolic and systolic function with pacing in the RVOT compared to traditional RVA pacing.

Various explanations may be offered for the differences among the findings from the studies carrying out comparative evaluation of RVOT and RVA pacing. There are likely to have been differences between the patient populations in the various studies and in the atrioventricular delays used, which may not always have been optimum, while the RVOT is not a precise anatomical site and we do not know whether pacing was performed at the same location in each case.

However, leaving the above differences aside, the rather encouraging results of RVOT pacing in the acute studies do not appear to apply in the long-term. Victor et al. [26], in a unique and extremely well designed study, examined the possible benefits of long-term RVOT pacing compared with RVA. In this prospective, randomised, crossover study no symptomatic improvement or haemodynamic benefit was noted after 3 months of RVOT pacing in comparison with RVA pacing.

In addition, it should be noted that RVOT pacing, at least as far as the acute studies have shown, has no place in the treatment of patients with heart failure and prolonged atrioventricular and/or interventricular conduction time [27, 28]. These patients can benefit from biventricular pacing or pacing from the left ventricle.

In conclusion, although the findings from most acute studies seem to be in favour of RVOT pacing, it has not been proven superior to RVA in the long term, as regards the haemodynamic result and any improvement in symptoms, in patients with either normal or impaired left ventricular function. Multisite pacing may prove to be a more satisfactory solution for the treatment of patients with bradyarrhythmias and for those with drug-refractory heart failure.

References

1. Furman S, Schwedel J (1959) An intracardiac pacemaker for Stokes-Adams seizures. N Engl J Med 261:943-948
2. Wiggers CJ (1925) The muscular reactions of the mammalian ventricles to artificial surface stimuli. Am J Physiol 73:346-378
3. Rosenqvist M, Isaaz K, Botvinnick E, Dae M, Cockrell J, Abbot J, Schiller H, Griffin J (1991) Relative importance of activation sequence compared to atrioventricular synchrony in left ventricular function. Am J Cardiol 67:148-156
4. Leclercq C, Gras D, Le Helloco A, Nicol L, Mabo P, Daubert C (1995) Hemodynamic importance of preserving the normal sequence of ventricular activation in permanent cardiac pacing. Am Heart J 129:1133-1141
5. Vardas PE, Simantirakis EN, Parthenakis FI, Chrysostomakis SI, Skalidis EI, Zuridakis EG (1997) AAIR versus DDDR pacing in patients with impaired sinus node chronotropy: an echocardiographic and cardiopulmonary study. Pacing Clin Electrophysiol 20:1762-1768
6. Lee MA, Dae MW, Langberg JJ et al (1994) Effects of long-term right ventricular apical pacing on left ventricular perfusion, innervation, function and histology. J Am Coll Cardiol 24:225-232
7. Tse HF, Lau CP (1997) Long-term effect of right ventricular pacing on myocardial perfusion and function. Am J Cardiol 29:744-749
8. Adomian GE, Beazell J (1986) Myofibrillar disarray produced in normal hearts by chronic electrical pacing. Am Heart J 112:79-83
9. Karpawich PP, Justice CD, Cavitt DL, Chang CH (1990) Developmental sequelae of fixed-rate ventricular pacing in the immature canine heart: an electrophysiologic, hemodynamic, and histopathologic evaluation. Am Heart J 119:1077-1083
10. Prinzen FW, Augustijn CH, Arts T, Allessie MA, Reneman RS (1990) Redistribution of myocardial fiber strain and blood flow by asynchronous activation. Am J Physiol 254:300-308
11. Prinzen FW, Cheriex AC, Delhaas T, van Oosterhout FM, Arts T, Wellens HJJ, Reneman RS (1995) Asymmetric thickness of the left ventricular wall resulting from asynchronous electrical evaluation: a study in dogs with ventricular pacing and in patients with left bundle branch block. Am Heart J 130:1045-1053
12. Jeanrenaud X, Goy JJ, Kappenberger L (1992) Effects of dual-chamber pacing in hypertrophic obstructive cardiomyopathy. Lancet 339:1318-1323
13. Fananapazir L, Cannon RO III, Tripodi D, Panza JA (1992) Impact of dual-chamber permanent pacing in patients with obstructive hypertrophic cardiomyopathy with symptoms refractory to verapamil and beta-adrenergic blocker therapy. Circulation 85:2149-2161
14. Fananapazir L, Epstein ND, Curiel RV, Panza JA, Tripodi D, McAreavey D (1994) Long-term results of dual-chamber (DDD) pacing obstructive hypertrophic cardiomyopathy. Evidence for progressive symptomatic and hemodynamic improvement and reduction of left ventricular hypertrophy. Circulation 90:2731-2742
15. Kappenberger L, Linde C, Daubert C, McKenna W, Meisel E, Sadoul N, Chojnowska L, Guize L, Gras D, Jeanrenaud X, Ryden L (1997) Pacing in hypertrophic obstructive cardiomyopathy. A randomized crossover study. PIC Study Group. Eur Heart J 18:1249-1256
16. Simantirakis EN, Kanoupakis EM, Kochiadakis GE, Kanakaraki MK, Parthenakis FI, Manios EG, Markianos E, Vardas PE (1998) The effect of DDD pacing on ergospirometric parameters and neurohormonal activity in patients with hypertrophic obstructive cardiomyopathy. Pacing Clin Electrophysiol 21:2269-2272

17. Simantirakis EN, Kochiadakis GE, Kanakaraki MK, Marketou ME, Parthenakis FI, Kanoupakis EM, Vardas PE (1999) Impact of chronic DDD pacing on time-domain indexes of heart rate variability in patients with hypertrophic obstructive cardiomyopathy. Pacing Clin Electrophysiol (in press)
18. Gadler F, Linde C, Juhlin-Dannfeldt A et al (1996) Influence of right ventricular pacing on left ventricular outflow tract obstruction in patients with hypertrophic obstructive cardiomyopathy. J Am Coll Cardiol 27:1219-1224
19. Barin ES, Jones SM, Ward DE, Camm AJ, Nathan AW (1991) The right ventricular outflow tract as alternative permanent pacing site: long-term follow-up. Pacing Clin Electrophysiol 14:3-6
20. Giudici MC, Thornburg GA, Buck DL, Coyne EP, Walton MC, Paul DL, Sutton J (1997) Comparison of right ventricular outflow tract and apical lead permanent pacing on cardiac output. Am J Cardiol 79:209-212
21. Ishikawa T, Sumita S, Kikuchi M, Kosuge M, Sugano T, Shigemasa T, Endo T, Kuji N, Kimura K, Tochikubo O, Ishii M (1997) Hemodynamic effects of right ventricular outflow pacing. J Cardiol 30:125-130
22. De Cock CC, Meyer A, Kamp O, Visser CA (1998) Hemodynamic benefits of right ventricular outflow tract pacing: comparison with right ventricular apex pacing. Pacing Clin Electrophysiol 21:536-541
23. Alboni P, Scarfo S, Fuca G, Mele D, Dinelli M, Paparella N (1998) Short-term hemodynamic effects of DDD pacing from ventricular apex, right ventricular outflow tract and proximal septum. G Ital Cardiol 28:237-241
24. Buckingham TA, Candinas R, Schlapfer J, Aebischer N, Jeanrenaud X, Landolt J, Kappenberger L (1997) Acute hemodynamic effects of atrioventricular pacing at differing sites in the right ventricle individually and simultaneously. Pacing Clin Electrophysiol 20:909-915
25. Buckingham TA, Candinas Attenhofer C, Van Hoeven H, Hug R, Hess O, Jenni R, Amann FW (1998) Systolic and diastolic function with alternate and combined site pacing in the right ventricle. Pacing Clin Electrophysiol 21:1077-1084
26. Victor F, Leclercq C, Mabo P, Pavin D, Deviller A, de Place C, Pezard P, Victor J, Daubert C (1999) Optimal right ventricular pacing site in chronically implanted patients: a prospective randomized crossover comparison of apical and outflow tract pacing. J Am Coll Cardiol 33:311-316
27. Blanc JJ, Etienne Y, Gilard M, Mansourati J, Munier S, Boschat J, Benditt DG, Lurie KG (1997) Evaluation of different ventricular pacing sites in patients with severe heart failure: results of an acute hemodynamic study. Circulation 96:3273-3277
28. Leclercq C, Cazeau S, Le Breton H, Ritter P, Mabo P, gras D, Pavin D, Lazarus A, Daubert JC (1998) Acute hemodynamic effects of biventricular DDD pacing in patients with end-stage heart failure. J Am Coll Cardiol 32:1825-1831

Treatment of Severe Heart Failure: Is Left Ventricular Pacing Alone Enough or Do We Need Biventricular Pacing?

J.J. Blanc, Y. Etienne, J. Mansourati and M. Gilard

In patients with severe heart failure in spite of "optimal" drug treatment, interventions remain limited. Adjustment of drug treatment may be helpful but its benefit is generally of short duration and the problem is merely delayed; heart transplant is restricted to a few patients due to the small numbers of donors and other non-pharmacological treatments remain investigational (mechanical assistance device) or questionnable (cardiomyoplasty). Since the beginning of the 1990s, many efforts have been directed toward the use of pacing in such situations. After a brief period of hope [1], it has been demonstrated that right apical pacing has no or little effectiveness in patients with severe heart failure [2-4]. In fact, only some of those with a very long PR interval achieved significant improvement of their symptoms with this pacing site [5]. Other right ventricular pacing sites were evaluated but in most of the patients remained unsuccessful [6, 7]. In 1994, a brief paper was published reporting that the adjoining of a left ventricular pacing site to the right one led to significant improvement in patients with end-stage heart failure [8]. This observation gave the impetus for a flourishing field of research. It was initially thought that hemodynamic improvement was exclusively a direct consequence of the resynchronization of the two ventricles, as this procedure was only effective in patients with left bundle branch block [9]. It rapidly appeared that this explanation was totally insufficient, as we demontrated in acute hemodynamic studies that left ventricular pacing alone was at least as effective as biventricular pacing [10]. The aim of the present paper is to summarize our present knowledge on left ventricular pacing alone. However, we should remained cautious, as developments in this field are coming quickly and it is difficult to assume that the present data will be confirmed by ongoing studies.

Acute Studies

As previously mentioned, the concept of left ventricular pacing alone (as compared to biventricular) is based on acute hemodynamic data. To summarize our

---

Department of Cardiology, Brest University Hospital, France

first study on 23 patients, we observed that, when compared to baseline hemodynamic status, right apical or right outflow tract pacing did not improve cardiac index, "V" wave, mean capillary wedge pressure (CWP) or aortic systolic blood pressure (SBP). But when the lateral part of the left ventricle was paced (in all these evaluations the AV delay was maintained at 100 ms) a significant and sometimes dramatic improvement in these parameters was observed [10]. Interestingly these improvements were similar in biventricular (right ventricular apex - left lateral wall) and left ventricular pacing [10]. A recently published series ends with similar results concerning biventricular pacing but did not evaluate left ventricular pacing alone [11]. Kass et al. [12] studied acutely the behaviour of an accurate left ventricular function parameter: the DP/DT max. They reported, in accordance with the previous papers, that right ventricular pacing did not modify the left ventricular function but that left ventricular alone improved the DP/DT max significantly more than biventricular pacing [12]. This observation lends support to our work as it was obtained with a different approach and provides the evidence that resynchronization of right and left ventricles is not the main explanation for acute improvement during biventricular pacing.

In order to disclose whether some subgroups of patients benefitted more from one than from the other pacing procedure (biventricular versus left ventricular alone), the procedures were compared in patients with sinus rhythm and atrial fibrillation. In these two groups of patients, the magnitude of improvement in acute hemodynamic parameters with both pacing procedures was identical [13]. A similar result was obtained when we compared patients with ischemic cardiomyopathy versus patients with dilated cardiomyopathy.

The conclusion drawn from these acute hemodynamic studies is that left ventricular pacing alone provides an improvement in severe heart failure patients with long QRS duration which is similar to that provided by biventricular pacing.

Results with Permanent Pacing

Only one series has been reported in a supplement of PACE on the long-term results of biventricular permanent pacing in patients with the above-mentioned characteristics, i.e severe NYHA class III or IV and left bundle branch block. This nonrandomized study, which included 68 patients, concluded that this pacing mode improves significantly the mean subjective and objective status of the cohort [14]. This result is in accordance with orally reported results based on a more limited number of patients who originated from other groups. Well-designed studies comparing biventricular pacing to "no pacing" have either been submitted for publication or are ongoing. There are no published data on the long-term evaluation of left ventricular pacing alone. In our series, the results obtained after a 12-month follow-up period are similar in patients paced simultaneously in both ventricles and in those paced in the left ventricle alone. This very preliminary result, although in accordance with acute studies, should be taken with caution as it is based on a limited number of patients not randomly assigned to the two pacing modalities.

Theoretical Advantages of Left Ventricular Pacing Alone

It is evident that biventricular pacing needs the insertion of one more lead than left ventricular pacing alone. This means three leads versus two in patients with sinus rhythm. Although this is not a crucial technical issue, the venous access is more complicated, and the long-term thrombosis rate of subclavian or even superior vena cava is higher. In case of infection, extraction of one more lead in the right ventricle will prolong the time and increase the risk of the procedure.

Pacing two ventricular sites simultaneously enhances the pacemaker current consumption, and the battery duration in patients who are permanently paced will be shorter. This has no serious consequences in patients with severe heart failure and a limited life expectancy duration, such as those implanted at the present time, but may be relevent if patients with less severe disease become candidates for this pacing modality.

Finally the technical requirements of biventricular pacing provide a significant increase in cost (one more lead and a triple- versus dual-chamber pacemaker) when compared to left ventricular alone.

These arguments, together with the results of acute hemodynamic studies, are sufficiently incentive not to exclude left ventricular pacing alone in patients with heart failure until it has been demonstrated that biventricular pacing is clearly more effective in these patients. If only a trend in favor of biventricular pacing is shown, the ratio between adverse events and benefits would have to be calculated for every patient before choosing bi- or single-ventricular pacing implantation.

References

1. Hochleitner M, Hörtnagl H, Ng CK, Hörtnagl H, Oschnitzer F, Zechmann W (1990) Usefulness of physiologic dual-chamber pacing in drug-resistant idiopathic dilated cardiomyopathy. Am J Cardiol 66:198-202
2. Innes D, Leitch JW, Fletcher PJ (1994) VDD pacing a short atrioventricular intervals does not improve cardiac output in patients with dilated heart failure. Pacing Clin Electrophysiol 17:959-965
3. Gold MR, Feliciano Z, Gottlieb SS, Fisher ML (1995) Dual-chamber pacing with a short atrioventricular delay in congestive heart failure: a randomized study. J Am Coll Cardiol 26:967-973
4. Linde C, Gadler F, Edner M, Nordlander R, Rosenqvist M, Ryden L (1995) Results of atrioventricular synchronous pacing with optimized delay in patients with severe congestive heart failure. J Am Coll Cardiol 75:919-923
5. Nishimura RA, Hayes DL, Holmes DR, Tajik AJ (1995) Mechanism of hemodynamic improvement by dual-chamber pacing for severe left ventricular dysfunction: an acute Doppler and catheterization hemodynamic study. J Am Coll Cardiol 25:281-288
6. Victor F, Leclercq C, Mabo P, Pavin D, Deviller A, De Place C, Pezard P, Victor J, Daubert C (1999) Optimal right ventricular pacing site in chronically implanted patients. A prospective randomized cross over comparison of apical and outflow tract pacing. J Am Coll Cardiol 33:311-316

7. Gold MR (1999) Optimization of ventricular pacing: where should we implant the leads? J Am Coll Cardiol 33:324-326

8. Cazeau S, Ritter P, Bakach S, Lazarus A, Limousin M, Henao L, Mundler O, Daubert JC, Mugica J (1994) Four chamber pacing in dilated cardiomyopathy. Pacing Clin Electrophysiol 17:1974-1979

9. Cazeau S, Ritter P, Lazarus A, Gras D, Backadach H, Mundler O, Mugica J (1996) Multisite pacing for end-stage heart failure; early experience. Pacing Clin Electrophysiol 19:1748-1757

10. Blanc JJ, Etienne Y, Gilard M, Mansourati J, Munier S, Boschat J, Benditt D, Lurie K (1997) Evaluation of different ventricular pacing sites in patients with severe heart failure. Circulation 96:3272-3277

11. Leclercq C, Cazeau S, Le Breton H et al (1998) Acute hemodynamic effects of biventricular DDD pacing in patients with end-stage heart failure. J Am Coll Cardiol 32:1825-1831

12. Kass DA, Chen CH, Curry C et al (1999) Improved left ventricular mechanics from acute VDD pacing in patients with dilated cardiomyopathy and ventricular conduction delay. Circulation 99:1567-1573

13. Etienne Y, Mansourati J, Gilard M, Valls-Bertault V, Boschat J, Benditt DG, Lurie KG, Blanc JJ (1999) Evaluation of left ventricular based pacing in patients with congestive heart failure and atrial fibrillation. Am J Cardiol 83:1138-1140

14. Gras D, Mabo P, Tang T, Luttikuis O, Chatoor P, Pedersen AK, Tscheliessnigg KH, Deharo JC, Puglisi A, Silvestre J, Kimber S, Ross H, Ravazzi A, Paul V, Skehan D (1998) Multisite pacing as a supplemental treatment of congestive heart failure: preliminary results of the Medtronic Inc. In Sync Study. PACE 21 (pt II):2249-2255

Multisite Biventricular Pacing to Treat Refractory Heart Failure: Why and How?

J.C. Daubert, C. Leclercq, C. Alonso and P. Mabo

Despite pharmacological advances, in particular the introduction of ACE-inhibitors and β-blockers, the prognosis of patients with severe heart failure (grades III and IV of the NYHA classification) remains pejorative and their quality of life is poor. A number of nonpharmacological treatments have been proposed for this type of patients: heart transplantation remains the reference treatment although its application is restricted by donor shortage, among other factors. Left ventricular (LV) support devices are still at the evaluation stage and the results of cardiomyoplasty are highly controversial. In the early 1990s, standard dual-chamber pacing with short AV delay was proposed as a supplementary treatment for drug-resistant heart failure. Initial results were encouraging but were never confirmed. These studies, however, made it possible to select a population of potentially responsive patients, especially those with a prolonged PR interval reflecting major atrioventricular asynchrony in the left heart. That relative failure of standard dual-chamber pacing could be linked to the fact that by capturing the ventricle from the right apex, it increases, or at least it cannot correct the marked asynchrony of activation, contraction and relaxation which characterizes a number of patients with chronic LV dysfunction. Such is the case in particular in patients with important QRS enlargement linked to major intraventricular conduction delay. Biventricular pacing, which simultaneously activates both ventricles, may contribute to correcting the asynchrony and thus improve cardiac performance.

Rationale of Biventricular Pacing: Electromechanical Correlates in Chronic Heart Failure

The purpose of multisite biventricular pacing is to correct the sometimes major electromechanical abnormalities that result from conduction disorders associated with chronic LV systolic dysfunction.

Département de Cardiologie et Maladies Vasculaires, Centre Cardio-Pneumologique, Hôpital Pontchaillou CHU, Rennes, France

Conduction Disorders in Chronic LV Systolic Dysfunction

PR Interval Abnormalities

Wilensky's pathologic-clinical study of 34 patients who died as a result of anatomically proven dilated cardiomyopathy (DCM) confirmed that major changes in PR interval occurred during the progression of disease in patients who remained in sinus rhythm [1]. He noted a significant increase after a mean follow-up duration of 3 years (180 ± 30 ms vs 210 ± 30 ms; $p < 0.01$). At the end of follow-up, 60% of patients in sinus rhythm had a PR interval > 200 ms. Xiao et al. [2] compared ECG findings from 77 patients with DCM at various stages of progression and in 15 matched healthy controls. The PR interval was significantly longer in DCM patients (185 ± 30 ms vs 150 ± 15 ms; $p < 0.05$).

Intraventricular Conduction Delay

Wilensky's study analyzed the evolution of QRS duration over a mean follow-up period of 30 months [1]. He observed a significant increase in the course of follow-up (100 ± 30 ms vs 130 ± 20 ms; $p < 0.01$). In that study, more than 80% of patients developed conduction abnormalities and 27% of patients exhibited QRS duration over 150 ms with peaks above 200 ms on their last ECG preceding their death.

Xiao et al. [2] made the following similar observations: among 77 DCM patients, 70% presented with significant conduction abnormalities, mainly left bundle branch block or intraventricular conduction delay. The mean QRS duration was significantly higher than in the control group (127 ± 25 vs 101 ± 10 ms; $p < 0.05$).

Prognostic Implications of Abnormal Activation Sequence

Several studies have shown that the various electrocardiographic abnormalities noted on surface ECG of DCM patients were predictors of cardiovascular mortality. Thus, the existence of atrioventricular conduction disorders (1st and 2nd degree AVD) constitutes an independent risk factor of cardiac death in DCM patients [3]. Similar observations were made for intraventricular conduction disorders (IVCD or LBBB), especially in nonischemic DCM. Xiao [2] also showed that the association of AV conduction disorders and IV conduction disorders in DCM patients, as defined by a PR interval + QRS duration > 375 ms, constituted an independent mortality risk factor. The predictive value of intraventricular conduction disorders however is more controversial for other authors [4-7].

Electromechanical Consequences

These conduction disorders have a significant impact on cardiac performance. The lengthening of the PR interval, be it apparent or concealed, induces atrioventricular desynchronization, hence shorter ventricular filling time and reduced or even suppressed left atrial contribution to ventricular filling, as often reflected by the single-pulse aspect of the mitral Doppler flow resulting from the superimposition of wave A and wave E [8, 9].

The lengthening of QRS duration on surface ECG, reflecting the existence of intraventricular conduction disorders, is seen by some as a good rating marker of LV systolic dysfunction. In a series of 55 patients with ischemic DCM, Hamby et al. [10] demonstrated that prolonged QRS duration and LBBB aspect were related to a significant decrease in LV ejection fraction and a significant increase in endiastolic volume. Murkofsky et al. [11] showed recently that QRS width > 100 ms without any classic LBBB aspect on surface ECG was an excellent indicator of left ventricular dysfunction.

The hemodynamic consequences of abnormal LV activation in patients with DCM have been explored in depth by Xiao et al. [12, 13]. That study, conducted in 50 patients, revealed a positive correlation between QRS duration and Q wave delay at LV pressure peak and the interval between the Q wave and the peak + dP/dT. In contrast, QRS duration and the + dP/dT value were negatively correlated. These data showed that the longer the QRS duration, the longer the duration of LV isovolumetric contraction and relaxing time, hence the more altered the LV pump function was. Also, the increased isovolumetric contraction and relaxation times of the left ventricle induced a shortening of filling time in patients whose QRS duration was particularly long. The same authors have shown that in patients with DCM and complete LBBB or IVCD (as defined by a QRS duration > 120 ms and persistent septal Q wave), the ventricle was still activated from the upper part of the septum, but the start of mechanical systole was markedly delayed and symmetrical in both ventricles. The intervals between Q wave and the septal thickening, between septal thickening and that of the LV upper wall, between septum and the thickening of RV free wall were significantly increased in patients with conduction disorders.

Finally, mitral regurgitation is common in DCM patients. Several potential mechanisms have been evoked: enlargement of the mitral annulus, sub-valvular apparatus dysfunction, LV regional wall motion abnormalities and modification of the LV shape [14, 15]. Abnormal activation sequence may play a role in increasing mitral regurgitation: Xiao et al. [13] and Nishimura et al. [8] found a positive correlation between mitral regurgitation time and QRS duration on the one hand, and PR interval duration on the other hand. In addition, left diastolic atrio-ventricular gradient is a common occurrence in AV conduction disorders and may result in diastolic mitral regurgitation [16-18].

Acute Studies with Temporary Pacing

The first hemodynamic study of the acute effects of biventricular pacing was conducted postoperatively immediately following coronary bypass surgery in 18 patients with LVEF > 40%. Biventricular pacing significantly increased cardiac output and reduced systemic arterial resistance, by comparison with no pacing or right or left ventricular single-site pacing [19].

Cazeau et al. [20] reported an acute hemodynamic study conducted in 8 NYHA class IV patients with a mean LVEF of 22 ± 8%. The optimal biventricular configuration induced a significant increase in cardiac index from 1.8 ± 0.3 l/min/m² to 2.3 ± 0.3 l/min/m² with concomitant decrease in pulmonary capillary pressure from 31 ± 9 mmHg to 26 ± 9 mmHg ($p < 0.01$).

Our group [21] reported their experience in 18 patients in class III or IV with advanced DCM and intraventricular conduction delay (mean QRS duration = 170 ± 36 ms). All these patients were in sinus rhythm, with a mean PR interval of 224 ± 36 ms. Biventricular pacing induced a significant decrease in QRS duration on baseline (154 ± 18 ms vs 170 ± 37 ms; $p < 0.01$). The cardiac index was significantly improved by biventricular DDD pacing, when compared with no pacing or right ventricular, single-chamber DDD pacing (2.7 ± 0.7 l/min/m², 2 ± 0.5 l/min/m² and 2.4 ± 0.6 l/min/m², respectively; $p < 0.01$). In parallel, a significant decrease in mean pulmonary capillary pressure was observed with biventricular pacing.

Other authors studied the effects of left ventricular pacing. Blanc et al. [22] compared biventricular pacing, single-site left ventricular pacing, apical and outflow tract right ventricular pacing in 23 patients. Compared to baseline, biventricular pacing and LV pacing induced the same hemodynamic benefit, as assessed from the following criteria: systolic blood pressure, mean pulmonary capillary pressure and V-capillary wave; cardiac output was not considered in that study.

Recently Kass et al. [23] published the results of extensive hemodynamic studies aimed at assessing the acute effects of VDD pacing at varying sites (RV apex, RV midseptal, LV paced transvenously and biventricular) and AV delays in 18 heart failure patients. He showed that RV pacing at any site had negligible contractile/systolic effects. However, LV free-wall pacing increased dP/dT max by 23.7 ± 19% and pulse-pressure by 18 ± 18.4% ($p < 0.01$). Biventricular pacing yielded less change than LV pacing alone. In the same way pressure-volume curves analysis consistently revealed minimal changes with RV pacing but increased stroke work and lowered end-systolic volumes with LV and biventricular pacing. Finally, Kass et al. [23] showed that AV delay had less influence on LV function than pacing site.

Potential Mechanisms of Action of Biventricular Pacing

Several mechanisms can be evoked. Biventricular pacing permits electrical resynchronization of ventricles, as reflected by the significant reduction of QRS duration on surface ECG. Indeed, QRS duration was reduced by 20% on average by biventricular pacing in our study [24]. QRS axis also was improved by biventricular pacing.

Biventricular pacing also improves the mechanical re-synchronization of the two ventricles, as demonstrated by Cazeau et al. [20] in an angioscintigraphic study by phase analysis correcting the contraction asynchrony induced by major intraventricular conduction delay. This beneficial mechanical effect of biventricular pacing has also been demonstrated by Saxon et al. [25], who reported a significant improvement of LV function, secondary to a better coordination of right and left ventricular contractions.

Lastly, biventricular pacing probably has a beneficial effect on mitral regurgitation, as we were able to demonstrate in certain patients with an ON/OFF effect of biventricular pacing with instantaneous disappearance of pulmonary capillary V wave (Fig. 1). However, the exact mechanisms whereby mitral deficiency is reduced still remain to be elucidated.

Technical Requirements of Permanent Biventricular Pacing

How to Pace the Left Ventricle Permanently?

Among the technical difficulties of multisite biventricular pacing, one problem is to pace the left ventricle at the optimal site chronically and safely.

The first pacing experiments [20, 26] were conducted using the epicardial route, and thoracotomy or thoracoscopy. However, this method has two principal disadvantages. First, it incurs a non-negligible operative risk in such a severely diseased patient population. In the first seven patients in the French pilot study [25], one patient died during the operation, due to a non-terminable VF at the time of pericardial incision. Second, the epicardial technique is associated with a poor quality of acute pacing thresholds and a high rate of delayed exit blocks which result in LV pacing loss. However, this route has the theoretical advantage that the pacing electrode may be placed at the optimal site in each patient. In a preliminary experience of acute intra-operative hemodynamic testing with measurement of aortic pulse

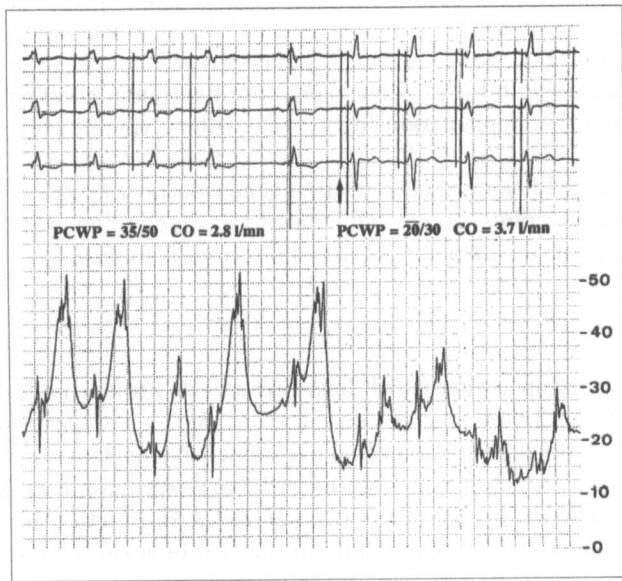

PCWP = 35/50 CO = 2.8 l/mn   PCWP = 20/30 CO = 3.7 l/mn

Fig. 1. Acute effects of DDD-biventricular pacing on mitral regurgitation. Switching the pacing mode from AAI (intrinsic conduction) to biventricular-DDD at the same pacing rate, results in instantaneous decrease in the mean pulmonary capillary wedge pressure from 30 to 15 mmHg while the V wave disappears. At the same time CO in-creases by 35% and the QRS reduction is shortened from 200 to 130 ms

pressure and LV + dP/dT in 25 patients, Auricchio et al. [27] showed that the observed benefit was primarily dependent on the LV pacing site. From the different sites to be tested, the mid-part of the LV free wall was the one to provide on average the greater hemodynamic benefit as compared with baseline, followed by the mid-part of the posterior wall, the LV apex, and finally the mid-part of the anterior wall. The LV base was not explored in that study. From these preliminary results, one can postulate that the target location is the LV lateral or posterolateral wall in most patients, probably at its mid-part.

To eliminate the need for general anesthesia and to minimize the operative risk, our group introduced from 1994 a transvenous approach using a lead inserted in a tributary vein over the LV free wall through the coronary sinus [28]. The target location was a lateral or posterolateral coronary vein. If lateral vein catheterization failed or in case of poor pacing thresholds, the LV lead was inserted into the great cardiac vein to pace the anterobasal wall, or in the mid cardiac vein to pace the inferoapical area. From the beginning of our experiment until 1996, non-specific models of unipolar, small-diameter and tine-free ventricular leads were used. The implantation success rate was low at only 54%. Since 1996, specifically designed coronary sinus leads (Medtronic models 2879, 2188 and 2187) have been used. The implantation success rate increased to 85% in the whole group and 92% in the last 50 patients. The target location i.e. a lateral or posterolateral vein in a mid position, could be reached in 72% of patients. No serious complications were observed during the implantation procedure, nor could be related to the coronary sinus lead during the follow-up. The mean acute pacing threshold was 1.15 ± 0.7 V. At the end of follow-up with a mean time of 10.2 ± 8 months, 97% of leads were fully functional with a mean chronic pacing threshold of 1.8 ± 0.7 V.

To improve the results of this implantation technique, some authors suggest using a long preshaped guiding sheath [29] to facilitate coronary sinus ostium catheterization and definitive positioning of the pacing lead, intra-operative coronary venogram to localize more precisely the target vein, and new lead technology, such as over-the-wire systems [27]. We can reasonably expect that in a near future improved technology combined with the growing experience (learning curve) will allow us to achieve a nearly 100% implantation success rate with acceptable procedure and fluoroscopy times.

Recently [30] LV endocardial pacing using a transeptal approach was proposed as an alternative to coronary venous pacing. This new technique is now under investigation with a special focus on the potential risk of thrombo-embolism.

RV Lead Placement

The optimal pacing configuration is that which best corrects electromechanical disorders. At the present stage of knowledge, our observations [31] encourage us to try to find the best RV and LV pacing sites according to patient, i.e., sites that would ensure the shortest QRS duration possible and optimal QRS axis normalization in each patient, during simultaneous pacing at the two ventricles. In practice, it is advisable to position the LV lead first, if possible in a lateral or posterolateral vein, and secondly to determine the best RV site, based on continuous surface ECG analysis during biventricular pacemapping. In most cases optimal electrical resynchronization is achieved by positioning the RV lead (screw-in lead) at the mid-septum or the mid-anterior wall, and not at the apex (Fig. 2). The best RV and LV pacing sites usually correspond to the earliest and latest activation sites during intrinsic conduction (Fig. 3) in the individual patient.

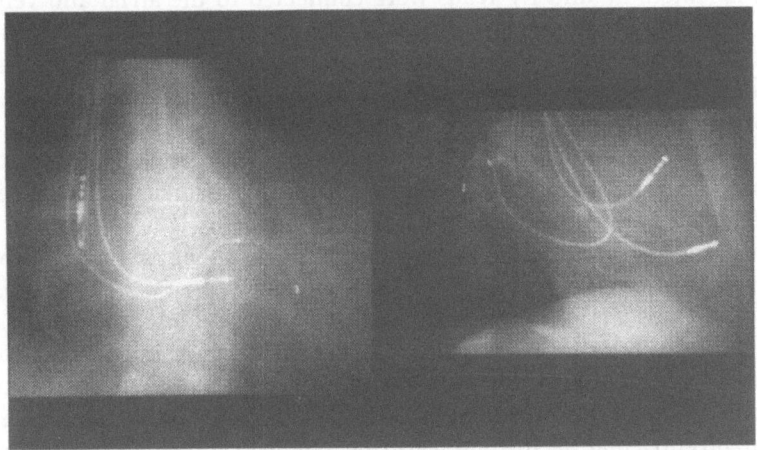

Fig. 2. Chest X-ray in frontal and sagittal views showing the ventricular leads positions in a long-term responder patient. The LV lead was inserted into a posterolateral vein through the coronary sinus. The RV lead was positioned anteriorly at the mid-part of the septum

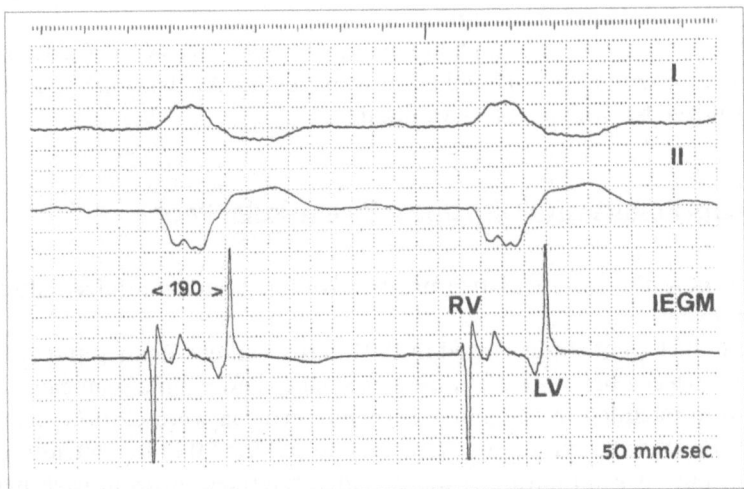

Fig. 3. Intraoperative ECG recording showing tha the two ventricular leads (same patient as in Fig. 2) were actually placed at the earliest (RV) and latest (LV) ventricular activation sites during intrinsic conduction. The interventricular conduction time was measured at 190 ms

Biventricular Pacing Systems

Three different types of biventricular pacing configurations have presently been described, and used according to each patient's electrophysiological characteristics, as collected before permanent implantation.

In patients with chronic atrial fibrillation, biventricular VVIR pacemakers were implanted. LV and RV leads were connected to the atrial and ventricular ports of DDDR pacemakers, respectively. The pacemakers were programmed in the DDDR mode with the shortest programmable AV delay (30 ms). To ensure full and permanent biventricular capture, the AV junction was systematically ablated (radiofrequency) at the time of implantation.

In patients with normal sinus rhythm, a biventricular VDD mode is usually recommended. In our early experience [25], conventional DDDR pacemakers were implanted with the atrial lead placed at the high right atrium and the two ventricular leads connected to the ventricular port of the pacemaker through a Y bifurcated, or a parallel unipolar or bipolar adapter. When a Y adapter was used, LV and RV leads were connected to the negative (cathode) and positive (anode) poles, respectively. In that series, the re-operation rate was high (34%). Nearly all re-operations were linked to a problem with the connector between the two ventricular leads. With the introduction of new, more sophisticated pacemakers dedicated to biventricular pacing and featuring a built-in connector inside the device, these technical difficulties should be considerably reduced.

Finally, in some patients with normal sinus rhythm but very long interatrial conduction time resulting in major electrical and mechanical asynchrony between the two atria, it was proposed to implant the so-called "four-chamber" pacemaker [32] aimed at ensuring biatrial synchronous pacing [33] plus DDD pacing plus simultaneous biventricular pacing.

In the patients who are implanted with a biventricular-VDD (or DDDR) four-pacemaker or with a "four-chamber" pacemaker, the AV delay has to be individually optimized by Doppler-echo technique.

Long-Term Results with Permanent Biventricular Pacing

Up until now, the results of two prospective but non-randomized studies have been reported.

The French pilot study started in 1994 in two centers, Rennes and Saint-Cloud [34]. Until December 1997, 50 patients, 45 males and 5 females, mean age 68 ± 8 years, were included in the study. Inclusion criteria were chronic heart failure class III or IV with symptoms refractory to medical therapy, including at least diuretics and ACE-inhibitors at the maximal tolerated doses in each patient, LV systolic dysfunction as assessed on LVEF < 35% and LV endiastolic diameter > 60 mm, and finally intraventricular conduction delay with a QRS duration > 150 ms during intrinsic conduction. At the time of inclusion, 34 patients were in NYHA class IV, including 17 in terminal phase, requiring permanent IV inotropic support, and 16 were in class III. The mean LVEF was 20 ± 6%. Heart failure was of ischemic origin in 24 patients and non-ischemic in 26, including 20 patients with idiopathic dilated cardiomyopathy. The mean QRS duration was 197 ± 32 ms.

Fourteen patients with chronic AF were implanted with a biventricular-VVIR pacemaker and had the AV junction ablated at the same time. The other 36 patients were in stable sinus rhythm and received a biventricular-DDD (R) pacemaker or a "four-chamber" device.

The mean duration of follow-up was 15.4 ± 10.2 months, ranging from 1 to 48 months. Twenty patients died during the follow-up period within a mean of 8 ± 7.2 months after pacemaker implantation. All deceased patients but two were NYHA class IV at the time of biventricular pacemaker implantation. Causes of death were progressive pump failure ($n = 11$), sudden cardiac death ($n = 6$), and non-cardiac factors ($n = 3$). At the end of follow-up period, 55% of patients were alive without heart transplant or any circulatory support. The survival rate differed significantly between patients who were NYHA class III or IV at the time of implantation (Fig. 4). In the course of follow-up, patient's functional status was significantly improved by permanent biventricular pacing. One month after implantation, the mean NYHA classification value was 2.37 ± 0.66 vs 3.7 ± 0.5 at the time of inclusion; $p < 0.001$. This functional improvement persisted henceforth to the end of follow-up, when the mean functional class was 2.2 ± 0.6. In the subgroup of 16 patients who were able to exercise before pacemaker implantation, a significant improvement in exercise tolerance was observed at 3 months, with significant increase in exercise duration (9 ± 3.4 min vs 6.3 ± 1.6 min; $p = 0.01$), in

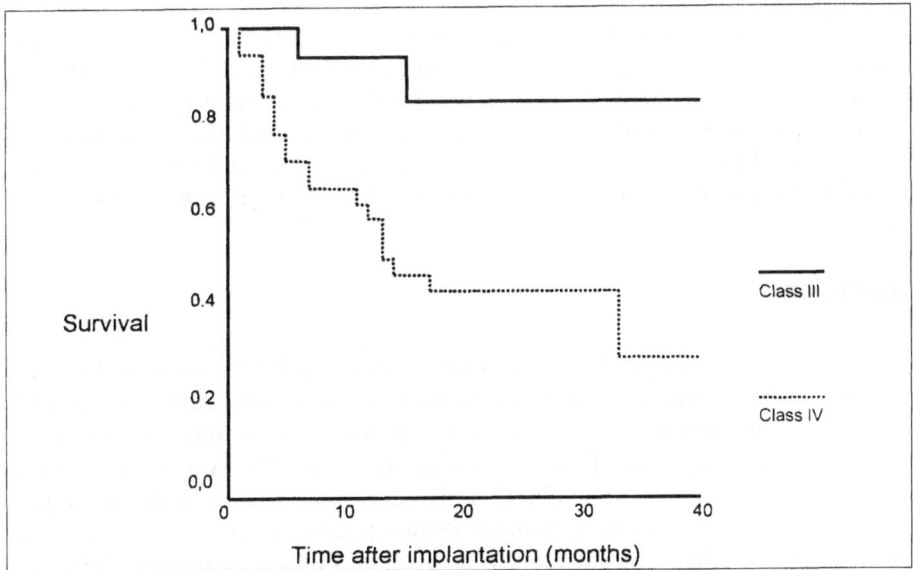

Fig. 4. Actuarial survival curves showing the survival rate in class III and in class IV patients in the French pilot study

sustained workload (73 ± 13 W vs 56 ± 19 W; $p < 0.01$) and in maximal oxygen consumption (15.5 ± 3.4 ml/kg/min vs 11.1 ± 3 ml/kg/ min; $p < 0.01$) when compared with pre-implantation period. Simultaneous biventricular pacing induced a significant decrease in QRS duration (162 ± 29 ms vs 197 ± 32 ms; $p < 0.001$). The variation in QRS axis was also significant with a clear trend to normalization. Finally echocardiographic data revealed a significant improvement of LVEF under biventricular pacing (24 ± 10 % vs 20 ± 6 %; $p < 0.01$).

The multicenter In-Sync study [34] involved 14 different centers in Europe and Canada, and was aimed at assessing the technical feasibility, the safety and the clinical efficacy of transvenous atrioventricular-biventricular pacing in heart failure patients with stable sinus rhythm. Inclusion criteria were identical to those of the French pilot study. Over a 10-month period, 81 patients were enrolled and 68 or 84% could be successfully implanted. The study population consisted of 52 males and 16 females, with a mean age of 66 ± 10 years. The etiology was ischemic in 28 patients and non-ischemic in 40. At the time of inclusion, 43 patients were in NYHA class III and 25 were in class IV. The mean 6-minute walking distance was 299 ± 121 m. The mean LVEF was 21 ± 9 % and the mean QRS duration was 177 ± 29 ms.

After the implantation, evaluations including symptoms (NYHA class), quality of life (Minnesota Living with Heart Failure questionnaire), exercise tolerance (6-min walking distance), 12-lead surface ECG recording and Doppler-echocardiography were planned at 1, 3, 6 and 12 months. During the follow-up period (1-12 months), seven patients died from cardiovascular causes including cardiac sudden death in four, between 11 and 127 days after pacemaker implantation. At 3 months follow-up, DDD biventricular pacing was associated with a significant improvement in symptoms (decrease of the mean NYHA class from 3.37 ± 0.5 to 2.05 ± 0.7; $p < 0.001$), in QOL (increase in MLHF score from 34 ± 10.4 to 55.2 ± 5.3; $p = 0.004$) and in exercise tolerance (increase in 6-min walking distance from 299 ± 16 m to 418 ± 20 m; $p = 0.04$) when compared with the pre-inclusion period. The mean QRS duration decreased from 177 ± 29 ms to 143 ± 18 ms; $p < 0.001$, and finally there was a non-significant trend to an increased LVEF (24 ± 6 % vs 21 ± 9 %; $p = 0.06$).

Conclusions

By correcting left ventricular asynchrony as well as left atrio-ventricular asynchrony, multisite biventricular pacing appears to significantly and durably improve the functional status, the quality of life and exercise tolerance of patients with drug-refractory heart failure secondary to chronic LV systolic dysfunction with major intraventricular conduction disorders. That technique appears highly promising as an adjuvant treatment for drug-refractory heart failure, in particular in class III patients, as mortality remains high in class IV patients. Technical advances should improve the accessibility of that treatment in the near future. However, controlled and randomized trials will be necessary to validate this novel concept and better define responding patients and assess the actual impact in terms of quality of life, exercise tolerance, mortality and cost-effectiveness ratio. The first cross-over trial (MUSTIC) is ongoing in Europe, to try to answer these questions.

References

1. Wilensky RL, Yudelman P, Cohen AI et al (1988) Serial electrocardiographic changes in idiopathic dilated cardiomyopathy confirmed at necropsy. Am J Cardiol 62:276-283
2. Xiao H, Roy C, Fujimoto S, Gibson D (1996) Natural history of abnormal conduction and its relation to prognosis in patients with dilated cardiomyopathy. Int J Cardiol 53:163-170
3. Schoeller R, Andresen D, Büttner P, Oezcelik K, Vey G, Schröder R (1993) First or second degree atrioventricular block as a risk factor in idiopathic dilated cardiomyopathy. Am J Cardiol 71:720-726
4. Cowburn P, Cleland J, Coast A, Komajda M (1998) Risk stratification in chronic heart failure. Eur Heart J 19:696-710
5. Aaronson K, Schwartz S, Chen T, Wong K, Goin J, Mancini D (1997) Development and prospective validation of a clinical index to predict survival in ambulatory patients referred for cardiac transplant evaluation. Circulation 95:2660-2667
6. Silverman M, Pressel M, Brackett J, Lauria S, Gold M, Gottlieb S (1995) Prognostic value of the signal-averaged electrocardiogram and a prolonged QRS in ischemic and non ischemic cardiomyopathy. Am J Cardiol 75:460-464
7. Likoff M, Chandler S, Kay H (1987) Clinical determinants of mortality in chronic congestive heart failure secondary to idiopathic dilated or to ischemic cardiomyopathy. Am J Cardiol 59:634
8. Nishimura RA, Hayes DL, Holmes DR Jr, Tajik AJ (1995) Mechanism of hemodynamic improvement by dual-chamber pacing for severe left ventricular dysfunction: an acute Doppler and catheterization study. J Am Coll Cardiol 25:281-288
9. Scanu P, Lecluze E, Michel L et al (1996) Effects of temporal Dual-Chamber cardiac pacing in refractory cardiac failure. Arch Mal Coeur 89:1643-1649
10. Hamby R, Weissman R, Prakash M, Hoffman I (1983) Left bundle branch block: a predictor of poor left ventricular function in coronary artery disease. Am Heart J 106:471-477
11. Murkofsky R, Dangas G, Diamond J, Mehta D, Schaffer A, Ambrose J (1998) A prolonged QRS duration on surface ECG is a specific indicator of left ventricular dysfunction. J Am Coll Cardiol 32:476-482
12. Xiao HB, Roy C, Gibson DG (1994) Nature of ventricular activation in patients with dilated cardiomyopathy: evidence for bilateral bundle branch block. Br Heart J 72:167-174
13. Xiao HB, Brecker SJD, Gibson DG (1992) Effect of abnormal activation on the time course of the left ventricular pressure pulse in dilated cardiomyopathy. Br Heart J 68:403-407
14. Kono T, Sabbah H, Rosman H, Alam M, Jaffri S, Goldstein S (1998) Left ventricular shape is the primary determinant of functional mitral regurgitation in heart failure. J Am Coll Cardiol 7:1594-1598
15. Boltwood C, Tei C Wong M, Shah P(1983) Quantitative echocardiography of the mitral complex in dilated cardiomyopathy: the mechanism of functional mitral regurgitation. Circulation 68:498-508

16. Panidis I, Ross J, Munley B, Nestico P, Mintz G (1986) Diastolic mitral regurgitation in patients with atrioventricular conduction abnormalities: a common finding by doppler echocardiography. J Am Coll Cardiol 7:768-774

17. Appelton C, Basnignht M, Gonzalez M, Carucci M, Henry C, Olajos M (1991) diastolic mitral regurgitation with atrioventricular conduction abnormalities: relation of mitral flow velocity to transmitral pressure gradients in conscious dogs. J Am Coll Cardiol 18:843-849

18. Ishikawa T, Sumita S, Kimura K et al (1994) Critical PQ interval for the appearance of diastolic mitral regurgitation and optimal PQ interval in patients implanted with DDD pacemakers. PACE 17:1989-1994

19. Foster AH, Gold MR, McLaughlin JS (1995) Acute hemodynamic effects of atrio-biventricular pacing in humans. Ann Thorac Surg 59:294-300

20. Cazeau S, Ritter P, Lazarus A et al (1996) Multisite pacing for end-stage heart failure: early experience. PACE 19 (part II): 1748-1757

21. Leclercq C, Cazeau S, Le Breton H et al (1998) Acute hemodynamic effects of biventricular DDD pacing in patients with end-stage heart failure. J Am Coll Cardiol 32:1825-1831

22. Blanc JJ, Etienne Y, Gilard M et al (1997) Evaluation of different ventricular pacing sites in patients with severe heart failure. Circulation 96:3273-3277

23. Kass DA, Chen CH, Curry et al (1999) Improved left ventricular mechanics from acute VDD pacing in patients with dilated cardiomyopathy and intraventricular conduction delay. Circulation 99:1567-1573

24. Leclercq C, Cazeau S, Victor F et al (1998) Long-term results of permanent biventricular pacing in refractory heart failure: comparison between class III and class IV patients. Eur Heart J 19:573

25. Saxon L, Kerwin W, Cahalan M et al (1998) Acute effects of intraoperative multiste ventricular pacing on left ventricular function and activation/contraction sequence in patients with depressed ventricular function. J Cardiovasc Electrophysiol 9:13-21

26. Auricchio A, Stellbrink C, Sack S et al (1999) The pacing therapies for congestive heart failure (PATH-CHF) study: rationale, design and endpoints of a prospective randomized multicenter study. Am J Cardiol 83:D130-D135

27. Auricchio A, Klein H, Tockman B et al (1999) Transvenous biventricular pacing for heart failure: can the obstacles be overcome? Am J Cardiol 83:D136-D142

28. Daubert JC, Ritter P, Le Breton H et al (1998) Permanent left ventricular pacing with transvenous leads inserted into the coronary veins. PACE 21:239-245

29. Blanc JJ, Benditt DG, Gilard M, Etienne Y, Mansourati J, Lurie K (1998) A method for permanent transvenous left ventricular pacing. PACE 21: 2021-2024

30. Jaïs P, Douard H, Shah DC, Barold S, Barat JL, Clémenty J (1998) Endocardial biventricular pacing. PACE 21:2128-2131

31. Alonso C, Leclercq C, Mansour H et al (1999) ECG-predicting factors of long-term improvement with multisite biventricular pacing in advanced heart failure. PACE 22:758 (abstr)

32. Cazeau S, Ritter P, Bakdachs et al (1994) Four chamber pacing in dilated cardiomyopathy. PACE 17:1974-1979

33. Daubert C, Leclercq C, Pavin D, Mabo P (1996) Biatrial synchronous pacing: a new approach to prevent arrhythmia in patients with atrial conduction block. In: Daubert C, Prystowsky E, Ripart A (eds) Prevention of tachyarrhythmias with cardiac pacing. Futura, Armonk, NY, pp 99-119

34. Gras D, Mabo P, Tang T et al (1998) Multisite pacing as a supplemental treatment of congestive heart failure: preliminary results of the Medtronic Inc. In Sync study. PACE 21:2249-2255

Biventricular Pacing: Is Acute Hemodynamic Evaluation Useful to Select Patients?

F. Di Pede, G. Gasparini and A. Raviele

Acute hemodynamic studies are currently performed to evaluate the effects of drugs or devices on cardiac performance and to understand the mechanisms by which they act. Cardiac pacing has been used to correct bradycardia. However, right ventricular pacing was found to worsen ventricular performance, and new pacing sites capable of preserving ventricular function have been studied. More recently, cardiac pacing has been used to treat congestive heart failure [1-5].

Patients with heart failure frequently have altered electrical activation which may lead to a dyssyncronous contraction of the heart and to a further impairment of their hemodynamic status. These data suggested the hypothesis that the resynchronization of the electrical activity of the heart may improve the mechanics and, consequently, the performance of the whole cardiovascular system [4, 5]. The results of the first attempt to improve the hemodynamic status in patients with congestive heart failure by pacing the heart were published in 1990 [1]. This study showed the potential benefits of shortening the atrioventricular sequence by a conventional P synchronous pacing of the right ventricular apex with short atrioventricular delay. However, other authors did not find the same benefits and the effects of this therapy remain controversial [2, 3]. In recent years attention has been focused on hemodynamic impairment produced by intraventricular and interventricular asynchrony and on the pacing techniques which may correct them [4, 5].

In this paper we will focus on the electrical and hemodynamic effects of bundle branch block, on the potential benefits of resynchronisation of ventricles and on the information that can be drawn from an acute hemodynamic study.

Activation of the Heart in Patients with Bundle Branch Block

The left ventricular performance is the main factor in the clinical manifestations of heart failure , and the activation sequence of the left ventricle (LV) is of clinical relevance. In patients with advanced heart failure, bundle branch block, mainly

Reparto di Cardiologia, Ospedale Umberto I, Mestre, Venice, Italy

left bundle branch block (LBBB), is a common finding. Experimental studies [6] have shown that activation in LBBB begins in the low right septal surface and spreads simultaneously to the endocardial surface of the right ventricle and to the high right ventricular septum. Then the septum is activated from the right to the left, first in the inferior and posterobasal portion (30-50 ms) and then to the superior and anterior portion (70-90 ms). The activation of the LV begins in the apex (40-60 ms) and spreads to the anterior wall (50-70 ms) and to the posterolateral region (65-105 ms). These experimental data demonstrate that the interventricular septum is activated very slowly, while the activation of the LV is faster [1].

However, in patients the activation pattern may be quite different due to specific heart disease. Left ventricular activation pattern was also studied by means of right ventricular stimulation and by endocardial mapping to determine the effects of myocardial infarction on LV activation. [7]. LV activation time was longer in patients with myocardial infarction than in patients without heart disease or with cardiomyopathy. Moreover, patients with anterior myocardial infarction have a longer activation time than patients with inferior myocardial infarction. The site of myocardial infarction is relevant to the site of latest activation. Whereas the site of initial activation of LV was always septal, the latest site was inferoposterior in most cases of patients without infarction or with inferior myocardial infarction; in patients with anterior myocardial infarction the latest site was variable [7].

Animal and clinical studies suggest that the site of block may be at different levels of the specialized conduction system (truncal or peripheral) and that the activation pattern may be profoundly influenced by the integrity of the distal specialized conduction system [6, 8]. When the block is in the His-Purkinje system or in the left bundle branch, the more peripheral left ventricular specialized conduction system is preserved. In this case the activation of the interventricular septum is very slow, but when the electrical activity enters the LV, the specialized conducting tissue may be engaged and the activation of the left free wall may occur near-normally.

In patients with more peripheral block the activation pattern may be quite different with a delayed activation of the whole ventricle. These different activation patterns may be relevant to the contraction pattern of the heart.

Acute Hemodynamic Study in Assessing Cardiac Function

Heart failure is commonly defined as the pathophysiological state in which an abnormality of cardiac function is responsible for the failure of the heart to pump blood at a rate commensurate with the requirements of the metabolizing tissues and/or to be able to do so only from an elevated filling pressure [9]. Therefore the main hemodynamic features of heart failure are high diastolic ventricular pressure and/or low cardiac output. In more advanced forms of heart failure both high diastolic ventricular pressure and low cardiac output are present. Heart failure is usually caused by a defect of myocardial contraction leading to pump dysfunction and to low cardiac output.

Cardiac function may be studied at several levels: myocardial function, left ventricular pump performance and integrated cardiovascular performance. Most variables useful to evaluate the cardiac function can be gathered from a hemodynamic study performed in a clinical setting: intracardiac diastolic and systolic pressures, cardiac output and derived parameters. Myocardial function is determined by four factors: preload, afterload, contractility, heart rate and cardiac rhythm.

Left ventricular preload reflects the initial sarcomere length before the contraction and can be assessed from the left ventricular filling pressure and the left ventricular end diastolic volume or the end diastolic stress. The end diastolic pressure is the pressure distending the LV immediately prior to the contraction. In absence of a disease of the mitral valve, it is equivalent to the pressure in the left atrium after the contraction of the left atrium and to the mean atrial pressure. When there is a vigorous atrial contraction the end diastolic pressure is higher than the mean left atrial pressure. Pulmonary congestion is related to mean left atrial pressure. Pulmonary capillary wedge pressure approximates the left atrial wave pressure. The A wave is a diastolic event and is produced by the atrial contraction. The V wave is a systolic event and is related to the systolic motion of the mitral valve, to the compliance of the left atrium, to the amount of blood flow from the pulmonary veins and to mitral regurgitation [9, 10].

Afterload is the load that the myocardium must bear to contract and can be represented by the systolic aortic pressure.

Contractility reflects the capacity for shortening of the myocardium. At constant preload and afterload increased contractility results in a greater extent and velocity of shortening. The extent and velocity of shortening are profoundly influenced by preload and afterload. Many indices have been proposed as measures of myocardial contractility: the maximum rate of rise of ventricular pressure (dP/dt_{max}) is an isovolumetric phase parameter of contractility, is not affected by aortic pressure but is sensitive to changes in preload [8]. It is very useful, can be used during acute studies but it requires high fidelity measurement of pressure.

The left ventricular pump performance depends on systolic and diastolic performance: systolic performance is the ability of the LV to empty and may be measured by ejection fraction; diastolic performance is the ability of the LV to fill. The evaluation of diastolic performance requires technologies not currently available in a clinical setting. Some information can be obtained from the end diastolic pressure. The most common cause of diastolic dysfunction is systolic dysfunction. However, diastolic dysfunction may occur without systolic dysfunction and may be due to obstruction of left ventricular filling, impaired left ventricular distensibility or external compression of the LV.

The integrated pumping function of the cardiovascular system results in cardiac output that can be easily measured in a routine hemodynamic study.

Thus the evaluation of cardiac function is a complex task and often requires technologies not currently available in a clinical setting. However, measurement of pressure, cardiac output and systolic and diastolic intervals can be easily obtained by routine cardiac catheterization and gives useful information concerning global cardiac function. Moreover, an acute hemodynamic study performed in the same patient during a short period of time without altering preload and afterload gives information concerning the effects of interventions on LV performance.

The effects of stimulation on activation and contraction pattern are immediate and intracardiac pressure changes from the first stimulated beats, while cardiac output requires a few minutes to be appreciated. Thus, to understand the effects of stimulation on hemodynamic parameters, an immediate evaluation of pressures and derived parameters and a steady state evaluation of pressure and cardiac output are useful.

Stimulation of the heart has been proposed to improve ventricular performance and therefore global cardiac function. The most useful hemodynamic parameters are cardiac output and aortic pressure as an index of global cardiac function; left ventricular end diastolic pressure, mean right atrium pressure, mean capillary wedge pressure, left ventricular and amplitude of V wave are useful to evaluate diastolic performance and mitral valve regurgitation. The simultaneous recording of capillary and LV pressure may be useful to understand the mechanisms of changes of capillary pressure. Systolic and diastolic intervals may be also useful: electromechanical delay, pre-ejection period, systolic ejection period, isovolumetric diastole, and diastolic filling period. An increase of cardiac output with or without a reduction of LV end diastolic pressure can be considered a positive effect of pacing. The analysis of the other parameters can help to understand the mechanisms and beneficial effects of pacing.

Hemodynamic Consequences of LBBB

LBBB produces an asynchronous contraction of the heart as a consequence of delayed activation. Left ventricular contraction is delayed comparing to the right ventricle (85 ms) and the interventricular septum has an abnormal motion during ventricular ejection [11, 12]. In brief, at the beginning of systole the interventricular septum exhibits a rapid dip towards the left ventricular cavity, followed by a gradual anterior displacement towards the right ventricular cavity throughout ventricular ejection, resulting in a reduced contribution of the interventricular septum to left ventricular ejection. The heterogeneity of activation of the LV can generate an overlap between diastole and systole with one portion of the LV contracting when other portions begin to relax. Moreover, as demonstrated by right ventricular pacing, asynchronous and delayed activation of the papillary muscles may result in functional atrioventricular valve regurgitation [13].

All these abnormalities lead to a reduction of systolic and diastolic performance [14-16]. In fact, electromechanical delay (time from the Q wave on surface ECG to the beginning of mitral regurgitation or to the beginning of left ventricular pressure), isovolumetric contraction (time from the beginning of mitral regurgitation or left ventricular pressure to aortic opening) and relaxation time

(time from aortic closure to mitral opening) are increased. Diastolic filling period and ejection fraction are reduced. QRS duration correlates positively with the time intervals from Q to peak pressure and to peak dP/dt, from the start of mitral regurgitation to peak aortic pressure and to peak dP/dt and with the duration of mitral regurgitation, but negatively with the rate of rise of LV pressure (dP/dt).

Hemodynamic Effects of Biventricular Stimulation

Biventricular stimulation was thought to improve hemodynamic state by promoting synchronous contraction of the heart in patients with advanced heart failure and major intraventricular block.

Based on animal data showing that one of the most effective stimulation sites was the anteroinferior paraseptal region, which is close to the native conduction system, Foster and co-workers [17] performed an acute hemodynamic study in patients undergoing elective aortocoronary bypass grafting during atrio-biventricular pacing compared to atrio-monoventricular pacing. Ventricular electrodes were placed epicardially on either side of the septum at the anterior distal third of the right and left ventricle. They found that atrio-biventricular pacing increased the cardiac index and decreased systemic vascular resistance compared with atrio-right ventricular and atrio-left ventricular dual chamber pacing. This was attributed to more effective contraction of the septum during biventricular pacing.

Blanc and co-workers [18] evaluated the acute hemodynamic effects of left ventricular pacing (lateral free wall) in comparison with right ventricular pacing (apex and outflow) and biventricular pacing (RV apex and LV) in patients with severe congestive heart failure and elevated mean capillary pressure (>15 mm Hg). Pressures were monitored throughout the study; while cardiac output was measured only at baseline, the LV was paced at its lateral free wall because in clinical studies the latest site of activation was found in this area. LV based ventricular pacing resulted in higher systolic blood pressure, and lower mean capillary pressure and V wave amplitude in comparison with baseline or RV pacing. LV pacing alone and biventricular pacing resulted in similar acute improvement. The substantial equivalence of LV and biventricular stimulation is not completely understood. Actually, while biventricular pacing can synchronize ventricular contraction, the stimulation of a single area of the LV free wall is unlikely to determine synchronization of the whole heart: in this case the activation wave starts from a single point, far from the His bundle, and spreads to the ventricles. However, it is possible that LV stimulation enhances LV synchrony in comparison with the activation occurring during LBBB. Experimental data have demonstrated that in LBBB the greatest delay occurrs when the activation wave crosses the interventricular septum, while the activation of the LV free wall is faster when the distal native conduction system can be engaged. Thus LV free wall stimulation may allow easier engagement of the native conduction system, resulting in a more synchronous contraction. However, this may occur only if the distal conduction system is preserved.

Leclercq and co-workers [19] performed a more detailed hemodynamic study in patients with NYHA class III or IV, severe left ventricular dysfunction and major intraventricular block to assess the potential benefit of biventricular pacing by comparison with no ventricular pacing and with conventional single site RV DDD pacing. Biventricular pacing was performed by temporary cardiac catheters inserted into the lateral or posterolateral vein through the coronary sinus ostium to pace the LV free wall, and at the RV apex or outflow tract to pace the RV. The LV lead was connected to the negative pole of ventricular entry and the RV lead to the positive pole. LV stimulation alone was not tested. Biventricular pacing significantly decreased QRS duration in comparison either with the reference mode or RV DDD pacing. Biventricular pacing resulted in a significant benefit in terms of cardiac output (+35% increase), mean PCWP (18.5% decrease) and V wave amplitude (21% decrease). Biventricular pacing was also better than conventional RV DDD pacing. However 33% of patients did not benefit from any stimulation [19]. Patients with lower ejection fraction exhibited the greatest improvement of hemodynamic parameters. The hemodynamic benefits were associated with a reduction of QRS duration.

Auricchio and co-workers [20] and Kass and co-workers [21] showed that pacing the LV free wall is associated with an increase of the rate of rise of LV pressure ($+dP/dt$) suggesting an improvement of LV systolic performance. Moreover Auricchio and co-workers [20] showed , in a retrospective analysis of PATH-CHF studies, that the hemodynamic benefits were greater when the midlateral epicardial site was paced.

All these data suggest that LV stimulation alone or biventricular stimulation improves acutely the hemodynamic state in patients with severe heart failure due to LV systolic dysfunction, by improving the LV systolic performance with an increase of cardiac output and a decrease of mean capillary pressure. This may be due to a synchronization of LV contraction. A clear demonstration of synchronization with appropriate imaging technique is still lacking. Synchronization of the LV may occur also with a single site stimulation, if the site is close to the native conduction system that can be engaged allowing a rapid activation of the LV. In fact the QRS duration may also become shorter with the lateral free wall stimulation. The lowering of mean capillary pressure may be a consequence of the improvement of LV systolic function but may also be a consequence of a reduction of mitral valve regurgitation. Some authors have shown that the amplitude of V wave decreases when LV stimulation is applied [18, 19].

Curry and co-workers [22] studied a small number of patients with cardiomyopathy and mechanical asynchrony due to intraventricular activation delay, by means of a sophisticated imaging technique (MRI). They found that stimulation of the left ventricle at the site of activation delay may produce a functional improvement.

However, intraventricular asynchrony is not completely abolished by LV free wall electrode or biventricular pacing. Thus, more studies to obtain a more physiological pacing are needed. This could be accomplished by adding more electrodes.

Only a few data are available concerning the role of hemodynamic data on prediction of the long term response to biventricular stimulation. Cazeau and co-workers [23] found that patients exhibiting an increase of cardiac output during an acute hemodynamic study had a favorable follow-up, while patients without this increase died early, suggesting that the acute hemodynamic response to biventricular pacing is predictive of clinical outcome.

What Is the Role of an Acute Hemodynamic Study?

An acute hemodynamic study can be considered as the first step in the evaluation of a new method of stimulation specifically designed to improve the hemodynamic state in patients with heart failure and to evaluate the best stimulation protocol. Multiple simultaneous recordings of intracardiac pressure and continuous measurements of cardiac output allow a more sophisticated analysis of mechanisms and time course of the hemodynamic effects. However, hemodynamic study is not a good technique for studying the synchronization of the heart contraction. Here, imaging techniques are more appropriate. For this purpose a combination of imaging and hemodynamic techniques could allow a complete analysis of the contraction pattern and of its hemodynamic consequences. On a theoretical basis the results of an acute hemodynamic study cannot be directly translated on a long term basis. Cardiac stimulation has consequences also on the systemic and local release of catecholamines, autonomic nervous system activation, release of vasodilator substances, and release of atrial natriuretic factors [17]. Therefore the effects of stimulation are more complex than a pure hemodynamic effect and may have unpredictable clinical consequences on the long term follow up.

To date, definitive proof of the long term efficacy of LV stimulation in patients with heart failure is lacking and, consequently, the predictive value of an acute hemodynamic study in selecting patients suitable for LV stimulation is under debate.

References

1. Hochlertner M, Hörtnagl H, Choi-Keung Ng et al (1990) Usefulness of physiologic dual-chamber pacing in drug-resistant idiopathic dilated cardiomyopathy. Am J Cardiol 66:198-202
2. Bercker SJD, Xiao HB, Sparrow J et al (1992) Effects of dual-chamber pacing with short atrioventricular delay in dilated cardiomyopathy. Lancet 40:1308
3. Saxon LA, Stevenson WG, Middlekauff HR et al (1993) Increased risk of progressive hemodynamic deterioration in advanced heart failure patients requiring permanent pacemakers. Am Heart J 125:1306-1310
4. Cazeau S, Ritter P, Bakdach S et al (1994) Four chamber pacing in dilated cardiomyopathy. Pace 17 (II): 1974-1979
5. Cazeau S, Ritter P, Lazarus A et al (1996) Multisite pacing for end-stage heart failure: early experience. PACE 19:1748-1757

6. Alboni P (1981) Bundle branch blocks. In: P Alboni (ed) Intraventricular conduction disturbances. Martinus Nijhoff, The Hague Boston London, pp 9-56

7. Vassallo JA, Cassidy DM, Miller JM et al (1986) Left ventricular endocardial activation during right ventricular pacing: effect of underlying heart disease. J Am Coll Cardiol 7:1228-1233

8. Piccolo E, Raviele A, Delise P (1981) I ritardi di attivazione ventricolare. In: Piccolo E (ed) Elettrocardiografia e vettorcardiografia. Piccin, Padua, pp 131-204

9. Little WC, Braunwald E (1997) Assessment of cardiac function. In: Braunwald E (ed) Heart disease. Saunders, Philadelphia, pp 421-444

10. Yang SS, Bentivoglio LG, Maranhão V, Goldberg H (eds) (1972) From cardiac catheterization data to hemodynamic parameters. Davis, Philadelphia, pp 157-201

11. Grines CL, Bashore TM, Boudoulas H et al (1989) Functional abnormalities in isolated left bundle branch block. Circulation 79:845-853

12. Feigenbaum H (ed) (1986) Echocardiographic findings with altered electrical activation. Echocardiography. Lea & Febiger, Philadelphia, pp 230-248

13. Lister JW, Klotz KH, Jomain SL et al (1964) Effect of pacemaker site on cardiac output and ventricular activation in dogs with complete heart block. Am J Cardiol 14:494-503

14. Xiao HB, Brecker SJD, Gibson DG (1992) Effects of abnormal activation on the time course of the left ventricular pressure pulse in dilated cardiomyopathy. Br Heart J 68:403-407

15. Xiao HB, Brecker SJD, Gibson DG (1993) Differing effects of right ventricular pacing and left bundle branch block on left ventricular function. Br Heart J 69:166-173

16. Xiao HB, Roy C, Gibson DG (1994) Nature of ventricular activation in patients with dilated cardiomyopathy: evidence for bilateral bundle branch block. Br Heart J 72:167-174

17. Foster AH, Gold MR, McLaughlin JS (1995) Acute hemodynamic effects of atrio-biventricular pacing in humans. Ann Thorac Surg 59:294-300

18. Blanc JJ, Etienne Y, Gilard M et al (1997) Evaluation of different ventricular pacing sites in patients with severe heart failure. Circulation 96:3273-3277

19. Leclercq C, Cazeau S, Le Breton H et al (1998) Acute hemodynamic effects of biventricular DDD pacing in patients with end-stage heart failure. J Am Coll Cardiol 32:1825-1831

20. Auricchio A, Klein H, Tockman B et al (1999) Transvenous biventricular pacing for heart failure: can the obstacles be overcome? Am J Cardiol 83:136D-142D

21. Kass DA, Chen CH, Fetics B et al (1998) Ventricular function in patients with dilated cardiomyopathy is improved by VDD pacing at left but not right ventricular sites. J Am Coll Cardiol 31:1015-1029

22. Curry CW, Fetics B, Wyman B et al (1998) Mechanical dyssynchrony at rest and with adrenergic stimulation in patients with dilated cardiomyopathy studied by MRI-tagging: can it help identify candidates for chronic VDD pacing therapy? Circulation [Suppl I]:302 (abstr)

23. Cazeau S, Ritter P, Lazarus A et al (1996) How to predict the hemodynamic benefit of multisite pacing for heart failure. Eur JCPE 6:544

Subject Index